# Conceptual Foundations of
# Professional
# Nursing Practice

# Conceptual Foundations of
# Professional Nursing Practice

*Edited by*

**JOAN L. CREASIA, PhD, RN**
Acting Chairperson, RN to BSN Program and
Assistant Professor
School of Nursing, University of Maryland
UMBC Campus, Baltimore, Maryland

**BARBARA PARKER, PhD, RN**
Coordinator, Off-Campus RN to BSN Program and
Associate Professor
School of Nursing, University of Maryland
UMBC Campus, Baltimore, Maryland

*with 46 illustrations*

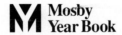
Mosby
Year Book

St. Louis  Baltimore  Boston  Chicago  London  Philadelphia  Sydney  Toronto

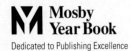
**Mosby**
**Year Book**
Dedicated to Publishing Excellence

Editor: N. Darlene Como
Developmental Editor: Laurie Sparks
Project Manager: Karen Edwards
Production Editor: Richard Barber
Book and Cover Design: Gail Morey Hudson

Mosby–Year Book, Inc.
11830 Westline Industrial Drive, St. Louis, MO 63146

**Library of Congress Cataloging in Publication Data**

Conceptual foundatiions of professional nursing parctice / edited by
    Joan L. Creasia, Barbara Parker.
        p.   cm.
    Includes bibliographical references and index.
    ISBN 0-8016-6148-X
    1. Nursing—Practice.   2. Nursing.   I. Creasia, Joan L.
II. Parker, Barbara, RN.
    [DNLM: 1. Nursing.   2. Nursing care.   WY 16 C744]
    RT86.7.C66   1991
    610.73—dc20
    DNLM/DLC
    for Library of Congress                          90-13675
                                                        CIP

CA/DC  9  8  7  6  5  4  3  2  1

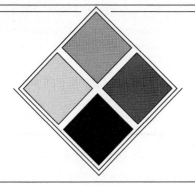

# Contributors

**ANNA C. ALT-WHITE, RN, PhD**

Associate Director of Nursing Service for Research
Nurse Researcher, Veteran Affairs Medical Center,
Washington, DC

**MARJORIE BEYERS, RN, PhD, FAAN**

Associate Vice President, Nursing & Allied Health
Services,
Mercy Health Services,
Farmington Hills, Michigan

**CARMELLE PELLERIN COURNOYER, RN,
MA, JD**

President, CRC Associates, Health Law Educator and
Consultant, and
Guardian-Office of Public Guardian,
Concord, New Hampshire

**LINDA LINDSEY DAVIS, PhD, RN, ANP**

Professor and Associate Dean, School of Nursing,
University of Alabama at Birmingham,
Birmingham, Alabama

**KAREN E. DENNIS, PhD, RN**

Associate Professor, School of Nursing,
University of Maryland,
Baltimore, Maryland

**JOYCE K. ENGEL, RN, MED**

Assistant Professor, University of Lethuridge,
Lethuridge, Alberta, Canada

**BETTY ROLLING FERRELL, PhD, FAAN**

Research Scientist, City of Hope National Medical
Center,
Duarte, California

**SARA T. FRY, RN, PhD, FAAN**

Associate Professor, School of Nursing,
University of Maryland,
Baltimore, Maryland

**HURDIS M. GRIFFITH, RN, PhD, FAAN**

Health Policy Researcher and Consultant,
Adjunct Associate Professor,
Vanderbilt University, University of Maryland,
University of Texas at Arlington
Schools of Nursing

**PATRICIA M. GRIMM, PhD, RN**

Assistant Professor,
The Johns Hopkins University School of Nursing,
Baltimore, Maryland

**LOUISE S. JENKINS, RN, PhD**

The Walter Schroeder Chair in Nursing Research,
School of Nursing, University of Wisconsin,
Milwaukee, Wisconsin

**JOYCE H. JOHNSON, RN, Phd**

Associate Professor, College of Nursing,
University of Illinois at Chicago,
Chicago, Illinois

**KATHRYN HOPKINS KAVANAGH, PhD, RN**

Assistant Professor, School of Nursing,
University of Maryland,
Baltimore, Maryland

**LORRAINE SPRANZO KELLER, RN, MS**

Instructor, School of Nursing,
University of Maryland,
Baltimore, Maryland

**GLENDA B. KELMAN, RN, MS, CS, OCN**

Doctoral Candidate, NYU
Nursing Consultant, Albany Medical Center,
Albany, New York, and Glen Falls Hospital,
Glens Falls, New York

**CONNIE J. LEEK, MS, RNC, OCN**

Nursing Instructor,
City of Hope National Medical Center,
Duarte, California

**DONNA M. MAHRENHOLZ, RN, PHD**

Faculty Research Associate, School of Nursing,
The Johns Hopkins University,
Baltimore, Maryland

**GAIL O. MAZZOCCO, EDD, RN**

Assistant Professor, School of Nursing,
University of Maryland,
Baltimore, Maryland

**ELEANORE L. MCCANN, MSN, RNC, GNP**

Assistant Professor, School of Nursing,
Indiana University,
Indianapolis, Indiana

**SUSAN MCCRONE, RN, PHD**

Assistant Professor, School of Nursing,
University of Maryland,
Baltimore, Maryland

**LONNA MILBURN, RN, PHD**

Consultant, Health Dynamics,
Austin, Texas

**SHIRLEY A. MURPHY, RN, PHD, FAAN**

Professor, Department of Psychosocial Nursing,
University of Washington,
Seattle, Washington

**BEVERLY A. OSBAND, RN, PHD**

Bereavement Counselor/Private Practice,
Associated Bereavement Services/Hospice of Tacoma,
Tacoma, Washington

**LESLEY A. PERRY, PHD, RN**

Associate Professor and Interim Executive Assistant
to the Dean,
School of Nursing, University of Maryland,
Baltimore, Maryland

**ROSANNE HARKEY PRUITT, PHD, RNC**

Assistant Professor, College of Nursing,
Clemson University,
Clemson, South Carolina

**C. FAY RAINES, RN, PHD**

Professor and Dean, School of Nursing,
University of Alabama in Huntsville,
Huntsville, Alabama

**JANE EHLINGER SHERMAN, PHD, RN, C**

Nurse Practitioner, Private Practice
Milford, Delaware

**LORRAINE M. SMITH, RN, MSN**

Assistant Professor, School of Nursing,
Indiana University,
Indianapolis, Indiana

**MARY E. SOJA, MSN, MA, RN**

Assistant Professor, School of Nursing,
Indiana University,
Indianapolis, Indiana

**SANDRA J. SUNDEEN, MS, RN, CNAA**

Chief Nurse, Mental Hygiene Administration,
Department of Health and Mental Hygiene,
Baltimore, Maryland

**CECELIA M. TAYLOR, PHD, RN**

Director of Nursing, Mohawk Valley Psychiatric
Center,
Utica, New York

**CONSTANCE R. UPHOLD, PHD, RN**

Assistant Professor, College of Nursing,
University of Florida,
Gainesville, Florida

**MARY ELLEN WEWERS, PHD, RN**

Assistant Professor, College of Nursing,
The Ohio State University,
Columbus, Ohio

**MARY ANN GNIADY WILKINSON, EDD, MSN, RN**

Assistant Professor, School of Nursing,
University of Maryland,
Baltimore, Maryland

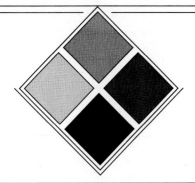

# Consultants

**SARA ARONSON, RN, BS, MPH**

Director, RN Pathway Program,
Hunter College/CUNY,
Hunter-Bellevue School of Nursing,
New York, New York

**DIANE M. BILLINGS, RN, EdD**

Professor of Nursing, Indiana University,
Indianapolis, Indiana

**MADOLYN J. CUTTER, RN, MS**

Assistant Professor, Texas Woman's University,
College of Nursing,
Denton, Texas

**JOANNE M. GORDON, RN, MA, MSN**

Associate Professor, Department of Nursing,
Southwest Missouri State University,
Springfield, Missouri

**PAULINE JOHNSON-HOFER, RN, EdD**

Nursing Department,
SUNY College at New Paltz,
New Paltz, New York

**ANN Z. KRUSZEWSKI, MSN, RN**

Assistant Professor, University of Michigan,
School of Nursing,
Ann Arbor, Michigan

**HELEN E. MINER, RN, PhD**

Assistant Professor,
Southeast Missouri State University,
Cape Girardeau, Missouri

**MARY ANN NOONAN, RN, MSN**

Assistant Professor, Medical Surgical Nursing,
Coordinator RN/BSN Programs,
Niehoff School of Nursing
Loyola University,
Chicago, Illinois

**JUDITH RYAN, PhD, RN**

Assistant Professor, University of Maryland,
School of Nursing,
Baltimore, Maryland

**MARY TEDROW, RN, EdD**

Associate Professor,
California State University, Dominguez Hills,
Carson, California

**MARY H. WILDE, RN, MS**

Assistant Professor,
SUNY Institute of Technology at Utica-Rome,
Utica, New York

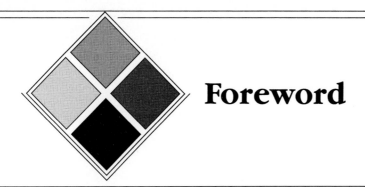

# Foreword

The authors of this text have developed a conceptual approach in exploring dimensions of practice and client care issues that are directly related to the professional practice of nursing. They have taken concepts that are most salient for professional nurses and presented them in a format that encourages both traditional and nontraditional modes of teaching and learning. The book's focus on the context, dimensions, and themes of nursing practice reflects a growing awareness of nursing's strategic position and ability to influence decisions and policy relative to the social, ethical, political, legal, and economic environments. Concepts related to client care emphasize nursing interventions that alleviate stressors and build on client strengths. Major life themes, such as parenting and aging, with associated health care needs, are also appropriately considered.

In addition to providing important information in a format that enhances and facilitates learning, this book acknowledges the maturity and previous knowledge base of the nurse. It will be useful for the professional nurse who needs current knowledge to improve practice, as well as for the nurse who is striving to enter the world of professional practice. Added values of this text include its readability, its application to clinical practice, and the integration of relevant research for each concept.

The authors carefully selected contributors who participate in nursing research, education, and practice and who are acknowledged authorities in particular content areas. As a result, the book is truly a reflection of nursing's growth in expertise, scientific inquiry, and professionalism and its ability to deal with vast amounts of complex knowledge in a succinct and informative manner. It is indeed a unique and comprehensive treatment of the most important concepts related to the professional practice of nursing. The knowledge acquired from this text will provide a useful framework for the practice of professional nursing in the health care environment of today and tomorrow.

**Rachel Z. Booth, PhD, RN**
*Dean and Professor*
*University of Alabama*
*School of Nursing*
*Birmingham, Alabama*

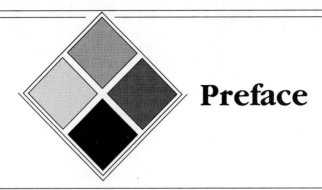

# Preface

Nursing has undergone significant changes and faced many challenges during the past few decades in its quest for professionalism in practice. One of the most influential forces has been the American Nurses' Association's (ANA) 1965 recommendation that the minimum educational preparation be at the baccalaureate level. Nursing educators have responded to this challenge by adapting and developing curricula to emphasize professional approaches to practice and to build on, rather than duplicate, education received in a basic nursing program. In addition, nursing no longer follows the traditional medical model but rather focuses on a conceptual and holistic foundation for independent and collaborative practice. Thus, it is appropriate to identify concepts that are broad in scope and applicable across a variety of client groups and clinical settings.

Changes in the health care delivery system also affect the practice and education of nurses. Both advanced technological developments and health policy issues play a major role in the planning and delivery of comprehensive nursing care. The focus on health promotion for individuals, families, and communities and efforts to control health care costs have given rise to alternative forms of health care delivery and innovative reimbursement models. In addition, increased acuity of hospitalized clients and limited hospital stays have resulted in a greater demand for home and community health services. These changes have political, legal, and economic implications that must be incorporated into the educational foundation and professional practice of nursing. We developed this book to provide students with the broad-based knowledge and skills needed to practice in this complex health care environment.

## ❖ ORGANIZATION

*Conceptual Foundations of Professional Nursing Practice* comprehensively explores issues and concepts that influence professional practice and the delivery of nursing care. The book is divided into two major parts: Concepts Related to Professional Nursing Practice and Concepts Related to Client Care. Part One begins with an exploration of the context of professional nursing practice. Subsequently, political, economic, legal, and ethical dimensions that have an impact on current practice are examined, and predominant themes that play an integral part in nursing care delivery are addressed. Concepts related to professional nursing practice were selected for inclusion in the book after reviewing the findings of a study conducted by The American Association of Colleges of Nursing. This study, *RN Baccalaureate Nursing Education, Special Report* (1988) identified concepts that are considered important to professional nursing practice by baccalaureate nurse educators and registered nurse students. Students assessed their knowledge of these concepts at both the beginning and completion of the program. A decision was made to include the concept in the book if the self-assessed beginning skill level was relatively low, the final skill level was relatively high, and emphasis on the content during the program was judged to be moderate to high.

Part Two, Concepts Related to Client Care, is divided into client/family stressors, strengths, and major life themes. Concepts were selected for inclusion in this part of the book if they were judged to be applicable across a variety of clients and clinical practice settings. Nursing interventions that alleviate stressors and build on client strengths are emphasized.

### ❖ APPROACH

With the trend toward advanced education in nursing, large numbers of nurses are returning to school after several years in practice. Older students with valuable life experience and students returning for renewed nursing careers are now commonplace in many nursing education programs. Since these nurses have varying amounts and types of clinical experience, the result is a highly diverse student population. For this group, as an adjunct to previously learned clinical skills and nursing knowledge, it is meaningful to develop a conceptual approach to nursing practice that is applicable across assorted client groups and clinical settings. This book offers such an approach and can be used effectively to teach nursing concepts to today's students.

As editors we have struggled with the terminology used to describe the recipients of nursing care. Although philosophically we prefer the term "client" with its connotations of partnership in nursing care, there were times when this terminology became cumbersome or inaccurate, as in reference to "patient classification systems," for example. Thus, the reader

will find the both the terms client and patient used, at times interchangeably. We believe the difficulty in determining the appropriate term is a reflection of the changing nature of nursing practice and the health care industry.

Individual, family, and community systems are included in the form of broad concepts and serve as the focus for clinical application of the concepts. However, frameworks and theories for family and community health nursing are not described in detail in this text because of the large amount of content in these areas. There are books devoted to those subjects that are more appropriate and comprehensive in covering content about family and community health.

### ❖ SPECIAL FEATURES

For the purpose of focusing the reader's attention, each chapter begins with learning objectives. Each concept is developed in a similar format. An overview of the concept is followed by definitions of key terms, an in-depth discussion of the concept, and application of the concept to clinical practice. Nursing care plans are used to further illustrate the clinical application of client strengths and stressors. Research on each concept is integrated throughout the chapter. Discussion questions reflecting application to clinical practice are found at the end of the chapter. A comprehensive and current reference list offers the opportunity to pursue further reading on the subject.

As each concept unfolds, the reader is challenged to discover new knowledge or reframe prior learning on a more conceptual and universally applicable level. Using this knowledge to enhance current and future nursing practice remains the final challenge.

**Joan L. Creasia**
**Barbara Parker**

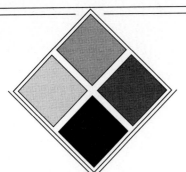

# Acknowledgments

We are deeply grateful to the many people who have helped us bring this work to completion. Our special thanks go to the talented contributors who shared their knowledge, experience, and expertise in a form that is of immeasurable value to professional nurses. We appreciate the efforts of anonymous reviewers and colleagues who graciously contributed their time to critique the manuscript and offer suggestions for refinement. Our colleagues at the University of Maryland School of Nursing, RN to BSN Program provided enthusiasm, intellectual challenges, and scholarly guidance. Dr.

Lesley Perry was particularly supportive of this endeavor. Our Senior Editor from Mosby, Darlene Como, offered encouragement, insight, and sound editorial sense to facilitate our efforts. The working relationship we shared as coauthors made writing this book a valuable and rewarding experience. Finally, we would not have been able to achieve our goal without the support and encouragement of our husbands, Dale Schumacher and Don Creasia, and our children, Peter, Andrea and Margret Schumacher, and Karen and Tracey Creasia.

Joan L. Creasia
Barbara Parker

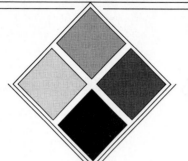

# Contents

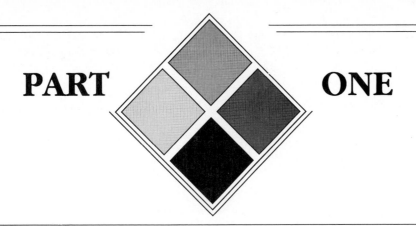

# PART ONE

# CONCEPTS RELATED TO PROFESSIONAL NURSING PRACTICE

CONCEPTS related to professional nursing practice are those elements, both internal and external to the nurse, that are integral to the delivery of nursing care. Several concepts are identified and described including the clients nurses serve, the setting where care is delivered, and the roles nurses assume. Also included are specific dimensions of the nurse's role and common themes in nursing practice, which are critical to the delivery of comprehensive nursing care.

Thus, professional practice concepts are divided into three categories: the context, dimensions, and themes of professional nursing practice. This classification scheme invites the reader to gain an appreciation of the surroundings where nursing care is delivered, obtain a new awareness of the extent of the nurse's role, and probe the common themes that cut across all areas of nursing practice. Critical analysis of these concepts can facilitate role expansion, encourage the use of effective intervention strategies, and further delineate the scope of practice. The expectation is that the reader will acquire a new appreciation of the magnitude of the nurse's role, which necessarily expands its depth and breadth, going beyond traditional boundaries and approaching new frontiers.

In this section, each concept is described and followed by definitions of key terms and an in-depth discussion of the theoretical components of the concept. Clinical examples illustrate application of the concept where appropriate, and current research findings are integrated throughout each chapter. Discussion questions are provided to further encourage application of the concept to clinical situations.

# UNIT I

# The Context of Professional Nursing Practice

**T**HE characteristics of the milieu within which nursing care is delivered constitutes the context of professional nursing practice. The frameworks used to design and implement nursing care, the clients nursing serves, the environment where nursing is practiced, and the roles nurses commonly assume are contextual variables inherent in the delivery of nursing care.

This unit begins with an overview of selected theories and frameworks for professional nursing practice followed by a discussion of individual, family, and community client systems. The environment where client care is delivered is presented from both a clinician's and an administrator's perspective. Finally, descriptions of roles nurses commonly assume, such as caregiver, teacher, and case manager, follow an overview of role theory. These contextual elements are further explicated and examined in this unit.

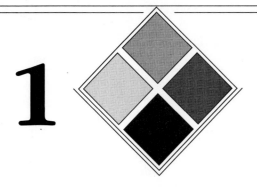

# 1 Theories and Frameworks for Professional Nursing Practice

Barbara Parker ◆ Joan L. Creasia

## OBJECTIVES

*At the completion of this chapter, the reader will be able to:*

◆ Differentiate between a concept, theory, conceptual framework, and model.

◆ Identify and define the four central concepts of nursing theories.

◆ Compare and contrast selected theories of nursing.

◆ Describe the nursing process and its application to client care.

Theories and conceptual frameworks provide direction and guidance for structuring professional nursing practice, education, and research. In practice, theories and frameworks assist nurses to describe, explain, and predict everyday experiences, and they also serve to guide assessment, intervention, and evaluation of nursing care. In education, a conceptual framework provides the general focus for curriculum design and guides curricular decision making. In research, the framework offers a systematic approach to identifying questions for study, selecting appropriate variables, and interpreting findings. The importance of theory in building a body of nursing knowledge is emphasized by Chinn and Jacobs (1987) who state "Nursing theory ought to guide research and practice, generate new ideas, and differentiate the focus of nursing from other professions" (p. 145).

Many nurse theorists have made substantial contributions to the development of a unique body of knowledge. Offering an assortment of perspectives, the theories vary in their level of abstraction and their conceptualization of the client, health, illness, and nursing. In this book, nursing theories are used to illustrate and assist in the development of some concepts, such as cultural influences on health, health promotion, sensory alterations, and stress. As a basis for understanding their incorporation in subsequent chapters, this chapter briefly describes some of the predominant theories in nursing and provides a synopsis of their essential components.

❖ **Table 1-1**

History of nursing theory development

| Events | Year | Nurse theorists |
|---|---|---|
| | 1860 | Florence Nightingale<br>Described nursing and environment |
| | 1952 | Hildegard E. Peplau<br>Nursing as an interpersonal process:<br>patients with felt needs |
| Scientific era: nurses questioned purpose of nursing | 1960 | Faye Abdellah (also 1965; 1973)<br>Patient-centered approaches |
| | 1961 | Ida Jean Orlando<br>Nurse-patient relationship; deliberative<br>nursing approach |
| Process of theory development discussed among professional nurses | 1964 | Ernestine Wiedenbach (also 1970; 1977)<br>Nursing: philosophy, purpose, practice,<br>and art |
| | 1966 | Lydia E. Hall<br>Core (patient), care (body), cure<br>(disease) |
| | 1966 | Virginia Henderson (also 1972; 1978)<br>Nursing assists patients with 14 essential<br>functions toward independence |
| Symposium: theory development in nursing | 1967 | Myra Estrin Levine (also 1973)<br>Four conservation principles of nursing |
| Symposium: nature of science and nursing<br>Dickoff, James, and Wiedenbach wrote<br>"Theory in a Practice Discipline," in<br>*Nursing Research* | 1968 | |
| Symposium: nature of science in nursing<br>First nursing theory conference | 1969 | |
| Second nursing theory conference | 1970 | Martha E. Rogers (also 1980)<br>Science of unitary man: energy fields,<br>openness; pattern, and organization |
| Consensus on nursing concepts:<br>Nurse/nursing, health,<br>client/patient/individual,<br>society/environment | 1971 | Dorothea E. Orem (also 1980; 1985)<br>Nursing facilitates patients' self-care |
| Discussion on what is theory: the elements,<br>criteria, types and levels, and the relation<br>to research | 1971 | Imogene King (also 1975; 1981)<br>Theory of goal attainment through<br>nurse-client transactions |
| NLN required conceptual frameworks in<br>nursing education | 1973 | |
| Borrowed theories from other disciplines<br>Expanded theories from other disciplines | 1974 | Sister Callista Roy (also 1976; 1980; 1984)<br>Roy's adaptation model: nurse adjusts<br>patient's stimuli (focal, contextual, or<br>residual) |

From Christensen, P.J., & Kenney, J. W. (1990) *The Nursing Process: Application of Conceptual Models.* St. Louis: C. V. Mosby, p. 11.

❖ **Table 1-1**
   History of nursing theory development—cont'd

| Events | Year | Nurse theorists |
|---|---|---|
| Recognized problems in practice and developed theories to test and use in practice | 1976 | Josephine Paterson and L. Zderad<br>Humanistic nursing |
| Second nurse educator conference on nursing theory | 1978 | Madeleine Leininger (also 1980; 1981)<br>Transcultural nursing<br>Caring nursing |
| Articles on theory development in *ANS, Nursing Research,* and *Image* | 1978<br>1979 | Jean Watson (also 1985)<br>Philosophy and science of caring; humanistic nursing |
| Books written for nurses on how to critique theory, how to develop theory, and describing application of nursing theories | 1980 | Dorothy E. Johnson<br>Behavioral system model for nursing |
| Graduate schools of nursing develop courses in how to analyze and apply nursing theories | | Betty Neuman<br>Health-care systems model: a total person approach |
| Research studies in nursing identified nursing theories as framework for study | 1981 | Rosemarie Rizzo Parse (also 1987)<br>Man-living-health: a theory of nursing |
| Numerous books published on analysis, application, evaluation, and/or development of nursing theories | 1982–present | |

Nursing theories can also be described from a historical perspective as they reflect increased sophistication and development of nursing ideas and the influence of the larger society. Table 1-1 describes a chronology of events related to the development of nursing theories.

## ❖ TERMINOLOGY ASSOCIATED WITH THEORETICAL PERSPECTIVES

For purposes of this discussion, it is necessary to differentiate between a concept, theory, and conceptual framework. A *concept* is a building block of theory. It is an idea or word that describes objects, events, or properties, bringing up a mental image of the phenomenon. A *theory* is a statement or group of statements that describes, explains, or predicts the relationship between concepts (e.g., objects,

events, or properties). Theories may be broad or limited in scope, thus varying in their ability to describe, explain, or predict. A *conceptual framework* provides the orienting scheme or world view that helps focus our thinking. A conceptual framework can be visualized as an umbrella under which many theories can exist. The major distinction between a conceptual framework and a theory is the level of abstraction, with a conceptual framework being more abstract than a theory. The term conceptual framework is often used interchangeably with conceptual model, although the term model is generally used to refer to a graphic illustration of relationships. Without attempting to justify the classification of individual theoretical perspectives included in this chapter, the term to which each is most commonly referred (i.e., theory, model, framework) will be used.

## ❖ COMPONENTS OF NURSING THEORIES

A nursing theory is a "relatively specific and concrete set of concepts and propositions that purports to account for or characterize phenomena of interest to the discipline of nursing" (Fawcett, 1989, p. 23). Four central concepts of interest to the discipline of nursing are person, environment, health/illness, and nursing. Persons are the recipients of nursing care and include individuals, families, or communities. Environment refers to the surroundings of the client as well as the setting where nursing care is delivered. Health and illness describe the client's state of well-being. Nursing is the discipline from which client care actions are derived. Most nursing theories define or describe the central concepts, either explicitly or implicitly. In addition to these concepts, many theories include assumptions about the nature of the client and the environment, propositions describing the relationships between the major concepts, and definitions of concepts specific to a particular theory.

In keeping with this organizational scheme, descriptions of the theoretical perspectives presented in this chapter include a brief overview, basic assumptions about the individual and the environment, definitions of health and illness, a description of nursing including the goal of nursing, and definition of concepts and subconcepts specific to each theory. Some theories are more amenable to this scheme than others because of their degree of specificity or stage of development. When the theorist does not explicitly detail the needed information, inferences are made based on what seems to be implicitly stated. Because most of the theories are quite global, condensing them into discrete and somewhat restrictive categories obscures some of the true essence of the relationships. Thus, the reader is encouraged to consult the primary source to gain a full appreciation of the depth, scope, and extent of the relationships put forth.

## ❖ OVERVIEW OF SELECTED NURSING THEORIES

Theories and frameworks selected for inclusion in this chapter are those used in the development of concepts in subsequent chapters as well as others that exemplify the evolution of nursing from early times (e.g., Nightingale) to more recent ones (e.g., Parse).

### Nightingale's Environmental Theory

Florence Nightingale conceptualized disease as a reparative process and described the nurse's role as manipulating the environment to facilitate and encourage this process. Her directions regarding ventilation, warmth, light, diet, cleanliness, variety, and noise are discussed in her classic nursing textbook *Notes on Nursing* (1859).

**Brief overview.** The environment is critical to health and the nurse's role in caring for the sick is to provide a clean, quiet, peaceful environment to promote healing. Nightingale's intent was to describe nursing and provide guidelines for nursing education.

**Assumptions about the individual.** Individuals are responsible, creative, in control of their lives and health, and desire good health.

**Environment.** The environment is external to the person but affects the health of both sick and well persons. The environment, one of the chief sources of infection, must include pure air, pure water, efficient drainage, cleanliness, and light.

**Health and illness.** Health is defined as a state of being well and using one's powers to the fullest. Illness or disease is the reaction of nature against the conditions in which we have placed ourselves. Disease is a reparative mechanism, an effort of nature to remedy a process of poisoning or decay.

**Nursing.** Nursing is a service to people intended to relieve pain and suffering. Nursing's role is to promote or provide the proper environment for patients to include fresh air, light, pure water, cleanliness, warmth, quiet, and appropriate diet. The goal of nursing is to promote the reparative process by manipulating the environment.

### Key concepts

*Environment*—Conditions external to the individual that affect life and development (e.g., ventilation, warmth, light, diet, cleanliness, and noise).

Three major relationships are identified: environment to the patient, the nurse to the environment, and the nurse to the patient. Examples of these follow.

The need for light, particularly sunlight, is second only to the need for ventilation. If necessary, the nurse should move the patient "about after the sun according to the aspects of the rooms, if circumstances permit rather than let him linger in a room when the sun is off" (p. 48).

Nursing's role is to manipulate the environment to encourage healing. Nursing "ought to signify the proper use of fresh air, light, warmth, cleanliness, quiet, and the proper selection and administration of diet" (p. 6).

The sine qua non of all good nursing is never to allow a patient to be awakened, intentionally or accidentally. "A good nurse will always make sure that no blind or curtains should flap. If you wait till your patient tells you or reminds you of these things, where is the use of their having a nurse?" (p. 27).

Variety is important for patients to divert them from dwelling on their pain. "Variety of form and brilliancy of color in the objects presented are actual means of recovery" (p. 34).

## Henderson's Complementary-Supplementary Model

Virginia Henderson viewed nursing as an art and a discipline separate from medicine. In *The Nature of Nursing* (1966), she indicated that the "unique function of the nurse is to assist the individual, sick or well in the performance of those activities contributing to the health or its recovery (or a peaceful death) that he would perform unaided if he had the necessary strength, will or knowledge" (p. 15).

**Brief overview.** The nurse's role is that of a substitute for the patient, a helper to the patient, and a partner with the patient. Fourteen basic patient needs comprise components of nursing care.

**Assumptions about the individual.** Since the mind and body are inseparable, a person must maintain physiological and emotional balance. An individual requires assistance to achieve health and independence or a peaceful death. Individuals will achieve or maintain health if they have the necessary strength, will, or knowledge (1966, p. 15). The individual and family should be viewed as a unit.

**Environment.** "The aggregate of all the external conditions and influences affecting the life and development of an organism" (1978, p. 829).

**Health and illness.** Health is a quality of life basic to human functioning. Although not specifically stated, health seems to be equated with independence. Conversely, it can be inferred that illness is a lack of independence.

**Nursing.** Nursing has a unique function of assisting sick or well individuals in a supplementary or complementary role. The goal of nursing is to help the individual gain independence as rapidly as possible.

**Key concepts.** Fourteen basic patient needs make up the components of nursing care:

1. Breathe normally.
2. Eat and drink adequately.
3. Eliminate body wastes.
4. Move and maintain desirable position.
5. Sleep and rest.
6. Select suitable clothes.
7. Maintain body temperature within normal range by adjusting clothing and modifying the environment.
8. Keep the body clean and well groomed to protect the integument.
9. Avoid dangers in the environment and avoid injuring others.
10. Communicate with others in expressing emotions, needs, fears, or opinions.
11. Worship according to one's faith.
12. Work in such a way that there is a sense of accomplishment.
13. Play or participate in various forms of recreation.
14. Learn, discover, or satisfy the curiosity that leads to normal development and health and use the available health facilities (1966).

## Johnson's Behavioral System Model

Originally presenting a paper at Vanderbilt University in 1968, Dorothy Johnson did not personally publish her theory of nursing until 1980. However, her early paper was widely cited, and published interpretations of it appeared in 1974 (Grubbs, 1974) and 1976 (Auger, 1976). Johnson views the individual as a behavioral system that is continually striving for balance. The nurse fosters "efficient and effective behavioral functioning ... to prevent illness and during and following illness" (1980, p. 207).

**Brief overview.** The individual is viewed as a collection of interrelated behavioral subsystems whose response patterns form an organized and integrated whole. The nurse serves as an external regulatory force to preserve and maintain system balance.

**Assumptions about the individual.** As a set of behavioral subsystems, the individual strives to attain and maintain behavioral system balance, sometimes requiring adaptation and modification to return to a steady state. The individual is characterized by organization, interaction, interdependency, and integration of the parts and elements (subsystems).

**Environment.** The natural forces impinging on the individual constitute the environment in which the behavioral system exists. There are both internal and external environments, but these are not defined.

**Health and illness.** It may be inferred that health is a state of balance in which the behavioral system is self-maintaining and self-perpetuating, and interrelationships between the subsystems are harmonious. Conversely, illness is a state of disorganization and dysfunction of the system.

**Nursing.** Described as an external regulatory force, the practice of nursing imposes external controls to fulfill the functional requirements of the subsystems. The goal of nursing is "to restore, maintain, or attain behavioral system balance and stability at the highest possible level for the individual" (1980, p. 214).

**Key concepts.** The concepts describe the individual as a set of subsystems that, together, form a behavioral system.

*Behavioral system*—composed of seven behavioral subsystems that are integrated and that characterize each person's life.

*Behavioral subsystem*—a formed set of behavioral responses that seem to share a common drive but that are modified over time through maturation or learning. The seven subsystems are:

Affiliative—security as a consequence of social inclusion, intimacy, and the formation and maintenance of a strong social bond.

Dependency—succoring behavior that calls for the response of nurturing and has as its consequence approval, attention, or physical assistance.

Ingestive—appetite satisfaction as it is governed by social and psychological considerations.

Eliminative—elimination of body wastes as a learned behavior, which strongly influences purely biological eliminative acts.

Sexual—procreation and gratification with responses originating with gender role identity and the broad range of behaviors dependent on one's biologic sex.

Achievement—mastery or control over some aspect of the self or environment; it includes intelligence, physical, creative, mechanical, care-taking, and social skills.

Aggressive—protection and preservation of self and society within the limits imposed by society.

## Rogers' Science of Unitary Human Beings

First presented as *The Theoretical Basis for Nursing* in 1970, Martha Rogers' conceptualizations dating back to the 1960s evolved into the current science of unitary human beings. She states that humans are dynamic energy fields who are integral with the environment and who are continuously evolving. She views nursing as a science and art that focuses on the nature and direction of human development and human betterment.

**Brief overview.** The individual is viewed as an irreducible four-dimensional energy field who is integral with the environment. The nurse seeks to promote symphonic interactions between humans and their environments.

**Assumptions about the individual.** The individual is a unified whole, manifesting char-acteristics that are more than and different from the sum of his or her parts, and is continuously evolving irreversibly and unidirectionally along a space-time continuum. Pattern and organization of humans are directed toward increasing complexity rather than maintaining equilibrium. The individual "is characterized by the capacity for abstraction and imagery, language and thought, sensation and emotion" (1970, p. 73).

**Environment.** The individual and the environment are continually exchanging matter and energy with one another, resulting in changing patterns in both the individual and the environment.

**Health and illness.** Health and illness are value laden, arbitrarily defined, and culturally infused notions. They are not dichotomous but are part of the same continuum. Health seems to occur when patterns of living are in harmony with environmental change while illness occurs when patterns of living conflict with environmental change and are deemed unacceptable.

**Nursing.** A science and an art, nursing is unique in its concern with unitary human beings as synergistic phenomena. The science of nursing should be concerned with studying the nature and direction of unitary human development integral with the environment and evolve descriptive, explanatory, and predictive principles for use in nursing practice. The art of nursing refers to the use of these scientific principles in the delivery of nursing care for human betterment. The goal of nursing is the attainment of the best possible state of health for the individual who is continually evolving by promoting symphonic interactions between humans and environments, strengthening the coherence and integrity of the human field, and directing and redirecting patterning of both fields for maximum health potential.

**Key concepts.** The concepts describe the individual and environment as energy fields, which are in constant interaction. The nature and direction of human development forms the basis for the principles of nursing science.

*Energy fields*—the fundamental level of unitary humans and the environment, they are dynamic fields having no real boundaries. Energy fields are of two types:

> Human energy field—more than the biological, psychological, and sociological fields taken separately or together, the individual possesses integrity and cannot be generalized from parts to whole.
> Environmental energy field—all that is outside a given human field.

*Openness*—as energy fields, the individual and environment are continuously open and extending to infinity.

*Pattern and organization*—characterize human and environmental fields and are continually changing, always becoming more diverse.

*Multidimensionality*—reality is multidimensional and "provides for an infinite domain without limit" (Manhart-Barret, 1990, p. 7).

*Principles of nursing science*—postulate the nature and direction of unitary human development; also called principles of homeodynamics, which are as follows:

> Helicy—"the continuous, innovative, probabilistic increasing diversity of human and environmental field patterns characterized by repeating rhymicities" (1989, p. 186).
> Resonancy—"the continuous change from lower to higher frequency wave patterns in human and environmental fields" (1989, p. 186).
> Integrality—"the continuous mutual human and environmental field process" (1989, p. 186).

## King's Theory of Goal Attainment

Although the foundation for her theory was developed in 1964, it wasn't until her 1971 publication *Toward a Theory for Nursing* that Imogene King presented her entire conceptual framework and identified the concepts of social systems, health, perception, and interpersonal relations. The theory was refined in *A Theory for Nursing: Systems, Concepts, Process* (1981) where King identified the focus of nursing as being on people interacting with their environments, leading to a state of health, which is the ability to function in roles.

**Brief overview.** The individual is viewed as an open system and as one component of a nurse-client interpersonal system whose interactions lead to the attainment of mutually agreed upon goals.

**Assumptions about the individual.** Human beings are open systems who interact with their environment and are conceptualized as social, sentient, rational, perceiving, controlling, purposeful, action-oriented beings.

**Environment.** As an open system, it is implied that the individual and the environment interact and that both the internal and external environments generate stressors.

**Health and illness.** Health is described as an individual's ability to function in social roles, which implies optimal use of one's resources to achieve continuous adjustment to internal and external environmental stressors. Illness is a deviation from the norm, an imbalance in a person's biological structure, psychological makeup, or social relationships.

**Nursing.** In a process of action, reaction, and interaction, the nurse and client communicate, set goals, and explore means to achieve those goals. "The domain of nursing includes promoting, maintaining and restoring health, caring for the sick and injured and caring for the dying" (1981, p. 4). The goal of nursing is to assist individuals to maintain their health so they can function in their roles.

**Key concepts.** Two sets of concepts are subsumed in the theory, one relating to the parties involved in the nurse-client relationship and the other pertaining to goal attainment.

*Personal system*—an individual

*Interpersonal system*—two or more interacting individuals

*Social system*—communities and societies

*Concepts of goal attainment:*

Interaction—a process of perception between the person and environment or one or more persons, represented by verbal and nonverbal behaviors that are goal-directed.

Perception—an individual's representation of reality.

Communication—process of giving information from one person to another.

Transaction—observable behavior or individuals interacting with their environment.

Role—a set of behaviors displayed by an individual who occupies a given position in a social system.

Stress—a dynamic state of interaction with the environment to maintain balance for growth, development, and performance.

Growth and development—"continuous changes in individuals occurring at molecular, cellular and behavioral levels" (1981, p. 148).

Time—a duration between one event and another.

Space—defined by "gestures, postures and visible boundaries erected to mark off personal space" (1981, p. 148).

## Neuman's Systems Model

Betty Neuman developed her systems model in 1970 in response to student requests to focus on breadth rather than depth in understanding human variables in nursing problems. First published in 1972, it was refined to its present form and published in *The Neuman Systems Model* (1989). Neuman believes that nursing encompasses a wholistic client systems approach to help individuals, families, communities, and society reach and maintain wellness.

**Brief overview.** This theory offers a wholistic view of the client system including the concepts of open systems, environment, stressors, prevention, and reconstitution. Nursing is concerned with the whole person.

**Assumptions about the individual.** The client is a whole person, a dynamic composite of interrelationships between physiological, psychological, sociocultural, developmental, and spiritual variables. "The client is viewed as an open system in interaction with the environment" (1989, p. 68). The client is in "dynamic constant energy exchange with the environment" (1989, p. 22).

**Environment.** Both internal and external environments exist, and the person maintains varying degrees of harmony between them. The environment includes all the factors affecting and affected by the system. Emphasis is on all stressors—interpersonal, intrapersonal, extrapersonal—that might disturb the person's normal line of defense.

**Health and illness.** "Health is equated with optimal system stability" (1989, p. 33). The wellness-illness continuum implies that energy flow is continuous between the client system and the environment" (1989, p. 33).

**Nursing.** Nursing is a "unique profession in that it is concerned with all of the variables affecting the individual's response to stress" (1982, p. 14). The major concern of nursing is in "keeping the client system stable through accuracy in both the assessment of effects and possible effects of environmental stressors and in assisting client adjustments required for an optimal wellness level" (1989, p. 34). Nursing goals are determined by "negotiation with the client for desired prescriptive changes to correct variances from wellness" (1989, p. 73).

**Key concepts.** The nurse is concerned with all the variables affecting an individual's response to stressors:

*Primary prevention*—reduces the possibility of encounter with stressors and strengthens the flexible lines of defense.

*Secondary prevention*—protects the basic structure by strengthening the internal lines of resistance.

*Tertiary prevention*—focuses on readaptation and stability. A primary goal is to strengthen resistance to stressors by reeducation to help prevent recurrence of reaction or regression. "Tertiary prevention tends to lead back, in a circular fashion, toward primary prevention" (1989, p. 73).

## Orem's Theory of Self-Care

Foundations of Dorothea Orem's theory were introduced in the late 1950s, but it was not until 1971 that the first edition of *Nursing: Concepts of Practice* was published. The second, third, and fourth editions were published in 1980, 1985, and 1990, respectively, and show evidence of continued development and refinement. Orem focuses on nursing as deliberate human action and notes that all individuals can benefit from nursing when they have health-derived or health-related limitations for engaging in self-care or care of dependent others.

**Brief overview.** The individual practices self-care, a set of learned behaviors, to sustain life, to maintain or restore functioning, and to bring about a condition of well-being. The nurse assists clients with self-care when there is a deficit in their ability to perform.

**Assumptions about the individual.** The individual is viewed as a unity whose functioning is linked with the environment and who, with the environment, forms an integrated, functional whole. "Human beings are capable of self-determined actions" (1990, p. 76) and function biologically, symbolically, and socially.

**Environment.** The environment is linked to the individual, forming an integrated and interactive system. It is implied that the environment is external to the individual.

**Health and illness.** Health, which has physical, psychological, interpersonal, and social aspects, is a state in which human beings are structurally and functionally whole. Illness occurs when an individual is incapable of maintaining self-care as a result of health-related limitations.

**Nursing.** Nursing involves assisting the individual with his or her self-care practices to sustain life and health, recover from disease or injury, and cope with their effects (1990, p. 41). The nurse chooses deliberate actions designed to bring about desirable conditions in persons and their environments. The goal of nursing is to move a patient toward responsible self-care or meeting existing health care needs of those who have health care deficits for purposes of maintaining, protecting, or promoting their functioning as human beings (1990, p. 49).

**Key concepts.** The concepts focus on self-care in terms of requisites, demands, and deficits and delineate the nurse's role in client care.

*Self-care*—learned activities and sequences of actions that individuals initiate and perform on their own behalf to maintain life, health, and well-being.

*Self-care requisites*—actions "performed by or for individuals in the interest of controlling human and environmental factors" (1990, p. 121). There are three categories of self-care requisites:

Universal—common to all human beings, they are concerned with the promotion and maintenance of structural and functional integrity.

Developmental—associated with conditions that promote known developmental processes at each stage of the life cycle.

Health-deviation—associated with genetic and constitutional defects and deviations that impair the individual's ability to perform self-care.

*Therapeutic self-care demands*—the totality of self-care actions performed by the nurse and/or self in order to meet known self-care requisites. *Self-care deficits*—gaps between known therapeutic self-care demands and the ability to perform self-care or dependent care.
*Nursing systems*—actions of nurses and patients that "regulate patient's self-care capabilities and meet patient's self-care needs" (1990, p. 73):

Wholly compensatory—the nurse compensates for the individual's total inability to perform self-care activities.
Partly compensatory—the nurse compensates for the individual's inability to perform some (but not all) self-care activities.
Supportive-educative (developmental)—with the individual able to perform all self-care activities, the nurse assists the client in decision making, behavior control, and acquisition of knowledge and skill (1985, pp. 154–157).

*Dimensions of nursing practice:*

Social—the complementary and contractual relationship between the nurse and client.
Interpersonal—the nurse-client interaction.
Technological—"diagnosis, prescription, and regulation as treatment and management of nursing care."

## Roy's Adaptation Model

Sister Callista Roy has continuously expanded her model from its inception in 1970 to the present. She focuses on the individual as a biopsychosocial adaptive system and describes nursing as a humanistic discipline that "places emphasis on the person's own coping abilities" (1984, p. 32). The individual and the environment are sources of stimuli that require modification to promote adaptation.

**Brief overview.** The individual is a biopsychosocial adaptive system, and the nurse promotes adaptation by modifying external stimuli.

**Assumptions about the individual.** The individual is in constant interaction with a changing environment and to respond positively to environmental change, that person must adapt. The person's adaptation level is determined by the combined effect of three classes of stimuli—focal, contextual, and residual. The individual uses both innate and acquired biologic, psychologic, or social adaptive mechanisms and has four modes of adaptation.

**Environment.** All conditions, circumstances, and influences surrounding and affecting the development and behavior of persons and groups constitute the environment. Having both internal and external components, the environment is constantly changing.

**Health and illness.** "Health and illness are one inevitable dimension of a person's life" (1989, p. 106). Health is a process of being and becoming an integrated and whole person. Conversely, illness is a lack of integration.

**Nursing.** An external regulatory force, nursing acts to modify stimuli affecting adaptation by increasing, decreasing, or maintaining stimuli. The goal of nursing is to promote the person's adaptation in the four adaptive modes, thus contributing to health, the quality of life, and dying with dignity.

**Key concepts.** The concepts describe and define adaptation in terms of the individual's internal control processes, adaptive modes, and adaptive level.
*Adaptation*—the individual's ability to cope with the constantly changing environment.
*Adaptive system*—consists of two major internal control processes:

Regulator—receives input from the external environment and from changes in the person's internal state and processes it through neutral-chemical-endocrine channels.

Cognator—receives input from external and internal stimuli that involve psychological, social, physical, and physiological factors and processes it through cognitive pathways.

*Adaptive modes*—ways a person adapts, which include four modes:

Physiological—determined by need for physiological integrity derived from the basic physiological needs.

Self-concept—determined by need for interactions with others and psychic integrity regarding perception of self.

Role function—determined by need for social integrity, it refers to the performance of duties based on given positions within society.

Interdependence—involves ways of seeking help, affection, and attention.

*Adaptive level*—determined by the combined effect of stimuli:

Focal stimuli—that which immediately confronts the individual.

Contextual stimuli—all other stimuli present.

Residual stimuli—beliefs, attitudes, or traits that have an indeterminate effect on the present situation.

## Leininger's Theory of Transcultural Nursing

Drawing from a background in cultural and social anthropology, Madeleine Leininger's contribution to nursing knowledge is related to transcultural nursing and caring. Her book, *Transcultural Nursing: Concepts, Theories and Practice* (1978), presented her conceptual framework for cultural care and health. She continues to explicate the linkages between nursing and anthropology as she identifies and defines concepts such as care, caring, culture, cultural values, and cultural variations (1984).

**Brief overview.** Transcultural nursing focuses on a comparative study and analysis of different cultures and subcultures in the world with respect to their caring behavior, nursing care, health-illness values, and patterns of behavior with the goal of developing a scientific and humanistic body of knowledge in order to derive culture-specific and culture-universal nursing care practices.

**Assumptions about the individual.** The social structure, world view, and values of people vary transculturally. Clients from different cultures perceive health, illness, caring, curing, dependence, and independence differently.

**Environment.** The environment is defined as a social structure, the "interrelated and interdependent systems of a society which determine how it functions with respect to certain major elements, namely: the political (including legal) economic, social (including kinship) educational, technical, religious and cultural systems" (1978, p. 61).

**Health and illness.** Perceptions of health and illness are culturally infused and therefore cannot be universally defined. World views, social structure, and cultural beliefs influence perceptions of health and illness and cannot be separated from them. For example, some cultures perceive illness to be largely a personal and internal body experience, while others view illness as an extrapersonal or cultural experience.

**Nursing.** Nursing is a learned, humanistic art and science that focuses upon personalized (individual and group) care behaviors, functions, and processes that have physical, psychocultural, and social significance or meaning. The goal of nursing is directed toward promoting and maintaining health behaviors or recovery from illness in a way that is culturally congruent.

**Key concepts.** Among the core concepts of transcultural nursing theory are:

*Care*—phenomena related to assistive, supportive, or enabling behavior toward or for another individual with evident or anticipated needs to ease or improve a human condition.

*Culture*—values, beliefs, norms, and lifeway practices of a particular group that guides thinking, decisions, actions, and patterned ways.

*Cultural care*—the cognitively known values, beliefs, and patterned expressions that assist, support, or enable another individual or group to maintain well-being, improve a human condition, or to face death.

*Cultural care diversity*—the variability of meaning, patterns, values, or symbols of care that are culturally derived for health or to improve a human condition.

*Cultural care universality*—common, similar, or uniform meanings, patterns, values, or symbols of care that are culturally derived for health or to improve a human condition.

## Watson's Science of Caring

Jean Watson's theoretical formulations focus on the philosophy and science of caring, the core of nursing. With an aim toward reducing the dichotomy between nursing theory and practice, the framework was first published in 1979 and further developed in her 1985 publication. Watson draws from multiple disciplines to derive carative factors that are central to nursing and describes concepts as they relate to the pivotal theme of caring.

**Brief overview.** Caring is central to nursing practice, but it is a moral ideal rather than a task-oriented behavior. An interpersonal process, caring results in the satisfaction of human needs.

**Assumptions about the individual.** Individuals (i.e., both the nurse and client) are nonreducible and are interconnected with others and nature (1985, p. 16).

**Environment.** The client's environment contains both external and internal variables. The nurse promotes a caring environment, one that allows individuals to make choices relative to the best action for himself or herself at that point in time.

**Health and illness.** Health is more than the absence of illness but, because it is subjective, it is an elusive concept (1979, p. 219).

**Nursing.** The practice of nursing is different from curing and consists of 10 carative factors as described below. The goal of nursing is to promote and restore health and prevent illness by offering a relationship that the client can use for personal growth and development.

**Key concepts.** Ten carative factors form the core of nursing and delineate the domain of nursing practice:

1. Formation of a humanistic-altruistic system of values.
2. Instillation of faith-hope to promote wellness.
3. Cultivation of sensitivity to self and to others.
4. Development of a helping-trust relationship.
5. Promotion and acceptance of the expression of positive and negative.
6. Systematic use of the scientific problem-solving method for decision making.
7. Promotion of interpersonal teaching-learning.
8. Provision for a supportive, protective, or corrective mental, physical, sociocultural, and spiritual environment.
9. Assistance with the gratification of human needs.
10. Allowance for existential-phenomenological forces.

### Parse's Theory of Man-Living-Health

Rosemarie Rizzo Parse developed a philosophical model that focuses on the inseparable concepts of Man-Living-Health as nursing's concern. Taking an existential approach, she derived three principles that center on the idea of Man-Living-Health always moving toward greater diversity and "becoming" (1981).

**Brief overview.** Always in the process of becoming, Man-Living-Health are inseparable. Nursing is a human science that focuses on Man and Health.

**Assumptions about the individual.** The individual is an open being, coexisting with the environment. Man freely chooses meaning in situations and bears responsibility for decisions. As life progresses, individuals become more complex and diverse, forming new patterns of relating.

**Environment.** The environment is inseparable from the individual.

**Health and illness.** Health is an open process of becoming and is a rhythmically coconstituting process of the man-environment interrelationship. Illness is not the opposite of health but rather a pattern of man's interrelationship with the world (1981, p. 41). Both health and illness are lived experiences.

**Nursing.** A human science, nursing focuses on man as a living unity and his participation in health experiences. The goal of nursing is to illuminate and mobilize family (human) interrelationships.

**Key concepts.** The concepts are incorporated into three major principles that focus on meaning, rhythmicity, and cotranscendence. Within each principle, succeeding concepts build on preceding ones.

*Meaning*—arises from man's interrelationship with the world and refers to happenings to which we attach varying degrees of significance.

> Imaging—structures the meaning of an experience.
> Valuing—process of confirming cherished beliefs.
> Languaging—expressing valued images.

*Rhythmicity*—the movement toward greater diversity.

> Revealing-concealing—disclosing of some aspects of self and hiding of others all at once.
> Enabling-limiting—the result of making choices; in choosing, one is both enabled in some things and limited in others.
> Connecting-separating—a simultaneous process; connecting with some phenomena results in separating from others.

*Cotranscendence*—the process of reaching out beyond the self.

> Powering—moving toward all future possibilities.
> Originating—distinguishing self from others.
> Transforming—an ongoing process of change; moving toward greater diversity by transcending the present.

● ● ●

It is evident that the theories and frameworks discussed here offer a variety of perspectives. For example, some are process-oriented and dynamic, such as King's theory of goal attainment, Rogers' science of unitary human beings, and Parse's Man-Living-Health. Others are more outcome-oriented, such as Roy's adaptation model, Johnson's behavioral system model, and Orem's theory of self-care. Rogers' and Neuman's models focus on the wholeness of the individual and conceptualize nursing as one component of the individual's life process. King's theory is directed toward the interaction between the nurse and the client, and they are inseparable. Leininger, Nightingale, and Henderson developed humanistic perspectives; they focus on personalized, individualized care for all. Johnson and Roy conceptualize the nurse as an external regulator whose function is to promote system balance or adaptation. Orem views the nurse as one who assists individuals with their self-care practices when they are unable to effectively care for themselves.

A more structured approach to nursing care than the conceptual frameworks, theories, and models previously discussed is the nursing process. Perhaps the most widely used framework in nursing, the nursing process offers a specific, organized, and systematic method for the delivery of nursing care within which many of the above theories can be accommodated. An overview of the nursing process is provided in the following section.

### ❖ THE NURSING PROCESS AS A FRAMEWORK FOR PRACTICE

The nursing process has been described as the core and essence of nursing. It is central to all nursing actions, applicable in any setting and within any conceptual reference. It is flexible and adaptable, yet sufficiently structured to provide a base from which all systematic nursing actions can proceed. It is organized, methodical, and deliberate (Yura & Walsh, 1988).

Most nurses are aware of the nursing process, and many use it in their daily practice. This chapter, therefore, gives only a brief overview of this framework to provide a common knowledge base for understanding its application in subsequent chapters that conceptualize client stressors, strengths, and major life themes. These chapters also include case studies (i.e., chronicity, crisis) and sample care plans, which apply the nursing process to selected dimensions of the concepts discussed. Nurses requiring more in-depth information are referred to textbooks devoted entirely to this topic such as *Nursing Process: Application of Theories, Frameworks, and Models* by Christensen and Kenney (1990) or *The Nursing Process: Assessing, Planning, Implementing, and Evaluating* by Yura and Walsh (1988).

### Overview of the Nursing Process

Nurses rely on interpersonal, intellectual, and technical skills to carry out client care. These skills are incorporated into a process to ensure safe, efficient care. The nursing process involves:

Assessing—identifying client strengths, health status, and concerns.
Analyzing—processing client data and identifying appropriate nursing diagnoses.
Planning—solving identified problems to build on client strengths.
Implementing—delivering the planned care.
Evaluating—determining the effectiveness of the care delivered.

As illustrated in Fig. 1-1, the nursing process is continuous and can accommodate changes in the client's health status and/or failure to achieve expected outcomes through a feedback mechanism. This mechanism allows the nurse to reenter the nursing process at the appropriate stage to collect additional data, restructure nursing diagnoses, design a new plan, or change implementation strategies.

More global nursing theories and frameworks can be accommodated within the framework of the nursing process, but the focus differs according to the specific theory that is guiding the care. For example, a nurse using Orem's theory would focus on the concept of self-care in all stages of the nursing process, assessing for self-care deficits, and planning interventions to compensate for or alleviate those deficits. Similarly, a nurse using Roy's adaptation model would assess biopsychosocial aspects of the individual and design interventions to modify stimuli to promote adaptation in the four adaptive modes. Regardless of the nursing theory or framework used, the distinct components remain identical: assessment, analysis and nursing diagnosis, planning including goals and objectives, implementation, and evaluation.

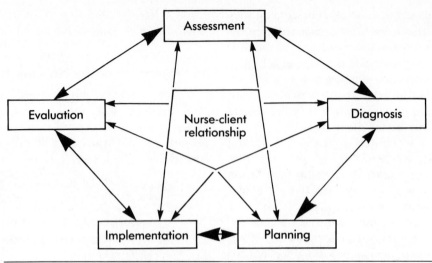

❖ **Fig. 1-1**   The nursing process feedback system. *(From Christensen, P.J. and Kenny, J. W.: Nursing process: application of conceptual models, St. Louis, 1990, The CV Mosby Co., p. 7)*

### Assessment

The first step of the nursing process, assessment, "is the deliberate and systematic collection of data to determine a client's current health status and to evaluate his present and past coping patterns" (Carpenito, 1989, p. 45). Sources of data are the client, family, health care record, and other health care providers. Assessment skills include the use of physical diagnosis instruments such as a stethoscope, otoscope, and cardiac monitor, active listening, observation, and the use of selected data collection measures and instruments such as those described in subsequent chapters.

Assessment begins by taking a nursing history. Many clinical areas have developed nursing history forms specific to the type of agency and clients served. However, all nursing histories include basic categories such as age, sex, presenting problem, health history, and current health status. The amount of detail may vary, as for example, the difference between a history obtained in an emergency department and one

taken in an extended care facility. The focus of the assessment and history may also vary based on the type of client served. For example, on an oncology unit, emphasis may be placed on assessment of pain, social support networks, and coping skills while in a prenatal clinic, the focus would be on assessment of fetal growth, knowledge of nutrition, and the need for community resources such as childbirth education classes or nutritional programs such as the women-infants-children (WIC) program. Beyond the areas of particular concern, however, it is important to assess all dimensions of the client including physiological, psychological, sociocultural, developmental, and spiritual aspects (Carpenito, 1989).

Data gathering in the assessment stage is time well-spent, since incomplete or inaccurate data will lead to an inappropriate diagnosis and a plan that will only serve to waste valuable time and frustrate the nurse and client. The assessment stage is also a time to establish the nurse-client relationship as the nurse becomes recognized as a caring but organized and purposeful resource for the client. Depending on the situation, the assessment stage may also be the time for the nurse to establish a relationship with the client's family and other supportive individuals who may be critical to effective discharge planning.

## Analysis and Nursing Diagnoses

Analysis involves processing the data by organizing, categorizing, and synthesizing the information. In the analysis stage, both objective and subjective data are "gathered together, shuffled, sorted, scrambled, and spit out in composite form" (Braden & Herban, 1976). Analysis gives meaning to the data as client strengths and actual or potential problems are identified. The data from the client are compared against known norms such as growth and development or disease-specific behaviors or expectations. Gaps or incongruities in data are identified, and patterns of behavior are ascertained. Analysis takes place with the client as the nurse is actively listening and questioning, and later as he or she processes the information to formulate a plan of care. Analysis is an ongoing process that is called forth when new information is obtained or changes in the client's health status occur. Analysis concludes with the identification of nursing diagnoses.

A nursing diagnosis is a "clear, concise, and definitive statement of the client's health status and concerns that can be affected by nursing intervention" (Christensen & Kenney, 1990, p. 159). The box on p. 22 lists nursing diagnoses approved by the North American Nursing Diagnosis Association (NANDA) Nursing diagnoses reflect actual or potential problems within 11 functional health patterns:

1. Health perception—health maintenance pattern
2. Nutritional and metabolic pattern
3. Elimination pattern
4. Activity-rest pattern
5. Sleep-rest pattern
6. Cognitive perceptual pattern
7. Self-perception—self-concept pattern
8. Role-relationship pattern
9. Sexuality-reproductive pattern
10. Coping-stress tolerance pattern
11. Value-belief pattern (Gordon, 1987).

The use of nursing diagnoses promotes comprehensive health care and facilitates communication among nurses by providing a common language. The identification of nursing diagnoses utilizes the nurse's knowledge, skills, and experience and sets the stage for the remaining steps of planning, implementation, and evaluation.

## Planning

Planning involves the development of a plan of action aimed at resolving nursing diagnoses to assist the client toward the goal of optimal wellness (Yura & Walsh, 1988). In the past, planning for client care was done *by* the nurse *for* the client. More recently, however, plans are often formulated and developed *with* the client. Nevertheless, as noted in Chapter 26 on empowerment, the client's readiness and willingness to mutually plan must be carefully assessed since individuals differ in their desire for involvement in the planning process. In addition, some clients want control over some aspects of care and not others. Periodic reassessment of the client's wish for mutual planning is important because the desire for mutual plans may change as the disease condition or circumstances change. Family members and significant others may also be incorporated into the planning process since they may be critical to effective discharge planning or may serve as support systems to clients who receive care in a community setting. The planning stage includes prioritizing the identified problems, developing long-term and short-term goals, and defining objectives to serve as measures of progress toward goal attainment.

## ❖ NANDA—APPROVED NURSING DIAGNOSES

Activity intolerance
Activity intolerance, potential
Adjustment, impaired
Airway clearance, ineffective
Anxiety
Aspiration, potential for
Body image disturbance
Body temperature, altered, potential
Bowel incontinence
Breastfeeding, ineffective
Breathing pattern, ineffective
Cardiac output, decreased
Communication, impaired verbal
Constipation
Constipation, colonic
Constipation, perceived
Coping, defensive
Coping, family: potential for growth
Coping, ineffective family: compromised
Coping, ineffective family: disabling
Coping, ineffective individual
Decisional conflict (specify)
Denial, ineffective
Diarrhea
Disuse syndrome, potential for
Diversional activity deficit
Dysreflexia
Family processes, altered
Fatigue
Fear
Fluid volume deficit (1)
Fluid volume deficit (2)
Fluid volume-deficit, potential
Fluid volume excess
Gas exchange, impaired
Grieving, anticipatory
Grieving, dysfunctional
Growth and development, altered
Health maintenance, altered
Health-seeking behaviors (specify)
Home maintenance management, impaired
Hopelessness
Hyperthermia
Hypothermia
Incontinence, functional
Incontinence, reflex
Incontinence, stress
Incontinence, total
Incontinence, urge
Infection, potential for
Injury, potential for
Knowledge deficit (specify)

Mobility, impaired physical
Noncompliance (specify)
Nutrition, altered: less than body requirements
Nutrition, altered: more than body requirements
Nutrition, altered: potential for more than body
   requirements
Oral mucous membrane, altered
Pain
Pain, chronic
Parental role conflict
Parenting, altered
Parenting, altered, potential
Personal identity disturbance
Poisoning, potential for
Post-trauma response
Powerlessness
Protective mechanisms, altered
Rape-trauma syndrome
Rape-trauma syndrome: compound reaction
Rape-trauma syndrome: silent reaction
Role performance, altered
Self-care deficit, bathing/hygiene
Self-care deficit, dressing/grooming
Self-care deficit, feeding
Self-care deficit, toileting
Self-esteem disturbance
Self-esteem, chronic low
Self-esteem, situational low
Sensory/perceptual alterations (specify) (visual,
   auditory, kinesthetic, gustatory, tactile,
   olfactory)
Sexual dysfunction
Sexuality patterns, altered
Skin integrity, impaired
Skin integrity, impaired, potential
Sleep pattern disturbance
Social interaction, impaired
Social isolation
Spiritual distress (distress of the human spirit)
Suffocation, potential for
Swallowing, impaired
Thermoregulation, ineffective
Thought processes, altered
Tissue integrity, impaired
Tissue perfusion, altered (specify type) (renal,
   cerebral, cardiopulmonary, gastrointestinal,
   peripheral)
Trauma, potential for
Unilateral neglect
Urinary elimination, altered patterns
Urinary retention
Violence, potential for: self-directed or directed
   at others

**Setting priorities.** Priorities may be conveniently categorized as high, medium, or low. In setting priorities, life-threatening client problems are addressed before other health concerns. Additional considerations in setting priorities are the need for early resolution of problems that have the potential to impair functioning or normal growth and development, the client's individual needs, values and overall health status, and constraints of time and resources.

With some clients, the setting of priorities may be influenced by the need to reinforce the nurse-client relationship through immediate goal attainment. In other situations where the client may be feeling helpless or hopeless, a consideration in setting priorities may be the need to select a problem with an easily achievable goal. This facilitates a sense of goal attainment and accomplishment for the nurse and client, demonstrates the value of the nurse to the client, and strengthens the relationship. This strategy may be especially useful with a client or family resistant to interventions or who may previously have had negative experiences with the health care system.

**Long-term and short-term goals.** Once priorities are established, long-term and short-term goals must be identified. A goal is a broad or abstract statement derived from the nursing diagnosis that reflects expected client outcomes to alleviate a concern or condition specified by the nursing diagnosis (McFarland & McFarlane, 1989). Goals reflect health restoration, maintenance, or promotion. Goals must be realistic and achievable, taking into account such factors as the client's strengths, limitations, lifestyle, and resources. As with setting priorities, goals are often mutually determined by the nurse and client. However, with a greater knowledge base than the client, the nurse may frequently need to assist the client to select appropriate goals.

**Objectives.** When goals have been estab-

lished, specific, measurable objectives must be developed. An objective describes the intended result of a particular nursing action or set of actions. In general, three to six objectives are needed for each goal (Christensen & Kenney, 1990) to reflect a logical, incremental progression toward goal attainment. To be truly measurable, an objective must be stated in behavioral terms and have three characteristics: performance, conditions, and criterion. Performance is the activity expected by the client, such as listing two sources of food high in calcium or demonstrating correct administration of insulin. Conditions describe the circumstances under which the client performs the activity, such as in the home setting, without assistance, or within a particular time frame. Criterion is the standard by which the performance is evaluated and may include measures such as speed, degree of accuracy, quality of the behavior (e.g., use of aseptic technique), or a criterion-reference such as according to the American Heart Association (Christensen & Kenney, 1990). An example of a measurable behavioral objective is presented in Table 1-2.

## Implementation

Implementation "is the initiation and completion of actions necessary to accomplish the defined goal of optimal wellness for the client" (Yura & Walsh, 1988, p. 154). During implementation the nurse uses intellectual, interpersonal, and technical skills to provide care that is client-focused, goal-oriented, and meets the physical and psychological safety needs of the

❖  **TABLE 1-2**
A measurable behavioral objective

| Objective | Characteristic |
|---|---|
| Mr. M. will walk | Performance |
| one half the length of the hall | Criterion |
| unassisted | Condition |
| on the second postoperative day. | Condition |

client. Implementation includes actions taken by the nurse, other members of the health team, and the client and/or family members. It involves executing the plan of care by undertaking nursing actions, supervising others in providing care, or both. The final stage of implementation includes careful documentation of the care delivered, observations made including new data that may have emerged, and the client's responses, which indicate progress (or lack of it) toward achievement of goals and objectives.

### Evaluation

Often the most neglected stage of the nursing process, evaluation serves several purposes. The primary purpose is to determine the client's progress toward goal attainment by measuring the extent to which objectives are achieved. Evaluation also serves to judge the appropriateness, adequacy, effectiveness, and efficiency of the plan of care and its implementation. Evaluation is an ongoing process and includes comparing current client responses to previous responses to similar interventions. If the outcomes are not as expected, the nurse needs to determine the reason. Questions that might be asked include:

1. Were the assessment data appropriate and complete?
2. Were the data interpreted correctly?
3. Were nursing diagnoses appropriate?
4. Were goals and objectives realistic, attainable, and measurable?
5. Was the nursing care plan directed toward resolution of nursing diagnoses?
6. Was the implementation of the plan individualized in accordance with the client's strengths and limitations?

Based on the answers to these questions, it may be necessary to reenter the nursing process at the appropriate point and try again.

### ❖ EVALUATING THE UTILITY OF NURSING THEORIES AND FRAMEWORKS

Not all theories and frameworks are equally comprehensive or equally useful in every situation. The definition of the client and the setting where care is delivered may limit the usefulness of some theories and frameworks described here. Before adopting a theory for use in practice, education, or research, it is important to examine its utility for the intended use and the consistency of its internal structure. The value and logical structure of a theory can be evaluated by asking questions proposed by Fawcett (1989) such as:

1. Are the assumptions inherent in the theory clearly stated?
2. Does the theory include the four concepts central to nursing?
3. Are the relationships between the concepts clearly explained?
4. Are there conflicting views within the structure of the theory?
5. Can relationships between concepts be tested in research and applied to practice?
6. Does the theory lead to nursing activities that meet societal expectations (social congruence)?
7. Does the theory lead to nursing activities that make important differences in the client's health status (social significance)?
8. Does the theory include explicit rules for use in practice, education, or research (social usefulness)?

### ❖ SUMMARY

The theories and frameworks presented in this chapter represent a wide range of perspectives. Varying in their degree of specificity, some have greater utility for direct application to practice than others. The more specific theories and frameworks can be readily adapted for use in any practice setting. The more global ones may better serve as frameworks for research, the findings of which can then be applied to practice. However, all have the potential to make substantial contributions to the nursing profession by enhancing the development of a unique body of nursing knowledge. Examples of their use are shown throughout this book.

## ❖ APPLYING KNOWLEDGE TO PRACTICE

1. Select a nursing theory presented in this chapter and apply the concepts to nursing practice in each of the following settings:
   a) A community mental health clinic
   b) An intensive care unit
   c) An extended care facility
   d) A well-baby clinic
2. Many nursing programs do not include Florence Nightingale in their basic curriculum. Have you been exposed to her ideas before? How do you think her ideas can be applied to nursing practice in the current health care system?
3. Discuss the advantages and disadvantages of the use of nursing diagnoses.
4. Discuss the type of nursing assessment instrument used in your current area of practice. Does it include questions specific to a particular clinical area? Could the tool be used in other clinical areas? Why or why not? Compare several tools from your classmates and list the advantages and disadvantages of each.
5. The evaluation component is the most neglected stage of the nursing process. Do you agree with this statement? Support your position with clinical examples.

## REFERENCES

Auger, J. R. (1976). *Behavioral systems and nursing*. Englewood Cliffs, NJ: Prentice-Hall.

Braden, C. & Herban, N. (1976). *Community health: A systems approach*. New York: Appleton-Century-Crofts.

Carpenito, L. (1989). *Nursing diagnosis: Application to clinical practice*. Philadelphia: J. B. Lippincott.

Chinn, P. & Jacobs, M. (1987). *Theory and nursing: A systematic approach*. St. Louis: C. V. Mosby.

Christensen, P. J. & Kenney, J. W. (1990). *Nursing process: Application of conceptual models*. St. Louis: C. V. Mosby Co.

Fawcett, J. (1989). *Conceptual models of nursing* (2nd ed.). Philadelphia: F.A. Davis.

Gordon, M. (1987). *Nursing diagnoses: Process and application*. New York: McGraw-Hill.

Grubbs, J. (1974). *An interpretation of the Johnson behavioral system model*. In J. P. Reihl & C. Roy (Eds.), *Conceptual models for nursing practice* (pp. 160-197). New York: Appleton-Century-Crofts.

Henderson, V. (1966). *The nature of nursing: A definition and its implications for practice, research, and education*. New York: Macmillan.

Henderson, V. & Nite, G. (1978). *The principles and practice of nursing*. New York: Macmillan.

Johnson, D. E. (1980). *The behavioral system model for nursing*. In J. P. Reihl & C. Roy (Eds), *Conceptual models for nursing practice*, (2nd ed.), (pp. 207-215). New York: Appleton-Century-Crofts.

King, I. (1971). *Toward a theory for nursing*. New York: John Wiley & Sons.

King, I. (1981). *A theory for nursing: Systems, concepts, process*. New York: John Wiley.

Leininger, M. (1978). *Transcultural nursing: Concepts, theories and practices*. New York: John Wiley & Sons.

Leininger, M. (Ed.). (1984). *Care: The essence of nursing and health*. Thorofare, NJ: Slack.

Manhart-Barret, E. (1990). Visions of Roger's Science based nursing. New York: National League for Nursing.

McFarland, G. K. & McFarlane, E. A. (1989). *Nursing diagnosis and intervention*. St. Louis: C. V. Mosby.

Neuman, B. (1982). *The Neuman systems model: Application to nursing theory and practice*. Norwalk: Appleton-Century-Crofts.

Neuman, B. (1989). *The Neuman systems model*. (2nd ed.). Norwalk: Appleton and Lange.

Nightingale, F. (1946). *Notes on nursing: What it is and what it is not*. Philadelphia: Edward Stern. (Original work published 1859)

Orem, D. (1971). *Nursing: Concepts of practice*. New York: McGraw-Hill.

Orem, D. (1980). *Nursing: Concepts of practice*, (2nd ed.). New York: McGraw-Hill.

Orem, D. (1985). *Nursing: Concepts of practice,* (3rd ed.). New York: McGraw-Hill.

Orem, D (1990). Nursing: Concepts of practice. (4th ed.). St. Louis: C.V. Mosby.

Parse, R. (1981). *Man-living-health: A theory of nursing.* New York: John Wiley.

Rogers, M. (1970). *An introduction to the theoretical basis of nursing.* Philadelphia: F. A. Davis.

Rogers, M. (1989). *Nursing: A science of unitary man.* In J. P. Reihl-Sisca (Ed.), *Conceptual models for nursing practice,* (3rd ed.). (pp. 181-188). New York: Appleton and Lange.

Roy, C. Sr. (1970). *Adaptation: A conceptual framework for nursing. Nursing Outlook. 18,* 254-257.

Roy, C. Sr. (1984). *Introduction to nursing: An adaptation model* (2nd ed.). Englewood Cliffs, NJ: Prentice-Hall.

Roy, C. Sr. (1989). The Roy Adaptation Model. In J. P. Reihl-Sisca (Ed.), *Conceptual models for nursing practice,* (3rd ed.). (pp. 105-114). Norwalk: Appleton and Lange.

Watson, J. (1979). *Nursing: The philosophy and science of caring.* Boston: Little-Brown.

Watson, J. (1985). *Nursing: Human science and health care.* Norwalk, Appleton-Century-Crofts.

Yura, H. Walsh, M. (1988). *The nursing process: Assessing, planning, implementing, and evaluating,* (5th ed.). Norwalk: Appleton and Lange.

# 2 Client Systems

**Gail O. Mazzocco**

## OBJECTIVES

*At the completion of this chapter, the reader will be able to:*

◆ Define and describe the elements of General Systems Theory.

◆ Apply those elements to the assessment of the individual, family, and community.

◆ Analyze data, implement nursing care, and evaluate that care based on General Systems Theory.

Nursing today combines its enduring concern for clients with a more recent awareness of the role of science and technology in improving health care. Unfortunately, those two perspectives are difficult to fuse. Because the assumptions underlying each are often contradictory, nurses are frequently frustrated as they attempt to be compassionate and technically expert practitioners. General Systems Theory, when combined with the nursing process, successfully joins humanistic and scientific perspectives into a single model—one that can direct nursing practice. This chapter focuses on three types of client systems: the individual, the family, and the community. All three are typical of living systems, since they are goal-directed and display complex behaviors.

## ❖ GENERAL SYSTEMS THEORY
### Overview

General Systems Theory was developed in response to the tendency of modern science to analyze complex phenomena by breaking them into their component parts. While that approach worked reasonably well in the physical sciences, it was less successful when used to explore behavior. Bertalanffy (1956), with the assistance of a number of other scientists, developed General Systems Theory as a new analytical approach; one that has as its central concepts integration and holism.

"General Systems Theory is a set of related definitions, assumptions, and propositions which deal with reality as an integrated hierarchy" (Miller, 1978, p. 9). Systems Theory focuses on each *system* as a whole, but pays particular attention to the interaction of its parts or *subsystems.* This dual perspective makes Systems Theory particularly helpful in dealing with complex problems and relationships (Lazlo, 1972). Because it is so widely applicable, the theory also has the potential to improve communication between physical and behavioral scientists. These general attributes make systems theory particularly helpful to nursing.

27

Most nurses are employed in institutions that use a body systems or "medical model" approach to health care. A client's health problems are identified and treated based on a health history, a review of systems, and a physical examination. The specific body system or systems that are malfunctioning are then treated in an attempt to improve the client's health status. While education and social support may be provided, these are distinctly secondary services.

Consider the effect of this approach on the most typical of clients, a 74-year-old woman who enters the hospital with congestive heart failure. Although her immediate problems may be well-served by treating her cardiovascular and respiratory symptoms, long-term success is rarely the result of intervention with either of those systems. In fact, a common outcome of this approach would be repeated readmissions to the hospital to stabilize her condition. Most nurses are all too familiar with this in-and-out phenomenon.

A General Systems perspective is much more likely to be helpful. This method considers the functioning of the individual as reflected by body systems, psychosocial and educational needs. Because it attempts to meet those needs as a whole, it can help this client improve her health, both in the hospital and after discharge. Many nurses intuitively recognize the need for such a holistic approach, but lack experience in using one. This lack of familiarity, when combined with experience using the medical model, often discourages nurses from trying this global approach, regardless of its potential usefulness.

The nurse who uses Systems Theory evaluates the individual, family, or community as a whole, but simultaneously considers the relationship between parts. For that reason, the theory serves as the foundation for a comprehensive assessment and analysis of human systems (La Monica, 1985). Because the theory is general, information is easy to share with nurses in a variety of settings as well as with other health professionals. Moreover, when it is fully tested, the theory may allow the practicing nurse to make more accurate predictions about client behaviors (Ryan, 1979).

## Components of a System

A *system* is a group of elements that interact with one another in order to achieve a goal (Bertalanffy, 1956). Matter, energy, and information that enter that system are called input. The system's parts or *subsystems* use that input in a process that is referred to as *throughput,* and release matter, energy, and information into the *environment* as *output.* While most of the output remains in the environment, part of it is returned to the system as *feedback.* Feedback allows a system to monitor its own output over time and to attempt to move itself closer to a steady state known as *equilibrium* or *homeostasis.* Every system is surrounded by a *boundary,* which separates it from its environment and determines what enters the system. Outside that boundary is the *suprasystem,* which is the next larger organized entity of which that system is a part. Beyond the suprasystem is the environment, composed of all the other systems, which either influence or are influenced by the system under study (Fig. 2-1).

An individual is a system because he or she takes matter, energy, and information in the form of food, fluids, oxygen, data, and sensations into the body as input, and then uses biologic, psychologic, and sociocultural subsystems to process that input. The individual then returns matter, energy, and information to the environment in the form of both physical and psychosocial behaviors. Some of that output returns to the human system as feedback, which allows the individual to determine how well he or she is functioning. In the case of a person, the amount of feedback that is accepted is partially controlled by that individual (Yura & Walsh, 1978).

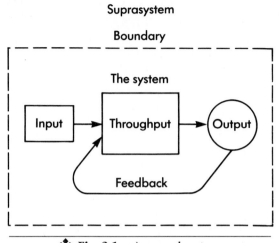

Suprasystem

Boundary

The system

Input → Throughput → Output

Feedback

❖ **Fig. 2-1**  A general system.

In the human, the boundary extends beyond the skin to an area of personal space and separates the individual system from that of the family, which is usually the immediate suprasystem. Surrounding that suprasystem is the larger environment, including the community, with which the individual also interacts.

## Operational Characteristics of Systems

All systems have common characteristics that influence their ability to operate. The first of these is related to the system's structure and function. Structure refers to the arrangement and organization of a system's visible physical parts, while function represents those operations that a system carries out to maintain itself or to achieve its goal (Helvie, 1981). Every system is composed of interacting elements that are related (Miller, 1978). The elements have common structural and functional properties that make it possible for them to work together to process input. Structure and function are not separate entities, however. Rather, they are so closely related that a change in one causes a change in the other. For example, a person has physical structures that process all input. Those

structures include relatively complex nervous and endocrine systems, which function together to coordinate and mediate both physical and psychosocial behaviors. A structural change in the nervous system will alter the functioning of both systems.

A second characteristic is related to boundary permeability. Each system is surrounded by a boundary, which may range from being completely open to the environment to being completely closed to it. However, few systems are found at the extremes, since most require some manageable amount of environmental input in order to function. Without that input, a system becomes increasingly disordered or *entropic.* In order to avoid this, most systems have semipermeable boundaries and are classified according to their degree of openness to external input. For example, the pituitary gland is quite sensitive to releasing factors from the neurosecretory cells of the hypothalamus, but less so to the neurotransmitter acetylcholine (boundary permeability). In fact, without the feedback loop between the hypothalamus and the pituitary, the endocrine system becomes entropic and functions erratically, as does the individual of whom the system is a part.

Finally, systems are hierarchically arranged within an environment (Christensen & Kenney, 1990). In other words, there is an organizational scheme in which simple systems precede those that are more complex. As a result, most systems are part of larger, more complex systems and have smaller, simpler systems that are a part of them. For example, a child is a part of a family system, and that family is a part of a community. However, the child also has biological subsystems that work as systems themselves (Fig. 2-2). Surrounding the system and suprasystem is an environment composed of all those elements that have an impact on the system being studied. While it may be more accurate to think of the environment as a series of increasingly complex systems, it is generally simpler to view it as a unit.

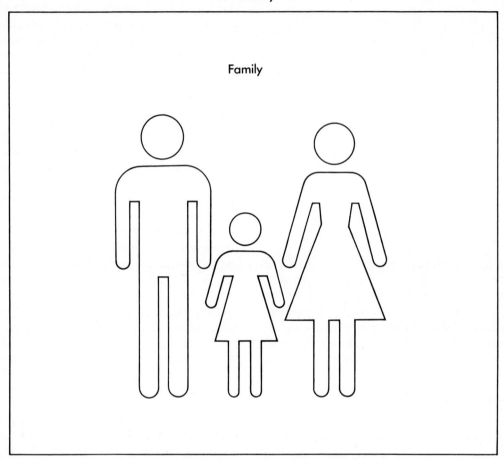

❖ **Fig. 2-2**  A family system.

## Characteristics of Behavioral Systems

The generalizations made thus far apply to all systems, closed or open, living or nonliving. However, the nurse is primarily concerned with living or behavioral systems. These systems have some additional characteristics that reflect their vital nature.

Perhaps because they have the physical and chemical characteristics of life, behavioral systems operate as more than just a collection of specialized systems. As the parts work together

to achieve the system's goals, the subsystems become an efficient and functional team. Therefore, living systems perform as unified wholes rather than as merely the sum of their parts (Byrne & Thompson, 1972). A common purpose is the fuel for this cooperative effort.

Because common purpose is so important, living systems must be goal-directed. The specific goal varies with the system, but that goal must direct the functional and structural elements of that system (Ryan, 1979). Individuals, because they are complex behavioral systems, may select and later alter some of their goals. Those alterations require the system to overcome the homeostatic forces that operate to maintain the system's status quo.

Living systems continually take in matter, energy, and information from the environment, and so they never reach true equilibrium. Instead, they achieve homeostasis, a condition of balance within the range of normal activities (Bertalanffy, 1956). In order to maintain that balance, living systems must adapt to environmental changes. Homeostatic regulators must sometimes be overcome in order to stimulate alterations in the system's internal processes, and to change its level of functioning (Kast & Rosenzweig, 1981). This process is not easy, particularly when the system's goals and those of the environment are at odds. For example, an individual may be totally committed to life in a small town, where employment is unavailable. If he or she is to survive economically, it may be necessary to move to a less desirable location. In spite of the environmental pressure, that move may be impossible if the individual's homeostatic mechanisms cannot be overcome.

Fortunately, living systems are always open to their environments (La Monica, 1985). The continual intake of new matter, information, and energy combined with feedback provides ample opportunity for a system to become aware of the need to change its goals. Equally importantly, input allows the system to become increasingly complex and organized. This increasing organization, which is derived from the importation of energy, is called *negentrophy* (Flynn & Heffron, 1988). The ability to absorb input is essential both for system elaboration and for goal achievement. In fact, open systems will become entropic if they are unable to obtain sufficient energy.

A final characteristic that is also related to goal achievement is *equifinality*. This refers to a living system's ability to reach the same goal from different initial conditions and by different routes (Bertalanffy, 1956). It was initially difficult for systems theorists to explain how open systems, which began with differing resources and in different environments, could achieve similar goals. Bertalanffy suggests that this ability results from the dynamic interaction of the subsystems involved, which allows for creative and novel approaches to goal achievement.

## ❖ SYSTEMS THEORY AND THE INDIVIDUAL

Systems theory can help the practicing nurse deliver humane, clinically proficient health care. However, that goal will be reached more easily if that nurse keeps several suggestions in mind. These hints will help one who is new to Systems Theory to use it more easily and effectively. They will also help the more experienced user avoid some of the pitfalls that can result when any theory is applied in a practical setting.

1. Clearly define which system is being assessed and work with the system that seems to be the source of the problem. The divisions between subsystem, system, and suprasystem are sometimes arbitrary. For example, in a tightly knit or fused family, the family group may carry on some functions that commonly belong to the individual. Infants and small children are very dependent on their families for basic needs. In these and similar cases, it may be difficult to decide where the individual ends and the family begins. In such situations, assess the system in which the problem's solution is likely to reside and work with that system.

2. As was indicated earlier, Systems Theory is a general theory that can be used across disciplines. Therefore, the systems approach is most helpful in dealing with problems broadly and in attending to the relationships that are central to the theory. In fact, because the theory is so broad, the attempt to apply its concepts directly to specific nursing problems may be counterproductive. For example, an assessment form that contains all the questions that could be suggested by the Theory is likely to contain more questions than anyone could possibly ask. Therefore,

use Systems Theory as a general guide rather than as a blueprint for nursing action.

3. It is essential to remember that general approach for another reason. Systems Theory is an attempt to bring a holistic perspective to the progressive method of the nursing process. Fusion of the two approaches is difficult and, if the nurse does not work to maintain that balance, it may be lost. It is particularly easy to focus on the system's parts and to lose sight of the whole. It is also possible to take an overly global view of the client, although this lapse is far less common.

4. An important limitation of Systems Theory has to do with its elements and characteristics. They do not apply equally well to every system being analyzed (Kast & Rosenzweig, 1981). In some situations, it may be impossible to use every element of the theory to analyze a situation. However, it should be possible to employ the major components and to omit only those aspects that are not appropriate to a particular client system.

## Assessment

The greatest challenge in completing a systems-based client assessment is to focus on the system as a whole, rather than on its parts. Always gather data concerning the system's parts in an attempt to better understand how the entire system is functioning. The following approach may facilitate this process.

◆ **Assess the individual's input.** Identify the quantity and quality of the substances that the individual takes in. This consists of, but is not limited to, foods, fluids, and essential nutrients, medications, oxygen, love, social support, family and community values, information, and verbal and nonverbal communication. It may also include toxic materials such as chemicals, some medications, allergens, pathogens, and social isolation (Helvie, 1981). Pay particular attention to the age and developmental stage of the client since both physical and psychosocial needs vary with age. Because the list of potential inputs is long, it may seem necessary to ask

the client a series of detailed questions to cover them. As was noted earlier, it is more practical to ask general questions about broad topics until a client's response suggests that more detailed information is needed.

◆ **Assess the individual's output.** Evaluate the individual's observable behaviors, both physical and psychosocial. These include the end products of metabolism (carbon dioxide, perspiration, urine, feces, etc.) heat, immune responses, skin integrity, coordination, and symptoms that suggest health problems. Carefully observe appearance, habit patterns, verbal and nonverbal communication, tension-relief, and defense mechanisms. Ask about employment; relationship patterns including family and friendships; sexual, cooperative, and competitive bonds; and participation in the community. Again, focus on general questions except when specific problems arise.

◆ **Assess the individual's throughput mechanisms.** The way in which the system processes matter, energy, and information may be suggested by system output and the relationship between input and output. For example, an individual may have signs or symptoms of illness, such as shortness of breath or edema (output), or may be losing weight in spite of eating adequately (imbalance between input and output). It is sometimes possible to directly visualize internal structures, although nurses more commonly depend on indirect indicators to assess structure and function. For example, intellectual functioning is often evaluated by having the client perform simple mathematics.

◆ **Assess the individual's feedback mechanisms.** Consider both the physiologic and psychosocial output that returns to the individual as feedback. Pay particular attention to the individual's ability and willingness to accept feedback. Problems with the sensory subsystem, such as poor hearing, may make it impossible for some feedback to reenter the system. A client may also have difficulty monitoring his or her own behavior when an accurate perception of feedback is frightening or would require a change in a valued behavior. For example, a 39-year-old man who has a strong family history of heart disease may ignore episodes of chest pain (feedback) because he is so afraid of having a "heart attack."

♦ **Assess the individual's boundary.** Determine whether the boundary is effectively screening input and output. The boundary must be selectively permeable if the system is to function adequately. Selective permeability refers to the ability of the boundary to determine which substances can enter or leave the system. Since those substances are physiological and psychosocial in origin, both areas must be considered. For example, an individual may be unable to take in sufficient food either because he or she has esophageal atresia or because he or she has an eating disorder.

It is equally important to consider the integrity of the boundary. In some instances, system boundaries completely break down. Because they are unable to monitor input or output in any way, major system failures result. Physiologically, boundary failure is often the result of the failure of a subsystem. For example, when one's kidneys fail, the entire system loses the ability to monitor some output. Psychosocial boundary failures are more difficult to describe. Certainly, the schizophrenic client who cannot tell where he or she ends and the outside world begins has a problem with boundary integrity.

Finally, consider the age and developmental stage of the client as you assess the boundary. Permeability is affected by both these factors, and some predictions can be made based on them. Certain nutrients are absorbed best at certain ages or stages (i.e., calcium during the growth years, and in women, before menopause). There also seems to be crucial ages during which certain learning occurs most easily. In fact, if it does not happen at that time, it is far more difficult to achieve later. Adolescents are typically more resistant to parental input than are either younger children or adults. This kind of variation in boundary permeability is normal and should be expected in most clients.

♦ **Assess the individual's environment.** The environment includes both the immediate suprasystem (usually the family) and the larger world. While the family and community systems will be covered in considerable detail later in this chapter, resource assessment will be reviewed here. It is particularly important to assess the resources available in the client's environment. In some instances, problems that seem to belong to the client are actually not a part of the client's system. Rather, too few, too many, or inappropriate resources within the larger environment may be causing a problem in the client's system. Since the difficulty did not arise within the client, it cannot be solved there. Instead, a solution to the problem must be found in the system in which those problems arose.

Remember that even as the necessary data are being gathered, that information is being interpreted and analyzed. For example, the specific questions you ask are, to some degree, determined by your analysis of previous answers. Therefore, while assessment and analysis are described separately here, they actually occur almost simultaneously.

### Analysis

Analysis is the process of drawing inferences based on the raw data that have been gathered. It is a process that requires the nurse to apply nursing knowledge and experience to a particular client. According to Benner (1983), experience is the central element in the development of an expert practitioner. That experience, when combined with education, allows the expert to comprehend a situation as a whole and to avoid considering the irrelevant. In fact, the ability to combine knowledge, experience, and client and sensory cues into a unified sense of the client's condition is the mark of a skilled nurse (Pyles & Stern, 1983). It is clear that, in spite of the difficulties involved, a holistic analysis is essential to the provision of competent nursing care.

The process of analyzing data is not simple. However, the following approach can make the course more direct. As each concept is considered, the focus on the whole person, which has been emphasized throughout this chapter, must be maintained.

Consider first how well the individual is meeting both his or her biologic and psychosocial goals. Begin by determining whether the individual's subsystems are operating in a way that contributes to goal achievement and whether the subsystems are operating in a coordinated manner. Both must be occurring if the individual is to maintain or improve health status. Pay special attention to the interaction between the biologic and psychosocial subsystems. General Systems Theory, as well as most nurses' experiences, indicate a direct relationship between feelings and health status. Describe and evaluate the interaction between the subsystems.

Next, indicate how well the individual is able to maintain homeostasis. Is the individual taking in sufficient matter, energy, and information to achieve health goals? If a person is committed to following an extremely limited diet, or if he or she lacks essential health information, it may be impossible to learn about and follow a healthier diet. This may be true in spite of having a goal that is directed at improving nutrition. One potential nursing diagnosis would be altered nutrition less than body requirements.

A disparity between input and output may suggest a problem with maintaining a steady state. Is the individual able to effectively balance the matter, energy, and information that enters the system with that which leaves? A number of physiologic and psychological difficulties, such as fluid volume excess or deficit,

ineffective breathing patterns, or some appetite disorders fall into this category. In some instances, internal processes are working so inefficiently that they prevent effective use of environmental input.

How well is the individual adapting to internal and external change? The process of change requires energy, which must either be imported or diverted from elsewhere. How well is the individual doing this? There may be problems in dealing with situational change or with finding the energy to manage developmental change (impaired adjustment or ineffective coping).

## Planning, Implementation, and Evaluation

The remaining steps of the nursing process, which are planning, implementation, and evaluation, will be considered together. These three steps will be combined for two reasons. First, because Systems Theory is general, the following suggestions apply equally well to all three phases. Second, a systems approach encourages the nurse to see the nursing process as more than a mere collection of steps. Instead, it emphasizes their linked and interrelated nature. Because this chapter assumes that the reader has a basic knowledge of the parts of the nursing process, the interactive nature of that process can be demonstrated by integrating these steps (Ryan, 1979).

In general, a systems approach is similar to other theoretical approaches to planning, implementation, and evaluation. The nurse and client together determine which nursing diagnoses are amenable to nursing intervention and then develop goals and objectives that focus on those diagnoses and plans that will help to achieve the objectives. During implementation, the client and nurse execute the plans that have been developed and evaluate their success at all stages of the nursing process. Planning, implementation, and evaluation all reflect the nurse's knowledge and experience. In spite of those similarities, there are some unique features in a systems approach.

**Characteristics of open systems.** There are four characteristics of open systems that are particularly helpful to the nurse who is planning, implementing, and evaluating nursing care. All four strengthen traditional approaches to those phases, while retaining what is best of more commonly used models. These characteristics include *holism, equifinality, homeostasis,* and *adaptation.*

*Holism.* A focus on the whole individual emphasizes the uniqueness of that individual. Although nursing has almost universally emphasized the need for individualized client care, personalized care occurs relatively rarely in practice settings. Systems Theory reminds the nurse of the importance of looking at the client as more than just a collection of parts. In fact, if the nurse does not consider the client as a whole, the systems approach suggests that planning and intervention will be less than effective.

*Equifinality.* A second characteristic allows the nurse to be flexible in responding to a client's unique needs during the development and implementation of plans of care. Equifinality suggests that a client's health care goals may be reached by a number of different routes. Therefore, planning and implementing care can be an accommodative process; one that meets the needs of the client but recognizes reasonable limits in the health care system. In fact, as one evaluative criteria, the nurse should consider the degree to which the plan is responsive to client needs.

*Homeostasis.* Planning and implementation should focus on maintaining or improving homeostatic mechanisms. While this may sound complex, it actually reflects a traditional nursing role. A client who has unmet health needs is likely to have difficulty maintaining a stable energy supply. This may occur either because the demands that are made on the system as a result

of illness require increased energy, or because normal energy sources (food, oxygen, etc.) are unavailable. Therefore, the nurse and client should develop, implement, and evaluate plans that attempt to reduce energy needs or to increase available energy, both biological or physiological.

*Adaptation.* Maintaining homeostasis does not preclude adapting to new circumstances, however. Many common health problems require increased energy merely to maintain a steady state. Positive changes, such as gathering new information or altering habit patterns, require even more energy. Adapting to internal or environmental change means that energy must either be imported by the system or transferred from some other activity. Plans that center on adaptation or change should always include some consideration of how the energy required for the change will be obtained. If this is not done, nursing actions aimed at adaptation are likely to be unsuccessful.

It is clear that the nursing process will be more successful if used in conjunction with Systems concepts. These concepts strengthen assessment, analysis, planning, implementation, and evaluation for any nurse. They are particularly helpful to the experienced practitioner, however. That person has the experience to apply those concepts in the workplace in a flexible, realistic way. Rather than approach client care in a step-by-step manner, the nurse can see the process as a whole. As a result, the nursing process becomes a real process, one that deals with the client as an individual who functions best in a system that is humane and scientifically sound.

**Applied research.** Research that applies General Systems Theory to the care of the individual is limited. This is the result of several factors. Any theory is difficult to test in the workplace, and because Systems Theory is so general, it is particularly difficult to test in its pure form. However, the Theory has served as a source for many nursing theorists. For example, Johnson, King, Orem, Rogers, and Neuman all base their theoretic models at least in part on General Systems Theory. Although elements of these theories have been tested, the tests that were used rarely meet all the evaluation criteria for theory testing. Between the years of 1952 and 1985, Silva (1986) found that only 9 of 62 studies that purported to test nursing theories actually met those criteria.

A second problem is related to the fact that clinical nurse researchers do most of their applied research in areas other than theory testing (Knafl, Bevis, & Kirchhoff, 1987). In spite of these difficulties, a number of authors have been successful in applying systems theory directly to the care of clients. For example, Johnson developed a reliable and valid instrument that evaluates behavioral change in cancer patients (Derdiarian, 1983).

Finally, because Systems Theory is especially good at examining the relationship between parts, even studies of individuals tend to have a family focus. For example, studies may explore feedback between a mother and child (Anderson, 1981), or mothers' perceptions during childbirth (Mercer, Hackely, & Bostrom, 1983). As a result, applied research supports the use of General Systems Theory in family-centered health care settings.

## ❖ FAMILY SYSTEMS

Most of us are born into, live out our lives, and die within families, but in spite of that experience, we rarely examine how these families operate. General Systems Theory provides a framework that helps the nurse assess a family, draw conclusions about how that family operates, and plan, implement, and evaluate nursing interventions. General Systems Theory is sufficiently broad to include within it the perspectives of a number of family theorists. These viewpoints are particularly helpful during family assessment, since they focus on family char-

acteristics and behaviors that influence family functioning.

The family is defined as "... an open system of interacting personalities composed of inter-related positions and roles" (Fawcett, 1975). It is a living system in which there are "... a series of interlocking ... subsystems (where) a change in one part will produce a change in another" (Bowen, 1974). The family system takes in matter, energy, and information as input, processes it, and either retains it or releases it into the environment as output (Christensen & Kenney, 1990). The family uses feedback to determine whether it is meeting its goals. Feedback includes activities as simple as monitoring the savings account balance, or as complex as monitoring the children. Every family has a boundary that, since it is emotional rather than physical, may be difficult to identify. Finally, the family exists within an environment, usually the community.

The same suggestions that help the nurse use Systems Theory to care for an individual client apply to the care of the family. Be certain to clearly define the boundaries of the family with which one is working. Then, focus attention on the way in which the defined family system operates. During the assessment phase, pay particular attention to the relationships between the family's subsystems, rather than to the subsystems themselves. Finally, while one need not use every component of the Theory, consider at least the major elements.

### Assessment

♦ **Assess the family's input.** Identify the matter, energy, and information that the system takes in. Input that provides the system with resources includes income, social support from friends and neighbors, and help from family members who are outside the defined family system. The community may furnish educational, spiritual, recreational, and social support to the family. Stressors are inputs that require that the family use resources and include lack of sufficient assets as well as demands from the environment. Pay particular attention to situational stressors, such as the loss of a job, divorce, disease, or a disaster. Ask general questions about these areas unless the family's responses suggest that follow-up is required.

♦ **Assess the family's output.** Evaluate the family's observable behaviors, both short-term and long-term. Consider first the activities in which they engage. In what type of educational, spiritual, social, and recreational activities do they participate? How committed are they to these activities? How do they meet their health care needs? Do they receive preventive health care or is care limited to emergencies? What can you see of their value system? For example, how to parents respond to their children's misbehavior? Do they encourage their children to actively interact with their environment? Pay particular attention to family behavior patterns. When conflicts arise, how do family members handle them? Do they address problems directly or avoid them? Is any particular member used as a scapegoat in order to relieve tension (Bowen, 1974)?

Describe the behavior you see rather than your conclusions about that behavior. Try to avoid using terms like "difficult," "childish," or "irresponsible." Instead, identify the actions that suggest that those terms are accurate.

♦ **Assess the family's throughput mechanisms.** As was true with the individual, the way in which a system processes information is suggested by the relationship between the system's input and output. However, there are specific areas that directly influence system functioning. Each of these should be considered individually.

The first of these are family set factors. Set factors are those enduring family characteristics that predispose a family to behave in a particular way. These include religion, educational level, socioeconomic class, ethnocultural back-

ground, and values. Pay particular attention to the relationships between these characteristics, since many of them seem to be interconnected. For example, education, socioeconomic class, and values tend to be related and may sometimes predict one another.

Next, determine which of the following structural forms best describes the defined family system:

♦ the nuclear family, which includes a husband, wife, and their minor children. If only a husband and wife are present, this family type is referred to as a nuclear dyad.
♦ the extended family, which includes more than two generations of a family living in the same household. These members may include aunts, uncles, cousins, etc.
♦ the single parent family, which includes one parent with his or her children.
♦ the single adult living alone.
♦ the blended family, which is composed of a divorced or widowed person, his or her spouse, and children of either or both spouses.
♦ the kin network, which is composed of two or more related families who live near one another and share goods and services.
♦ nontraditional relationships, which include common law or group marriages, homosexual or communal relationships, or others (Helvie, 1981; Stanhope & Lancaster, 1988).

Now, identify the developmental stage of the family. Developmental theorists suggest that families change in predictable ways over time (Friedman, 1986). These normal changes result from internal and environmental experiences, which typically occur as a family matures. Until quite recently, developmental stage was based on childbearing and rearing responsibilities. DuVall (1985) identifies eight stages of family growth. These include:

Stage I—Beginning families during which the family is established.
Stage II—Early childbearing families (oldest child 30 months or less) during which a family adjusts to the presence of an infant.

Stage III—Families with preschool children (oldest child 6 years old or less) when families learn to nurture children.

Stage IV—School-age families (oldest child 6 to 13) when families both socialize and educate children.

Stage V—Teenage families (oldest child 13 to 20) when families help children learn to balance freedom with responsibility.

Stage VI—Launching families (from first to last child leaving home) when families release their children and readjust their marriages.

Stage VII—Middle-aged families (empty nest through retirement) when families reestablish the marital dyad and maintain family links.

Stage VIII—Aging families (retirement to the death of both spouses) when families adjust to aging, loss, and death.

Because some families do not include children, theorists have also described less child-oriented stages, which can apply to all families. Generally these stages focus on: (1) the initiation of family, (2) the formation of a family identity, (3) increasing family integration with or without childbearing, and (4) an actualizing period when the focus is on the mature, adult family (Stanhope and Lancaster, 1988). Regardless of which approach is used, attempt to determine whether the family is carrying out the functions appropriate to its developmental stage.

Finally, assess the way in which the family functions. Family function, which is strongly influenced by structure, refers to the way in which the family operates as a unit. As family functioning is evaluated, consider the following areas:

◆ How well is the family able to carry out those activities, which are traditionally its responsibility? Specifically, how does it meet its members' biologic, psychologic, social, and economic needs? Gather information about income, housing, health care, family relationships, goals, and values. Consider specifically how the family operates as a unit. This will be influenced by the family's developmental stage.

◆ What patterns of communication does the family use? Is communication dominated by certain members of the family or do all members actively participate? How is that participation encouraged? Are family members able to change their responses to one another as their circumstances change? Are there identifiable dysfunctional communication patterns?

Pay particular attention to the way families communicate when they are under stress, since that is when communication is likely to break down. According to Satir (1972), four common patterns in such circumstances include blaming others when things go wrong; placating other family members by accepting the blame for others; computing, which involves a member acting as if he or she is in great control; and distracting by attending to something unrelated to the stressor. Note whether any particular family member seems to be a scapegoat or operates as a tension reducer by acting out (Bowen, 1974).

◆ How are decisions made within the family? Who participates in the process? How much input does each family member have? How is a final decision made when there is conflict? Pay special attention to the way individual family members influence the decision-making process. Do they accommodate themselves to the wishes of others, manipulate others, bargain, or compromise as they attempt to decide?

Decisions can be made using variations of three basic decision-making styles. A family in which nearly all decisions are made by one member with relatively little input from others is using an autocratic style. When parents take a leadership role, but decisions are discussed by the family members and arrived at by consensus, a family is using democratic decision-making. If family members make decisions without any leadership, a family has a laissez-faire style (Lewin, Lippet, & White, 1939). It is unusual for a family to use a single approach to decision-making. Most families combine styles and, in our society, even authoritarian families commonly allow some participation in the decision process.

Decision-making patterns usually reflect the way power is distributed in the family. However, that relationship is not direct. For example, a family in which power is shared between members is also likely to share decision-making responsibilities. In times of stress, however, that family may use a decision-making style, which requires less effort in order to accelerate the process. In fact, a change in decision-making style may suggest that a family is experiencing an increase in stress.

◆ What roles do individual family members play in the family? Roles refer to the behavior expected of an occupant of a particular position and include both rights and responsibilities, (Hein & Nicholson, 1982). Since roles within a family influence how the family functions, information about how a family operates can be obtained by assessing those roles.

Consider formal roles (mother, father, child, etc.) that family members fill. Are role expectations clearly stated and accepted by the occupants of each role? Are these roles flexible or are they fairly fixed? Try to determine how the family alters roles as the family grows and changes. Notice whether those changes are managed easily or with difficulty. Certain developmental stages require that a family make major role changes. For example, a family with young adolescents has to realign role expectation in order to increase the responsibilities of the teen-age members. How does the family make those changes? What is the effect on overall family functioning?

As you observe the family, remember that functioning is the result of a combination of factors. Family structure, developmental stage, communication, and decision-making patterns, as well as roles, all influence the way a family works together. Rather than focusing on each factor individually, consider how they operate cooperatively within a family. Sometimes a weakness in one area is compensated for by strengths in another. It is often true that a family with multiple weaknesses suffers from severely compromised functioning. A systems approach is a practical way to consider how these factors together influence family functioning. At least one assessment tool, the Feetham Family Functioning Survey, which measures the ability of the family to function as an open system, has been found to be reliable and valid (Roberts & Feetham, 1982).

◆ **Assess the family's feedback mechanisms.** How does the family monitor its own functioning? What kind of information does it accept as evidence that it is meeting its goals? While individuals commonly use both physical and psychosocial data as they evaluate themselves, families primarily use psychosocial measures. In some families, goal accomplishment is determined mainly by external measures of success, such as income or status, while others measure success internally, based on personal values. Notice how a family handles feedback. This suggests that a cherished goal is not being achieved.

◆ **Assess the family's boundary.** Determine first where the family's boundary is located. While an individual's boundary may be easy to identify, a family's may be more difficult to find (Helvie, 1981). Does it surround only the family members, or does it also include the home in which they live? Is there agreement about who is included in the family and who is not? For example, are adult children who no longer live at home still a part of the family?

How permeable is the family's boundary? Do members purchase most of what they require or do they prefer to make or grow what they need? Are others welcome in their home or do they limit visitors to members of the immediate family? What messages do they send to others about the boundary permeability? Do they lock their gate and pull down their shades as a clear message to visitors, or is the "keep out" message more subtle? How welcome is the nurse in their home?

Finally, is the boundary intact? One of the

functions of a boundary is to exclude matter, energy, and information that the system doesn't need. In some families, that function is severely compromised. If substances that could be harmful to members are allowed to enter freely, then the boundary is not functioning effectively. Notice whether the family is able to exclude such substances from the family system.

♦ **Assess the family's environment.** Consider the family's immediate suprasystem, which is normally the community in which the family lives. Many of the resources on which the family depends must be obtained from the suprasystem. What type and quality of resources are available in the community? Consider the specific needs of the family that is being served. Often the developmental stage helps determine what resources are most significant to the family. An elderly family may be particularly concerned about health care services, but care little about schools, while a family with growing children may have different priorities. A mixed age community requires a balance of services, which can meet the needs of all residents.

Consider the access to resources that the community provides. Must some member of the family drive in order to reach the services that they need, or is public transportation available? In some communities, specialized transportation is available at no charge to those within the area who have special problems. Are such services available to those families who need them?

Because family assessment is the basis for planning, intervention, and evaluation, it must be comprehensive. In addition, the family must be considered as a whole, rather than as a collection of members. General Systems Theory, with its holistic focus, facilitates this process.

## Analysis

Analysis is the process of making sense of the information about the family that the nurse

has gathered. The nurse must make inferences that are based on adequate data and that arise from a strong nursing knowledge base. Experience is also a valuable component in the process. Although many nurses have developed their own approaches to analysis, the following method may make the inferential process easier.

Consider first how well the family is meeting its goals. Family goals include the functions that the society asks all families to carry out and those more personal family decisions about how time, money, and energy should be spent. Use the gathered data to make a statement that reflects your sense of how well the family is functioning. Be sure to include the strengths and weaknesses that the family demonstrates as it operates (Reinhardt & Quinn, 1980). Notice how family set factors, developmental stage, communication, decision-making patterns, and roles influence the family's ability to function. According to Johnson and colleagues (1988), ethnic background influences the elderly family's ability to cope with the inevitable stresses and strains in life. Attempt to trace the strengths and weaknesses that exist to one or more of these functional areas. Try to draw conclusions about why a family is successful in achieving its goals. Are there ways to explain why a family is less than successful?

Next, indicate whether the family is able to maintain homeostasis. For a family to maintain a steady state, it must take in enough matter, energy, and information to balance what it uses with what it returns to the community. How well is the family doing that? Since it is the boundary that regulates what enters and leaves the system, consider the information that was gathered about the boundary. A family that is relatively closed to its environment may have difficulty in obtaining what it needs to maintain homeostasis. On the other hand, a family may give so much to the community that it has insufficient energy to meet its own needs.

A large disparity between input and output may also suggest that a family is having difficulty maintaining its balance. When a family absorbs many resources and still has difficulty functioning, something may be wrong with its internal processes. Stressors such as illness or a developmental or role change may either demand increased resources or may impair the family's ability to effectively use those they have. Consider nursing diagnoses such as altered family processes or ineffective family coping.

Consider the meaning of any entropic forces in the family (Helvie, 1981). Is scapegoating consistently used to reduce stress between members? Are parent-child relationships poor? Has the family limited access to needed resources? Forces that cause the family to be increasingly chaotic often have significant environmental components that must be addressed. More importantly, unless countered, they lead to an extremely negative outcomes for individual family members, for the family, and for society.

Finally, consider how well the family is able to adapt to change. Begin by focusing on the family's specific developmental stage. While each of these stages requires that the family alter its functioning, some of them are particularly challenging. Beginning families, early childbearing families, families with teenage children, and aging families all face role changes that may sap their adaptive energies.

Families in which the first child is less than 30 months old are in the process of identifying new parental roles and of redefining the relationship between members. Particular family behaviors have the potential to make this change easier. Parents who provide a great deal of direct care to their child find the transition easier than do noncare-giving parents (Roberts, 1983). Men who attend prepared childbirth classes are more satisfied with their marital relationships after the birth of their infants than are others (Moore, 1983). Interestingly, formal education, age, and parent education classes seem to be unrelated to either acceptance of the parental role or to marital satisfaction (Moore, 1983; Perry, 1983).

Families with teenage children face a similar set of challenges as they deal with the "dependence-independence" dilemma (Leiman & Strasberger, 1985). The majority of families do not experience major disturbances as their children grow into adulthood (Hill, 1985). Certain families are at a particular risk to have problems during these years, however. These include parents who are young themselves (38 years old or younger) and those whose oldest child is entering adolescence (Cohen, Adler, Beck, & Irwin, 1986). Difficulties are also more likely if the adolescent is a male, since females seem less vulnerable to negative peer pressure (Steinberg & Silverberg, 1986).

Consider whether the family has the adaptive energy that is required by its developmental stage. Look carefully at those families who fit into categories that research suggests are high-risk. Attempt to determine whether they are actually having difficulty.

Consider as well the environmental stressors with which the family must deal. Because the environment is less predictable than normal development, environmental stressors may require an excess of adaptive energy. How well has the family dealt with problems like unemployment, illness, or death in the past? Are there currently stressors in the family that would affect their ability to manage new problems?

## Planning, Implementation, and Evaluation

Planning, implementation, and evaluation are based on the family nursing diagnosis and represent the action segments of the nursing process. They give the nurse who is working with a family the opportunity to cooperatively and thoughtfully develop, carry out, and evaluate that process. Because the three steps are so closely connected that they are often reciprocal, they will be discussed together.

A systems approach to planning, implementation, and evaluation has some unique features. Because the family as a functioning unit is goal-directed, its participation is essential to achieve health-related goals. The family should clearly identify the goals that it is willing to pursue and, with the nurse, determine how to meet them. While the nurse may be aware of particular strategies that may be helpful, a range of possible approaches, any of which may achieve the goal, should be considered (equifinality).

Nursing actions should focus on supporting or improving the family's homeostatic mechanisms. When a family is overwhelmed by demands, it is often necessary to identify and attempt to reduce the number of stressors with which they are dealing. More commonly, the family must actually change its behavior in order to return to or maintain a steady state. It is during periods of stress that the family has the opportunity to experiment with new approaches to problems in order to make permanent adaptations. The nurse should encourage healthy changes that increase family stability.

Additionally, the nurse may help the family adapt to change or increase the permeability of its boundary. Adaptation requires that the family alter its internal processes in specific ways. Changing patterns of communication may allow suppressed problems to emerge. Rational problem solving may then help to identify potential solutions to those problems (Friedman, 1986). The nurse may also help the family to identify ways to increase role flexibility within the family, which may reduce the stress on particular family members. Increasing boundary permeability has a dual purpose: to help the family identify external resources and then to actually use them (Miller & Janosik, 1980).

Finally, seek out nursing research that suggests useful strategies for a specific family. The family-based research discussed includes a number of specific suggestions about the kind of family that would benefit from intervention and what kind of intervention might be helpful. These findings can be used to help the family achieve its goals more effectively.

## ❖ COMMUNITY SYSTEMS

The community is the last of the living systems with which this chapter deals. A community is a system because it has a goal and is made up of components or subsystems that interact with one another (Stanhope & Lancaster, 1988). Many people think of a community as a living environment with physical or political boundaries. The definition is broader than that, however, since it also includes situational communities that have only conceptual boundaries. The alumni of a college or the League of Women Voters are examples of situational communities. General Systems Theory provides the nurse with a framework that is broad enough to consider both the private and public health services available to both types of communities.

### Assessment

The primary reason to assess a community is to determine its health needs by identifying those functional patterns that affect its health status. Community assessment requires the nurse to gather data from a variety of sources in order to provide an accurate and comprehensive picture of the community. This process can seem overwhelming to the nurse who is new to community practice. A systematic approach can help make the process more manageable.

♦ **Assess the community's input.** Consider the matter, energy, and information that influences the community's health status. Begin by identifying the type of people who live in the community. Gather demographic information that describes the people who choose to live there and that suggests the area's predominant health needs. How are members distributed by age, sex, race, and socioeconomic class? Is the community heterogeneous or homogeneous in composition? What are the community's resources, particularly as they affect health care? Communities may lack the resources to provide adequate health services or may choose to spend available resources in other areas.

Finally, consider how and what type of information enters the system. Newspapers, radio, and television all reflect and influence public opinion. Pay particular attention to the effect of local media on the community. Be aware of the influence of state and national policy as they influence the community.

◆ **Assess the community's output.** Consider the community's goals and the degree to which they are achieved. Goals usually reflect both the needs of the current inhabitants and the past history of the community. Regardless of the unique features of the community, two goals are nearly always present. All communities work to ensure their own survival and to achieve self-fulfillment for themselves and for their members. How successful is the community in achieving good health? Pay particular attention to health statistics, since they both reflect community health outcomes and suggest potential problem areas. Note whether there are particular illness patterns or public health problems that are unique to the community. In some communities rabies is a serious problem, while other areas are more concerned about teenage pregnancy.

Assess the state of the community. Describe its physical characteristics, particularly as they affect community health. Are buildings, homes, and other structures in good condition or do they pose risks to health and safety? Consider biologic and chemical characteristics that affect the community. Are there toxic materials or pollutants that are potential health hazards?

◆ **Assess the community's throughput mechanisms.** Consider the social characteristics of the community. How is information communicated between members? Are there formal communication networks, or do informal systems predominate? Are there local community

newspapers or newsletters? What about radio or television stations? What recreational opportunities are there? Are there a variety of other interactional opportunities for residents? Do they take advantage of them? Again, pay particular attention to health-related data, including wellness programs and health education programs.

What activities is the community involved in to ensure that it will remain healthy, both physically and economically? What opportunities are there for members to gain a sense of themselves within the community. Does the community have a sense of its own uniqueness?

Finally, what social services are available within the community? Do the schools and industries have the health personnel they need? Consider as well the social welfare, economic, and religious services available.

◆ **Assess the community's feedback mechanism.** How does the community interpret its own output? Does it attempt to realistically evaluate feedback and then make an effort to respond to the data appropriately? Pay particular attention to how the community responds to its health-related outputs.

◆ **Assess the community's boundary.** Does the community have a clearly defined boundary that surrounds it? Does that boundary reflect the area's political boundary or does it overlap with the surrounding communities? Notice whether the boundary allows necessary matter, energy, and information to enter the region, as well as the boundary's ability to exclude what is unnecessary. Remember that most communities are not self-sufficient and must interact with their environments to function effectively.

◆ **Assess the community's environment.** How are services provided to those in need? Are health care services readily available

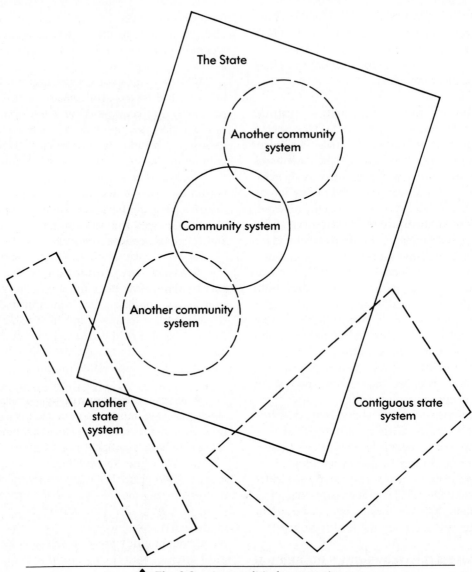

The State

Another community system

Community system

Another community system

Another state system

Contiguous state system

❖ **Fig. 2-3**    A geopolitical community.

or must they be obtained from the environment? What other services must be obtained from the larger environment? Is the community isolated, either physically or geographically, so that it must provide for most of its own needs? Although suburban communities can often depend on their neighbors or urban nucleus for support, a rural community far from other service areas must often provide for itself. If physical and political boundaries differ, how are those differences dealt with? In the case of health services, it may be necessary to consider the immediate suprasystem and the one beyond it, since both may have an impact on the community (Fig. 2-3). Most community health nursing texts contain community survey tools that cover the preceding information. They may be helpful to the nurse who undertakes a community assessment (Stanhope & Lancaster, 1988).

### Data Analysis

The purpose of analyzing community data is to identify community health needs. To do this, the nurse must draw conclusions about the data that have been gathered. There are a number of approaches to data interpretation, which can facilitate the inferential process. The functional approach used here focuses on how well the community operates. Both community strengths and weaknesses emerge from this type of analysis, as well as the functional areas from which each arise. There are five functional areas that should be analyzed.

1. Evaluate how well the community is producing and distributing the goods and services that its members require. Goods refer to personal property and moveable possessions, while services include activities that are required by the public, such as health care and public utilities. Are the goods and services that the community requires readily available? Is their quantity and quality sufficient to meet the members' needs? For example, are there sufficient numbers and types of health care providers to meet the needs of the specific population that the community serves? Is there adequate health care for those unable to pay for it?

2. Determine how well the community socializes its members. How effectively are prevailing knowledge, values, beliefs, and customs transmitted to members? Does the community seem able to alter its values and beliefs in response to environmental change, or are they relatively fixed? Again, pay particular attention to the effect of socialization on community health care. Is preventive health care valued by the community? Communities that are quite heterogeneous may also be quite flexible about these value-laden issues. However, heterogeneity may also make transmission of common values, beliefs, and customs difficult.

3. Analyze how the community exerts social control over its members. Does it effectively control proscribed behavior and encourage prescribed activities? Be sure to consider the role of the suprasystem, which can legally limit the power of the community to enforce its own norms.

4. Determine whether the community provides adequate opportunities for social participation. Are there a broad array of activities available to meet the needs of all community members? Are there sufficient opportunities for informal participation?

5. Finally, evaluate the mutual support system within the community. Although this system is usually informal and is, therefore, quite difficult to evaluate, data that indicate how connected and involved members feel within their community may help. How adequate are the voluntary agencies that serve the community? Throughout the analysis, be certain to draw conclusions about the data that have been gathered, rather than merely restating the information.

## Planning, Implementation, and Evaluation

The same skill and knowledge that helps the nurse to plan, implement, and evaluate care with the individual and the family is used in the community. However, there are some special abilities essential to the community-based nurse. This is true because resolving a community health problem is rarely accomplished by one person. Instead, it requires the concerted action of all those in the community who are concerned about health care. As a result, the nurse must work cooperatively with other professional groups, as well as with governmental and voluntary agencies and organizations. This cooperative planning requires a great deal of patience, negotiation, and compromise. The outcome is a plan that reflects community input and that is therefore more likely to be successfully implemented. It may, however, be quite different from what the nurse originally envisioned.

Evaluation is the weak link in many community health plans. Because the planning and implementation process require so much energy, there is often little inclination to rework those steps when they are ineffective. Therefore, evaluation that begins early in the process (when alterations are less costly) is helpful. However, because many of these plans address complex problems, it remains necessary to measure long-term outcomes in spite of the difficulty involved.

In spite of the challenges that are a part of addressing community health problems, it can be an extremely rewarding process for the nurse. It encourages the development of new skills that can be used to help clients in a wide variety of settings. More importantly, the process can improve the private and public health care of large numbers of community members.

## ❖ SUMMARY

General Systems Theory is a broad theory that encourages the nurse to evaluate the individual, the family, and the community as a whole, while paying particular attention to the interrelationship of the system's parts. Because it is used by professionals in a variety of disciplines, it has the potential to improve interprofessional communication.

Systems Theory may be used in conjunction with the nursing process to provide care that is both holistic and methodical. This combined approach is particularly helpful as the nurse deals with living systems. Assessment, planning, analysis, implementation, and evaluation are carried out with a systems perspective. A focus on the entire client is maintained and is coupled with a concern for maintaining the client in a homeostatic state. Client participation in all phases of the nursing process is essential if the nurse is to respond to the client's unique needs.

A systems approach can be used as the nurse works with an individual, a family, or a community. While it may be necessary to make minor alterations, most of the theory can be applied in the same way with all types of clients. This makes it reasonably easy for nurses in a variety of settings to share information and to plan cooperatively with each other.

## ❖ APPLYING KNOWLEDGE TO PRACTICE

1. What are the major advantages to using General Systems Theory as a basis
for your client care?
2. Describe the following terms as they
apply to a living system: input,
throughput, output, boundary, environment, homeostasis, suprasystem.
3. List and define three operational characteristics of a system.
4. Describe the six components of an assessment of an individual.
5. Describe the process of developing a
system-based data analysis.
6. One of the most challenging parts of
family assessment is assessing the family's throughput. What are six of the
structural forms that may influence
how the family processes information?
7. What are two goals present in most
communities?
8. How can research help the nurse implement a systems-based plan of care
with a client?

## REFERENCES

Anderson, C. (1981). Enhancing reciprocity between mother and neonate. *Nursing Research, 30*(2), 89-93.

Benner, P. (1983). Uncovering the knowledge embedded in clinical practice. *Image, 15*(2), 36-41.

Bertalanffy, L. von (1956). General systems theory. In B. D. Ruben & J. Kim (Eds.), *General systems theory and human communication* (pp. 7-16). New Jersey: Hayden Book Co., Inc.

Bowen, M. (1974). Bowen on triangles. *Workshop Monograph,* Center for Family Learning.

Byrne, M. & Thompson, L. (1972). *Key concepts for the study and practice of nursing.* St. Louis: C. V. Mosby.

Christensen, P. & Kenney, J. (1990). *Nursing process: Application of theories, frameworks, and models (3rd ed.).* St. Louis: C. V. Mosby.

Cohen, M., Adler, N., Beck, A., & Irwin, C. (1986). Parental reactions to the onset of adolescence. *Journal of Adolescent Health Care, 89*(7), 101-106.

Derdiarian, A. (1983). An instrument for theory and research development using the behavioral systems model for nursing: The cancer patient. *Nursing research, 32*(4), 196-200.

DuVall, E. & Miller, B. (1985). *Marriage and family development.* (6th ed.). New York: Harper & Row.

Fawcett, J. (1975). The family as an open, living system: An emerging conceptual framework for nursing. *International Nursing Review, 22,* 113-116.

Flynn, J. & Heffron, P. (1988). *Nursing: from concept to practice,* (2nd ed.) Norwalk, Appleton & Lange.

Freidman, M. (1986). *Family nursing: Theory and assessment.* New York: Appleton-Century-Croft.

Hein, E. & Nicholson, M. (1982). Assessing organizational structure. In E. Hein, & M. Nicholson (Eds.), *Contemporary leadership behavior,* Boston: Little, Brown, & Co.

Helvie, C. (1981). *Community health nursing.* Philadelphia: Harper & Row.

Hill, J. (1985). Family relations in adolescence: Myths, realities, and new directions. *Genetic, Social, and General Psychology Monographs, 11*(2), 233-248.

Johnson, F., Foxall, M., Kelleher, E., Kentopp, E., Mannlein, E., & Cook, E. (1988). Comparison of mental health and life satisfaction of five elderly ethnic groups. *Western Journal of Nursing Research, 10*(5), 613-628.

Kast, F. & Rosenzweig, J. (1981). General systems theory: Applications for organizations and management. *Journal of Nursing Administration, 81*(8), 32-40.

Knafl, K., Bevis, M., & Kirchhoff, K. (1987). Research activities of clinical nurse researchers. *Nursing Research, 36*(4), 249-252.

La Monica, E. (1985). *The humanistic nursing process.* California: Wadsworth Health Science Division.

Lazlo, E. (1972). The origins of general systems theory in the works of von Bertalanffy. In E. Lazlo (Ed.). *The relevance of general systems theory.* New York: Brazeller.

Leiman, A. & Strasberger, V. (1985). Counseling parents of adolescents. *Pediatrics,* 85 (Suppl.) 664-667.

Lewin, K., Lippitt, R., & White, R. (1939). Patterns of aggressive behavior in experimentally created "social climates". *Journal of Social Psychology, 10,* 271-299.

Mercer, R., Hackley, K., & Bostrom, A. (1983). Relationship of psychosocial and perinatal variables to perception of childbirth. *Nursing Research, 32*(4), 202-207.

Miller, J. (1978). *Living systems.* New York: McGraw-Hill.

Miller, J. & Janosik, E. (1980). *Family focused care.* New York: McGraw-Hill.

Moore, D. (1983). Prepared childbirth and marital satisfaction during the antepartal and postpartum periods. *Nursing Research, 32*(2), 73-79.

Perry, S. (1983). Parent's perceptions of their newborn following structured interactions. *Nursing Research, 32*(2), 208-212.

Pyles, S., & Stern, P. (1983). The discovery of nursing gestault in critical care nursing: The grey gorilla syndrome. *Image, 15*(2), 51-57.

Reinhardt, A. & Quinn, M. (1980). *Family-centered community nursing.* St. Louis: C. V. Mosby.

Roberts, F. (1983). Infant behavior and the transition to parenthood. *Nursing Research, 32*(2), 213-217.

Roberts, C., & Feetham, S. (1982). Assessing family functioning across three areas of relationships. *Nursing Research, 31*(4), 231-235.

Ryan, B. (1979). Nursing care plans: A systems approach to developing criteria for planning and evaluation. In A. Marriner (Ed.) *The nursing process* (2nd ed.) (pp. 249-258). St. Louis: C. V. Mosby.

Satir, V. (1972). *Peoplemaking.* California: Science and Behavior Books.

Silva, M. (1986). Research testing nursing theory: State of the art. *Advances in Nursing Science, 9*(1), 1-11.

Stanhope, M. & Lancaster, J. (1988). *Community health nursing.* St. Louis: C. V. Mosby.

Steinberg, L. & Silverberg, S. (1986). The vicissitudes of autonomy in early adolescence. *Child Development, 57,* pp. 841-851.

Yura, H. & Walsh, M. (1978). *The nursing process.* New York: Appleton-Century-Croft.

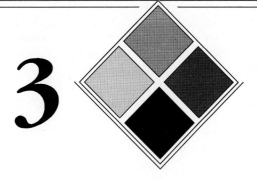

# 3

# The Professional Climate for Nursing Practice

## Perspectives of Hospital Nurses

Louise S. Jenkins

## OBJECTIVES

*At the completion of this chapter, the reader will be able to:*

- ◆ Discuss key issues involved in creating a professional climate for nursing practice.
- ◆ Identify characteristics of a professional practice climate as proposed by the American Nurses' Association.
- ◆ Describe the "real" and "ideal" professional climate for nursing practice from the perspective of a sample of hospital-based nurses.

Professional nursing practice occurs in an ever-expanding diversity of settings, both inpatient and outpatient. One commonality across inpatient settings is that the delivery of care, whether in tertiary, rehabilitation, or long-term care settings, takes place within highly complex organizations. Over the years, continued attempts have been made to design nursing care delivery models, which purport to be effective and efficient. Less emphasis has been placed on the relationship between the nurse and the organization or the environment in which nursing is practiced. Thus, despite the emergence of innovative models designed to enhance professional practice, such as shared governance or variations on the theme of primary nursing, case management, and others, theoretical and empirical attention given to the actual professional climate for nursing practice has been comparatively small. Recently, however, there seems to be an increased interest in identifying and structuring a professional climate that can facilitate the practice of nursing. In addition to empowering the nurse, Orsolits' (1989) discussion, drawn from a review of the 1988 recommendations from the Department of Health and Human Services Commission on nursing, posits that enhanced organizational environments or climates for nursing may also benefit the clients for whom we care.

What exactly is the professional climate for nursing practice? Is it structure, such as the organizational hierarchy of a health care institution or a model of shared governance? Is it process, such as decision making? Is it the same across an organization as a whole? Or, are there core elements of the professional climate specific to the type of unit, clients being cared for, or care delivery system in place? Can the overall professional climate, or selected core elements of it, be assessed across institutions? Regardless of our role in nursing, we each have an opportunity, and indeed, a responsibility, to address these questions and participate in ongoing assessment and definition of a professional climate for nursing practice.

In this chapter, key issues in creating a professional climate for nursing practice are identified, and three professional governance models are described. Identification of the characteristics of the professional climate for nursing practice is shown as being an evolutionary process, spanning the past decade and continuing even today. Initial approaches to measure this construct are described. The findings from a new study of the perceptions of a sample of hospital nurses regarding the characteristics of a professional climate for nursing practice are presented, highlighting the importance and relevance of this concept to the practicing nurse. Discussion questions that follow offer the reader an opportunity to consider the professional climate for nursing practice from highly individual perspectives.

## ❖ CREATING A CLIMATE FOR PROFESSIONAL PRACTICE

According to Porter-O'Grady (1986), there are five key issues involved in creating a professional practice climate. The nurse must have:

1. The freedom to function effectively
2. A sense of support from peers and leaders
3. Clear expectations of the work environment
4. Appropriate resources to practice effectively
5. An open organizational climate

To practice as professionals, nurses must have control over the practice environment so that clinical judgments and interventions can reflect the uniqueness of each client. Lateral communication and dialogue among peers al-

lows nurses to validate clinical judgments according to standards of professional practice. Through peer-based quality evaluation and assurance, nurses can maintain high standards of client care. When nurses have a defined role in governance, policies that could have a negative impact on high quality care can be averted.

A number of contemporary client care delivery models were developed to facilitate the practice of nursing as a professional discipline (Mayer, Madden & Lawrenz, 1990). Many of the models address the issues cited by Porter-O'Grady with systems such as shared governance, self-governance, case management, or cooperative care. While specific organizational designs may vary, all can be classified as professional practice models because they focus on autonomy over and accountability for nursing practice.

## Overview of Professional Governance Models

An accountability-based governance system is a predominant feature of professional practice models. Responsibility and authority are established in specified processes rather than in particular individuals who, in turn, determine the placement of accountability. The nurse is central to the organization and is supported by major service components such as standards, quality, assurance, continuing education, and peer process. Nursing management has no legitimate role in practice-related decisions; rather, management facilitates, integrates, and coordinates nursing operations to support the practitioner. Organizational administration is concerned with system-wide operations and serves as a link to the external environment (i.e., consumers). These elements, which comprise a framework for professional governance, are illustrated in Fig. 3-1.

There are three prevailing models of professional governance in current use (Porter-O'Grady, 1987). The *councilor* model uses elected councils to structure staff and manage-

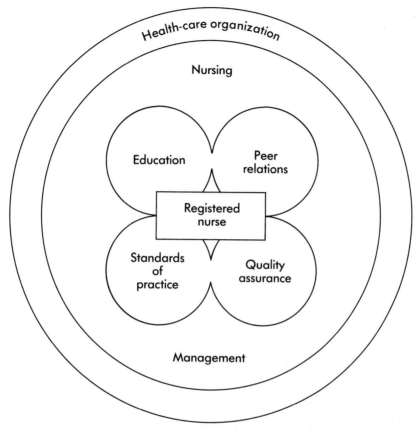

❖ **Fig. 3-1**    Model for professional governance. *(Adapted from Porter-O'Grady T: Shared governance and new organizational models, Nurs Econ 5(6):284, 1987. Reprinted with permission.)*

ment governance processes. Councils on practice, quality assurance, and education are composed primarily of practicing nurses, with management having minority representation. These councils make decisions related to clinical practice. The management team has a management council, with clinical staff having minority representation, where decisions regarding system operations are made. A second model, the *congressional* format, consists of a president and cabinet of officers who are elected from the staff of the organization and who oversee the operations. Cabinet members are

a mixture of clinical and management representatives. There may be equal representation from each group or, consistent with the belief that the organization is a clinical service, it may be weighted with more clinical representatives. Committees, often chaired by cabinet officers, are empowered with certain responsibilities and accountabilities and report back to the cabinet. The third model, the *administrative* model, is perhaps the least professionally structured. Although a management and a clinical forum are the basic structural units, each forum is more typically aligned in a hierarchical fashion, and the nurse executive often has a mechanism for vetoing considerations of the various decision-making groups.

## ❖ CHARACTERISTICS OF A PROFESSIONAL CLIMATE FOR NURSING PRACTICE

While the foregoing governance models describe the structural design of the professional environment, what are the distinctive characteristics that identify a professional climate for nursing practice? In other words, what combination of structure and process elements would need to be put into place to establish a professional climate? Over the past decade, various individuals and groups have been instrumental in defining and refining the characteristics of a professional climate. The following section illustrates this evolutionary process.

### Identification of Initial Characteristics

Initial work in identifying aspects of a professional climate for nursing practice was reported in 1979 when an American Nurses' Association task force published *The Fourteen Characteristics of a Professional Practice Climate for Nursing* (Commission on Nursing Services, 1979). Working toward the goal of shared accountability for nursing services between nursing staff and nursing administration in an institution/agency, the following statements describing the characteristics of a professional climate were developed:

1. A system of shared governance (including either contracted agreements or officially approved bylaws, rules, and regulations) within the nursing department provides means for accountability to the governing body of the institution and to the patient/client.

2. Planning of program and budget reflect variable levels of patient needs and requisite levels of staff competence.

3. Institutional policies administered by nursing assure shared responsibility between the institution and the individual nurse for development and maintenance of practitioner competence.

4. Support is given to experiments in staff utilization that have likelihood of improving the quality of care and containing costs.

5. The compensation system for nurses recognizes educational preparation, prior professional experience and level of competence, as well as length of service.

6. Nursing policies and practices are congruent with the following:
   a. ANA Code for Nurses.
   b. ANA Standards for Nursing Service.
   c. ANA Standards for Nursing Practice.
   d. State nurse practice act.
   e. Standards of voluntary accrediting body appropriate to the agency.
   f. Requirements of regulatory body appropriate to the agency.

7. Administrators are appointed whose preparation and practice are consistent with the roles, responsibilities and qualifications for nursing administrators identified by the ANA Commission on Nursing Services.

8. Practicing nurses have individual accountability for the care of each patient/client.

9. Provision is made for nurse-to-nurse consultation within the facility and between agencies and institutions.

10. A program of evaluation assesses practitioner performance and administrative effectiveness, as well as patient outcomes.

11. Nurses receive administrative support in the role of patient advocate.

12. Staff and administrative support are provided for nursing studies and research.

13. Nursing administration and staff activities result in a sense of accomplishment and commitment to professional practice.

14. A joint practice committee promotes collegial relationships between physicians and nurses (ANA, 1979).

These characteristics had significant appeal, some perhaps being very idealistic for the time, and others seeming idealistic to varying degrees even today. A logical question was the potential usefulness of each characteristic in creating a professional climate for nursing practice. To address the issue of usefulness, and also to begin working toward consensus on the components of the professional practice climate, Parrish and Cleland (1981) surveyed a group of 71 top-level nurse administrators.

The questionnaire used in this study asked the administrators to use a 5-point Likert-type scale to rate each of the above 14 characteristics for: (1) *value* as indicated by the extent to which they would like to see the characteristic in their setting; (2) *appropriateness* to their institution and staff; and (3) *likelihood* of being able to implement the characteristic in their institution. Responses indicated that *all* 14 characteristics incorporated into the questionnaire were valued by the nurse administrators. The most valued characteristic (the one they would most like to implement) was number 13, "Nursing administration and staff activities result in a sense of accomplishment and commitment to professional practice." The least valued was number 1 relating to shared governance.

When rating the appropriateness of the characteristics for their respective institutions, the administrators again gave high rankings to *all* the characteristics. Receiving the highest ranking was number 9 relating to nurse-to-nurse collaboration. Once again, characteristic number 1 relating to shared governance received the lowest ranking. (It must be noted that this "low" ranking was still high with a mean item score of 4.0 on a 5-point scale.)

With regard to the likelihood of implementing the characteristics, numbers 2, 12, 6, 9, 10, and 11 received the highest scores. Not surprisingly, characteristic number 14 referring to establishing a joint practice committee was rated as the least likely to be implemented.

While Parrish and Cleland acknowledged

the limitations of using a convenience sample of registrants at a nursing administration conference, their work provided the first systematic study of possible characteristics of a professional climate for nursing practice. Their findings described the perspectives of nursing administrators across diverse hospital settings. The similarity of the administrators' responses suggested that many anticipated barriers to the implementation of the characteristics could be minimized.

## Characteristics Refined and Extended

Further work on articulating the characteristics of the professional climate for nursing practice was done by the American Nurses' Association's Commission on Nursing Services. In 1981, this work was incorporated into components of a professional nursing system by the Task Force on Nursing Practice, which listed 19 characteristics. Besides coming up with five additional characteristics, some of the original ones were refined. For example, the first characteristic relating to shared governance was expanded to become:

> The Division of Nursing communicates directly with the Board of Trustees and has mechanisms for shared governance, including contracted agreements, nursing staff bylaws approved by the Board of Trustees and/or rules and regulations which provide for clinical privileges and for accountability to the governing body and to the patient (ANA, 1982, p. 8).

In this later listing, the numerical order of the characteristics was also altered and the following five characteristics were added:

2. The Division of Nursing has sufficient autonomy and budgetary control to be able to assume accountability for the quality of nursing practice and the outcomes of nursing care.
3. A nursing management information system and other resources are used to develop and

manage divisional planning, budgeting, and monitoring the quality of nursing care.

4. Nursing administration participates fully, by title and action, in top-level administrative decision making and with the governing body.

8. Effective around-the-clock services are available to support the practice of nurses.

12. Nurses effectively recommend decisions on admissions, placement, and discharge of patients (ANA, 1982, pp. 8-9).

It is of interest to note that many of these characteristics have at least two commonalities; they address organizational structure and reflect emphasis on the need for a formal structure of shared governance, including specific functions and responsibilities.

## The Need for Continued Refinement

In the following years, a number of events occurred that underscore the need to intensify efforts toward defining and implementing a climate for professional practice. For example, there have been at least two cycles of nursing "shortage" with explanations ranging from low salaries to lack of control over nursing practice to increased demands for nursing services. In addition, the implementation of Diagnosis Related Groups (DRGs) and new reimbursement structures have changed the face of health care institutions/agencies in many ways, not the least of which have been issues related to financial status. Shorter hospital stays and declining access to health care have contributed to increased acuity levels in hospitalized patients. The need to optimize nursing resources has continuously challenged nurses, staff, and administrators to be able to deliver high-quality patient care in a cost-effective manner. A recent review of standard nursing models (i.e., team, modular, total patient care, and primary) concluded that there is no single nursing model that is most cost-effective (Glandon, Colbert &

Thomasma, 1989). Studies of quality of nursing care also remain less than definitive today, consistent with a previous review provided by Lang and Clinton (1984).

The professional climate for nursing practice remains no more clearly defined today than it was in the early 1980s. While various models of professional governance have been established in some health care agencies, there has been little validation of the distinctive characteristics that constitute a professional climate by nurses who practice in those settings. Thus, it is not surprising that until recently, research studies have not addressed the characteristics of the professional climate for nursing practice, and few instruments for measuring this important construct exist.

## Measuring the Professional Climate for Nursing Practice

Three instruments either directly or indirectly purport to measure components of the professional climate for nursing practice. The one direct approach actually builds on the characteristics of a professional climate articulated by ANA groups as described above. Miller and Polentini (1985) developed the *Professional Practice Climate Tool (PPCT),* which was designed for use with professional nurses in hospital settings. This instrument lists 50 characteristics of the professional climate. Using a 5-point Likert-type scale, nurses are instructed to rate each characteristic for: (1) perceived value and (2) the extent to which it is perceived to be present in their practice setting.

Two scores are produced from these ratings: "ideal" and "current" perceptions of the professional climate. Each score can range from 50 to 250; the higher the score, the greater the extent to which the group of characteristics of the professional climate is perceived as valued (ideal) or present (current).

In related efforts, two studies describe instruments claiming to measure the broader construct of the "hospital work environment." Dennis (1989) conceptualized "real" and "ideal" perspectives and incorporated characteristics from three work environment dimensions (personal, interpersonal, and system) and three environmental influences (professional attributes, motivational incentives, and physical comfort). Kramer and Hafner (1989) developed the Nursing Work Index for use in a national study, which includes perceptions of an environment supporting quality nursing care.

Instruments such as these offer the ability to identify aspects of the professional climate for nursing practice as perceived by practicing nurses. Two of these (the *PPCT* and the work by Dennis) allow for comparison of two dimensions: "ideal" and "real." As the environment for professional nursing practice becomes more clearly defined, the need to develop additional instruments can be anticipated in order to capture evolving viewpoints and to identify elements.

### ❖ HOSPITAL NURSES' PERSPECTIVES ON THE PROFESSIONAL CLIMATE

Work continues on the effort to identify and define the characteristics of a professional climate for nursing practice. The following section illustrates the usefulness of studying the professional climate from the perspective of practicing nurses. Several issues are addressed, such as the role of shared governance, the perspectives of nurses in different roles and on different patient care units, and the relationship of a professional climate to nurse job satisfaction.

### Role of Shared Governance

Does the presence of shared governance in a hospital guarantee an optimal professional climate for nursing practice? This question is logical considering the focus on shared governance that was pervasive in the early work of defining the professional climate. Jacobson et al (1987) used the *PPCT* in a hospital (Hospital A,

below) where shared governance had not yet been implemented. Jenkins (1989) and Jenkins and Kosmoski-Goepfert (1989 a, b) used the *PPCT* in a hospital (Hospital B) where a model of shared governance had been in place for nearly 6 years. The mean scores obtained in these studies were:

|  | HOSPITAL A (N = 179) | HOSPITAL B (N = 374) |
|---|---|---|
|  | No shared governance | Shared governance |
| Current | 154.88 | 154.73 |
| Ideal | 199.79 | 209.88 |

These findings suggest that there is far more to the professional climate for nursing practice than the existence of a shared governance model. Despite the absence or presence of shared governance, the scores from the two hospitals were highly similar.

### Diverse Perspectives by Nursing Roles

As previously discussed, Parrish and Cleland's (1981) study provided baseline data on characteristics of the professional climate from the viewpoint of nursing administrators. Since it was primarily those in administrative roles who worked in the groups to identify and refine these characteristics, it is relevant to determine whether nurses in different roles share their perceptions. More specifically, do nurses in various roles perceive the professional climate for nursing practice differently?

To answer this question, mean item scores on the "current" and "ideal" scales of the *PPCT* obtained in the Jenkins study were examined (Practice Philosophy Ad Hoc Committee & Jenkins, 1989; Jenkins & Cieslak-Duchek, 1989). Data from 395 nurses were reviewed. Staff nurses comprised nearly 90 % (n = 352) of the sample; 10 were nurse managers or directors and 33 were nursing students enrolled in an elective nurse intern program.

Indeed, staff nurses, managers, and nursing students all valued the professional climate characteristics listed on the *PPCT,* as evidenced by the high item scores obtained on the "ideal" scale. However, there was a wider disparity of scores on the "current" scale as illustrated below:

|  | CURRENT | IDEAL |
|---|---|---|
|  | Range of scores | |
| Staff nurses | 2.08 - 4.10 | 3.73 - 4.63 |
| Managers/directors | 2.30 - 4.30 | 3.30 - 4.60 |
| Nursing students | 3.67 - 4.61 | 3.88 - 4.93 |

A graphic comparison of the perceptions of these groups is illustrated in Fig. 3-1.

Recalling that *PPCT* item responses could range from a low of 1 to a high of 5, it is clear that:

1. Nursing students perceived the characteristics of the professional climate to be present to a greater extent than did either staff nurses or managers/directors.
2. As indicated by the broader range of scores, the responses from staff nurses and managers/directors were more variable than were those from nursing students.

Using the mean item scores for each group on each of the 50 characteristics, the numerical rankings of the characteristics on the "ideal" and "current" scales were obtained. Only eight characteristics were common to more than one group: these are displayed in Table 3-1.

As can be seen in Table 3-1, only one ideal characteristic ranked among the top 10 across all three groups: registered nurses have control over the quality of nursing care provided. This characteristic was ranked first by staff nurses and manager/directors and ninth by nursing students. Four characteristics were common to the top 10 list of staff nurses and managers/directors, though as seen, rankings were different for each

group. Three characteristics were common to staff nurse and student groups. Again, rank order varied. No characteristics were unique only to managers/directors or nursing students.

Likewise, the top 10 ranked characteristics by each group on the "current" scale were examined. Again, eight characteristics were common to two or more groups. As seen in Table 3-2, this list is somewhat different from that for the characteristics of the "ideal" professional climate (Table 3-1). Five characteristics were common across all groups, though the rank order differed. Two characteristics were found to be common to staff nurses and managers and only one between students and managers.

The highest ranked characteristic (i.e., that perceived to be most characteristic of nursing within the institution) was different for each group. For staff nurses, it was that nurses had individual accountability for their patients; for the managers/directors, it was goal-directed nursing based on the nursing process; for students, it was that nursing was responsive to the needs of the patient.

**Discrepancy between "ideal" and "current" scores.** Of related interest was the size of the difference between total "current" and "ideal" scores in these three groups. For the staff nurse group, the difference was 57.88; for managers/directors, it was 37.25; and for students, the difference was only 6.30. The marked variation in this discrepancy across groups further underscores the differing perceptions of nurses in diverse roles.

## Diversity of Perceptions Across Nursing Units

As perceptions of the professional climate vary among nursing roles, do they also vary across nursing units? This question could be addressed from at least two perspectives: type of governance structure of the unit and type of patient care unit.

Focusing on the governance structure of

**Table 3-1**
Highest rated characteristics and rankings of characteristics of the "ideal" professional climate

|  | Staff nurses | Managers/ directors | Students |
|---|---|---|---|
|  | | Rank | |
| RNs have control over quality of patient care | 1 | 1 | 9 |
| Administration supports RN as advocate | 5 | 2 | |
| RN influences treatment program | 3 | 8 | |
| Plan for continuing education for increased RN competency | 6 | 9 | |
| Assignments commensurate with nurse qualifications | 8 | 4 | |
| Nursing practice responsive to patient needs | 2 | | 1 |
| Administration supports formal education | 10 | | 8 |
| RNs integrate theory with practice | 9 | | 10 |

❖ **Table 3-2**
Highest rated characteristics and rankings of characteristics of the "current" professional climate

|  | Staff nurses | Managers/ directors | Students |
|---|---|---|---|
|  | | Rank | |
| Practice goal directed/nursing process | 7 | 1 | 2 |
| Practice responsive to patient needs | 2 | 2 | 1 |
| Nursing diagnosis used | 3 | 5 | 3 |
| Practice responsive to family needs | 9 | 3 | 2 |
| Philosophy reflecting ethical obligations | 6 | 6 | 8 |
| RNs being individually accountable for care | 1 | 4 | |
| Having a forum for exploration of ethical issues | 10 | 7 | |
| Activities producing a sense of accomplishment | | 8 | 5 |

units within another hospital setting, Dennis (1989) studied nurses from two units: a newly opened unit with a form of "professional" governance and critical care units with "traditional" governance. Perceptions of "real" and "ideal" work environments were considered. Results indicate that the nurses from the critical care units perceived the "real" and "ideal" work environments as distinctly different from one another with little overlap. Responses from nurses on the professional practice unit indicated much overlap between their perceptions of the "real" and "ideal" work environments.

While the differences in perceptions of the hospital work environment found by Dennis crossed several units, no systematic study of the difference in views of nurses in different types of patient care units has been reported to date. This remains a fertile area for further study.

## Professional Climate and Job Satisfaction

In the studies by Jenkins and colleagues, *PPCT* scores from the "current" and "ideal" scales were correlated with scores from a measure of job satisfaction, which was administered at the same time. While the relationships between both "current" and "ideal" *PPCT* scores and job satisfaction scores were both statistically significant, the robust size of the relationship between the "current" score and job satisfaction score was marked. The higher the "current" score, or the greater the extent to which the characteristics on the *PPCT* were present, the greater the job satisfaction score. In the series of multiple regression analyses carried out on data from this study, nurse perceptions of the "current" environment were consistently the most potent predictor of job satisfaction.

This finding has particular importance in times of shrinking nursing resources. For example, at the hospital where this study was conducted, over two thirds of the nurses had been employed for 6 years or more and were at the top two levels of a four-tiered career ladder system. To retain these valued employees at the institution, and perhaps even within the nursing profession, it would seem logical that interventions designed to enhance the environment for professional nursing practice would be beneficial. Improved nurse retention is cost-effective and contributes directly to the delivery of high-quality patient care.

## ❖ CONCLUSIONS

While much of this discussion has been drawn from individual studies reflecting the perspectives of hospital nurses at one point in time, the differences in perspectives point to the importance of nurses in all types of roles being involved in continuing definition of the key elements of the professional climate for nursing practice. Further research in this area should include nurses other than nurse administrators; indeed, all professional nursing roles should be appropriately represented for a given setting.

Ongoing work aimed at defining and measuring the key elements of the professional climate must continue. Such efforts may lead to the development of interventions aimed at enhancing the professional climate, or minimizing the discrepancy between "real" and "ideal" perceptions. If minimizing this discrepancy proves to be a key factor in nurse retention by institutions and agencies as well as the profession at large, we may be successful in proactively dealing with the challenges of "shortage." Elimination of these recurring cycles can free nursing to move ahead as a vital force, capable of determining its own future in the health care system, and progressing in its continuing emergence as a profession. Considering the key role that perceptions of the professional climate played in predicting job satisfaction in one hospital, further explication of the professional practice environment poses challenges across nursing roles and provides an exciting arena for collaboration among clinicians, administrators, and researchers.

## ❖ SUMMARY

In this chapter, issues involved in creating a professional climate for nursing practice are identified, and three governance models in current use are described. Identifying the characteristics of the professional climate is shown to be an evolutionary process that continues to the present time. A study of the perspectives of hospital nurses represents a continuing effort to identify "real" and "ideal" characteristics of a professional climate for nursing practice, to determine the differences in perceptions of nurses in various nursing roles and across different types of patient care units, and to identify some positive outcomes (such as nurse retention) associated with a professional practice climate. A professional climate that builds trust, enhances communication, and develops staff nurse autonomy and accountability shows promise for improving the quality of care for the patient and increasing job satisfaction for the nurse.

## ❖ APPLYING KNOWLEDGE TO PRACTICE

1. Considering the characteristics of the professional climate for nursing practice discussed in this chapter, identify those which you value the most and provide a rationale for your choice.
2. To what extent do you think each of these characteristics or elements is present in the:
   a. client care unit
   b. nursing department and
   c. hospital/institution/agency
   with which you are most familiar? Support your answers with examples.
3. If you were to serve on a committee to identify strategies to improve the professional climate for nursing practice in the hospital/institution/agency with which you are most familiar, what would you suggest?
4. Why might one anticipate that perceptions of nursing students about the environment for professional nursing practice would differ from those of staff nurses?

## ❖ ACKNOWLEDGMENTS

◆ I acknowledge the efforts of the many people who have provided support for the content of this chapter. Particular appreciation is extended to Michelle Miller for permission to use the *PPCT*, the Practice Philosophy Task Force and nurse respondents at St. Luke's Medical Center, Milwaukee, Wisconsin, Kerry Kosmoski-Goepfert for collaboration and consultation on aspects of job satisfaction, and Thelma Riederer and Denise Christopher for assistance in carrying out related data analyses.

### REFERENCES

American Nurses' Association (1982). *Standards for organized nursing services.* Kansas City: American Nurses' Association.

Commission on Nursing Services (1979). Final report of the Task Force on Nursing Practice Climate. Kansas City: American Nurses' Association.

Commission on Nursing Services and the Task Force on Nursing Services (1981). *Components of a professional nursing system.* Kansas City: American Nurses' Association.

Dennis, K. E. (1989, October). *The real and ideal hospital work environments in juxtaposition.* Paper presented at the Fifth International Conference for the Scientific Study of Subjectivity, Columbia, MO.

Glandon, G. L., Colbert, K. W., & Thomasma, M. (1989). Nursing delivery models and RN mix: Cost implications. *Nursing Management, 20*(5), 30–33.

Jacobson, A., Hartmann, B., Johnson, K., McQuide, P., Talsky, J., & Kalt, J. (1987, November). *A professional practice climate: Attitudes and ratings of the professional nurse.* Paper presented at the 10th Annual Research Day, School of Nursing, University of Wisconsin, Milwaukee.

Jenkins, L. S. (1989, October). *The environment for professional nursing practice: A key factor in job satisfaction.* Paper presented at the Third Annual National Shared Governance Conference: Pathway to Autonomy and Professionalism in Nursing, Milwaukee, WI.

Jenkins, L. S. & Cieslak-Duchek, M. (1989). *Impact of elective nurse intern programs in medical-surgical and critical care nursing.* (Technical report). Milwaukee, WI: St. Luke's Medical Center.

Jenkins, L. S. & Kosmoski-Goepfert, K. (1989a, November). *A measure of the professional practice environment: Factor structure.* Paper presented at the Scientific Sessions of Sigma Theta Tau International Honor Society of Nursing's Thirtieth Biennial Convention, Indianapolis, IN.

Jenkins, L. S. & Kosmoski-Goepfert, K. (1989b, April). *Operationalizing the environment for professional nursing practice: The PPCT.* Paper presented at the Thirteenth Annual Conference of the Midwest Nursing Research Society, Cincinnati, OH.

Kramer, M. & Hafner, L. P. (1989). Shared values: Impact on staff nurse satisfaction and perceived productivity. *Nursing Research, 38*(3), 172–177.

Lang, N. M. & Clinton, J. F. (1984). Assessment of quality of nursing care. In H. H. Werley and J. J. Fitzpatrick (eds.), *Annual review of nursing research* (vol. 2, pp. 135–163). New York: Springer Publishing Co.

Mayer, G. G., Madden, M. J., & Lawrenz, E. (1990). *Patient care delivery models.* Rockville, MD: Aspen Publishers.

Miller, M. & Polentini, A. (1985). *Professional practice climate.* Unpublished paper, Measurement of Clinical and Educational Nursing Outcomes Project.

Orsolits, M. (1989). Organizing nursing for the future: Nursing commission recommendations and research implications. *Applied Nursing Research, 2*(2), 64–67.

Parrish, D. M. & Cleland, V. S. (1981). Characteristics of a professional nursing practice climate: A survey. *Journal of Nursing Administration, 11*(4), 40–45.

Porter-O'Grady, T. (1986). *Creative nursing administration: Participative management into the 21st century.* Rockville, MD: Aspen Publishers.

Porter-O'Grady, T. (1987). Shared governance and new organizational models. *Nursing economics, 5*(6), 281–287.

Practice Philosophy Ad Hoc Committee and Jenkins, L. S. (1989). Impact of changes in patient care delivery. *Interchange, 9*(3), Special Supplement, 1–4.

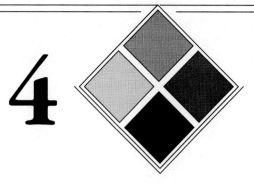

# 4

# Enabling Professional Nursing Practice

## An Administrator's Perspective

Marjorie Beyers

## OBJECTIVES

*At the completion of this chapter, the reader will be able to:*

- ◆ Describe the influences of nursing administration on nursing practice.
- ◆ Discuss major aspects of the practice environment that affect the practice of nursing.
- ◆ Identify and apply a framework for creating and sustaining an environment conducive to professional nursing practice.

Growth of nursing administration theories, frameworks, and concepts has not kept pace with the growth of nursing as a profession. Systematic development of the knowledge base for effective nursing administration is now receiving attention as a result of several recent national studies of the nursing shortage. (National Commission on Nursing, 1983; Secretary's Commission on Nursing, 1988). These study findings indicate that the effectiveness of nursing administration is a major factor in client and staff nurse satisfaction. Effective nursing administration practices are associated with professional practice models of nursing care delivery (Clifford, 1988; Ethridge & Lamb, 1989). It is now recognized that the nursing administra-

tor's primary role is to establish an environment that enables professional nursing practice.

## ❖ CLARIFYING THE DISCIPLINE OF NURSING

Establishing clear relationships between nursing practice and nursing administration is timely. The contribution that nursing, as a clinical discipline, makes to health care is being scrutinized for several reasons. Public attention has been drawn to health care and its cost, its quality, and its importance to societal well-being. Society identifies *health status* as a measure of the effectiveness of the health care system. Health status is expressed in productivity;

the wealth of a country; the fulfillment of human potential; the status of the dependent disabled, elderly, and the chronically ill; and the ability to grow and develop to full potential of physical and cognitive human capabilities. Nursing, as one component of the health care system, contributes to aggregate societal health by caring for individuals, families, and groups throughout the entire continuum of health care—from wellness to hospice care. This contribution has not always been recognized because nursing services have traditionally been hidden in organizationally provided health care services. The specific contribution nursing makes to the attainment of health status is often poorly understood. It is time to ensure that the practice of nursing as a clinical discipline makes nursing's contribution to health status more visible. To accomplish this, the theories, frameworks, and concepts of nursing administration must be the same as or compatible with those used to explain or define nursing practice.

Another dimension in this discussion is whether management is integral to nursing practice. It may be useful to examine the issues using the term *management* rather than *administration,* since management seems to be the more commonly used term. It should be noted that administration and management are often interchangeable in common usage. Asking important questions using the term *management* rather than *administration* is also useful because in some traditional as well as emerging models of nursing practice, management is used to describe the staff nurse function, as in management of client care or as in case management. In fact, as the nursing process was being conceptualized, one of the debates was whether the nursing process was a management approach for decision making or not. If management is integral to nursing practice, then every nurse is a manager. Yet, in another sense, nurses in practice are managed. Does a professional nurse in practice need a manager? Or does the practice of nursing incorporate management in the delivery of care?

## Professional Nursing Practice

Professional nursing practice has its own logic and content. The nursing process is used to express the logic of nursing. Essentially, the logic of a profession refers to the way its members learn to think and make decisions: to use professional knowledge in practice. The content of nursing refers to the knowledge base for practice: the facts and principles that have been tested through research and experience and found to be useful in practice. Professional nursing requires that its knowledge base is continually questioned and developed through practice and research.

Professional nursing practice is also characterized by use of theories of nursing to define and explain the relationships among concepts for purposes of uncovering and examining newly identified phenomena associated with nursing practice. Theories allow consideration of relationships such as those between the nurse and the individuals and families the nurse cares for, or between the client/family and environmental factors influencing health status. In professional nursing practice, theories are developed and tested to expand the knowledge base through research. In addition, the interventions nurses use in providing care can be organized into a theoretical framework for discussion and explication. Orem's self-care theory, for example, relates the client's need for care to the nurse's role in meeting that need. Roy's adaptation theory likewise describes and relates the client's need for care to nursing functions. Rogers' theory relates nursing to the broader environment and societal influences *of* nursing and *on* nursing.

Professional nursing practice requires that nurses make decisions using principles, concepts, and nursing theories. The way a nurse "processes" this information for outcomes is the logic of nursing. In professional nursing practice, the nurse assesses the client's condition, develops and implements an individualized nursing care plan, evaluates outcomes, and manages the use of the organizational resources to deliver that care. Learning to practice nursing begins in the basic educational program and continues through experience. This learning is maintained, sustained, and further developed through continuing nursing education as well as through continuous questioning of the practice phenomenon.

## The Nursing Administration Specialty

Nursing administration is often defined in terms of the roles and functions of nurses involved in managing or administering the delivery of nursing care in the context of the patient care unit, hospital, or other health care agency rather than in the context of nursing's relationships with clients and families. In some instances, nursing administration has become more like general administration than a specialized field in nursing. In these instances, a basic question is being raised—does one have to be a nurse to effectively manage nursing services?

Nursing administration is a specialty within nursing; it can also be considered a specialty within the field of administration. In either case, it is a specialty grounded in and focused on the clinical discipline. In this sense, is the nurse administrator a practicing nurse (a peer), an administrator who has a nursing background, or both?

These differences are not self-evident. On the one hand, one could argue that administration is administration. On the other hand, one could claim the administrator of nursing services must be a nurse. The difference may be in the mind-set, knowledge base, or in relative values. If so, do these differences matter in the real world? To answer these questions, a pragmatic approach to examining the relationship between the practice of nursing and its administration is needed. The answers require a useful model for professional nursing practice, which will facilitate the necessary alignment of nursing practice and administration.

## ❖ CLARIFYING THE RELATIONSHIPS
## The Relationship Between Nursing Education, Practice, and Administration

During the past several decades, there has been considerable concern about the relationship between nursing practice and nursing education. Recruitment and retention problems, among others, have been attributed to dissonance between education and practice. Yet the relationship between administration and practice is even more basic than the relationship between education and practice. The necessary linkages between nursing education and practice cannot be achieved until the issues between nursing practice and its administration are satisfactorily resolved.

The dissonance between nursing education and practice is well documented in the literature and is the subject of many discussions about the future of nursing. More realistic nursing education is often advocated. A common statement is that students should be ready to take care of clients in the hospital setting soon after graduation and orientation. Determination of what is "realistic," however, depends on relating nursing practice to nursing administration in ways to more effectively enable the practice of nursing. If, for example, the new graduate is well-prepared to take care of clients, the administration should enable that care. Professional nursing practice models now being developed and strengthened have proven to be more effective in encouraging quality nursing care as well as nurse satisfaction than previous traditional models of nursing care delivery. These traditional delivery models often focused on hospital routines rather than on client care. Consideration of key aspects of the practice-administration relationship reveals the differences between the professional and traditional models.

**Employment expectations.** Consider, for example, the phenomenon of employment. Since the majority of nurses are employees of health care organizations, employment expectations play a major role in the practice-administration relationship. Both the nurse employees and the employing organizations have expectations about nursing practice. The nurse expects to provide care to clients based on the standards of practice learned in his or her basic education. As employees, however, nurses are often expected to practice according to organizationally designed roles and functions, which may not match the roles learned in the educational setting (Kramer & Schmalenberg, 1988a; 1988b). In dysfunctional practice-administration relationships, nurses' expectations regarding their practice have not been met. Models of professional nursing practice are more effective because they require professional competence and because nurses' expectations for clinical nursing practice are aligned with the organization's expectations for performance.

## Relationship Between Nursing Practice and Nursing Administration

What premises, assumptions, theories, or frameworks best serve to explain the desired relationships between nursing practice and administration? To answer this question, it is useful to examine the influence of nursing administration on the outcomes of nursing practice. What effect does administration have on practice? Why do we need nursing administration? Does a practicing nurse have sufficient autonomy to practice; to use knowledge and skills to deliver a service to the public? How would the practice of nursing be affected by the absence of nursing administration? Very simply stated, is nursing administration necessary and if so, why?

Administration of nursing services should enable professional nursing practice. Descriptions of nursing administration may be generally placed in two different categories. One category is organizationally based and defined by

the organization. In this view, the nursing administrator manages nurses and the functions of nursing care. The second category is based in the discipline of nursing. In this view, nursing administration exists to enable professional practice. The nursing administrator manages the environment for professional nursing practice and ensures the required resources.

## Relationship Between Nursing Practice and Organizations

Because nursing care is most frequently delivered under the auspices of a health care organization, the relationship of nursing to the organization must be considered. Organizational structures place administrators or managers in positions to carry out their expected functions. Managers in organizations garner and use scarce resources to produce an outcome valued by the organization. Practitioners in such an environment rely on effective administration/management to ensure resources adequate for effective practice. Supplies, equipment, appropriate facilities, support services, and other resources are needed. Could nurses in practice effectively procure necessary resources in the absence of nursing administration?

During the past 10 years, the effects of nursing management on practice have been debated and studied. The basic assumption is that managers are necessary to set forth the day's activities that nurses are expected to undertake. Necessary management activities include developing and ensuring implementation of nursing department policies and procedures, nursing unit policies and procedures, standardized care plans, and appropriate staffing. Supervision and oversight are commonly emphasized by directors, head nurses, or clinical managers.

Nursing practice is thought to benefit from effective management. The question is whether it is the practice or the people or both that need to be managed. Retrospective studies of the effects of nursing management practices on the effectiveness of nursing practice could provide important insights. If management is integral to nursing, theories incorporating management would be integral to nursing science. On the other hand, if management is adjunctive to nursing, or enabling of nursing practice, management theories for nursing would be complementary but not integral.

## The Evolution of Practice-Administration Relationships

What happens to nursing practice with and without management? Examining nursing in the early 1900s, a time when nursing management and health care organizational management was minimal, provides a view of how the practice-administration relationship could be shaped today. Did nursing thrive in this time? In the early 1900s nursing management essentially fulfilled two main functions: placement of nurses (i.e., staffing) and support for practitioners who mostly cared for clients in their homes. In addition to placement and support of nurses, administrative functions also included basic nursing education, which was experiential and incorporated delivery of nursing services. These nursing administrators' functions thus required an integration of education, service delivery, continued support of graduates, and ongoing service to clients and families in their homes. After completing the educational program, nurses were placed in home settings by matching them to a client/family. Effective nursing practice then depended on two factors: the competence and interactive skills of the practitioner and the compatibility of the nurse and client, both personally and environmentally.

What, if any, aspects of this situation could be applied or used to develop a framework for contemporary professional nursing practice? Competence and effective interaction are two factors that continue to be critical in today's environment. In fact, the interpretation of these two as-

pects of nursing has remained relatively constant over time. Isolating these constants is one way to use known information to develop new frameworks that allow further study of the relationship between practice and administration.

Further development of a framework is aided by examining findings of previous studies of nursing administration. The single most extensive study on administration was conducted in 1950 to 1952 by Finer (1952). This remarkable work was funded by the Kellogg Foundation Nursing Service Administration Research Project. In this study, several premises were set forth. One premise was that the "primary duty of nurses" occurred through mastery and sufficient practice of the clinical elements of patient care, both basic and specialized. A second premise was that administration "follows only on clinical competence." The study explored the similarities and distinctions between public health nursing and nursing in hospitals. It is interesting that relationships between public health and hospital nurses are now being revisited in today's health care environment. At any rate, the Finer study did not draw distinctions between hospitals and public health, believing that nursing administration followed practice in whatever setting the care was delivered. The principles of administration were thought to be similar. Practice differences were explained as variations in complexity rather than in substance of care.

Finer described eight organizational elements of nursing administration that were used to analyze nursing service. These eight elements were (1) aims, policies, organization; (2) staffing; (3) planning and directing nursing care; (4) coordination of interdepartmental activities; (5) community health planning; (6) plant, supplies, and equipment; (7) budgeting; and (8) records and reports. Administrative functions depicted for nursing surrounding these elements were human relations; communications; teaching; research; and personal professional development.

### ❖ REINTEGRATING BASIC ELEMENTS FOR PRACTICE

Throughout its history, nursing service administration has remained fairly consistent in the elements cited in Finer's study, but the ways these elements were interpreted have changed. Significant changes in elements of staffing, planning and directing nursing care, community health planning, and plant supplies and equipment are worth mentioning. Compared to 1952 levels, recent nurse staffing practices have changed to incorporate increasing numbers of registered nurses and fewer numbers of assisting staff (Aiken, 1983). Planning and directing nursing care has been interpreted over the years in functional definitions of nursing duties and as aspects of nursing care delivery models. These models of nursing care delivery dominated the literature in the past 30 years. Team nursing, cluster, group, or total nursing care or primary nursing care are examples.

Work to define nursing practice within the organization and to restore clinical practice has been accomplished. One major contribution was the definition of the nursing process. This definition allowed nurses to see the logic of nursing practice more clearly. Unfortunately, the nursing process became institutionalized in some settings by developing standard care plans or lists of tasks to be completed during each shift rather than individualized plans for care. The nursing process was thus superimposed on rather than integrated into nursing practice.

A second influential effort was the development of patient classification systems. These systems were developed to identify and set standards for appropriate staffing for care, usually on a unit level. The intent was to ensure that clients received appropriate care and to provide a mechanism through which nurses could communicate client care requirements with hospital management more systematically and objectively. Unfortunately, patient classification systems were often reduced to the level of nursing tasks. In the initial development, cer-

tain nursing care tasks had been identified as indicators of intensity, acuity, or more recently, severity of illness. For example, basic hygienic care, medications, treatments, and other measures were reduced to lists of tasks. Time and motion studies were used to determine the numbers and types of nursing staff needed to care for patients as "classified" by the tasks to be performed. The intent of the classification system was lost. In early systems, patient teaching was considered adjunctive to care and "not counted."

Likewise, models of nursing care delivery were developed to make nurses more efficient and in some models, such as team nursing, to spread the registered nurse's work to encompass care of a greater number of clients. Models of nursing care delivery, nursing process, and patient classification systems, although each a potentially excellent method for supporting management and clinically related decision making by nurses, were not used in an integrated fashion to fulfill their intended purpose. The purpose of these management tools was to help nurses make decisions about care. Rationalizing staff mix through a model of nursing care delivery and monitoring nursing productivity by use of a patient classification system have been viewed as discrete activities. Only recently has the nursing process been integrated into realistic expectations of nurses in practice. Only recently have we begun to examine nursing productivity in light of client care outcomes.

### ❖ ESTABLISHING A FRAMEWORK FOR RELATING NURSING ADMINISTRATION TO NURSING PRACTICE

Establishing a framework for the relationship between nursing administration and nursing practice must take into account both the practice and the organization. Health care organizations and nursing practice are much more

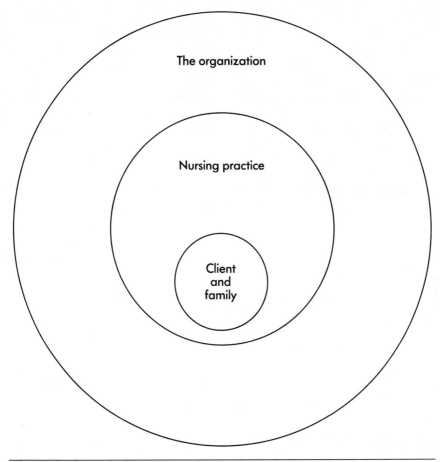

**❖ Fig. 4-1**     Three elements in a framework for nursing administration.

complex today than in the early 1900s. The framework, defined as the structure of a set of concepts and relationships among the concepts, must illustrate how aspects relate, such as the nurse to the organization or nursing practice to organizational dynamics.

An example of such a framework for nursing administration is offered for consideration. This framework includes three main elements: *the client and family; the nursing practice;* and *the organization* (Fig. 4-1). The first element, client and family, is the basic unit of analysis in nursing practice, since the need for nursing services is derived from the client and family.

Nursing practice, the second element, consists of the role and function of nurses to meet that demand. The third element, the organization, is a dynamic structure that exists to allow or enable the practitioner to meet the needs of the client and family. The organization contains all services, both clinical and support, needed to provide total care to the client and family.

## ❖ THE THREE ELEMENTS IN THE FRAMEWORK

The *client and family element* is the central unit of analysis for both nursing practice and nursing administration. This element in the framework forms the basis on which nursing care is evaluated from (1) the perspective of an individual nurse's performance; (2) the perspective of nursing service; and (3) the perspective of the organization's ability to serve clients. Concepts used in assessment and subsequent planning are those that are important to evaluate client needs such as pain, stress, self-care, social support, family, and health status. The ensuing plan of care is the written expression of nursing interventions derived from the assessment that must be accomplished to achieve the desired outcomes. Concepts depicting these client outcomes might include coping, adaptation, hope, empowerment, and functional dependency.

The client-family unit is the focus of the nurse in professional nursing practice. A given nurse relates to multiple client-family units and manages care in appropriate sequences. An overriding concept is individualized care, which means that each care plan is specifically designed for a given client. Another is continuity of care. Continuity of care incorporates not only discharge planning but also ensures that referrals are completed, that the client knows how to carry out self-care, how to use resources, and where to go for help. A simple example is teaching regarding a particular outpatient procedure (Barsevick & Lauver, 1990). The framework connects these concepts as they are incorporated to guide decision making for client care (Zwolski, 1989). The nurse assesses the client's present need, response to care, and potential future needs. Systematic planning for continuous care emphasizes the client's particular needs at a given point in time for aspects such as physical care, psychosocial care, emotional care, and education that may be provided in a sequence of hospital, home, and ambulatory care settings.

The client-family unit is defined not only as the population of a nursing care unit, but also as a continuum of client encounters in an ambulatory care clinic or as a member of a group receiving counseling or education. In a broader sense, client populations can be defined as persons served within a community such as in elderly day care or adolescent programs. Nursing practice must also reflect the environment in which nursing care is provided. The current emphasis on client participation in health care influences nursing practice because it implies a demand for knowledge and education for self-care. Now a high degree of decision making with the client, physician, and others is inherent in professional nursing practice.

The *nursing practice element* incorporates the knowledge base and skills nurses must have to be effective. Nursing practice, like client care, must be viewed holistically. Professional nursing practice is sustained through mechanisms such as quality assurance, continued nursing education, and professional advancement. The focus of all nursing activities at every level in the organization is individualized client-/family care or, in some instances, group care. The knowledge base of nursing related to this individualized care is applied in specific nursing interventions. The logic through which the assessment is made and appropriate interventions are selected is the nursing process. In professional nursing practice, all care is developed from the nursing assessment and systematically organized in the care plan. The care plan is the record that serves to document the nurse's decision making. Interventions employed by the nurse in care and the client's responses to them are also recorded and used in the evaluation component of the process. Table 4-1 depicts the major elements of nursing care that can be described as functions or interventions; the client-family unit participation in care and the other disciplines involved in total health care.

In continuity of care models, the nurse works with health professionals from other disciplines to plan and evaluate care. Nursing case conferences are expanded to include members of other disciplines to become client care con-

❖ **Table 4–1**

Individualized client care planning and nursing care accountability

| Registered nurse accountability | Care aspects accepted by client/family | Care aspects delegated to Supportive Services | Integration |
|---|---|---|---|
| Pre- to post-hospital sequence of care: | | | Care provided by other health professionals integrated into total plan of care |
| Nursing care elements | | | Groups nursing works with most consistently: |
| Nursing assessment | | | • Physicians |
| Nursing care plan | | | • Clinic/office staff |
| • Pre-admission testing | | | • Dietician |
| • Education | | | • Pharmacist |
| • Information | | | • Laboratory technician |
| • Counseling/guidance | | | • X-ray technician |
| • Referral | | | • Rehabilitation therapist |
| • Discharge plan | Accountabilities are defined | | • Social worker |
| • Comfort/hygiene | based on the nursing assessment | | • Pastoral ministry |
| • Nutrition | and physician plan of care in | | |
| • Elimination | cooperation with other caregivers | | All health professionals |
| • Exercise | listed in last column | | involved in a given client's |
| • Rest | | | care integrate their |
| • Pain control | | | participation through: |
| • Medications | | | • Case conferences |
|    Admininstration | | | • Chronologic documenta- |
|    Monitoring | | |   tion of care |
| • Diagnostic tests, | | | • Evaluation of the client's |
|   treatments and therapy | | |   progress |
|    Preparation | | | • Quality assurance |
|    Administration/coordination | | | • Design/improvement of |
|    After care | | |   service sequence |
| • Monitoring/assessing | | | |
|   client status and progress | | | |
| • Evaluation | | | |
| • Follow-up by appropriate | | | |
|   caregivers: physicians, | | | |
|   home care, long-term care | | | |

ferences. Nurse-physician rounds are expanded from informing the physician of the client's progress and special needs to a planning session in which both the physician and nurse participate with the client in discussing the ongoing plan of care. In some settings, the nursing care plan is now part of the permanent record. This rightfully changes the care plan from a vehicle for assigning duties to an integral part of the permanent record. Use of integrated charting formats in which personnel from every involved discipline record their notes reflects the integration of care in interdisciplinary team interaction. The nurses' decision making stands out as a major component of this care because nurses often direct and coordinate all care in the hospital, the home, or the long-term care facility. Nurses are almost always present, while persons from other disciplines come and go according to their functions in the overall care process.

The *organization element* in the framework includes aspects of organizational structure, interdisciplinary interactions, human resource management and productivity, and resource acquisition and utilization, such as supplies, staff, and facilities. Organizations are administered/managed by decision makers who ensure appropriate resources through procurement, selection, and evaluation processes; activate the organizational mission and set goals for performance; and design the structure that aligns people, resources, plant/facilities to accomplish the work (i.e., undertake the eight activities identified by Finer). For nursing, the usual link between the professional nurse employee and the organizational decision makers is nursing administration. The nurse administrators participate in executive management committees, planning panels, and in clinical group meetings to represent nursing (Balasco, 1989; Brett & Tonges, 1990).

The organization is also the entity that relates to the community as a whole as well as segments of the community. A number of for-

mal activities take place in this relationship. Planning for health services that meet community demand; communicating the organizational mission and goals to promote community understanding; mutual learning between community members and health professionals; acknowledging and promoting leadership within the community on health related matters; marketing services; and providing opportunities for employment are some of the major ways that organizations relate to communities.

As nursing is recognized for its practice, nurses also reach out into the community to work with community groups in a variety of ways. One way is to provide education to community organizations about health. Another way is to provide a service to a specific population such as through an outreach clinic in a nursing home or church. Nurses also serve as committee members in various community groups and as decision makers in local, state, and national planning and policy groups concerned with health care. In many ways, nurses market the hospital or health care services through these interactions with the community, since health care organizations are designed to serve the public.

## ❖ ENABLING NURSING PRACTICE

The framework for professional nursing practice exists in an environment that influences both the construction of the framework and the key relationships between and among its elements. Health care services are provided in both public and private sectors. In both sectors, federal, state, local, and sometimes regional policy determines or highly influences health care services. Services are derived from public demand or need and regulated to ensure public safety and welfare. Nursing practice is sanctioned by the public, and each licensed nurse has a duty to protect the public safety and welfare in the performance of nursing care.

Professional nursing requires that every practicing registered nurse has sufficient autonomy to carry out his or her responsibilities and to use knowledge and skills to safely deliver a service to the public. In professional nursing practice, nursing administration recognizes practice requirements and the administrator's duty is to garner and use scarce resources to produce a positive outcome. Practitioners rely on effective administration/management because professional practice depends on adequate resources.

Two main functions—staffing and budgeting—are critical in nursing administration decisions that relate to public accountability for practitioners. The care of clients and effective interactions between the client and nurse require appropriate staffing with clear roles and functions and sufficient budget to ensure adequate resources to meet professional nursing practice standards. This administrative support is an essential environmental factor in the framework for professional nursing practice.

Nurses now view their work and world differently. Health care during this century first became strongly institutionalized and now is becoming "deinstitutionalized." Shifts in public use of health care from inpatient to ambulatory care focuses nursing more clearly on the human condition and the influence of society on health care. Clearly, nursing administration must be closely aligned with the way society perceives and uses services, because nurse recruitment and retention is colored by these perceptions. Nursing administration must enable nurses to develop, disseminate, and use nursing knowledge, which is the substance of all care.

## ❖ SUMMARY

This chapter explores the relationship between nursing practice and nursing administration and discusses strategies for enabling professional nursing practice. The role of nursing administration is developed from a historical perspective, and the interaction between nursing practice, nursing education, and nursing administration is explored. A model for the analysis of the interaction between the client and family, nursing practice, and administration is presented.

## ❖ APPLYING KNOWLEDGE TO PRACTICE

1. This chapter asks the question "Does one have to be a nurse to effectively manage nursing services?" What is your answer to this question? Provide rationale for your response.
2. In your experience does nursing administration help or hinder the daily practice of nursing care? Provide examples.
3. Does a professional nurse require a manager? Why or why not? Do other professional disciplines in the health care setting have the same number of managers as nursing?

**REFERENCES**

Aiken, L. H. (1983). Nursing's future: Public policies, private actions . . . shortage or surplus? . . . federal aid to nursing education, *American Journal of Nursing, 83*(10), 1440–1440.

Balasco, E. M. (1989). The nurse executive: Finally, it's time, *Journal of Professional nursing, 5*(4), 174.

Barsevick, A. M. & Lauver, D. (1990). Women's informational needs about colposcopy, *Image, 22* (1), 23–26.

Brett, J. L. & Tonges, M. C. (1990). Resource allocation in managing the nursing shortage, *The Nursing Shortage: Opportunities and Solutions,* AONE and ANA monograph.

Clifford, J. C. (1988). Will the professional practice model survive? (editorial), *Journal of Professional Nursing, 4* (2), 77, 141.

Department of Health and Human Services (1988). Secretary's Commission on Nursing, Final Report, Vol. 1.

Ethridge, P. & Lamb, G. S. (1989). Professional nursing case management improves quality, access and costs, *Nursing Management, 20* (3), 30–35.

Finer, H. (1952). *Administration and the Nursing Services.* New York: MacMillan.

Kramer, M. & Schmalenberg, C. (1988a). Magnet hospitals: Institutions of excellence, Part I & II (research), *Journal of Nursing Administration, 18* (1), 13–24 and *18* (2), 11–19.

Kramer, M. & Schmalenberg, C. (1988b). Magnet hospitals talk about impact of DRGs on nursing care, Part I & II (survey), *Nursing Management, 18* (9), 38–42 and *18* (10), 33–36, 38–40.

National Commission on Nursing Summary Report and Recommendations (1983), National Commission on Nursing, Chicago, Illinois.

Zwolski, K. (1989). Professional nursing in a technical system, *Image, 21* (4), 238–242.

# 5 Professional Nursing Roles

Joan L. Creasia

## OBJECTIVES

*At the completion of this chapter, the reader will be able to:*

- ◆ Differentiate between the structural-functional and symbolic interactionist perspectives as theoretical foundations for the study of nursing roles.
- ◆ Discuss common role stressors as they relate to the role of the nurse.
- ◆ Describe selected roles commonly assumed by the professional nurse and the responsibilities associated with each.

## ❖ OVERVIEW

As the health care system continues to grow in size and complexity, health care delivery becomes less traditional and more innovative. The traditional structure of provider roles is challenged as the professional disciplines are called on to provide expanded and more diverse health care services in a wide variety of settings. Nursing is responding to the challenge by examining the structure of the professional role, identifying its component parts, and adapting it to better meet the needs and changes of a dynamic health care system.

This chapter focuses on role taking in nursing by examining theoretical foundations of roles, the types of roles nurses commonly assume, the impact of multiple roles, and common role stressors. Finally, selected nursing roles and associated responsibilities are discussed.

## ❖ THEORETICAL FOUNDATIONS OF ROLES

Individuals assume roles that define their position in society. Although the concepts of role and position are often used interchangeably, it is important to differentiate the two. *Roles* are sets of patterned behaviors unique to a given position (Biddle, 1979) and may reflect personal, social, or occupational domains. The behavior patterns are manifested in the performance of duties and tasks and the assumption of certain responsibilities. *Position*, on the other hand, denotes status or a place within a specified context such as a health care organization. An organizational chart is used to illustrate the placement of positions within the organization and to depict vertical and horizontal relationships. Thus, roles are classifications of behavior, while positions are classifications of people (Biddle, 1979).

The expected behaviors of those who occupy a social position determine how a person in a given role should act (Kramer, 1974). A social position refers to an identity that is widely known and held by persons who behave in a characteristic way. Roles, then, are associated with social positions and are shaped by the expectations of others in an individual's social network, often referred to as socializing agents (Biddle, 1979). Either explicitly or implicitly, socializing agents communicate the values and norms that are associated with a certain role. Subsequently, the values and norms are assimilated by the person assuming that role and develop into a behavior pattern.

The context in which the social position exists also contributes to role expectations. Context may be defined as a setting (e.g., community), an organization (e.g., hospital), or a social situation (e.g., discussion group). While one person could theoretically hold an identical position in all three contexts (e.g., a nurse), it is clear that the expected behavior patterns would vary markedly. Thus, role behaviors are limited by the physical, environmental, or temporal boundaries of the context. Applying these concepts of role theory to professional nursing roles, the expected behaviors or roles of the nurse are determined by the nurse's social position and the context in which nursing care is delivered.

## Role Theories and Paradigms

There are two competing theoretical perspectives used to study roles. The first perspective is the *structural-functional approach,* which links the individual to the social structure and focuses on the division of labor within that context (Hardy & Conway, 1988). There are formal prescriptions for actions, which result in appropriate behavior. For example, this perspective might focus on the job description of the nurse who holds a staff nurse position in a large teaching hospital. An additional assumption of the structural-functional perspective is that norms and values attached to the position are handed down from generation to generation (Berger & Luckman, 1966). As the social structure changes over the years, the values and norms of a given position adapt to that change.

The second perspective is the *symbolic interaction approach,* which focuses on the interaction between people in the social system. Specifically, the meaning that is given to acts and symbols forms the basis upon which behaviors are selected and roles are constructed. Symbols must have the same meaning for each person in the interaction if they are to communicate effectively (Hardy & Conway, 1988). Mutual understanding of the meaning of symbols controls role-related behavior by either supporting or suppressing it. The responses of others serve to validate behavior. This perspective explains the concept of professional socialization of nurses, for example, who learn the role of a professional nurse by observing other nurses' actions, understanding the meaning of their actions, and responding to their reactions. More specifically, a new graduate who orients to a position with a preceptor learns the staff nurse role by observing the preceptor's actions and responding to the preceptor's feedback regarding his or her own performance.

In nursing, both perspectives are valid. Nurses, for the most part, function in highly structured settings. A great deal of formalization exists in the form of policies, procedures, job descriptions, evaluation mechanisms, and classification systems. Thus, the structural-functional perspective can be a useful approach to study the formalized aspects of a nurse's role.

As nurses assume caregiver and administrative roles, however, they interact with a variety of people. As the symbolic interaction perspective suggests, meaning is given to the various interactions as perceived by the individuals involved. This perspective is useful to study the interdependent nature of nursing roles and the process of acquiring behaviors specific to a given nursing role.

## ❖ TYPES OF ROLES

As discussed earlier, all roles evolve from social positions and the context in which they are enacted. Examination of the content of roles reveals that they are derived from personal, social, and occupational domains. Nurses commonly assume positions in all three domains, often simultaneously. For example, a nurse may be a mother or father, a leader in a civic organization, and a nurse educator. Although these roles are not mutually exclusive, they reflect a primary orientation to what we refer to as our personal life, social life, or occupational life.

In most societies, the social structure consists of positions that are reciprocal, meaning they are dependent on one or more persons for appropriate enactment of the role. Such positions include the roles of mother, father, wife, husband, teacher, nurse, breadwinner, or politician. Each of these positions brings to mind an image of the person assuming the role along with the associated set of expected behaviors, and other people in the social system who are critical to the enactment of the role. Thus, the nurse who holds positions in all three domains develops behavior patterns for each role and interacts with a wide range of people with whom interdependent relationships are established. The result is a complex pattern of overlapping social positions and roles, each demanding certain unique behaviors and relationships.

## ❖ THE PROFESSIONAL NURSING ROLE

How do these concepts apply to the role of the professional nurse? McClure (1989) describes the role of the nurse as consisting of two subroles: caregiver and integrator. Caregivers attend to clients' needs. Integrators coordinate services of other specialized departments as patients' needs warrant. The nursing role is a reciprocal one because it is interdependent with others in the role constellation such as patients, physicians, and ancillary health care workers

for its enactment. The responses of these people contribute to the behavior patterns of the professional nursing role when they send messages that sanction some behaviors and enhance others. Additionally, the role is circumscribed by the context within which it is enacted and by the formalized role prescription designed by the organization.

As previously mentioned, the performance of duties and tasks and the assumption of certain responsibilities form the pattern of behaviors that characterize the professional nurse. But the professional role is unique because it is influenced by a *Code of Ethics* that helps shape professional behavior and frame role expectations. For instance, the nurse is expected to provide high quality nursing care "with respect for human dignity and the uniqueness of the client, unrestricted by considerations of social or economic status, personal attributes or the nature of the health problem" (American Nurses' Association, 1985, p. 1). The *Code of Ethics* also specifies dimensions and responsibilities of the role such as accountability, advocacy, competence, delegation, and collaboration. And because nurses are licensed, there are also legal dimensions to the role as specified in state nurse practice acts. These influences serve to add to the complexity of the professional nursing role by identifying multiple subroles and dimensions of the role, which are bounded by organizational, ethical, and legal constraints.

## ❖ IMPACT OF MULTIPLE ROLES

People in today's society typically assume multiple roles, and nurses are no exception. A women may be a wife, mother, daughter, daughter-in-law, student, nurse, and teacher. Similarly, a man may be a husband, father, son, son-in-law, and brother and still hold several occupational roles. In addition, each may participate in religious or civic organizations by taking membership or leadership roles that demand another set of role behaviors.

Often multiple roles are assumed within different contexts. However, it is possible to assume multiple roles within the same context. Such is the case with the role of the professional nurse who may be a caregiver, case manager, teacher, or advocate. When a person holds several roles with a similar focus, they are referred to as subroles. Each subrole may be equally critical to the focal role, or one may be more dominant. For instance, a staff nurse who practices in a setting that employs a number of nonprofessionals to assist with nursing care might see management and supervision of these caregivers as the dominant subroles. As the number and type of roles and subroles held by an individual increases, the risk of role strain also increases.

### Role Stress and Strain

Role stress and strain are common phenomena among individuals with multiple roles. *Role stress,* generated by the social structure, is said to exist when role obligations are vague, irritating, conflicting, or unrealistic. These conditions are external to the individual, but they may result in role strain, an internal response. *Role strain* is described as an emotional reaction to role stress that may be experienced as feelings of frustration, anxiety, irritability, or distress. When an individual encounters major difficulty in meeting role obligations, role strain is apt to occur (Hardy & Conway, 1988).

What conditions are likely to contribute to role stress and strain in nursing? A number of factors are identified by Hardy and Conway (1988) including changes in the organization and delivery of health care, generation of new nursing roles, economic conditions (which result in redefining patient-provider roles), and technological advances. As a result of one or more of these factors, nurses may experience feelings of frustration or anxiety as their role perception and competence are threatened.

However, the severity of role stress and strain is individually determined and is dependent on the perception of the difficulty encountered by the person assuming the role.

### Common Role Stressors

Role conflict, role ambiguity, role incongruity, and role overload are stressors common to nursing. A discussion of each follows.

**Role conflict.** When role expectations within or among roles are incompatible with one another, *role conflict* may result. An early study by Corwin (1961) identified alienation in nurses who had a high professional and a high bureaucratic orientation. This has become known as the professional-bureaucratic conflict, whereby professional norms and values dictate behaviors that may be in conflict with organizational norms and values. The result is a strain that, if not reconciled, can result in what is known as "burnout." Kramer (1974) addresses a similar issue when she discusses reality shock, the impact felt by recent nursing graduates who assume positions in highly bureaucratic settings. Explaining professional and bureaucratic role orientations of professional nurses continues to be an area of research interest, and associations between selected personality variables (Kinney, 1985), moral behavior (Ketefian, 1985), and role concept have been found.

The nurse in middle management is a prime candidate for role conflict because of incompatible staff and administration expectations, such as those identified by Langenfeld (1988). Areas of potential conflict are evident when the manager is expected to "operate from a management perspective, seeing the broad picture in terms of impact for the entire institution" [management expectation] (p. 79) and "understand problems from the employee's point of view, creating 'win-win' situations" [employee expectation] (p. 78). Additional areas of possible role conflict include the base of loyalty (e.g., the organization vs. the profession) and the cost-quality dichotomy, (e.g., cost-cutting measures that decrease nursing time with clients) in terms of what is ideal and what is realistic (Nyberg, 1988).

Research does not consistently support the contention that nurses experience a high level of role conflict, however. Rosse and Rosse (1981) conducted a study of role conflict with a sample of nursing personnel, 220 of whom were registered nurses. Contrary to expectations, they found low levels of role conflict, defined as incompatible demands from various role senders or from multiple roles held simultaneously. There was a significant relationship, however, between role conflict and job stress, organizational commitment, job satisfaction, and intentions to quit.

Role conflict is often thought to be common to the registered nurse returning to school for advanced education. This individual probably holds a job, has personal and family responsibilities, and additionally assumes the student role (Creasia, 1989). Behavior patterns for each role have already been established, and now a new role is added. Expected behaviors associated with the new role may compete with the established behavior patterns, resulting in role conflict. Contrary to these notions, however, a study by Campaniello (1988) found that for a sample of registered nurses returning to school, the occupancy of multiple roles did not increase their perceived role conflict. For this group, the role of parent more than any other role was a major source of conflict.

Personality orientation was used to explain the lack of role conflict in a sample of 167 nurses returning to school (Rendon, 1988). The findings suggested that when interpersonal orientation was compliant, rather than detached or aggressive, there was role congruence rather than conflict. Areas of stress and dissatisfaction identified by this group related mostly to economic burden and disruptions of social and family life.

**Role ambiguity.** When role expectations are unclear, the stressor is termed *role ambiguity*. Possibly more problematic for nurses than role conflict, "ambiguity for nurses has been related to their diversity of role partners, the lack of clarity in role expectations and to an uncertainty as to how to initiate subroles of the nursing role" (Hardy & Conway, p. 202). In addition, the uncertainty associated with professional practice contributes greatly to role ambiguity. Clinical decision making is one example of uncertainty in which action is taken, possibly based on incomplete information, without assured knowledge of the outcome. Role ambiguity was also identified as a stressor for the nurse executive and was significantly correlated with job dissatisfaction (Burke & Scalzi, 1988). Although the health care organization may be designed to minimize structurally generated ambiguity, professionals are expected to deal with role ambiguities related to their area of expertise and scope of practice (Hardy & Conway, 1988).

Although role ambiguity has been identified as a construct separate from role conflict, much of the role-related research examining role conflict also measures role ambiguity (Lambert & Lambert, 1988). In several studies of nurses and organizations, the findings indicated that role ambiguity is more detrimental to role performance, satisfaction, and commitment than is role conflict (Hardy & Conway, 1988).

**Role incongruity.** *Role incongruity* occurs when values are incompatible with role expectations. Refer to the prior example of the staff nurse who spends much of the time supervising and directing nonprofessional caregivers as a dominant subrole. If the nurse's value system embraces the belief that nursing care should be provided by a nurse rather than by nonprofessionals, then there is a potential for role strain because of role incongruity.

Role transition is a form of role incongruity familiar to nurses. Kramer and Schmalenberg (1977) describe professional socialization of the graduate nurse who, upon assuming a new social position in a health care organization, must assimilate the values and norms of that position as set forth by the organization. A problem arises when these are not in concert with the values and norms the nurse was exposed to as a student. To further complicate the issue, the new graduate must learn the professional nursing role and internalize professional norms and values. Hardy and Conway (1988) note, however, that the strain resulting from role incongruity in this situation may be a prerequisite to learning a new role and may actually facilitate it.

**Role overload.** Finally, when too much work is expected in the allotted time or the role becomes too complex, *role overload* is experienced. This is a common problem for nurses that may be attributed to structural, contextual, or role-related factors. Take, for example, the nurse who practices in an acute care hospital. Since the beginning of the cost containment effort in 1983, hospitalized clients as a group are much more acutely ill. Combined with the shortage of professional nurses, the rapid advances in technology and additional consumer expectations, hospital-based nurses have more responsibilities today than ever before. They often carry a caseload of clients who are more acutely ill and who have very complex care requirements. In addition, they may have to oversee the work of nonprofessionals or professionals who are unfamiliar with the setting. They may also be required to perform a variety of nonnursing tasks. By the time the shift is over, nurses are often exhausted, frustrated, and distressed that the quality of care they were able to deliver was less than optimal. Not exclusively the problem of staff nurses, nurse executives in hospitals also reported a high level of role overload (Burke & Scalzi, 1988).

Role overload is a serious problem in other health care settings as well. As hospitalized patients are discharged earlier, the use of home health services is escalating. Not only do community-based nurses have an increased caseload, but home care is more intense and technologically oriented. As the government has become more involved in health care financing, the amount of paperwork has also increased. And the shortage of nurses is no less acute in community settings than it is in hospitals.

## Strategies to Resolve Role Stress and Strain

Modifying contextual or structural conditions and negotiating one's role with others are some of the methods used to relieve role stress and strain. Contextual conditions that can be modified include the environment in which care is delivered, the organization of nursing care delivery, and the control and allocation of resources in the form of money, space, time, materials, or personnel. As these contextual conditions are favorably modified, there is an indirect effect on the type and amount of role strain experienced.

Role redefinition is a more direct strategy used to relieve role strain due to role conflict, ambiguity, or overload. This may be accomplished on either a formal or informal basis. In other words, the role may be redefined in writing or it may be negotiated with others. While a change in the formal job description is more permanent, negotiating changes in the role is usually a more immediate solution. This latter strategy, derived from the symbolic interactionist perspective, involves mutual understanding between role partners, which results in reprioritizing role expectations, reallocating the workload, and redefining adequate role performance.

The appropriate strategies selected to resolve stress and strain are situation-specific and are influenced by the availability of resources, the flexibility of the setting, and/or the position of the nurse in the organization. For example, a middle manager who seeks to resolve role overload may delegate some managerial functions to an assistant. This strategy can also be used at the staff nurse level to delegate nonnursing functions to available personnel. However, it may be that resources are not sufficient to delegate part of the workload to others. In that case, it becomes necessary to set priorities to make the workload more manageable, recognizing that less important tasks will not get done.

Perhaps role ambiguity is best addressed by rewriting the job description so that expectations are clearly presented. Other solutions include setting one's own performance expectations in writing and sharing these with the supervisor for approval or developing written goals and objectives as part of the performance appraisal mechanism.

Eliminating some of the demands of multiple roles is one strategy to reduce role conflict. For example, a nurse who works full-time and maintains home and family responsibilities is likely to experience role conflict when additional roles are added, such as the role of student. As one continues to add new roles, adjustments in ongoing roles must be made to make the role constellation manageable (e.g., delegating household chores to spouse or children). This involves changing the behavior pattern associated with a specific role to a more realistic set of behaviors, given the situation. A frequent roadblock to using this strategy is that it usually involves changing the expectations of oneself, a notion that presents major difficulties for some people.

To resolve role incongruity, it is necessary to negotiate aspects of the role so the conflicting situations can be avoided. Finally, if no middle ground can be reached, assuming a position where role expectations are more compatible with the values of the nurse may be the only recourse.

## ❖ PROFESSIONAL NURSING ROLES

Professional nurses assume a number of roles and subroles concurrently as they seek to provide comprehensive care to clients with multiple disorders in a variety of health care settings. The nurse, drawing from the functional, cognitive, and affective domains, uses skills, abilities, knowledge, judgment, attitudes, and values to develop sets of appropriate nursing actions. Nursing care is modified by the setting where care is delivered and the subrole(s) being assumed by the nurse. Fig. 5-1 illustrates these relationships.

Certain role patterns may be operationalized differently across various client care settings or they may be unique to a given setting. Keeping in mind that the setting where care is delivered tends to shape the content of the role, the following section describes selected roles common to nursing practice and identifies some specific responsibilities associated with each.

### Caregiver

A fundamental nursing role is that of caregiver. Nurses provide care within three types of nursing systems: wholly compensatory, partly compensatory, or supportive/educative (Orem, 1985). Nursing actions are selected to provide a complete care for the client who is totally dependent, either physically or psychologically, to provide partial care when the client cannot fully assume self-care, and to provide supportive/educative care to assist clients in attaining or maintaining the highest possible level of health. The goal of nursing is to move clients toward responsible self-care at the highest point on the health-illness continuum of which they are capable.

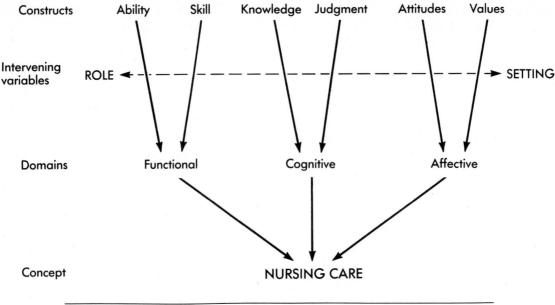

❖ **Fig. 5-1**  Model for nursing care.

With the client viewed as a biopsychosocial system (Roy, 1989), caregiving is directed toward addressing identified physiological, psychological, social, and spiritual needs. The nurse draws from a repertoire of skills derived from the functional, cognitive, and affective domains to develop nursing interventions appropriate to the caregiver role. Subsumed within the caregiver role are a number of subroles such as teacher, counselor, and case manager, some of which will be subsequently discussed in greater depth.

**Role responsibilities.** McClure (1989) describes the caregiver role as meeting the following client needs: dependency, comfort, monitoring, therapeutic, and educational. Whether the client is defined as the individual, family, or community, nursing care proceeds along similar lines. Using the nursing process, the nurse:

1. Assesses the client
2. Analyzes the data
3. Identifies the nursing diagnoses
4. Develops the nursing care plan
5. Implements the plan
6. Evaluates the outcomes

Nursing responsibilities can include the provision of direct nursing care or the delegation and supervision of care to other caregivers. Coordinating efforts of the multidisciplinary health team, teaching, counseling, discharge planning, and referral are additional responsibilities that fall into the realm of the caregiver role. The nurse also makes use of self by exhibiting caring behaviors such as empathy, comfort, and compassion.

## Teacher

As clients attempt to execute complex treatment regimens in an effort to cope with chronic disease over extended periods of time, the nurse in both inpatient and outpatient settings frequently assumes the role of teacher. A subrole of the caregiver role, teaching is also a primary focus of specialized positions such as diabetic educator, cardiac rehabilitation nurse, and ostomy specialist. Health teaching is the process whereby information is imparted to clients for the purpose of altering cognitive, affective, or psychomotor behavior. A goal of health teaching is to assist individuals in attaining and maintaining healthful practices and life-styles by preventing, promoting, or modifying a number of health-related behaviors (Redman, 1988). Thus, teaching activities are aimed at promoting self-care behaviors such as adherence to a prescribed treatment regimen, maintenance of a healthful life-style and appropriate use of health care services. It is important for the nurse to have a thorough understanding of the teaching-learning process to facilitate successful client teaching.

**Role responsibilities.** The nurse may either assume an active teaching role or coordinate the teaching efforts of others. When the nurse assumes the role of teacher/evaluator, responsibilities include:

1. Identifying teaching-learning needs
2. Developing individual goals and objectives
3. Planning the teaching-learning experience
4. Providing information, using appropriate teaching strategies
5. Evaluating outcomes of teaching-learning interaction

When several disciplines are involved in educating the client, the nurse may also serve as coordinator of the multidisciplinary approach, a subrole identified by a majority of the nurses in a study by Honan and colleagues (1988). Responsibilities include referring teaching-learning needs to appropriate disciplines, scheduling teaching sessions to enhance learning, reinforcing information provided by others, and evaluating outcomes.

## Client Advocate

The role of client advocate is one that lies at the heart of nursing's value system (see Chapter 9). When the nurse assumes the advocacy role, the primary emphasis is on supporting the client emotionally, physically, spiritually, and socially. Curtain (1979) describes advocacy as the philosophical foundation of nursing and not the concept implied in the client's rights movement or in the legal system. Rather, it is based on mutual understanding between nurses and clients as human beings, taking into account our common needs and our common rights. Corcoran (1988) argues that, although advocacy has been well developed conceptually, it has not been thoroughly operationalized for nursing.

The role of client advocate has three major themes: (1) protector of the client's self-determination, (2) mediator between the client and persons in his or her environment, and (3) actor on the client's behalf (Nelson, 1988). Nursing actions are performed solely to benefit the client. The nurse may provide material necessary for informed decision-making, encourage clients to make health care decisions that they believe are in their best interest or directly act on behalf of clients. Thus, the client advocate runs the risk of conflict with others in the patient's personal and/or health care environment.

**Role responsibilities.** Within each component of the advocacy role, specific responsibilities have been identified. As protector of the client's self-determination, the nurse assists the client to make autonomous and informed decisions by:

1. Ensuring that relevant information is available to the client
2. Helping the client examine and prioritize values and goals
3. Supporting the client in whatever decision is made

As mediator between the client and the environment, the nurse is responsible for:

1. Coordinating health care services
2. Clarifying communication between the client and community, family, other disciplines, and/or medical services
3. Explaining the roles and relationships between various health care providers

As one who acts on the client's behalf, the nurse may directly intervene by:

1. Altering the environment to safeguard the client's welfare
2. Protecting the client against receiving inadequate care
3. Championing clients' rights in the health care, social, and political arenas

### Quality of Care Evaluator

Providing comprehensive and high quality care has long been a basic value of nursing. Attempts to assess health care quality in nursing and other disciplines, however, have been minimally successful, in part, because quality of care is an evolutionary concept that is multidimensional, value-laden, dynamic, and changing in response to consumer expectations and technological advances. In addition, many studies lack scientific rigor. There has been little attempt to relate the process of care to client outcomes, an approach often recommended by nurse researchers. Despite these and other shortcomings, efforts to evaluate the quality of care have gained momentum in recent years because of the increased involvement of the government in health care financing (Scearse, 1989), concern for accountability rising out of the consumer movement, proliferation of health care organizations, and the swift pace of advances in health care (Baker, 1983).

As a result, some health care organizations have created a position for a quality assurance coordinator to design and implement studies, review findings, make recommendations for improvement, and coordinate the reevaluation effort. More often, however, nurses in various positions across the organization assume the responsibilities of quality of care evaluator as a nursing subrole. In this situation, the evaluation effort is coordinated by a task force composed of representatives from various nursing units. With the current emphasis on unit-based monitoring, the task force structure can be a fairly effective approach. Quality of care evaluation becomes more meaningful when nurses are involved in quality monitoring on the unit where they work. It is expected that they will have a vested interest in demonstrating high-quality care if they are involved in evaluating it.

**Role responsibilities.** The quality assurance model proposed by the American Nurses' Association (1977) guides the quality of care evaluation process, which determines the responsibilities of the nurse evaluator. The nurse involved in unit-based evaluation is first responsible for identifying relevant problems for ongoing monitoring. The task force may assist with selecting criteria for evaluation, setting standards of care against which actual performance will be judged, and identifying measures to use for data collection (Schroeder, 1988). How the study proceeds from this point depends on how the evaluation program is designed. Frequently, it is the responsibility of the unit-based nurse evaluator to develop a method of sampling, identify a time frame for the study, and determine the frequency of monitoring. At the end of the study, the evaluator tabulates the data and compares actual performance against the performance standard. If remedial action needs to be taken, the quality of care evaluator may be responsible for identifying possible courses of action, developing the plan, and setting a time for reevaluation.

### Manager

All nurses function as managers to some degree, and nurses occupy management positions in health care organizations, which command roles that vary in breadth, scope, and homogeneity. Positions whose roles are primarily managerial include clinical manager (head nurse), nursing supervisor, clinical director, and vice-president for nursing. Other positions such as staff nurse and assistant clinical manager are usually mixed. In other words, the position includes aspects of the caregiver role as well as the management role.

Nursing management positions demand many different behaviors and strategies for proper role enactment. The set of expected behaviors depends on the perspectives of the people in the role constellation, the placement of the position on the organizational chart, and the relevant issues with which it is concerned. For example, a staff nurse who manages and supervises nonprofessional caregivers as a primary nursing subrole uses strategies related to personnel management but does not necessarily deal with issues related to the broader organization such as finances and information technology. Nurses at higher levels of management are involved with issues such as resource allocation and labor relations and make liberal use of problem-solving and decision-making skills.

**Role responsibilities.** Because of the variety of management positions in nursing, it is difficult to come up with a single set of responsibilities that would equally apply. Not only are manager roles highly differentiated within a single organization, but manager roles at the same administrative level can also vary across organizations (Miller & Heine, 1988). Thus, the responsibilities outlined below generally relate to positions in middle management such as clinical manager or supervisor and are listed in no particular order.

Responsibilities of the manager:

- Establishes operating goals and objectives
- Manages a budget
- Concerns self with staffing and productivity
- Hires personnel
- Evaluates performance
- Delegates effectively

- Serves as a clinical resource
- Resolves conflict
- Promotes high-quality client care
- Facilitates communication, both formally and informally
- Serves as role model and mentor for future managers
- Monitors interpersonal relations within and between departments
- Enforces organizational policy
- Serves on committees to develop policies, procedures, and standards of care
- Uses problem-solving and decision-making skills
- Initiates and manages change

## Researcher

The *Code of Ethics* specifies that the nurse participate "in activities that contribute to the ongoing development of the profession's body of knowledge" (American Nurses' Association, 1985, p. 1). In concert with this mandate, nurses are assuming an increasingly active role in research. In recent years, some hospitals and other health care delivery organizations have created the position of nurse researcher. Typically, a doctorally prepared nurse assumes this role for the purpose of coordinating institutional approval of research studies, writing grants, and directing research programs. In addition, the researcher spearheads the involvement of clinical nurses in the research process. The expanding body of research builds the theoretical basis for nursing practice and assists in the understanding of specific client issues related to health and illness, nursing issues related to the professional nursing role, and a broad range of health care delivery issues.

**Role responsibilities.** Responsibilities of the nurse researcher vary according to the level of research expertise and, frequently, level of education, as outlined by the American Nurses' Association (1981). All nurses can be consumers of research, however, by critically evaluating research studies for their quality and relevance to nursing and by applying the findings to clinical practice. For those who wish to take a more active role in research, responsibilities include identifying nursing problems for study, participating in nursing research under the guidance of a senior investigator, or directing the scientific investigation of nursing problems.

The research process serves as a framework for identifying specific responsibilities related to the researcher role:

1. Identifying the problem
2. Reviewing related literature
3. Formulating hypotheses
4. Determining a suitable research design
5. Delimiting the setting and sample
6. Selecting and testing measures for data collection
7. Collecting data
8. Analyzing data and interpreting the results
9. Reporting findings

A senior nurse researcher can be fully involved in the entire research process, while less experienced nurses can participate in many of the activities under the direction of the senior investigator.

## Consultant

As nurses develop specialized areas of expertise, they are often called on to serve as consultants. A consultant draws from personal expertise to advise others, validate current practices, or provide specialized knowledge. Of 270 nurse consultants surveyed, 63% were in independent practice, 30% were employed by business organizations, and 7% were employed by consulting firms (Flaherty & DeMoya, 1989). Consultants can be contracted for such varied services as assisting with research design and data analysis, evaluating new health care products, advising health care professionals and other caregivers on complex client care procedures, designing and evaluating new programs,

developing curricula for nursing education, or reviewing records for legal cases. In addition, nurse consultants also serve as expert witnesses in legal cases involving malpractice, environmental hazards, or pharmaceuticals.

**Role responsibilities.** To ensure its success, marketing must be a major responsibility of the consultant role. This is especially critical for nurses in independent practice. Marketing involves identifying the groups who can use the consulting service and then developing a market mix: defining the service, promoting the service, identifying the place where the service will be delivered, and setting a price (Camunas, 1985).

Contracting is a second major responsibility of this role. Contracting should be a formal process that involves outlining the services to be performed, determining a time frame, and setting a fee. If expenses such as transportation, lodging, food, and supplies are to be paid by the contractor, it should be indicated in the contract. To prevent unforeseeable future problems, it is recommended that legal counsel be obtained to go over the contract.

## Case Manager

An outgrowth of the need for cost-effective and high-quality care in an increasingly complex health care system, the role of professional nurse case manager is rapidly evolving. "Case management is a new approach to balancing the needs of patients and their families with those of the health care industry and society" (Conti, 1989, p. 58). In contrast with primary nursing where a nurse *provides* total care for a group of clients, the case manager *administers* the care of a caseload of clients but does not necessarily provide it (Loveridge, Cummings, & O'Malley, 1988). As case manager, the nurse uses professional expertise to ensure coordinated and cost-effective care alternatives throughout the course of treatment. A key factor in the case management approach is the identification of outcomes, which are specific and time-based. This allows continuous tracking of the client and ongoing evaluation of progress toward expected outcomes, including postdischarge outcomes (Bair et al., 1989). The case management approach to care increases both caregiver and client satisfaction, while maintaining cost-effective accountability (Olivas et al., 1989).

Health care delivery organizations are not the only ones using this approach. Third party payers are becoming increasingly aware of the value of using the case management system to ensure high quality and cost-effective care. In this situation, the case manager serves as a gatekeeper and either approves or denies care as professional expertise warrants, or suggests alternatives that might be more cost-effective.

**Role responsibilities.** The case manager is responsible for assessing clients and families, identifying nursing diagnoses, developing a nursing care plan, delegating care to nursing personnel as appropriate, activating interventions, coordinating and collaborating with the interdisciplinary health care team, and evaluating outcomes of care (Ethridge & Lamb, 1989). An additional responsibility is that of providing counseling to clients and their families and exploring options for care (Conti, 1989). The case manager is accountable for achieving outcomes within an appropriate length of stay, using resources efficiently, and establishing standards of care (Zander, 1988).

## ❖ SUMMARY

The practice of nursing involves assuming a number of diverse roles, some of them simultaneously, in a variety of settings. Role theory is useful in understanding the professional nursing role and the problems generated by the social system in which the nurse practices. Accordingly, this chapter focused on role-taking in nursing and the multiple roles nurses routinely assume. Theoretical foundations of roles were discussed, including two perspectives for studying roles, which can be useful for nursing. The impact of assuming multiple roles was explored, and common role stressors that contribute to role strain were identified. Finally, selected nursing roles were described, and responsibilities related to those roles were identified.

## ❖ APPLYING KNOWLEDGE TO PRACTICE

1. Select a nursing role of your choice and:
   a. Analyze it according to the symbolic-interactionist perspective and/or the structure-functionalist perspective.
   b. Describe the role stressors that may be an integral part of the role.
   c. Identify strategies that can be employed to reduce role strain.
2. What sources of role conflict are you currently experiencing? What can *you* do to reduce this conflict? What can *others* do?
3. Describe a situation where you experienced role overload. What were the consequences? How did you resolve it? Are there any additional strategies that might have been useful?
4. Describe a situation related to the professional nursing role where role incongruity might be an issue for you. What alternatives can you identify that would result in a satisfactory resolution?

## REFERENCES

American Nurses' Association (1985). *Code of ethics with interpretative statements*. Kansas City, Mo.: American Nurses' Association.

American Nurses' Association (1981). *Guidelines for the investigative function of nurses*. Kansas City, Mo.: American Nurses' Association.

American Nurses' Association (1977). *Quality model: A plan for the implementation of the standards of nursing practice*. Kansas City, Mo.: American Nurses' Association.

Bair, N. L., Griswold, J. T., & Head, J. L. (1989). Clinical RN involvement in bedside-centered case management. *Nursing Economics, 7*(3), 150-154.

Baker, F. (1983). Quality assurance and program evaluation. *Evaluation and the Health Professions, 6*(2), 149-160.

Biddle, B. J. (1979). *Role theory: Expectations, identities and behaviors*. New York: Academic Press.

Berger, P. & Luckman, T. (1966). *The social construction of reality*. New York: Free Press.

Burke, G. D. & Scalzi, C. C. (1988). Role stress in hospital executives and nursing executives. *Health Care Management Review, 13*(3), 67-72.

Campaniello, J. A. (1988). When professional nurses return to school: A study of role conflict and well-being in multiple-role women. *Journal of Professional Nursing, 4*(2), 136-140.

Camunas, C. (1985). Marketing as a nursing skill. In Mason, D. J. & Talbot, S. W., *Political action handbook for nurses* (pp. 205-212). Menlo Park, Calif.: Addison-Wesley Publishing Company.

Conti, R. (1989). The nurse as case manager. *Nursing Connections, 2*(1), 55-58.

Corcoran, S. (1988). Toward operationalizing an advocacy role. *Journal of Professional Nursing, 4*(4), 242-248.

Corwin, R. (1961). The professional employee: A study of conflict in nursing roles. *American Journal of Sociology, 66*(6), 604-615.

Creasia, J. (1989). Reducing the barriers to RN educational mobility. *Nurse Educator, 14*(4), 29-33.

Curtain, L. (1979).The nurse as advocate: A philosophical foundation for nursing. *Advances in Nursing Science, 1*(3), 1-10.

Ethridge, P. & Lamb, G. (1989). Professional nursing case management improves quality, access and costs. *Nursing Management, 20*(3), 30-35.

Flaherty, Sr. M. J. & DeMoya, D. (1989). An entrepreneurial role for the nurse consultant. *Nursing & Health Care, 10*(5), 259-263.

Hardy, M. E. & Conway, M. E. (1988). *Role theory: Perspectives for health professionals* (2nd Ed.). Norwalk, Conn.: Appleton & Lange.

Honan, S., Krsnak, G., Peterson, D., & Torkelson, R. (1988). The nurse as patient educator: Perceived responsibilities and factors enhancing role development. *Journal of Continuing Education in Nursing, 19*(1), 33-37.

Kramer, M. (1974). *Reality shock*. St. Louis: C. V. Mosby Co.

Kramer, M. & Schmalenberg, C. (1977). *The path to biculturalism*. Wakefield, MA: Contemporary Publishing Co.

Lambert, C. E. & Lambert, V. A. (1988). A review and synthesis of the research on role conflict and its impact on nurses involved in faculty practice programs. *Journal of Nursing Education, 27*(2), 54-60.

Langenfeld, M. L. (1988). Role expectations of nursing managers. *Nursing Management, 19*(6), 78, 80.

Loveridge, C. E., Cummings, S. H., & O'Malley, J. (1988). Developing case management in a primary nursing system. *Journal of Nursing Administration, 18*(10), 36-39.

McClure, M. L. (1989). The nurse executive role: A leadership opportunity. *Nursing Administration Quarterly, 13*, (3), 1-8.

Miller, M. & Heine, C. (1988). The complex role of the head nurse. *Nursing Management, 19*(6), 58-59, 62-64.

Nelson, M. (1988). Advocacy in nursing: A concept in evolution. *Nursing Outlook, 36*(3), 136-141.

Nyberg, J. (1988). Roles and rewards in nursing administration. *Nursing Administration Quarterly, 13*(3), 36-39.

Olivas, G. S., Del Togno-Armanasco, V., Erickson, J. R., & Harter, S. (1989). Case management: A bottom-line care delivery model, Part I: The concept. *Journal of Nursing Administration, 19*(11), 16-20.

Orem, D. (1985). *Nursing: Concepts of practice* (3rd ed.). New York: McGraw Hill.

Redman, B. (1988). *The process of patient education* (6th ed.). St. Louis: C. V. Mosby.

Rendon, D. (1988). The registered nurse student: A role congruence perspective. *Journal of Nursing Education, 27*(4), 172-177.

Rosse, J. G. & Rosse, P. H. (1981). Role conflict and ambiguity: An empirical investigation of nursing personnel. *Evaluation & the Health Professions, 4*(4), 385-405.

Roy, C., Sr. (1989). The Roy adaptation model. In Riehl-Sisca, J. P. *Conceptual Models for Nursing Practice* (3rd ed.). (pp. 105-114.) New York: Appleton-Century-Crofts,

Scearse, P. (1989). Quality of care: Another look. *Journal of Professional Nursing, 5*(5), 245, 293-294.

Schroeder, P. (1988). UBQA: The system revisited. In Pinkerton, S. & Schroeder, P., (Eds.), *Commitment to excellence: Developing a professional nursing staff* (pp. 33-41). Rockville, MD: Aspen.

Zander, K. (1988). Nursing case management: Strategic management of cost and quality outcomes. *Journal of Nursing Administration, 18*(5), 23-30.

# UNIT II

# Dimensions of Professional Nursing Practice

CONCEPTS that extend across and influence the full range of nursing activities are referred to as dimensions. In this regard, nursing is a multidimensional discipline because it consists of political, economic, legal, and ethical influences, which have an impact on nursing care delivery and guide nursing practice.

The political dimension of nursing practice reflects the nurse's concern for and response to health policy legislation as it affects the health care of individuals, families, and communities. Additionally, understanding the short-term and long-term implications of health policy legislation is fundamental to taking a pro-active position on issues that positively or adversely influence nursing and health care. The economic dimension of nursing practice is grounded in the use of scarce resources, which ultimately affects payment for nursing services and the delivery of nursing care. An understanding of the relationship between the economic concepts of the supply of, demand for, and cost of health care services can assist the nurse in analyzing health care delivery problems, propose solutions, and articulate the nursing role as the health care system is restructured. The legal dimension of nursing practice includes legal concepts, expectations, and consequences that surround the practice of nursing. While it is beyond the scope of this book to examine all these areas in depth, an overview of the relationships that underlie the practice of nursing (including the nurse/state relationship, the nurse/employer relationship, and the nurse/patient relationship) are presented. Finally, the ethical dimension of nursing practice embraces both moral reasoning and ethical decision making. Since nurses are constantly faced with ethical dilemmas, which they are expected to resolve, an awareness of principles and frameworks that guide ethical decision making can facilitate rational and intelligent decisions. These dimensions are further defined and explored in the following unit.

# 6 Political Influences on Health Care and Nursing

Donna M. Mahrenholz

## OBJECTIVES

*At the completion of this chapter, the reader will be able to:*

◆ Demonstrate knowledge about terms and processes used in formulating health care policy.

◆ State how nurses have influenced health care policy.

◆ Discuss how nurses can have an impact on health care policy.

◆ Use policymaking terms when discussing health care policymaking.

Before the twentieth century, health care in the United States was viewed as a responsibility of individuals or private organizations. During the eighteenth and nineteenth centuries, the scourge of epidemics related to impure foods, contaminated water supplies, inadequate sewage disposal, and poor housing conditions impelled local governments to respond with measures to protect the health of their citizens. These recurring epidemics also led to the first public health effort by the United States federal government: a national port quarantine system. After the yellow fever epidemic of 1873, Congress established the Marine Hospital Services to regulate and enforce this quarantine. Thus, out of group need, the precedent of intervention by the government at the local, state, and federal level was established (Hyman, 1982).

According to Feldstein (1988) health legislation, especially on the federal level, follows the principle of self-interest paradigm. This principle assumes that individuals act according to self-interest, not necessarily the public interest. Individuals, as legislators, voters, or health care providers, are assumed to act in pursuit of their own interests. Organized groups that are able to deliver greater political support are expected to have greater political influence than other less organized groups. Feldstein writes that organized groups seek to achieve through legislation what they cannot achieve through the marketplace. Massive redistribution of wealth in the health care arena has benefited two groups: health care providers, such as physicians, whose incomes have risen more than would otherwise have occurred, and the aged, who have received health care services that exceed the value of the payments they have made. These two groups provided the necessary organized political support to politicians in order to

89

get legislation enacted in their favor.

Policy decisions are affected by the legislative process, economics, individuals, and special interest groups, which in turn shape legislation and policies regulating health care. Nurses, as the largest group of health care providers, can have an impact on nursing and health legislation and policies. In order to have an impact, an understanding of the terms and process, past successes and failures, and areas for potential impact is needed. This chapter will explore these issues.

## ❖ LEGISLATIVE TERMS AND PROCESS

To understand how the political system influences health care, it is necessary to understand how health care policies are made. Policies can be either informal or formal. *Formal policies* are written, such as rules, regulations, and laws. *Informal policies* are customs or traditions and usually are more difficult to change. Most of the time, these informal policies are changed after long battles or they are changed incrementally, a little at a time. Before any action is taken, an issue should be put on the *public agenda.* Placing an issue on the public agenda requires actions that bring a concern to the attention of policymakers and the public, so that people other than those affected by the situation are aware of the issue and its consequences.

For example, the elderly have been effective in putting their concerns about costs of health care services for the aged with fixed incomes on the public agenda. They have banded together in groups such as the American Association of Retired Persons, Gray Panthers, and even groups within their condominium complexes to publicize their issues. They endorse and work for political candidates who support their concerns, give newspaper interviews, and contact legislators (local, state, and federal). In turn, other segments of the public adopt their concerns and contact policymakers in an attempt to influence these programs. In the past, these activities produced changes in the Medi-

care program, and today there are attempts to amend that program to cover home care and nursing home care.

First and most important, in order to influence policies, one needs to know the *issue,* that is, the questions and problems including some potential solutions to those problems. As nurses, we are experts about health care problems in the areas in which we practice. It is important to know not only how the legislative process works, but also what actors are involved: opponents and potential opponents, as well as the proponents and those who will remain neutral on the issue. It is also necessary to identify and become familiar with the arena in which the action will take place as well as the socioeconomic climate of the times. For example, financial support from the federal government for nursing education programs will not be a priority in Congress during a stock market crisis or a legislative battle to balance the budget by cutting funds. The arena can be at the local, state, or federal level and can involve the legislature, courts, or the bureaucracy. This assessment of the players, arena, and climate will help the astute nurse know whether the time is appropriate to push for activity on the issue or to maintain a "holding pattern." These same principles apply whether nurses want to influence federal, state, or local policies.

### The Legislative Process

Formal health policy is determined by legislation, rules and regulations, and judicial rulings by courts. Legislation has become the glamour component of health care policymaking for the nurse. But many times after the law has been passed, rules and regulations determine not only the shape of the legislation but also if that legislation will be implemented. Close monitoring of this process is needed.

How a bill becomes law is a similar process, whether it is in a state legislature or in Congress (Fig. 6-1). The process can be influenced anywhere from the formation of the bill to the sign-

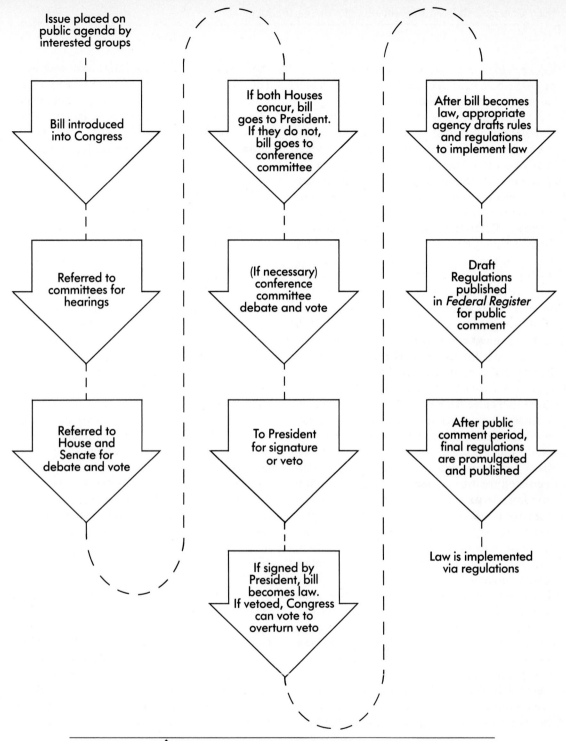

❖ **Fig. 6-1**  Formal health care policy process.

ing or veto by the executive. The key times are at committee hearings, markup of the bill, and during floor debates and votes.

Since the process of legislation in the 50 states is similar to that at the federal level, with a few differences such as the length of the legislative session. Therefore, discussion of legislation will concentrate on Congress and the federal level. Congress is in session for 2 years. Thus a bill remains "alive" until passed or killed for the 2 years. The 102nd Congress starts in January 1991 and ends December 31, 1992. The federal fiscal year begins October 1 and ends September 31. A fiscal year is called by the year in which it ends. For example, fiscal year 1991 begins October 1, 1990 and ends September 31, 1991.

Two types of bills are needed to establish and implement a legislative program: authorization and appropriations. A program must first be authorized by Congress. In other words, there must be authority for the program to exist. These bills give broad outlines of the program with the maximum amount of dollars authorized for the fiscal year. Typically, this authorization will be for 2 or 3 fiscal years. But for each fiscal year there must also be appropriations legislated for the authorized program. Appropriation bills passed by Congress permit federal agencies to incur obligations and result in payments out of the Treasury for the programs' specified purposes. Programs can be authorized without any funds appropriated or with a much lower amount than authorized. For example, in 1986, the 99th Congress authorized a program to compensate for injuries resulting from vaccinations. A no-fault compensation program was passed by Congress and signed by the President, but no funds were appropriated from the federal budget, and no other method was established to collect monies to fund the program. The 100th Congress in 1987 approved an excise tax on several child vaccines ranging from 6 cents to $4.56 per dose to fund a compensation pool. Thus, even though the authorizing legislation was passed in 1986, the appropriating legislation was not passed until the next year. This type of program where money is raised by additional taxes instead of coming out of the operating budget is called budget neutral. In today's economic climate, programs have a better chance of passing if they are budget neutral.

## Fiscal Appropriations

Thirteen appropriations bills are required to be passed by Congress and signed by the President by the beginning of each fiscal year. These 13 bills represent the amount of monies the 13 Cabinet departments can spend that year. The 13 departments are the Departments of Agriculture, Commerce, Defense, Energy, Health and Human Services, Housing and Urban Development, Interior, Justice, Labor, State, Treasury, Education, and Transportation. These Cabinets are generally combined into a general appropriation bill sometimes called the *omnibus spending bill.* There are two specialized types of appropriation bills: continuing and supplemental. When a fiscal year begins and if Congress has not yet enacted the regular appropriation bills for that year, Congress will pass a joint resolution continuing appropriations for government agencies at rates based on their previous year's appropriations. This bill is referred to as the continuing resolution. The continuing resolution, which can be a substitute for one, two, or all 13 appropriations bills, is in effect until a specific date or until a specific appropriation is enacted. Supplemental appropriation bills are passed when unanticipated or emergency funds are needed after the general or regular omnibus appropriation bill has been enacted. The President does not have line item veto and therefore must accept or veto each appropriation bill in its entirety even if he disagrees with a program within the bill. Therefore, because appropriation or budget bills are required for the functioning of the government, they are often used as vehicles to which other pieces of legislation and programs are attached.

The budget cycle is an important part of the federal legislative process. The President presents the administration's budget proposal in January along with current services estimates. This budget proposal, formulated from all the Cabinet departments and prepared by the Office of Management and Budget (OMB), outlines the President's estimates of tax receipts and budget outlays with a detailed recommendation for the ensuing fiscal year's appropriations. These estimates, based on continuation of existing levels of service, are called current services estimates and reflect the anticipated costs of continuing federal programs and activities at the current spending levels without policy changes. In other words, this means ignoring all new initiatives, presidential or congressional, that are not yet law. These estimates are accompanied by the underlying economic and programmatic assumptions upon which they are based, such as the rate of inflation, the rate of the real economic growth, the unemployment rate, program case loads, and pay increases. The President's budget, with its inherent policy priorities, serves as the starting point for Congress as it begins its budget deliberations. Congress debates the president's budget proposal as it develops its own proposal called a budget resolution. Budget resolutions are passed by the Senate and the House of Representatives setting forth levels and functional allocations for a fiscal year. If these two resolutions are different, negotiations occur until an acceptable resolution by both Houses is achieved. This concurrent resolution, which must be developed by Congress by April of each year, is not signed by the President and does not have the force of the law. Essentially, this is Congress' budget plan similar to what the President submits at the beginning of the year. The reconciliation process is how Congress brings revenues, expenditures, and entitlements into conformity with the levels set in the budget resolutions.

## Types of Health Care Programs

There are two types of health care programs: controllable and uncontrollable. *Controllable* health care programs are those subject to annual appropriations by Congress and consist primarily of categorical health services, training, and research programs called discretionary programs. *Uncontrollable* programs are called entitlements because members are entitled to their benefits by law because of age, disability, or economic status. The federal government is obligated to pay these benefits regardless of cost. The only way these costs can be controlled is by changing the authorizing legislation. Examples of health care entitlement programs are Medicare and Medicaid; Social Security, veteran's compensation, and pensions are examples of income entitlement programs (Kalisch & Kalisch, 1982). Approximately two thirds of the Department of Health and Human Services' budget is for entitlement programs, which means that only 33% of the amount appropriated by Congress for this department can be controlled.

In 1985, Congress passed the Gramm-Rudman-Hollings law (PL 99-177), which requires the federal budget to meet annual deficit reduction targets that would result in a balanced budget by 1991. This was amended in 1988 to extend the time to achieve a balanced budget to 1993. The measure sets maximum permissable budget deficits so that there will be no deficit in 1993. Initially, the act contained an automatic mechanism for making across-the-board spending cuts (sequestration) if the deficit targets were not met. This automatic mechanism was struck down in 1986 by the Supreme Court. Now Congress is mandated to pass a joint resolution to make the cuts.

After a bill is passed and signed into law, rules and regulations to implement that law are written and published for public comments. Initial rules and regulations as well as any changes are published by the executive branch of the government at both the federal and state level. These proposals are published in a government document called the Federal Register at the national level and in a similar register at the state level. After a period of time in which public comments can be submitted, the rules and regulations are promulgated, either published or revised. Laws are written in broad language; the rules and regulations to implement the law are written more specifically. Rules and regulations can be revised without changing the original law.

## ❖ POLITICS, HEALTH, AND NURSING

Nurses are not only the largest group of health professionals in the health care system but also are the most diverse in terms of education and practice. This "depth and breadth" of the nursing profession gives the nurse extraordinary potential to influence the health care delivery system. Nurses can influence health care policy as individuals and as professionals. Nurses as citizens should not abandon their rights to influence legislation and politics; as professionals, nurses are obligated to ensure that the public has access to quality health care at controlled costs. Armed with information on how to influence health care policy, nurses can become advocates for patients and become true participants in the formulation of effective health care policy. Policy decisions regarding financial resources influence the type of nursing staff, the number of nurses, the amount and type of management and support services, and supplies—all of which affect the quality of nursing care.

The need to control costs of health care without diminishing its quality or accessibility is becoming increasingly important. The public needs to ask continually if its money is being well-spent for health care. Nurses are well-placed and well-equipped to help with this analysis. Nurses cannot afford to assume that the

public—even in their local communities or institutions—understands how health care policies are made, unless they take some responsibility for helping formulate them.

Because 40% of health care monies are spent by state and federal governments (Division of National Costs Estimates, 1987), the government controls spending as well as influencing the quantity and quality of health care. Most of this spending involves Medicare and Medicaid programs. Governmental policies determine not only the accessibility and the type of health care available but also who will deliver it, in what setting, and how much will be paid for it. This control dictates the parameters within which nursing care is delivered, the type of nursing personnel, and how much nurses are paid to deliver that care.

Influencing a change or a creation of a new policy begins when there is a familiarity with the way laws, rules, and regulations are made, and with the players, the arena, and the socioeconomic political climate surrounding the issue. Nurses can influence legislators by testifying as experts on the issue, by lobbying governmental officials, and by building coalitions with other groups interested in the issue. To do this, it is important for nurses to be knowledgeable clinicians. But clinical expertise alone will not influence policy. Nurses also have expert interpersonal skills that they exercise with clients; these skills can be used in the policy arena as well.

Policies are changed incrementally rather than in one massive step. In the past, nurses have accepted these incremental changes, without analyzing the additive effect of all the small changes. Alert nurses will recognize the effects of the incremental changes and will support or influence their direction. Nurses are responsible for the policies affecting nursing care.

Legislation of interest to nurses is of two types: (1) funding bills that provide monies for education, research, innovative projects, or delivery methods, and payment for services that have a direct impact on the nursing profession and (2) legislation that creates advisory committees, task forces, and commissions that provide opportunities for nurses to become visibly active participants in the deliberations of health care policies.

## Nursing's Influence on Nursing Education Legislation

The Nurse Education Act is traditionally the most important piece of federal legislation to nurses. It generally is authorized for 3 years with appropriations set each year. The present act started with the first Nurse Training Act of 1964, although this was not the first time the federal government appropriated money for nursing education. In 1798, the federal government created the Marine Hospital Service, the antecedent of the present U.S. Public Health Service (PHS) with the eventual development of the Division of Nursing within PHS. World War II helped bring about the trend of federal support for nursing education (Abdellah, 1987).

Federal support for nursing education began with the passage of PL 74-271, which contained a provision for stipends for special postgraduate short courses and long-term training in public health nursing (Burke, 1983). In 1940, the National Council for National Defense was created by nursing leaders from the national nursing organizations and several government agencies to help prepare American nursing for war services. This council conducted a large survey, one of the first to determine nursing resources and to plan the expansion of basic nursing education to cope with the demands of the war for nurses. The Nurse Training Appropriations Act of 1941 (PL 77-146) provided some monies to schools to increase their enrollments and to improve their programs. This was significant because it was the first time the federal government provided money for basic nursing education. The initial appropriation was for $1.2 million for FY 1942 to cover tuition and subsistence for students in basic nursing education programs and some advanced programs (Abdellah, 1987; Eastaugh, 1985; and Kalisch & Kalisch, 1982).

Following the attack on Pearl Harbor in 1941, military recruitment of nurses diminished, and drafting nurses into the armed forces was seriously considered as a means to avert a shortage of nurses in the military. Since the principal source of nurses for the military was hospitals, this drafting potentially threatened nursing care in civilian hospitals. Nursing leaders, according to Kalisch and Kalisch (1982), "steadfastly opposed conscription and also opposed any effort to reduce the student nurse training period (suggested to accelerate the entry of young women into the profession) because they feared a massive collapse of the already meager educational standards" (p. 173). This opposition to drafting nurses remains today.

It became apparent that some type of accelerated training program was needed in order to produce an adequate number of nurses for the war. Nursing coalesced behind the plan called the U.S. Cadet Nurse Corps, which would provide free tuition, maintenance, uniforms, and a monthly stipend for 65,000 new cadets in either a 24-month or 30-month program. The program was authorized to begin in 1943 and was administered by the Public Health Service. The Division of Nursing Education was created within the PHS to administer this program. This was the largest federally subsidized nursing education program up to that time. This Act helped nursing schools in several ways. Probably the most profound was the need for the nursing schools to establish their own budgets separate from hospitals, since that was where most of the schools were housed. The growth of personnel within the PHS during this period included nurse consultants who were scattered throughout many of the government offices. The PHS was streamlined into four divisions:

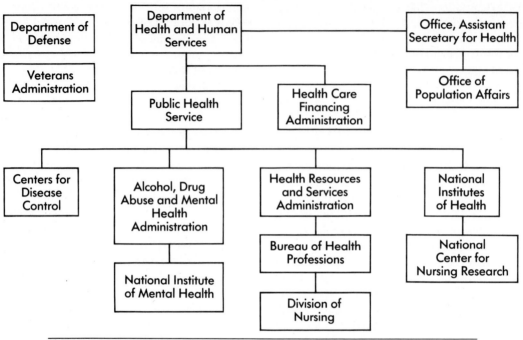

❖❖ **Fig. 6-2**    Selected agencies in federal government that administer programs supporting nursing education and research. *(Adapted from Jacox, A. (1985). Science and politics. Nursing Outlook 33(2), p. 80.)*

Office of the Surgeon General, the National Institute of Health, the Bureau of Medical Services, and the Bureau of State Services. Pearl McIver, Director of Public Health Nurse Consultants, recommended a plan to create a Division of Public Health Nursing within the Bureau of State Services to be responsible for all nursing activities in that bureau. This arrangement met its demise with the end of the war. See Fig. 6-2 for locations of nursing programs in the federal government today.

The Division of Nursing was authorized in the Public Health Service Act of 1944, but the Cadet Nurse Corps and postwar aid to nursing education and services including the Division of Nursing Education was phased out after the war. Nursing leaders found the change back to prewar funding and support to be unaccept-

able. So they worked together and found a funding source, the Carnegie Corporation, and a director, Esther Lucille Brown of the Russell Sage Foundation, to conduct an extensive survey of the current state of nursing education. This 1948 study was entitled "Nursing for the Future" and recommended the closing of weak schools and the development of nursing programs in universities and colleges. The report gained tremendous popular support (Kalisch & Kalisch, 1982).

Admissions to nursing schools declined after the war, and with the termination of the cadet corps, severe shortages of nurses in hospitals occurred. The American Medical Association (AMA) conducted a survey among physicians that indicated dissatisfaction with the quality and quantity of nurses. The AMA created a Committee on Nursing Problems in 1948, which after consultation with nursing leaders, recommended that the nursing profession be divided into professional and practical nurses with increased emphasis on baccalaureate education for the professional nurse and upgrading of the practical nurse training (Kalisch & Kalisch, 1982).

During the 1950s, several bills were introduced in Congress for funds to support nursing education, but they all failed because of opposition from the AMA and hospitals, who feared interference with the operation of their nursing schools. A liberal majority was established in Congress after the congressional elections in 1958. This more receptive political climate and the impact of a report, "Physicians for a Growing America" caused nursing leaders to become more optimistic about the chances of federal funding for nursing education. The leaders in the Division of Nursing convened a nursing consultant group in 1961 to study federal assistance for nursing. This group included representatives from national organizations of professional nursing, practical nursing, nursing education, physicians, medical educators, hospital administrators, and leaders from areas of education, labor, and civil rights.

This group published a report in 1963, "Toward Quality in Nursing," which recommended several actions. To increase recruitment, the group recommended increasing the amount of federal aid to students as well as expanding coverage to include schools of professional and practical nursing. This support would expand programs and would enable construction of more facilities. The group recommended that funds be used for consultative services and for project grants to strengthen in-service and continuing education programs. Graduate study and nursing research was to be stimulated through fellowships, traineeships, and research grants.

This report, and the more liberal climate in Congress along with President John F. Kennedy's recognition of the shortage of health care personnel in his initiative to improve the nation's health, helped the health professions including nursing with the enactment of the Health Professions' Educational Assistance Act. This act provided funds for the construction of facilities for health professionals' education and training. This was the first successful program since the war that nursing was able to get passed. This piece of legislation led to the Nurse Training Act of 1964, which was engineered by the Division of Nursing staff. It incorporated many of the recommendations of the Consultant Group on Nursing. This Act was the beginning of continuous federal funds at varying levels and for different education programs. It has evolved into the present Nurse Education Act.

Nursing is the only one of the various health professions to be able to retain a separate funding law with a separate national advisory committee for education. Although every President since President Nixon has not included nursing education in their budgets, Congress, at nursing's request, has funded nursing education even over Presidential vetoes. This attests to the skill and wisdom of the nursing leaders and the nursing community during these 25 years. Between 1965 and 1971, more than $380 million dollars were spent on nursing education for both students and institutions. Doctoral students and programs started receiving more emphasis and support during the mid-1970s. Programs also were established to educate nurse practitioners (Kalisch & Kalisch, 1982; Scott, 1972).

## Nursing's Influence on Nursing Research Legislation

Nursing research funding has been included in most of the nurse education acts. Although this research has been funded by the federal government and has been conducted by nurse researchers, nursing leaders argued that nursing research should be "integrated into the mainstream of science if it is to flourish and be better understood by other scientists and the public and that creation of a National Institute of Nursing would help accomplish these goals" (Jacox, 1985, p. 78). Jacox stated that the quality of nursing care could be greatly improved by research, that the promotion of strong nursing research programs could best occur in the mainstream of science, and that this justified the creation of a separate institute of nursing within the National Institutes of Health.

Nurses in research coalesced under the guidance of the Cabinet of Nursing Research of the American Nurses' Association (ANA). After the Institute of Medicine (IOM) issued its report on nursing in 1983 acknowledging nursing research and recommending that a federal entity for nursing research be established in the mainstream of science, three organized nursing groups, ANA, National League for Nursing, and the American Association of Colleges of Nursing, agreed in June 1983 to work with nurse researchers to accomplish this goal.

As stated earlier, since every administration since Nixon did not request money for nursing in the President's budget, it was assumed that there would be considerable resistance from the executive branch to the establishment of an institute for nursing. In spite of this strong resistance, the nursing organizations were successful in 1983 in getting legislation introduced in the House of Representatives to create a National Institute of Nursing. This bill passed unanimously by voice vote in November 1983. In October 1984, it was successfully considered by the Senate and House Conference Committee and was reported out as part of the National Institutes of Health reauthorization bill. This bill, passed by both Houses, was vetoed by President Reagan who said, in his veto message, that it was an example of "unnecessary, expensive new organizational entities" (Reagan, 1984). In January 1985, the Secretary of Health and Human Services (HHS) announced the establishment of a

Center for Nursing Research in the Division of Nursing, saying that this was the best approach to implementing the IOM's recommendation regarding nursing research. This initiative added six new positions for a total of twelve positions. All this did was add additional personnel positions to an already existing research program within the Division of Nursing. It did nothing to move nursing research into the mainstream of scientific research.

So the nurses tried again! Learning from their experience and initiating actions that would ensure that the "grass roots" of nursing would respond by contacting their legislators, the bill was reintroduced. The opposition to the bill continued to be not only the Administration, but also scientists in other Institutes within the NIH. These scientists saw the addition of a nursing institute as another slice of the fiscal pie with possible reduction in funds for their own research. Nurses working in the Division of Nursing's Center for Nursing Research were also reluctant to support an entity that would take away their work and funding. But with careful planning and enthusiastic support by others in nursing and Congress, the fight was on. This time a compromise was worked out when a senator who had consistently supported the idea but at a center level rather than at an institute level refused to budge.

A center is one level below an institute at NIH. The sponsor of the original bill and the new bill counseled compromise to the nursing organizations when it became clear that the NIH bill would be vetoed unless it was a center. Republican leaders supporting the bill believed they had reached a compromise with the White House in that there would be no veto if it was a Center for Nursing rather than an Institute for Nursing. Much to their surprise, President Reagan vetoed the bill on November 8, 1985. Congress then overwhelmingly voted to override the presidential veto to establish a National Center for Nursing Research (NCNR) (Nurses win battle, 1986).

## Nursing's Influence on Nursing Practice Legislation

The most important legislation affecting nursing practice is the nurse practice acts (NPAs) enacted in each state. The United States governs under the principle of states' rights. This principle gives individual states the right under the doctrine of police power to regulate anything that affects the health, welfare, and safety of its citizens. These laws are designed to protect the public, not to control entry into practice. Consequently, all states have nurse practice acts (NPA) that license nurses. Some states have NPAs with "sunset" provisions or laws automatically terminating a licensure statute after a designated period of time. It then is up to the profession to show the state legislature that the profession needs to be licensed to protect the public. This "proving" requires intensive and widespread political effort from nurses within that state to convince the legislators to license nurses (Wilson & Neuhauser, 1982).

Each state under practice acts mandates what qualifications the health professionals should possess in order to be licensed to practice their profession in that state. These statutes establish the requirements for licensure, which generally consist of necessary educational experiences, including the requirement of successful completion of an examination. The first practice act for nurses was passed by North Carolina in 1903. By 1923 all states and the District of Columbia had such laws. At first, licensure was not mandatory for the practice of nursing, but rather prohibited any unlicensed person from using the title of "registered nurse." Nurse practice acts define and regulate the entry to nursing practice and are administered by state boards of nursing. These boards are given the charge to promulgate the rules and regulations necessary to implement the nurse practice statute.

Much of the federal legislation affecting nursing practice has centered around payment for services. The first legislation affecting payment to nurses was the Rural Health Clinics Act of 1977 (PL 95-210). This law amended Title XIX (Medicaid) of the Social Security Act to include rural health clinic services by nurse practitioners within the definition of "medical assistance" eligible for payment under the Title. It also amended Title XVIII (Medicare) of the Social Security Act to provide payment for rural health clinic services under the supplementary medical insurance program and required the states to establish a plan for medical assistance and payment of rural health services.

This law was the first recognition of nurses as providers receiving third-party payment by the federal government. Senator Barbara Mikulski, a Democrat from Maryland, related that because she was a supporter of this bill when she was a Congresswoman and that she refused to retract her support for third-party payment for nurse practitioners, she lost financial support of the AMA when she campaigned for her Senate seat in 1986 (Personal communication, May 1986). Nurse practitioners (NPs) have consistently been the pioneers in receiving payment for their services from the federal government. Nurse anesthetists and nurse midwives receive payment, though often at a lower percentage rate of the fee received by the physician.

The first session of the 101st Congress flip-flopped over the issue of whether to change Medicare and Medicaid to provide for direct and/or indirect payment for nurse practitioners. This issue has been opposed by organized medicine for the last several years. So Congress compromised and passed legislation in November 1989 that provides direct payments from Medicaid to pediatric and family NPs for family health services. Specifically, as of July 1, 1990, states are required to cover the services of these two types of NPs regardless of whether the services are provided under the supervision of or associated with a physician. Other restrictions imposed by state laws still apply. As part of nursing home reform, indirect payments for nurse practitioners' services were included along with the authorization of nurse practitioners to certify and recertify patients in long-term care facilities. These small victories are the result of many years of political lobbying by organized nursing groups and the constant education of legislators and consumers as to the value of nurse practitioners. A report on nurse practitioners and others by the Office of Technology Assessment (OTA) has helped convince government officials of the worth and cost-effectiveness of nonphysician providers (U.S. Congress, Office of Technology Assessment, 1986).

## Political Influences on Health Legislation

The selected example of political influences on health legislation to be discussed is the amendments to the Social Security Act that created Medicare (Title XVIII) and Medicaid (Title XIX) in 1965. This law (PL 89-97) established health insurance for the aged and grants to states for medical assistance. This law occurred because of a combination of factors such as increased medical competence, heightened consumer expectations and use, and rising costs. These factors shaped the environment for the demand of this public policy. The United States was the slowest of the Western countries to develop some form of government action regarding the insuring of health care. In 1883, Bismarck in Germany initiated a health insurance plan for industrial workers and in 1911, England included health insurance for low-income workers in its social security program, which provided pensions. By 1940, no Western European country was without some type of government health insurance program, at least for low-income workers. The benefits of these various programs varied widely. The restriction

to the aged in the United States' plan was unique, unlike the European plans that covered low-income workers.

Although the issue of government-sponsored health insurance was raised during the 1930s, Roosevelt's New Deal programs generally were concerned only with social security income proposals. In order to correct the unequal distribution of medical services, a proposal submitted during Truman's administration attempted to remove financial barriers to the accessibility to health care. The underlying belief behind this proposal was that health services varied with income and not simply with illnesses resulting in regions where charity care was not available. Truman's proposal in 1949 to remove the financial barriers to care through government action failed in Congress. The American Medical Association was not placated by the attempt in Truman's plan to make physicians' participation voluntary. AMA started the campaign to educate the public that "socialized medicine" was not a good thing for the American people. Truman submitted similar proposals in 1950, 1952, and 1953, all of which failed.

Although these proposals failed, several shifts occurred in order to trim the all-encompassing plan. The recommendations given to Truman by his staff were: "softpedal the general health issue; push some peripheral programs in the area but not general insurance; or appoint a study commission to go over the whole problem" (Marmor, 1973, p. 14). A commission was established and charged to find the "right people" as well as a simultaneous push for "some peripheral programs." The administration attempted to come up with a proposal that would meet one of the major objections to Truman's proposal, which was that general medical insurance was a "give-away" program that made no distinction between the deserving poor and the undeserving poor. Thus the shift turned to focus on the aged. As a group it was believed that the aged could be presumed to be both needy and deserving because it was through no fault of their own that they had lower earning capacity and higher medical expenses than any other adult age group. Because the proponents wished to avoid an income means test to determine eligibility that would look too much like welfare, they limited eligibility to those over 65 who had contributed to the social security systems during their lifetime with a limit on the days in the hospital. This limitation on days in the hospital was added to show that the program was not a giveaway. Physicians' services were excluded in order to reduce their hostility toward the plan.

Different plans with Truman's compromises were introduced at various times throughout the following years. The political climate in Congress remained somewhat conservative with no opportunity for passage of such a proposal. With the election of John F. Kennedy as President in 1961, a shift toward a more liberal climate in Congress occurred. Also during this time several organizations and groups were becoming active supporters and opponents of such a proposal (Table 6-1). Among the supporters was organized labor. Organized labor was asking more and more for health benefits in collective bargaining agreements for their members.

Even though the political climate in Washington became increasingly liberal, Congress generally responded to the conservative Southern Democratic legislators, but the 1965 elections changed the composition of Congress. With this shift in Congress, Kennedy's assassination, and liberal Lyndon Johnson's assumption of the presidency, the political climate was changed. The time became ripe for the passage of a national health insurance plan. President Johnson took advantage of this, and Medicare was passed and signed into law on July 30, 1965.

**Catastrophic Amendments Debacle.** In the 1980s, during President Reagan's administration, a debate on the effect that catastrophic illnesses would have on the elderly led to a commission to study these effects. This commission developed a plan that was submitted to Congress by President Reagan. Congress debated the issue and proposed several plans of its own. Several areas of debate centered on how to pay for the added benefits. Congress, in an attempt to control the spiraling deficit of the federal budget, attempted to make the added benefits budget neutral by developing a plan that included an income surtax on approximately 40% of the beneficiaries. This surtax would pay for catastrophic benefits for this 40% and for the poorer 60%. Less than 5% of the

❖ **Table 6-1**
Supporters and opponents of the establishment of Medicare

| Supporters | Opponents |
|---|---|
| American Nurses' Association | American Medical Association |
| AFL-CIO | American Hospital Association |
| Council of Jewish Federations and Welfare Funds | Life Insurance Association of America |
| American Association of Retired Workers | National Association of Manufacturers |
| National Association of Social Workers | National Association of Blue Shield Plans |
| National Farmers Union | American Farm Bureau of Federation |
| The Socialist Party | The Chamber of Commerce |
| American Geriatrics Society | The American Legion |

Adapted from Marmor, T. R. (1973). *The Politics of Medicare.* New York: Aldine Publishing Company.

beneficiaries would pay the full amount, $800, during the first year. This amount was planned to rise every year as more of the benefits were phased in. The concept had support from many people and a variety of organizations, including the American Association of Retired Persons and the American Nurses' Association. Several complaints were voiced that the elderly also needed coverage for nursing home care. But, since it was estimated that the average annual cost of nursing home care in the 1980s was $25,000, this was a prohibitive cost to the federal government at this time.

Several factors delayed the passage of a bill (e.g., the stock market crash in October 1987, the balancing of the budget, and objections from several Congressmen). Congressman Claude Pepper, a Democrat from Florida, introduced a proposal to increase coverage for home health care for the elderly and other disabled persons. Since he was chairman of the rules committee, he ruled that his bill should go directly to the floor of the House of Representatives for debate, thus bypassing the two health committees with extremely powerful chairmen. These two influential chairmen were angered by Pepper's maneuver and vowed to defeat his bill. This procedural and turf battle defeated Pepper's bill and assisted the passage of the catastrophic bill, which mandated unlimited hospital care, limited out-of-pocket expenses for physician bills, and partial payment for prescription drugs. The aftermath of this legislative battle was an addition to the final bill to create a commission to examine the problem of long-term care and possible solutions. This commission is commonly referred to as the Pepper Commission and was set up to study the issue of long-term care for the elderly.

The Medicare Catastrophic Protection Act (PL 100-360) was signed into law on July 1, 1988. It was heralded by Congress, the Administration, elderly consumer groups, and others including health care providers. Rules and regulations were written to implement the law in-

cluding the precedent-setting financial method of income surtaxes. As the details of the rules and regulations were disseminated to the public, a backlash from the elderly, mainly middle class, occurred over the surtax. They felt they were being asked to pay more taxes than other nonelderly citizens for benefits they were paying for in private insurance plans called Medigap plans. Their vehement opposition generated such an uproar that Congress in November 1989 repealed most of the measures contained in the catastrophic bill passed the year before. *Not* only were the catastrophic amendments the largest expansion since the inception of the Medicare program, but this was also the first time that a large health benefit program had been repealed before it was fully implemented. The aftermath of this debacle is the reluctance of Congress to consider in the near future any health insurance plan for the elderly. The final report of the Pepper Commission is still to be acted on.

Other health landmark laws passed by Congress that had some indirect and direct effect on nursing were the Social Security Act of 1935 (PL 74-241), which for the first time provided grants-in-aid to states for maternal and child care, aid to crippled children, blind persons, the aged, and other health-impaired persons. The Hospital Survey and Construction Act (PL 79-725) enacted in 1946, commonly called the Hill-Burton Act, which supported surveys, plans, and new facilities such as hospitals, was a turning point in the delivery of health care. During this time, health care delivery shifted into hospitals with nurses becoming predominantly salaried employees of the institutions.

## ❖ SPHERES OF NURSING INFLUENCE

The nurse has the opportunity to make an impact on policies in four spheres of influence as identified by Talbott and Mason (1988). These spheres are (1) government, (2) workplace, (3) organizations, and (4) community.

Since the community encompasses the other three spheres, only government, organizations, and workplace will be discussed here.

### Government

Laws, with their accompanying rules and regulations, control nursing practice and health care. Nurses have been more involved in federal and state governments, although local governments provide many health care services. Local governments control school health programs, local public hospitals, and home and community health care. Several books detail how nurses can influence governments (Goldwater & Zusy, 1990; Mason & Talbott, 1985; Archer & Goehner, 1982; and Kalisch & Kalisch, 1982). In general, the nurse first must be a registered voter. Nurses can join collective actions by working with political action committees (PACs). These committees support deserving candidates who support nursing and health care issues. The ANA political action committee is called ANA-PAC and supports candidates favorable to nursing issues. ANA and ANA-PAC depend on nurses at the grass roots level not only to contribute money but also to work in endorsed candidates' campaigns for national offices. Goldwater and Zusy (1990) discuss in detail how nurses can participate in campaigns as well as run for elective offices. Most states have state nurses' association PACs for state and local candidates. Contact your state nurses' association on how you can get involved. Most of these organizations are set up to instruct novices on how to become involved. Other ways to become involved include joining your local branch of a political party and becoming involved in local political clubs. This type of involvement enables nurses to be involved in issues other than health care as well as developing nonnurse support for health issues.

Another way to become involved at the governmental level is to work for an elected official either as a paid employee or as a volunteer expert consultant. Elected officials have numerous bills or reports to review and to respond to—a nurse can be influential in molding the official's position on issues. For example, a nurse volunteering in Mayor Koch's New York City campaign was asked to write his position paper on health care. Increasing in importance is for the nurse to run for elected office or to assume a political appointment. These political appointments can be on task forces, committees, or positions in the local and state health department.

### Workplace

Since most nurses work in bureaucratic organizations, they should take advantage of the opportunity to influence the policies of their workplace. Over 66% of nurses work in hospitals and should be influential in setting hospital policies, especially regarding patient care. Nurses can influence how quality care is delivered with controlled costs, ensuring that cuts do not diminish the amount and type of care needed. Most hospitals currently require that many nonnursing tasks be done by nurses. Through collective action, nurses serving on committees in the institution can help eliminate these tasks. Nurses working with other providers on interdisciplinary committees can have an impact on how nursing is viewed and used. Nurses can even serve on the board of trustees of the institution. Nurses who successfully practice the politics of change in their place of employment can influence the type and quality of patient care (Talbott & Mason, 1988).

### Organizations

Important influences include professional organizations such as the American Nurses' Association (ANA) and many specialty organizations. ANA members have an impact not only on legislation at the federal and state level, but they also have the capacity to monitor many issues and can alert nurses when to support or oppose issues. The organizations work in coalitions with other health groups to support or oppose issues. Nursing organizations are often approached to recommend nurses for appointments on task forces and committees. By joining and being active in a professional organization, an individual nurse has access to a wider range of tools and information to use in order to influence health care policies.

### ❖ IMPACT OF NURSING RESEARCH ON HEALTH POLICY

Historically, research and reports on nurses and nursing have resulted in policy changes. Studies, such as the 1948 survey entitled "Nursing for the Future" resulted in legislation to financially assist the training of nurses by providing funds for nursing scholarships and general support for nursing schools. Selected examples of how nursing research, reports, or studies influenced changes in policy will be presented.

### Nursing Practice

The Department of Nursing Resources of the PHS published its study, "Patients and Personnel: A Method of Studying Patient Care in Hospitals," in 1957 designed to determine whether satisfaction with nursing care was related to nurse staffing. This exhaustive survey study of some 20,000 patients and staff members was conducted to show hospitals how to incorporate patients' needs into their studies. Studies such as this and others done by the Department of Nursing Resources helped improve the use of nursing resources. For example, Kalisch and Kalisch (1982) reported that in one typical hospital the time spent on nonnursing activities by the nursing staff had been markedly reduced as a result of these studies.

As reported earlier, the 1963 study, "Toward Quality in Nursing," recommended an increase in the number of nurses and established goals that resulted in the first nurse training act in 1964. The Department of Nursing has completed several National Sample Surveys of Registered Nurses, which have affected the amounts of monies appropriated by Congress as well as the types of education programs that receive these funds.

Fagin (1982) wrote a classic article identifying studies that demonstrated the economical use of nursing care for cost-effective patient care.

### Nursing Research

Several studies were used to demonstrate the need for a separate entity within the National Institutes of Health (NIH) for nursing research. Besides the 1983 Institute of Medicine's (IOM) report on their study of nursing, a study sponsored by the ANA Council of Nurse Researchers was used to demonstrate that many nursing studies did not fit into the National Institutes of Health research programs. The study, conducted by Joanne Stevenson (1983), reviewed 111 draft research proposals written by nurses and submitted to the federal government for funding. Of the 61 directed to the National Institutes of Health, NIH determined that 12 were relevant to NIH's mission, 24 were of potential interest, and 25 were clearly outside the research focus of NIH. These 25 deemed not in NIH's domain were in the following areas: development of knowledge in the domain of care, rather than cure; studies of the family as the target of health care; studies of the interpersonal processes, especially verbal and nonverbal communication as intervention techniques; and health promotion directed toward the chronically ill and healthy persons. These four areas are the core of nursing research, yet did not fit within the scope of research done at NIH at that time (Jacox, 1985, 1986; Stevenson, 1983). Jacox (1985) cited several studies conducted by the federal government, which had implications for the location of nursing research in the federal government.

## Nursing Economics and Finances

When the Medicare program was implemented in 1966, an extra payment of 2% of Medicare costs was paid to hospitals for the care of elderly patients. It was assumed that there were more costs in delivering care to the aged than to non-aged patients. This bonus was eliminated in 1969. In response to this loss of revenue, hospitals complained that Medicare patients required more nursing care than non-Medicare patients because of their age. A study of 55 hospitals conducted by the American Hospital Association in 1966 was used by hospitals in their successful persistent lobbying to get enacted a per diem hospital inpatient routine nursing salary payment of an additional 8.5%. This differential was eliminated by the government with a subsequent reinstitution after a successful lawsuit brought by the American Hospital Association. Several studies were conducted in the ensuing years, but none were successful in changing policy until a study was conducted using 1979 Medicare data. As a consequence of this study the routine nursing salary cost differential was eliminated in 1983 (Fitzmaurice, 1983).

## ❖ SUMMARY

This chapter defined the terms and processes used in influencing health care policies. Looking at how nursing has influenced nursing education legislation, nursing research legislation, nursing practice legislation, and health legislation provides success stories on which nurses of the future can build. Nurses should incorporate the desire and the practice of influ-

ence into their clinical practice whether they become involved at the hospital, organizational, or governmental level, because nurses are responsible for the quality of care delivered to clients.

---

## ❖❖ APPLYING KNOWLEDGE TO PRACTICE

1. What types of legislation have nurses influenced? Discuss health care issues of particular importance in your local community.
2. Where and how can nurses influence health care policies?
3. Why should nurses become involved in the policymaking process?
4. How can nursing research have an impact on health care policies?

### REFERENCES

Abdellah, F. G. (1987). The federal role in nursing education. *Nursing Outlook. 35*(5), 224–225.

Archer, S. E. and Goehner, P.A. (1982). *Nurses: A Political Force.* Monterey, CA: Wadsworth Health Sciences Division.

Burke, S. (1983). The nurse training act: A history of support. *Imprint. 30*(3), 47–52.

Division of National Cost Estimates. (1987). National health expenditures. *Health Care Financing Review. 8*(4), 1–36.

Estaugh, S. R. (1985). The impact of the nurse training act on the supply of nurses, 1974–1983. *Inquiry.* (22), 404–417.

Fagin, C. (1982). The economic worth of nursing research. *American Journal of Nursing. 82* (12), 1844–1849.

Feldstein, P. J. (1988). *The Politics of Health Legislation.* Ann Arbor, MI: Health Administration Press Perspectives.

Fitzmaurice, J. M. (1983) A statistical analysis of the Medicare hospital routine nursing salary cost differential. *Health Care.*

Goldwater, M. and Zusy, M. J. L. (1990). *Prescription for Nurses: Effective Political Action.* St. Louis: C. V. Mosby Company.

Hyman, H. H. (1982). *Health Planning: A Systematic Approach.* Rockville, MD: Aspen Publication.

Jacox, A. (1985). Science and politics. *Nursing Outlook. 33*(2), 78–84.

Jacox, A. (1986). The coming of age of nursing research. *Nursing Outlook. 34*(6), 276–281.

Kalisch, B. J. and Kalisch, P. A. (1982). *Politics of nursing.* Philadelphia: J. B. Lippincott.

Mason, D. J. and Talbott, S. W. (1985). *Political Action: Handbook for Nurses.* Menlo Park, CA: Addison-Wesley Publishing Company.

Marmor, T. R. (1973). *The Politics of Medicare.* Chicago: Aldine.

Nurses win battle for research center at NIH; Congress rebukes Reagan and overides his veto. (1986). *American Journal of Nursing. 86* (1), 75.

Reagan, R. (Oct. 30, 1984). Memorandum of disapproval. Washington, D.C. Office of the Press Secretary, White House.

Scott, J. M. (1972). Federal support for nursing education 1964–1972. *American Journal of Nursing. 72*(10), 1855–1861.

Stevenson, J. (1983). *New investigator federal sector grantsmanship project: Final report. ANA Pub. D-75.* Kansas City, MO: American Nurses' Association.

Talbott, S. W. and Mason, D. J. (1988). Chapter 18, Power and professional influence. In B. Kozier and G. Erb. *Concepts and Issues in Nursing Practice.* Menlo Park, CA: Addison-Wesley Publishing Company.

U.S. Congress, Office of Technology Assessment. (1986). *Nurse practitioners, physicians' assistants, and certified nurse-midwives: Policy analysis.* Washington, D.C.: U.S. Government Printing Office.

Wilson, F. A. and Neuhauser, D. (1982). *Health services in the United States, 2nd Edition.* Cambridge, MA: Ballinger Publishing Co.

# 7

# Economic Issues in Health Care and Nursing

Lonna T. Milburn ◆ Hurdis Griffith

## *OBJECTIVES*

*At the completion of this chapter, the reader will be able to:*

◆ **Define the basic elements of health economics.**

◆ **Identify the major health economic issues of the 1990s.**

◆ **Apply health economic principles to nursing practice, education, and research.**

## ❖ OVERVIEW OF ECONOMICS

Economics represents the study of allocating scarce resources among competing needs. Allocating resources refers to how each good produced is distributed to its consumers. When resources are limited, as most are, and individual or societal desires for these resources appear to be limitless, then a scarcity of the resource exists. Simply stated, economics becomes the intellectual liaison between nature and technology on the *supply* side and the preferences and desires of consumers and overall society on the *demand* side (Byrns & Stone, 1987; Fuchs, 1976; Phelps, 1985; Robbins, 1935).

The economics involved with health care is important on both sides of the *supply- demand* equation. Regardless of the affluence or productivity of a society, it cannot provide its citizens with all the health care and technology that they might wish to consume. Decisions must be made about who will be the recipients for these

scarce resources. In the decision-making process, economics provides an evaluative framework with several questions:

1. What health care will be produced? Society wants health care that prevents, treats, and rehabilitates.
2. How will the goods be produced? The health care system reacts to the incentives created by society to produce the services, weighing the relative benefits and costs of providing services in alternative ways.
3. How much health care will be produced? Services are delivered as long as the perceived benefits outweigh the perceived costs.
4. Who will get the goods produced? This is a value-laden decision that must be made by the given society (Hicks & Boles, 1984).

Thus, economics provides a systematic mechanism to obtain information about the availability, potential, and results of the health care system. Also, economics can be used to

**107**

trace relationships among the health of the population, the size and productivity of the work force, and the demand for health care. Forecasts based on economic models can pave the way for informed, pro-active decision making on alternatives for efficiently using resources. In today's unstable economy, period of rapidly changing societal expectations, era of cost containment in health care, and volatile environment where health care is everchanging, nurses must be prepared to substantiate their delicate, caring and coordinating responsibilities of client care with sound economic and management principles. Then nurses can actively turn the key for dramatic changes in the health care system.

## ❖ ECONOMIC INDICATORS OF HEALTH CARE

Several economic indicators reflect changes in the health care system (Health Insurance Association of America, 1989). Among the most common are the following:

*Consumer Price Index (CPI):* measures the average change in prices of all types of consumer goods and services purchased by urban wage earners and clerical workers. The index measures only the effect of price changes on the cost of living. It does not measure changes in the total amount families spend. This index is computed monthly by the Federal Government.

*Hospital Status:*
*Admissions, Cost Per Inpatient Day, Length of Stay, Outpatient Visits, Occupancy Rates, and Staffed Beds* indicate consumption and costs of consumption for hospital care. These data are available on an annual basis from the American Hospital Association in Chicago.

*National Health Expenditure (NHE):* includes both private and public expenditures for personal health care, medical research, the construction of medical facilities, program administration, insurance costs, and government-sponsored public health programs. It covers spending for health care over the 12-month calendar year and is issued annually by the Federal Government.

*Personal Consumption Expenditure (PCE):* represents private payments for medical care. Monies from three government programs (Medicare, Worker's Compensation, and Temporary Disability Insurance) are treated as transfer payments and are included. It is computed as an annual average by the Federal Government. Basic categories of expenditures constitute the PCE for medical care and the PHCE portion of the NHE figure; different accounting practices are used for each.

*Personal Health Care Expenditure (PHCE):* indicates expenditures for consumers, whether insured or not. Included are expenses for nonprescribed drugs and medicines, household supplies, and other items not covered by insurance. Issued annually by the Federal Government.

*Professional Status:*
*Office Visits:* indicate the number of office calls consumers make to a physician. Data are available from the American Medical Association in Chicago.
*Physician Fees* reflect charges for office and other physician visits. Data are available from the American Medical Association in Chicago.
*Surgical Charges* indicate the fee for common surgical procedures and emergency medical procedures across the United States. Data are available from the American Medical Association in Chicago and the Health Insurance Association of America in Washington, D.C.

## ❖ ECONOMIC CONCEPTS IN HEALTH CARE

The three basic concepts of *supply, demand,* and *cost* are intricately related in economics. Each of these concepts is explored as they relate to health care.

### Supply of Health Care

The *supply* of health care refers to the amount of resources currently available for delivering health services. Resources include health care facilities, manpower, and financing.

Among health care facilities, hospitals still serve as the hub for client care activity, but the emergence of other facilities such as managed care organizations (i.e., Health Maintenance Organizations (HMOs) and Preferred Provider Organizations (PPOs), home health units, and ambulatory care centers in the 1980s) created a very different health care system. During the 1980s, financial woes created by inequities in third-party reimbursements (i.e., health insurance companies, Medicare, Medicaid), declining admissions, and high levels of uncompensated care resulted in the closure of 40 to 80 hospitals annually. Most of these hospitals were located in large inner-city markets and in rural areas (Hendershot, 1988; Huge Gain in Health Care Jobs, 1989). The number of hospital beds, however, increased as hospitals diversified beyond the traditional medical, surgical, obstetric, and pediatric units.

Managed care organizations also experienced some instability while experimenting with their products, their marketing strategies, and their target clients. As HMOs and PPOs attempted to stabilize their operations, their enrollment rates increased, while the number of new and operating HMOs and PPOs decreased. Interstudy (1989) identified 643 HMOs in the United States in 1988 with total enrollments of 31 million members. At the same time, 692 PPOs contracted with physicians, hospitals, nursing homes, home health care agencies, and other providers. A Marion Laboratory survey (1989) found that a total of 12.9 million workers were covered by 449 of the PPOs. Based on these figures, it was estimated that between 28 and 29 million Americans were eligible for the PPO option. In the 1990s, managed care organizations will continue to wrestle with issues such as limitations in enrollments and extent of coverage options.

Ambulatory care centers serve as an alternative to hospitalization by providing outpatient surgical and emergency care. The growth in this industry is evident as the number of centers increased from 600 to 3800 between 1982 and 1986 (Health Insurance Association of America, 1989).

During the 1980s, health care provider levels increased in terms of numbers of active personnel and in new professions. To illustrate, payroll jobs in the health services sector rose by 480,000 (41%) in 1988, bringing the overall employment in the health sector to 7.46 million from 6.98 million 1 year earlier and from 1.8 million 5 years earlier (Huge Gain in Health Care Jobs, 1989). Table 7-1 depicts the changes that occurred in the supply of health care providers. While physician numbers increased, the number of physicians per 100,000 population grew almost three times faster for the entire United States than for rural areas. In 1985, the United States had physician population ratios of 165 per 100,000 as compared to ratios of 30 per

❖ **Table 7-1**
A comparison of health providers by totals and number/100,000 population for 1980 and 1986

| Health provider | 1980 | | 1986 | |
|---|---|---|---|---|
| | Total | Number/100,000 population | Total | Number/100,000 population |
| Physicians | 409,917 | 182.0 | 545,000 | 228.0 |
| Nurses | 1,272,900 | 560.0 | 1,592,600 | 661.0 |
| Hospitals | 6,229 | 2.8 | 6,035 | 2.5 |
| Hospital beds | 1,080,164 | 480.0 | 1,660,611 | 689.0 |

From USDHHS. *Health,* United States - 1988.

100,000 in counties having less than 2500 people and 54 per 100,000 in counties having populations between 5000 and 9999 (Kindig & Movassaghi, 1989). Distributional inequities also existed for nurses and allied health personnel, but the largest problem in 1989 was the nationwide, short supply of these health professionals. According to the American Hospital Association, the supply of nurses and allied health personnel was inadequate, with vacancy rates of 16% for physical therapists, 15% for occupational therapists, 11% for registered nurses, 10% for certified registered nurse anesthetists, 10% for clinical perfusionists, and 9% for speech pathologists (Glenn, 1989a).

Today, subsidization of health care comes from a variety of public and private third-party payers. Public financing from the federal level is dominated by two well-known entitlement programs: Medicare and Medicaid. Both programs were established in 1965 as a mechanism to ensure that Americans had equal access to health care. Medicare, as part of the Social Security system, is entirely federally funded. It provides uniform health care coverage to all individuals age 65 and older who receive Social Security benefits. It also covers those who have been determined permanently disabled for 2 years or more and those with endstage renal disease. Medicaid, a joint federal-state program, was designed as a health insurance program for the poor, especially poor mothers and children. For the poor elderly, Medicaid serves as an important supplement to Medicare by paying Medicare's premiums, deductibles, and co-insurance and supplementing Medicare's limited benefit package for prescription drugs, hearing aids, and preventive services. Medicaid also covers long-term care services excluded by Medicare, and rarely covered by private insurance plans. The federal government pays slightly more than half the program costs. Because each state establishes eligibility criteria, benefit packages, and reimbursement policies,

the program varies widely from state to state. Other federally sponsored health plans include:

1. Treatment for military personnel and their dependents at Department of Defense Medical facilities and an insurance program called CHAMPUS (Civilian Health and Medical Program of the Uniformed Services) for treatment in nongovernment medical facilities.
2. Insurance programs for civilian employees who work for the federal government.
3. Health care coverage for veterans in 170 Veterans Administration sponsored medical centers and 232 outpatient clinics.
4. Medical care and health services provided for 2 million Native Americans and Alaskan natives.

At the state and local levels, public programs for health care are located in the state and local health departments. Usually, four primary program areas exist: personal health, environmental health, health resources, and laboratory services.

Private programs from commercial health insurance companies such as Blue Cross/Blue Shield issue two basic categories of coverage: medical expense insurance and disability income insurance. Medical expense insurance provides broad benefits that can cover virtually all expenses connected with hospitals, medical care, and related services. Disability income insurance provides periodic payments when an insured individual is unable to work as a result of sickness or injury. Other private programs come through HMOs and PPOs that provide comprehensive health care services to their members for a fixed premium. In these plans, groups of physicians and auxiliary health personnel deliver care as specified in the contract provided to subscribers (Health Insurance Association of America, 1989).

The supply level is influenced by developments in technology, changes in the cost to produce goods and services, the prices of comparable goods and services, and consumer expectations. Also, the number of producers in the market, the level of taxes, the subsidies and government regulations affect how many resources exist and are produced (Byrns & Stone, 1987).

## Demand for Health Care

The *demand* for health care refers to the amount and type of health care the consumer requires and is willing to purchase (Feldstein, 1983). The realities of health care are such that today the most important factor affecting the demand for health care is how it is subsidized. Federal and state tax codes encourage employer supported health insurance coverage by allowing business deductions, exactly as any other wage expense.

In 1987, more than 205 million Americans, 86% of the civilian noninstitutional population, were covered with a third party payer for health insurance. Of this number, 181 million individuals were covered by private health insurance. Claims for medical care or disability paid for those having private coverage amounted to $139 billion, an 8.2% increase over 1986, and more than three times the amount paid 10 years earlier. Public expenditures increased at a level of 9.7% in 1987. Contributing to that figure were the 33 million Medicare recipients and 23 million Medicaid recipients who consumed $80 billion and $45 billion, respectively, for health care (Health Insurance Association of America, 1989).

A glimpse at the use of health care gives some perspective on the demand for health services. In 1987, there were 32 million hospital admissions, 245 million outpatient hospital visits (indicating an increased use of new facilities for the treatment of medical and psychiatric clients on an outpatient basis), 60 million visits to ambulatory care centers, and 730 million visits to physicians' offices. Consumer demands reflected some distinct trends for hospitalization:

1. Women were hospitalized more often for surgery.
2. Clients under 15 years were most often hospitalized for pneumonia, acute respiratory infections, asthma, and chronic diseases of the tonsils and adenoids.
3. Clients between 15 and 44 years of age were most often hospitalized for psychoses, fractures, abortions, and ectopic pregnancies and deliveries.
4. Clients 45 to 64 years of age were most often hospitalized for heart disease.
5. Clients over 65 years were hospitalized most often for heart disease and malignant neoplasms (Health Insurance Association of America, 1989).

The use of physicians' services can best be documented by physicians' office visits. In 1987, there were 5.4 visits per capita to physicians' offices. Blacks, aged 45 years or older, visited their physician more than whites with an average of 7.3 visits per capita in the 45 to 65 age group and 9.4 per capita for those over 65 years. By income, individuals earning less than $10,000 per year averaged nearly two more visits per capita than individuals with incomes of $10,000 to $19,999 (Health Insurance Association of America, 1989), but the lower income individuals were hospitalized less frequently by their physician (Hendershot, 1988).

With the advent of AIDS in the 1980s, the demand for new laboratory tests, new drugs, new social support modalities, innovative financing arrangements, and treatment programs has become evident. According to the Centers for Disease Control (CDC), over 146,000 cases of AIDS have been reported. CDC estimates that the disease is at epidemic rates with 1.5 million Americans infected with the AIDS virus (Health Insurance Association of America, 1989).

The demand for health care is affected by consumers' illnesses, their tastes and preferences, their income, and their knowledge about health care. Also, the price and cost of health care, the prices of related health care products, and the health care providers' choices for treatment modalities affect the demand for health care. On a societal level, demographic changes such as an aging population, the population's awareness of health risks, or a population inflicted with AIDS alters the health care demand (Sorkin, 1984).

## Costs for Health Care

The *costs* for health care refer to the amount a provider pays to produce health-related goods and services, as well as the amount a consumer pays to purchase these goods and services.

Since the passage of Medicare and Medicaid legislation in 1965, health care costs have risen rapidly. Increases in the per capita costs for health care reflect these quantum leaps with Americans spending $217 per capita in 1965, $590 in 1975, $1620 in 1985, and $2395 in 1989. Each year, more U.S. dollars are spent for health care ( $498.9 billion in 1987 and $618.4 in 1989). Correspondingly, a greater percentage of the Gross National Product (GNP) (i.e., the overall output of goods) represents health care expenditures, with 6.2% in 1965, 10.6% in 1985, and 11.4% in 1989. (See Table 7-2.)

Between 1980 and 1987, personal health care expenses increased 101% from $219.7 to $442.6 billion. The largest increases were in other professional services (184%); physicians services (119%); and dentist services (113%), while the smallest increases were in drugs/medical sundries (81%); eyeglasses/appliances (86%), and hospital care (93%) (USDHHS, 1988).

Subsidizing the nation's health care bill in 1987 were private sources (59% or $293 billion) and public sources (41% or $207.3 billion). Further analysis of the private payers reveals that consumers directly paid 42% or $123 billion of the bill, and private insurers paid 54%

 **Table 7-2**
Aggregate and per capita national health expenditures selected calendar years, 1929-1988

| Calendar Year | Total Health Expenditures | | |
|---|---|---|---|
| | Amount* | Per Capita | % of GNP |
| 1929 | $  3.6 | $  29 | 3.5 |
| 1935 | 2.9 | 23 | 4.0 |
| 1940 | 4.0 | 30 | 4.0 |
| 1950 | 12.7 | 82 | 4.5 |
| 1955 | 17.7 | 105 | 4.4 |
| 1960 | 26.9 | 146 | 5.3 |
| 1965 | 43.0 | 217 | 6.2 |
| 1970 | 74.7 | 359 | 7.6 |
| 1975 | 132.7 | 590 | 8.6 |
| 1980 | 248.0 | 1049 | 9.4 |
| 1985 | 425.0 | 1620 | 10.6 |
| 1986 | 458.0 | 1837 | 10.9 |
| 1987 | 498.9 | 2050 | 11.2 |
| 1988 | 558.7 | 2271 | 11.4 |
| 1989 | 618.4 | 2395 | 11.5 |
| 1990 estimates | 647.3 | 2511 | 11.6 |

*In billions of dollars
From USDHHS., Health Care Financing Administration, 1987a; U.S. Department of Commerce, 1989.

or $157.8 billion. Public or government assistance was predominantly from federal sources (70% or $144.7 billion), rather than from state or local sources. A comparison between private and public payers shows that public assistance was most prominent for hospital care (52%, $102.2 billion) and research/construction (63%, $10.8 billion), while private payers assumed a majority of the costs for physicians' services (69%, $70.9 billion); dentists' services (98%, $32.2 billion); drugs/medical sundries (88.8%, $30.2 billion); eyeglasses/appliances (76.8%, $7.3 billion); and Program Administration (72%, $18.7 billion). Nearly an equal percentage of the nursing home care was paid by private (51%, $20.4 billion) and public sources (49%, $19.9 billion). (See Table 7-3.)

❖ **Table 7-3**

National health care expenditures—1987 by type of expenditure and source of funds (in billions of dollars)

| Type of Expenditure | Total Expenditures | Private consumer | | | | Government | | |
|---|---|---|---|---|---|---|---|---|
| | | Total Private funds | Direct | Private insurance | Other | Total Government Funds | Federal | State and local |
| NHE | $500.3 | 293.0 | 123.0 | 157.8 | 12.2 | 207.3 | 144.7 | 62.7 |
| Health Services/supplies | 483.2 | 286.7 | 123.0 | 157.8 | 5.9 | 196.5 | 136.3 | 60.2 |
| Personal health care | 442.6 | 267.3 | 123.0 | 139.1 | 5.3 | 175.3 | 131.2 | 44.1 |
| Hospital care | 194.7 | 92.6 | 18.5 | 71.9 | 2.2 | 102.2 | 80.0 | 22.2 |
| Physicians' services | 102.7 | 70.9 | 26.3 | 44.6 | 0.1 | 31.8 | 25.7 | 6.1 |
| Dentists' services | 32.8 | 32.2 | 20.0 | 12.1 | — | 0.7 | 0.3 | 0.3 |
| Other professional services | 16.2 | 10.8 | 6.4 | 4.3 | 0.1 | 5.4 | 3.6 | 1.8 |
| Drugs/medical sundries | 34.0 | 30.2 | 25.5 | 4.7 | — | 3.9 | 1.9 | 2.0 |
| Eyeglasses/appliances | 9.5 | 7.3 | 6.3 | 1.2 | — | 2.1 | 1.9 | 0.2 |
| Nursing home care | 40.6 | 20.6 | 20.0 | 0.4 | 0.3 | 19.9 | 11.1 | 8.9 |
| Other personal health care | 12.0 | 2.6 | — | — | 2.6 | 9.4 | 6.7 | 2.7 |
| Program Administration/net Cost of private health insurance | 25.9 | 19.4 | — | 18.7 | 0.7 | 6.6 | 3.5 | 3.1 |
| Government public health activities | 14.7 | — | — | — | — | 14.7 | 1.6 | 13.1 |
| Research/construction | 17.1 | 6.3 | — | — | 6.3 | 10.8 | 8.4 | 2.4 |

From USDHHS, Health Care Financing Administration, Office of the Actuary, Division of National Cost Estimates, 1989.

Table 7-4 shows that government-sponsored personal health care totaled $175.3 billion in 1987, with Medicare accounting for 46% ($81.2 billion) and Medicaid accounting for 28% ($49.4 billion) of the health care expenditure. Government outlays for Physicians' Services amounting to $22.3 billion (70%) came predominantly from Medicare. The Medicaid Program, designed to supplement low income Americans of all ages, is becoming a program for the elderly with 59% of the nursing home bill paid by Medicaid and 3% of the bill paid by Medicare.

Between 1980 and 1987, the proportion of public and private payers remained constant. Private health insurers paid approximately 31% of the cost as compared to public insurers paying 40%. The remainder of the health care bill was borne by the self-paying consumer paying around 28%. (See Table 7-5.)

Increasing health care costs result from a number of factors affecting both the use and

❖ **Table 7-4**

Personal health care expenditures by type of payer and type of expenditure, 1987
(in billions of dollars)

| Source of payment | Total personal care | Hospital care | Physicians' services | Nursing home care | Other health services |
|---|---|---|---|---|---|
| Personal health care expenditures | $442.6 | $194.7 | $102.7 | $40.6 | $104.6 |
| Direct payments | 123.0 | 18.5 | 26.3 | 20.0 | 58.2 |
| Third party payments | 319.6 | 176.2 | 76.4 | 20.6 | 46.4 |
| Private health insurance | 139.1 | 71.9 | 44.6 | 0.4 | 22.2 |
| Other private funds | 5.3 | 2.2 | 0.1 | 0.3 | 3.0 |
| Government | 175.3 | 102.2 | 31.8 | 19.9 | 21.5 |
| Medicare | 81.2 | 53.3 | 22.3 | 0.6 | 5.1 |
| Medicaid | 49.4 | 17.8 | 4.4 | 11.8 | 6.0 |
| Other | 44.7 | 31.1 | 5.1 | 1.5 | 10.4 |

Detail may not add to totals due to rounding. From USDHHS, HCFA, *Health Care Financing Review,* Winter 1988.

❖ **Table 7-5**

Personal health care expenditures percent distribution by source of funds
(selected calendar years 1980-1987)

| Year | Total | Direct patient payments | Total third parties* | Private health insurance | Other private funds | Government Total | Federal | State and local | Medicare[†] | Medicaid[‡] |
|---|---|---|---|---|---|---|---|---|---|---|
| 1980 | 100.0 | 28.7 | 71.3 | 30.7 | 1.2 | 39.4 | 28.4 | 10.9 | 16.2 | 11.5 |
| 1983 | 100.0 | 28.2 | 71.8 | 31.1 | 1.3 | 39.4 | 29.5 | 9.9 | 18.3 | 10.8 |
| 1985 | 100.0 | 28.2 | 71.8 | 30.4 | 1.2 | 40.2 | 30.2 | 10.0 | 18.8 | 10.9 |
| 1987 | 100.0 | 27.8 | 72.2 | 31.4 | 1.2 | 39.6 | 29.6 | 10.0 | 18.4 | 11.2 |

*Total comes from private health insurance, other private funds and total government categories.
[†]Subset of federal funds.
[‡]Subset of federal and state and local funds.
From USDHHS, HCFA. Office of the Actuary and the Office of National Cost Estimates, 1988.

price components of cost. First, use has increased with the expanding elderly population, the rising supply of physicians, the increased use of medical technology, societal demands for access to care, and consumer separation from price concerns because of extensive health insurance coverage and pressure from the AIDS epidemic. Second, the price has risen because of the underlying inflation in the economy, purchaser indifference to price (until about 1981), increased intensity of services, and lack of some characteristics of other competitive markets, such as sufficient consumer information on costs.

## ❖ ECONOMIC TRENDS IN HEALTH CARE

Several intense pressures confront the economic dynamics of the health care system. Discussion follows on the inaccessibility of health care, the aging consumers, and cost containment efforts.

### The Inaccessibility of Health Care

In spite of the Great Society Programs designed to assist the nation's poor in the 1960s, the number of Americans without adequate health insurance has increased from 25 million in 1975 to nearly 40 million today (Pinkney, 1989; United Hospital Fund, 1986; Urban Institute, 1987). Of concern are the subgroups of the uninsured or underinsured population: 15 million women of reproductive age (The Alan Guttmacher Institute, 1987), 12 million individuals below the federal poverty line, (i.e., an annual income of approximately $12,000 for a family of four) (Chollet, 1987), 12 million individuals living in families with incomes of more than twice the poverty line (i.e., approximately $24,000 annually for a family of four) (Wilensky, 1988), 12 million children under 18 years (Johnson et al, 1988), and 29 million individuals working or residing in a home where someone

is working (Swartz, 1989; USDHHS, 1989). The uninsured and underinsured represent a diverse group including poor individuals ineligible for public benefits, unemployed or self-employed individuals who are uninsured, employees of small businesses that do not provide health insurance benefits, individuals over 65 years of age having health or long-term care costs exceeding Medicare reimbursement levels, others who have exhausted their health insurance benefits, and patients in high-risk categories who are uninsurable.

Several studies have further defined characteristics of the uninsured and underinsured population. The Urban Institute's study (1989) found that notable among the uninsured are those individuals who work. Seventy percent of the uninsured are full-time workers who earn low weekly wages and are employed primarily in the private sector, largely in the service, retail trade, construction, and agriculture, forestry, and fishing industries. The largest group of uninsured workers come from individuals aged 18 to 24 and 55 to 66 years. Haywood's comparison (1988) of the insured elderly (65 years or older) and working-age nonelderly found that the elderly had better access to medical care than the nonelderly. Among respondents with a medical illness, working-age nonelderly were 3.5 times as likely as the elderly to have needed supportive medical care, medications, or supplies and not to have received them, and 3.4 times as likely to have major financial problems because of their illness.

Solutions to this growing problem continue to challenge health care providers, consumers, and policymakers. Because access to health care is the problem of a diverse group, no one solution answers every need. Solutions must focus on individuals with incomes below the poverty level, on individuals having incomes between the poverty level and 200% of poverty, on individuals having no income restrictions, and on providers of health care who need adequate reimbursement for services (Glen,

1989b; Rich, 1990; Swartz & Lipson 1989; Wilensky, 1988). Prominent among suggestions for the access problem are the following:

Medicaid Reform: to create a national standard of uniform eligibility for all people below the federal poverty line and uniform minimum adequate benefits. Other proposals call for expanding Medicaid benefits for mothers and children, extending the Medicaid option for those leaving cash assistance programs to enter the work force, and creating a "buy-in" (i.e., low cost premium), to Medicaid for our nations near poor.

Formation of State Level Risk Pools: to provide coverage for consumers who find health care coverage unaffordable or unavailable.

Employer-Sponsored Coverage: to require that businesses offer health insurance to their employees.

Multiple Employer Trusts: to form coalitions of businesses and insurance companies, whereby health insurance premiums, especially for small businesses, may be reduced.

Raising the Minimum Wage: to provide those individuals who are working, but uninsured with more opportunity to purchase health insurance.

Subsidizing Hospitals for Care to Poor: to reimburse hospitals for the estimated $8 billion in uncompensated care they provide annually.

Earned Income Tax Credit: to supplement the salaries of those individuals who are working and unable to purchase health insurance.

Formation of a national health plan: to guarantee that all Americans would be insured by a public plan administered by the state and federal governments. Various proposals have been advanced by business, health, and legislative groups. The Canadian National Health Plan, a universal coverage program, has been proposed as a model. The Canadian Plan is attractive because this publicly funded program provides preventive, acute care and rehabilitative health care at a cost considerably lower than costs for these services in the United States.

Creation of special population programs: to provide direct care for those populations who are difficult to reach or who have special needs such as the homeless or high-risk, pregnant teenagers.

Until every American can have access to health care services, this issue will remain at the forefront of public policy debates. As supplies grow scarce, demand increases, and costs accelerate, the access problem will become even more complex.

## The Aging Consumers

By 2025, the number of individuals over 65 years will have doubled from its current level of 30 million. Already, our Medicare system is nearly buckling from the elderly's demands for health care costing our nation in 1986 some $74 billion (USDHHS 1987b; Cohen & Balanoff, 1987), but this amount represents less than half the health care bill for the elderly (National Health Policy Forum, 1987). The remainder is paid by Medicaid (13%), insurance providers (7%), other government programs (6%), and the individual in out-of-pocket costs (25%). Per capita, elderly Americans spent $4202 in 1986 with $1750 of that out-of-pocket for health and long-term care services (Dimond, 1989; National Health Policy Forum, 1987; U.S. Senate Special Committee on Aging, 1986).

With the elderly in 1986 consuming 29% of all personal health expenditures, that number will increase in the years ahead. A lengthening longevity has been accompanied by increases in the prevalence of chronic conditions among the elderly. Many older persons suffer from chronic, rather than acute illnesses. Between 1979 and 1985, the number of elderly persons reporting heart disease rose to 305.4 per 1000 from 274.4 per 1000. Increases were also experienced in other circulatory, respiratory, and digestive conditions (American Hospital Association, 1987). By 2003, the U.S. Department of Health (1987b) projects that individuals over 65 years will consume 26% of all physicians' services, 34% of the hospital care, and 90% of the nursing home care.

The burden on our nation in the 1990s is to define what role the public and private sectors will assume for health and long-term care of the elderly. Because a dramatic need exists for expanded health and long-term insurance plans for the elderly, their development is imminent. The hesitancy of public and private insurers to become involved in long-term care, however, will most likely remain until they can develop coverage plans that minimize the financial risk inherent in a most unpredictable population (i.e., length of life, type and intensity of illness and disability, and rehabilitative or supportive needs).

### The Cost Containment Efforts

In the three decades preceding 1980, demand for health care increased enormously, in part fueled by the spread of private health insurance plans that provided first-dollar coverage and cost-based reimbursement for hospital and physician care. Between the end of World War II and 1960, the number of individuals with hospital insurance increased from 32 million to 122 million, while coverage for physician's services leaped from fewer than 5 million to over 83 million individuals. In the 1960s, federal policymakers believed that the elderly and the poor should be entitled to the same kinds of health care as the middle class. The result was government-funded Medicare and Medicaid Programs for these special groups. Immediate changes on the demand side of health care were accompanied by substantial shifts in the supply of health care. To illustrate, the number of short-term hospital beds per 1000 population rose between 1950 to 1980 from 3.3 to 4.4 and the health care personnel ranks swelled from 1.8 to 2.1 per 1000. In addition, techno-

logical research and development were well-endowed by the National Institutes of Health, drug companies, and other private firms. Then, physicians in sharp control of health care used what hospital and specialists resources they deemed necessary for client care because the patient usually had insurance to cover these costs. The physicians had no financial incentives to use these resources efficiently since they did not lose money when unnecessary costs were incurred in treating the hospitalized client. As a result, spending for health care, which consumed 4.6 of the GNP in 1959 and 9.1 of the GNP in 1980, reflected that the highest quality of health care for all Americans dominated the health policy agenda (Fuchs, 1988).

Some uneasiness about health care costs crept into the mindsets of public and private sector policymakers during the 1970s. Then, a barrage of governmental controls dominated the health care scene with reductions in Medicare and Medicaid reimbursement, establishment of professional standards review organizations (PSROs) in 1972, and creation of health system agencies (HSAs) that planned and supposedly controlled health resources in 1974. At the federal level, the stage was set for competition with legislation in 1973 and 1977 supporting the expansion of the few existing HMOs (Brown, 1986). To counter the government-imposed regulations, a coalition of the American Hospital Association, the American Medical Association, and the Federation of American Hospitals in 1978 instituted the Voluntary Effort Plan to reduce hospital cost inflation to a level of 11.6% by 1979. The Plan was successful in 1978, but utterly failed by surpassing the target inflation rate in 1979 (Estaugh, 1981). As a result, cost containment fever was reaching a high. Other strategies needed to be introduced. Fueling a pro-competition strategy was a widespread dislike for national health insurance proposals that were surfacing and a belief that deregulation, which was working so well in the transportation, trucking, and banking industries, might work in the health care industry (Brown, 1983; Fuchs, 1988).

The 1980s brought forth a whole host of new activities in both the public and private sectors. Concern shifted from increasing access and raising quality to curbing the skyrocketing costs of health care. Even businesses and the insurance industry became involved in the cost war. Businesses, including health care providers, could no longer shift rising health care costs to their consumers because it was making them less attractive to consumers. Health insurance companies were caught in a similar bind, having to limit what costs they could pass on in premium increases (Tibbits, 1983).

The pervading philosophy called for stimulating competition to allocate health resources. Competition, it was believed, would curb the cost of health care by allowing the market place to dictate the cost and use of services. The aim was to keep businesses, insurance companies, and health care providers under constant pressure to provide care at lower costs (Estaugh, 1981; Sandrick, 1987). In the public sector, the initiatives to directly cut costs, increase competition, or both, included a number of Medicare and Medicaid cutbacks in 1981, creation of block grants (i.e., program-specific funding such as maternal-child grants) for certain health programs in 1981, Medicare's Prospective Payment System (PPS) based on Diagnostic Related Groupings (DRGs) (i.e., payment based on diagnosis) in 1983, enrollment of public program beneficiaries in capitated plans (i.e., payment of premium entitles policy holder to designated levels of health promotion, acute care, and rehabilitative services) in 1983, provisions of health insurance for the unemployed in 1983, and a Medicare physician fee freeze in 1984. Private sector activities included growing enrollments in HMOs and PPOs, increased cost sharing in private employment-based health insurance plans, and expanded utilization review.

Major corporations began managing their own insurance plans, rather than using insurance companies. Providers were asked to bid competitively for service contracts. A host of alternatives to inpatient hospitals such as ambulatory care centers, aftercare nursing facilities, hospices, and geriatric outpatient centers emerged (Brown, 1986; Long & Welch, 1988).

So what happened to costs? Not much. The overall growth of health expenditures per capita was more rapid after 1980 than in the previous decade. The growth in hospital expenditure rates, however, was curtailed, but expenditures for physicians' services grew at a faster rate from 1980 to 1986 than in the period following the introduction of Medicare and Medicaid. Spending for dental care, other professional services, drugs/sundries, and program administration also increased in the 1980s. A small curtailment in expenditures was noted for nursing home payments and government public health expenditures. Within the business community, health insurance premiums increased between 15% and 40% annually (Sandrick, 1987). Overall, it can be concluded that the cost-saving interventions mainly sought savings through reductions in waste and inappropriate use of health care services. The interventions did little about deeper cost-increasing forces such as demographic trends, technology, and consumers' patterns.

Cost containment efforts, however, had several major effects on the quantity of health care delivered. The number of hospital admissions decreased instead of rising rapidly like during the 1970s. Due to the expansion of HMOs and implementation of prospective payment systems initiated by Medicare, Medicaid, and some private payers, the length of stay in hospitals substantially declined. Also, admissions to hospitals declined to a level lower than during the 1970s. For the total U.S. population, the 1985 discharge rate of 148 per 1000 clients hospitalized in short-term general hospitals was the lowest since 1971 and represented a reduction of over 10% since 1980. Within the managed care arena, a greater proportion of the general population (from 5% in 1980 to 12% in 1986) enrolled in the HMO health plans. The impact of increased managed care membership had a significant effect on the delivery of health care because HMO members typically use only about two thirds as much hospitalization as non-HMO members. Group Health Association of America (1987) reports that in 1986, HMO members under 65 years were hospitalized 320 days per 1000 HMO enrollees as compared to 692 for the general population.

Also, the cost containment efforts affected the distribution of health care. To illustrate, the population can no longer gain access to new technologies at their demand. Clients insured with Medicare have become victims of the early hospital discharges associated with the Prospective Payment System. Some population groups such as the poor, the chronically ill, high-risk pregnant women, children, and residents in rural areas may be forced to postpone or avoid health care because costs have risen. Now, ethical decisions about containing costs may interfere with determining the choice, initiation, and cessation of treatment (Health Care Quality Alliance, 1988). Premiums are now tied more closely to one's health status instead of to cross subsidies, and use has been reduced by increasing deductibles and copayments (Fuchs, 1988). The impact on the quality of health care has been called into question (Office of Technology Assessment, 1988). Overall, consumers are theoretically more removed from quality health care than they were one decade ago.

In the future, cost containment efforts will continue in even broader and bolder directions. Because health care is becoming highly technologically driven, cost containment will be exceedingly difficult to achieve. In the long run, technology, more than anything else, drives the cost of health care. To slow spending, it is necessary to slow the growth of services. The demand for services by clients can be affected by

deductibles and coinsurance, since it is likely that third-party payments will always predominate. The major constraints on services must come from the supply side, the number of physicians, their specialty distribution, their training, the incentives they face, and most importantly, the facilities and technology at their disposal. As health care providers, policymakers, and consumers wrestle with these issues, one thing is certain: the decade of the 1990s, even more than previous decades, will present intense challenges to balance health care costs, quality of health care, and accessibility of health care for all Americans.

## ❖ APPLICATION OF ECONOMICS TO NURSING PRACTICE

The application of economic theory to nursing practice is one of the challenges nurses face as they become more active players in the health care policy arena. By applying economic concepts, we will become more proficient in analyzing health care delivery problems, proposing solutions, and articulating the nursing role in the restructuring of the health care delivery system.

Microeconomics would be a substantial addition to the baccalaureate curriculum in nursing education, because it could be readily applied in the practice setting as nurses deal with the rapidly changing system and struggle to define their role. With a basic understanding of economic concepts (such as scarcity, supply and demand, opportunity costs, substitutes and complements, and elasticity), nurses will be better equipped to analyze and respond to issues affecting their clinical practice, education, and research.

### Scarcity, Choice, and Rationing

"Economic theory is developed from basic postulates about how individual human beings behave, struggle with the problem of scarcity, and respond to change" (Gwartney, 1980, p. 3). The two fundamental ingredients of the economic approach are scarcity and choice. Because of high costs and limited availability, health care services are a scarce commodity, and therefore choices must be made about the types of services needed and the types of professionals to provide the services.

Nurses in the practice setting are often involved in these choices. "Wallet biopsies" are increasing before the delivery of services, and in some settings nurses may be inadvertently put in a position of denying care because the client does not have insurance coverage or out-of-pocket payment. Therefore, care is being rationed on the basis of ability to pay in this country, and nurses are often caught in the middle of this phenomenon. Karen Mitchell, PhD, RN (1989) stated, "I doubt any of us find the idea of rationing health care admirable or appealing. Yet our disjointed, expensive nonsystem of illness care does just that."

John Kitzhaber, MD, engineer of the proposed Oregon rationing plan, explains that "We blindly ration people while maintaining an increasingly rich benefit package for the shrinking number of people who remain eligible. And this constitutes rationing of the very worst kind—rationing that reflects no social policy, which has no ethical clinical basis, which is being done silently, implicitly, and by default" (Salzman, 1989, p. 1).

Nurses often experience the results of our system of "rationing on the basis of ability to pay" when they deal with complications that could have been prevented if the client had sought care earlier. This phenomenon is seen by nurses in the practice setting and is often the consequence of a client being uninsured or underinsured, a condition shared by an estimated 40 million people in the United States.

The 1987 decision by the state of Oregon to forego the funding of organ transplantation in favor of expanding Medicaid to include more people is an example of rationing based on social policy and health care priorities rather than the ability to pay. In 1989, the Oregon legislature passed Senate Bill 27, which formalized the process by passing legislation to provide health care for all low-income Oregonians. It established a Health Services Commission to recommend a prioritized list of health services, ranging from the most important to the least important, based on the positive effects each service has on the entire population, not just on a portion of it. "In this case, the rationing method is being changed from one that excludes patients to one that excludes services" (Welch, 1989).

Because of their familiarity with the needs of clients and the health care delivery system, nurses are in a unique position to help establish these priorities; fortunately, a public health nurse is one of the Oregon Health Services Commission members along with five physicians, four consumers, and a social worker. Too frequently, nurses are not represented on health policy commissions, such as the National Leadership Commission on Health Care and two health policy commissions recently established by the Bush Administration (the Social Security Advisory Committee and Health and Human Services Task Force). Although some may contend that the proportion of nurses to physicians is not adequate, the Oregon Commission is progressive in that there is nurse representation.

## Supply and Demand

The report of the Secretary's Commission on Nursing (USDHHS, 1988b) is a good example of the application of economic concepts to analyze and address one of nursing's pressing problems, the nursing shortage. The economic concepts of supply and demand were used to illustrate that the current shortage of RNs is primarily the result of an increase in demand as opposed to a contraction of supply. This analysis and conclusion by the Secretary's Commission on Nursing gave direction to hospitals and other agencies that had been increasing the demand by using registered nurses for nonnursing functions. Most hospitals have heeded the recommendation of the Secretary's Commission and are altering their use of nursing resources, preserving the time of the nurse for direct care of clients and families by providing adequate staffing levels for clinical and nonclinical support services (USDHHS, 1988a).

## Opportunity Costs

Opportunity costs, another economic concept, is applied by nurses, often unknowingly on a daily basis. "Opportunity costs are the highest valued benefits that must be sacrificed (foregone) as a result of choosing an alternative" (Gwartney, 1980, p. 22). It is what you give up to have something else. Because health care resources are limited, opportunity costs must be considered. The opportunity cost of maintaining and increasing highly technological, medical model services has been the sacrifice of the quantity or quality of primary care, preventive, and health promotion services. One of the major factors driving up medical costs in this country is the proliferation of expensive technology; in comparison, expenditures on prevention are very low, about 1% of the federal health budget. Nurses are traditionally proponents of prevention and health promotion, and nurses must continue to be the voice of reason by urging a redistribution of health care spending to provide more resources for health promotion.

In a similar manner under the rubric of opportunity costs, nurses as advocates of the "whole person" are appropriate providers to put health care spending in perspective to other domestic expenditures. Expenditures for medical care are particularly large as compared with other domestic expenditures that may ultimately have a greater impact on health, such as those for food stamps, housing, and education. Although they represent only 14% of federal outlays overall, medical expenditures now account for 126% of the income-security programs. If Social Security is excluded from the calculation, health care makes up a commanding 56% of the resulting "safety net" (Palmer, 1988). Nurses have fewer vested economic interests in preserving the status quo of medical spending in this country and therefore are in a better position than other medical providers to objectively evaluate and recommend changes in social services spending that do not reflect a special interest group bias but take into account a holistic approach to the needs of people. If additional funds come from other budgets (such as defense) or new revenues (such as taxes), it is important to consider that there are ways other than high-tech medical care to spend them—such as providing housing to the 100,000 children who are homeless (Institute of Medicine, 1988). Community health nurses frequently become frustrated when, for a poor family, they can access a CAT scan for a headache more easily than eliminating rats in a baby's crib at night. Nurses are often more able to see the "big picture" of human need because they are closer to the clients than other providers, and therefore policymakers may find them to be excellent resources and the voice of reason in helping prioritize the use of social resources.

The United States is spending over $600 billion yearly on medical care services. Most Americans think we are spending too much. They want greater value for the medical care dollar. In the explorations by the National Leadership Commission on Health Care, it was revealed that a substantial proportion of the medical dollar is not being used effectively. Dr. Arnold S. Relman, editor of *The New England Journal of Medicine* and a commission advisor, states: "It's a widespread impression and I'm convinced it's true that, as a conservative figure, 15% and maybe as much as 30% of what we now buy is not worth the money" (Knox, 1989).

Nurses are in a unique position to get involved in research exploring the effectiveness of medical and health care and to propose ways to increase the value of the health care dollar. Spending more on health care may not be the answer; exploring ways to redistribute spending to increase "the bang for the buck" is probably a more realistic approach.

### Substitutes and Complements

A related approach toward increasing the value of the health care dollar is to use health care providers more efficiently. "Evidence indicates that nurse practitioners, physician assistants, and certified nurse midwives have positive influences on quality of health care and access to services, and that they could increase productivity and save costs" (U.S. Congress, OTA, 1986).

However, how these health care providers and other nurse providers are used in the health care delivery system can increase or negate their cost-effectiveness. Griffith (1984) applied the economic concepts of substitutes and complements to the relationship between nurses and physical services to illustrate the importance of appropriate use of nurse providers in expanded roles. She demonstrated that if nursing services are seen as substitutes for physician services rather than complements, an increase in price of physician services will cause an increase in demand for nursing services. If nurses are reimbursed directly for their services by payers (including third party payers or insurers), the lower payment for services performed by nurses, as compared to the same services performed by physicians would result in lower costs for the same service. On the other hand, if other providers such as physicians received payment for the services performed by nurses, the cost in most cases would remain the same as if the physician performed the service. The

profit would be made by the middleman in this transaction, the physician.

### Elasticity

Elasticity is another concept that can be used as an example of how economics theory can be applied to nursing issues. When the demand for a product decreases substantially in response to a small rise in price, the demand is relatively elastic (elasticity coefficient is greater than 1). "Nearly all health economists believe that the price elasticity of demand for (medical) care is smaller than one, but none believes it is zero" (Fuchs, 1982, p. 79).

However, the elasticity of physician services may be increasing. Whereas in the past consumers perceived few options for physician services regardless of price, the recent demystification of medical services and availability of other types of care and self-care are causing some consumers to balk at rapidly increasing prices of medical services and to look for other types of care and providers when appropriate. Also because nursing services are increasingly viewed as substitutes for some physician services, elasticity of physician services may be increasing.

In a similar manner, demand for the services of registered nurses may be becoming more inelastic. A recent Health Care Financing study (Hartz, et. al., 1989) indicated that mortality rates were lower in hospitals with a greater percentage of registered nurses. As hospitals recognize that unregistered nurses cannot be substituted for registered nurses without jeopardizing quality of care, the demand for registered nurses will become more inelastic.

### ❖ NURSING RESEARCH ON ECONOMICS

Health services research, nursing systems projects, and studies on reimbursement for nursing services are three interrelated categories of nursing research on economics. The federal funding agencies most concerned with these areas of research are the National Center for Health Services Research and the National Center for Nursing Research.

According to the Institute of Medicine (1979, p. 14), health services research is "an inquiry to produce knowledge about the structure, processes, or effects of personal health services." Two criteria must be satisfied. Studies must relate to structure, process, or effects of personal health services and have a conceptual framework other than applied biomedical science. The National Center for Nursing Research categorizes nursing systems research as that which examines the environment in which nursing care is delivered and includes projects that investigate promising approaches to nursing management and nursing care delivery. Some examples are investigations of the outcome of home care, long-term care and/or hospital care; the identification of the mechanisms responsible for different outcomes in various care settings; the development and refinement of methods to improve the delivery of nursing care in underserved areas; the development of innovative approaches to the delivery of nursing care in nursing homes, including investigation of alternatives to nursing home care; factors underlying the quality of nursing care; assessment of the cost of providing nursing care; development of models to illustrate effective collaboration among nurses, physicians, and other members of the health team; the articulation of issues concerning the application of prospective payment systems as they relate to the provision of nursing care; and the use of automation to improve the effectiveness of nursing care.

## Health Services Research and Nursing Systems Projects

Prefacing remarks on nursing research, Aiken (1988) states that there are three strate-

gies that appear to dominate health care cost-containment: increasing productivity and efficiency, limiting the growth of wages and prices, and reducing the amount of care provided. She thinks that the third strategy has the greatest potential to cut costs. To reduce the amount of care provided without adversely affecting clients, we must target reductions in health care systems areas with types of interventions that do not adversely affect clients. So far, health care policymakers have been making across-the-board cuts, such as reducing hospital length of stay on all patients, rather than targeting any particular group of clients. "My question is whether nursing research can document some promising areas where reductions in length of stay might actually be good, and thus target more effectively our efforts to reduce hospital care which, of course, is the most expensive part of our health care system," states Aiken (p. 5). Brooten's (1986) study on the earlier discharge of low-birth-weight infants to a nurse home visiting program is an example of how we could target an area and save $20,000 per infant and improve outcome. Other studies of this type could further demonstrate how reductions in care could actually be targeted to achieve beneficial outcomes as well as protecting clients against iatrogenic outcomes. This could lead to rationing based on research and policy rather than on ability to pay.

There has been surprisingly little research done on nurse supply and demand considering the frequency and severity of nurse shortages that have plagued the health care system. Aiken and Mullinix (1987) demonstrated the inverse relationship between relative wages and hospital nurse vacancy rates over the past 25 years. However, Aiken (1988) also points out that the lack of wage response to the shortage during the last few years indicated that "nurses must be in a captured labor market, that the laws of supply and demand don't operate" (p. 9). Her first suggestion in this regard was for nursing research funding to support a cadre of researchers to study nurse labor market issues over the long run so that we will have more data the next time we have a cyclical shortage. Second, if nurses are in a labor market that's not adjusting, are there policy interventions that we should research that would minimize the adverse impact that creates this shortage? Third, Aiken suggests cross-industry studies to examine the solutions found by other 24-hour businesses to the kind of problems faced by hospitals.

Mullinix (1988) points out that most nurse labor market studies were based on data from the early 1970s (i.e., Bognanno, Hixon & Jeffers, 1974; Link & Settle, 1979, 1980, 1981a, 1981b; *Sloan & Richupan,* 1975) when the labor force participation of women was much less than today. In addition to updated studies in this area, she concurs with Aiken that long-term studies are needed. "No long-term sustained efforts exist to help explain remuneration effects on nurses' labor as exist for other labor markets" (p. 12).

The interrelationship between research and policy is demonstrated in the case of the elimination of the Medicare routine nursing salary cost differential (MRND). When Medicare was enacted, a 2% bonus was added to hospital cost reimbursement. This was discontinued in 1969. However, in 1971, hospitals convinced policymakers to reenact an 8.5% Medicare differential for nursing salaries to cover the additional care required by Medicare clients as compared to other patients; this restored about half the loss from the 2% bonus. However, considering Congress' subsequent desire to cut Medicare costs, they used as evidence a study conducted by Fitzmaurice (Mullinix, 1988) which did not support a MRND. Congress voted to eliminate it completely. Mullinix (1988) makes the case that since the enactment of the prospective payment system and DRGs, length of stay and admissions have dropped, Medicare clients are sicker and require more nursing care, and therefore, if the Fitzmaurice study were conducted today, it might support an MRND. The need for more nursing research to substantiate policy changes proposed by nurses is clear.

## Studies on Reimbursement for Nursing Services

More research related to nursing reimbursement is needed to assist policymakers as they deliberate reform of payment policies for health care providers. One of the areas currently being explored relates to the degree to which nurses perform services coded in the Current Procedural Terminology (CPT) manual (Griffith & Fonteyn, 1989). CPT codes are being used by policymakers involved in physician payment reform because payments made to physicians are coded using the CPT system. It is unknown at this time the degree to which nurses perform CPT coded services (e.g., the services for which physicians are paid). However, this information would be made available to policymakers as they consider physician payment reform. This should enable them to take all providers in consideration, not just physicians, when reforming payment policy (Griffith, 1989; Ott, Griffith, & Towers, 1989).

Research must be done on the ways in which various methods of reimbursing nurses in expanded roles affects client outcomes and costs (Jacox, 1988). Very few studies on reimbursement for nursing services by third party payers have been conducted in spite of the continuing efforts by the nursing profession in the legislative arena to enable direct third party reimbursement for nursing services. In a study conducted by Griffith (1986), four years after legislation was passed enabling direct third party reimbursement for nurse practitioner (NP) services in Maryland, 2% of NPs were being reimbursed on a fee-for-service basis, and less than 1% of eligible NPs had received direct third-party reimbursement. In Oregon, 7 years after enactment of similar legislation, 13% of NPs were being reimbursed on a fee-for-service basis, and 21% had received direct third-party reimbursement. The percentage of NPs responding that their charges were less than physician charges was three times greater in Oregon than in Maryland. In Oregon, clients and third-party payers were generally charged less for visits to NPs who received direct payment than for visits to salaried NPs. The difference between the charges for short initial visits and brief follow-up visits was statistically significant. These preliminary studies indicate that direct third-party reimbursement for nursing services may reduce health care charges without reducing quality of care since the Office of Technology Assessment (U.S. Congress, OTA, 1986) has concluded that the overall quality of care provided by NPs in their areas of expertise is comparable to that provided by physicians.

## ❖ SUMMARY

Economics in health care represents a delicate relationship among the supply, demand, and costs of health care. An understanding of these concepts as they relate to the past and present health care system can serve as a framework to project changes in the future health care system. Supply of health care refers to the amount of health care facilities, personnel, and financing available to consumers. Supply levels are constantly changing because of technological discoveries, costs for services, consumer demands, level of competition in the marketplace, and effect of government regulations. Demand for health care indicates what health care the consumer requires and is willing to purchase. The demand level revolves around consumer needs and desires, costs of health care, treatment selections ordered by health care providers, and general societal needs. Costs for health care reflect any financial expenditures contributed by consumers or providers to deliver and receive health care. Factors influencing the cost of health care are numerous, ranging from consumer demands to advancements in medical technology to the status of the nation's economy.

All these economic dynamics are changing.

The growing numbers of Americans lacking third-party insurance coverage has resulted in numerous public and private initiatives to solve this very complex, multidimensional problem. The access issue takes on new meaning when one considers that in the next century, the United States will have a very large elderly population. Concern arises about how health and long-term care will be made available to the elderly. As the nation wrestles with these and other issues, the need to contain health care costs becomes urgent. Plagued with soaring health care expenditures for the past two decades, the private and public sectors have implemented numerous regulatory and competition driven measures to ward off these escalating costs for health care. Except for some structural changes in the health care system such as the growth of managed health care plans, these cost containment approaches have had little effect on costs.

Greater application of economic theory to nursing practice could enable nurses to become more proficient in analyzing health care delivery problems, proposing solutions, and articulating the nursing care role. Examples of economic concepts that are relevant to nursing practice include scarcity, supply and demand, opportunity costs, substitutes and complements, and elasticity. Nurses are in a unique position to become leaders in policy related to rationing of health care resources and by targeting nursing research accordingly, they can also provide the scientific basis for some of those policy decisions. There are many situations in nursing practice that can be analyzed by using the economic concepts of supply and demand; some of the solutions of the nursing shortage proposed by the Secretary's Commission on Nursing used these and other concepts. The basic economic concept, opportunity costs, can be used by nurses as they help policymakers prioritize social resources and put health care in perspective. The concepts substitutes and complements help explain the relationship between nurses and physicians as well as ways to improve it. And elasticity can be applied to increase understanding of the relationships between the price of health care services and the demand for physician and nursing services as well as the relationship between supply of nurses and wages.

Nursing research on economic concepts, such as the above examples, will enable nurses to contribute to health economics theory and provide the basis for nursing proposals related to health care system restructuring. More health services research related to nursing issues, nursing systems projects, and studies on reimbursement for nursing services are needed to improve patient care and the health care delivery system by demonstrating the more cost-effective use of nursing care.

## ❖ APPLYING KNOWLEDGE TO PRACTICE

1. Discuss the economic concepts of supply, demand and costs of health care as they relate to nursing practice.
2. Do you think that nurses in practice ought to be concerned with economic issues related to health care? Why or why not?
3. What are the implications for the nursing profession of the issues of:
   a. health care inaccessibility
   b. aging consumers
   c. cost containment
4. How can nurses in clinical practice become involved in decisions regarding the rationing of health care delivery resources and services? What suggestions do you have for restructuring the health care delivery system to address problems associated with access to care, cost, reimbursement, and quality of care?

## REFERENCES

Aiken, L. (1988). Assuring the delivery of quality patient care: Keynote address. *State of the science invitational conference: Nursing resources and the delivery of patient care,* NIH Publication 89-3008, Bethesda, MD.

Aiken, L. H. & Mullinix, C. F. (1987). The nurse shortage: Myth or reality? *The New England Journal of Medicine, 317*(10), 641–646.

American Hospital Association (1987). *The aging U.S. population and its impact on health care use and expense.* Chicago: AHA.

Bognanno, M., Hixson, J., & Jeffers, J. (1974). The short-run supply of nurses' time: New evidence. *Journal of Human Resources, 9*(1), 80–94.

Brooten, D. et al. (1986). A randomized clinical trial of early hospital discharge and home following of very-low-birthweight infants. *The New England Journal of Medicine, 315,* 934–939, October 9.

Brown, L. (1983). Competition and health care policy: Experience and expectations. *Annals, AAPPS, 468,* 48–59.

Brown, L. (1986). Introduction to a decade of transition. *Journal of Health Politics, Policy and Law, 11*(4), 569–580.

Byrns, R. T. & Stone, G. W. (1987). *Economics.* Glenview, IL: Scott, Foresman.

Chollet, D. (1987). *Uninsured in the United States: The nonelderly population without health insurance.* Washington, DC: Employee Benefit Research Institutes.

Cohen, W. J. & Balanoff, J. H. (1987). Safeguarding our benefits. *Harvard Journal of Public Policy,* Winter Spring, pp. 24–26.

Dimond, M. (1989). Health care and the aging population. *Nursing Outlook, 37*(2), 76–77.

Eastaugh, S. R. (1981). *Medical economics and health finance.* Boston: Auburn House Publishing Co.

Feldstein, P. J. (1983). *Health care economics,* (2nd Ed.). New York: John Wiley and Sons.

Fuchs, V. R. (1976). Concepts on health, an economist's perspective. *The Journal of Medicine and Philosophy. 1*(3) 229–237.

Fuchs, V. R. (1982). Economics, health and post-industrial society. In R. Luke & J. Bauer (Eds.), *Issues in health economics.* Hagerstown, MD: Aspen Systems.

Fuchs, V. R. (1988). The "competition revolution" in health care. *Health Affairs, 7*(3), 5–24.

Glenn, K. J. (1989a). Coming up short: Hospitals seek workers. *Medicine and Health Perspectives,* June 12.

Glenn, K. J. (1989b). Uninsured take the spotlight. *Medicine and Health Perspectives,* February 13.

Griffith, H. (1984). Nursing practice: Substitute or complement according to economic theory. *Nursing Economics, 2,* 105–112.

Griffith, H. 1986. Implementation of direct third party reimbursement legislation for nursing services. *Nursing Economics, 4*(6), 299–304.

Griffith, H. (1989). Physician payment reform: Implications for nurses. *Nursing Economics, 4*(7), 231–233.

Griffith, H. & Fonteyn, M. (1989). Setting the payment record straight. *American Journal of Nursing, 89*(8), 1051–1058.

Group Health Association of America (1987). *HMO industry trends.* Washington, DC: GHAA.

Gwartney, S. (1980). *Microeconomics: Private and public choice.* New York: Academic Press.

Hartz, A. et al (1989). Hospital characteristics and mortality rates. *The New England Journal of Medicine, 321*(25), 1720–1725.

Haywood, R. A. (1988). Inequities in health services among insured Americans. *The New England Journal of Medicine,* June 9.

Health Care Quality Alliance (1988). *Quality health care: Critical issues before the nation.* Washington, DC: Health Care Quality Alliance.

Health Insurance Association of America (1989). *Source book of health insurance data—1989.* Washington, DC: HIAA.

Hendershot, G. E. (1988). Health status and medical care utilization. *Health Affairs, 7*(2), 114–121.

Hicks, L. L. & Boles, K. E. (1984). Why health economics? *Nursing Economics, 2*(3), 175–180.

Huge gain in health care jobs (1989). *Health Week,* February 6.

Institute of Medicine (1979). *Health services research.* (IOM Publication 78-06). Washington, DC: National Academy of Sciences.

Institute of Medicine, Committee on Health Care to Homeless People (1988). *Homelessness, health and human needs.* Washington, DC: National Academy Press.

Interstudy (1989). *The Interstudy Edge.* Minneapolis: Interstudy.

Jacox, A. (1988). Research on the influence of expanding clinical roles and opportunities on nursing resources. *State of the science invitational conference: Nursing resources and the delivery of patient care.* NIH Publication 89-3008. Bethesda, MD: USDHHS.

Johnson, C. M., Sum, A. M., & Weill, J. D. (1988). *Vanishing dreams: The growing economic plight of America's young families.* Washington, DC: Children's Defense Fund and Center for Labor Market Studies, Northeastern University.

Kindig, D. A. & Movassaghi, H. (1989). The adequacy of physician supply in small rural counties. *Health Affairs, 8*(3), 63–76.

Knox, R. (1989). Panel urges sweeping overhaul of US health care. *The Boston Globe,* January 31.

Link, C. & Settle, R. (1979). Labor supply responses of married professional nurses: New evidence. *Journal of Human Resources, 14*(2), 256–266.

Link, C. & Settle, R. (1980). Financial incentives and labor supply of married professional nurses: An economic analysis. *Nursing Research, 29*(4), 238–243.

Link, C. & Settle, R. (1981a). Wage incentives and married professional nurses: A case of backward-bending supply? *Economic Inquiry, 19,* 144–156.

Link, C. & Settle, R. (1981b). A simultaneous-equation model of labor supply, fertility and earnings of married women: The case of registered nurses. *Southern Economics Journal, 47,* 977–989.

Long, S. H. & Welch, W. P. (1988). Are we containing costs or pushing on a balloon? *Health Affairs, 7*(4), 112–117.

Marion Laboratories (1988). *Marion managed care digest—PPO edition—1988.* Kansas City: Marion Laboratories, Inc.

Mitchell, K. (1989). Editorial: Rationally rationing health care effectiveness research by another name? *Nursing Economics, 7*(6), 289.

Mullinix, C. (1988). Research on influences affecting availability of resources for patient care delivery. *State of the science invitational conference: Nursing resources and the delivery of patient care.* NIH publication 89-3008, Bethesda, MD: USDHHS.

National Health Policy Forum (1987). *Medicare beneficiary burdens: Out of pocket health care costs.* Washington, DC: The George Washington University.

Office of Technology Assessment (1988). *The quality of medical care.* Washington, DC: Government Printing Office.

Ott, B., Griffith, H., & Towers, J. (1989). Who gets the money? *American Journal of Nursing, 89*(2), 186–187.

Palmer, J. (1988). *Income security in America: Urban institute report 88-3.* Washington, DC: Urban Institute Press.

Phelps, E. S. (1985). *Political economy.* New York: W. W. Norton & Co.

Pinkney, D. S. (1989). Health care access for uninsured named a priority. *American Medical News,* December 15.

Rich, S. (1990). Unraveling the mystery of the working poor. *The Washington Post National Weekly Edition,* January 1–7, p. 38.

Robbins, L. C. (1935). *An essay on the nature and significance of economic science.* London: MacMillan.

Salzman, E. (1989). Oregon prescribes a cure for national health need. *Los Angeles Times,* part V, pp. 1, 6.

Sandrick, K. (1987). Will 1988 be the year of price competition? *Hospitals,* December 20.

Sloan, R. & Richupan, M. (1975). Short-run supply responses of professional nurses: A microanalysis. *Journal of Human Resources. 10*(2), 241–57.

Sorkin, A. L. (1984). *Health economics: An introduction.* Lexington, MA: Lexington Books.

Swartz, K. (1989). *The medically uninsured: Special focus on workers, a chartbook,* Washington, DC: The Urban Institute.

Swartz, K. & Lipson, D. (1989). *Strategies for assisting the medically uninsured.* Washington, DC: The Urban Institute.

Tibbits, S. J. (1983). *The future of health care delivery.* The Third Annual Lester Breslow Distinguished Lectureship, UCLA School of Public Health, Los Angeles.

The Alan Guttmacher Institute (1987). *Blessed events and the bottom line: Financing maternity care in the United States.* New York: The Alan Guttmacher Institute.

The Robert Wood Johnson Foundation (1987). *Access to health care, special report.* Princeton, NJ: The Robert Wood Johnson Foundation.

United Hospital Fund (1986). *Presidents' letter.* New York: United Hospital Fund.

Urban Institute (1987). Unpublished analysis of 1986 current population survey data. Washington, DC: Urban Institute.

Urban Institute (1989). *Workers without health insurance.* Washington, DC: The Urban Institute.

U.S. Department of Commerce (1989). *U.S. industrial outlook, 1989.* Washington, DC: Government Printing Office.

USDHHS (1989). *A profile of uninsured Americans.* Wash-

ington, DC: The National Medical Expenditure Survey, National Center for Health Services Research and Health Care Technology Assessment, Publication No. (PHS) 89-3443.

USDHHS (1987a). *1987 health care financing administration statistics.* Washington, DC: Health Care Financing Administration, Bureau of Data Management and Strategy, Pub. No. 03252.

USDHHS (1987b). *Changing mortality patterns, health services utilization, and health care expenditures: United States 1978–2003.* Washington, DC: Government Printing Office.

USDHHS (1988a). *Health care financing review, 9*(2).

USDHHS (1988b). *Secretary's commission on nursing,* final report, volumes I and II. Washington DC: U.S. Government Printing Office.

USDHHS (1989). National health care expenditures—1987. Washington, DC: Health Care Financing Administration, Office of the Actuary, Division of National Cost Estimates.

USDHHS (1989). *Health, United States—1988.* Washington, DC: Government Printing Office.

U.S. Congress, Office of Technology Assessment [OTA] (1986). *Nurse practitioners, physician assistants and certified nurse midwives: A policy analysis.* Washington, DC: U.S. Government Printing Office.

U.S. Senate Special Committee on Aging (1986). *Aging America: Trends and projections, 1985–86.* Washington, DC: The Senate.

Welch, H. (1989). Health care tickets for the uninsured— first class, coach or standby? *The New England Journal of Medicine, 321*(18), 1261–1264.

Wilensky, G. R. (1988). Filling the gaps in health insurance: Impact on competition. *Health Affairs, 7*(3), 133–149.

# 8

# Legal Relationships in Nursing Practice

Carmelle Pellerin Cournoyer

## OBJECTIVES

*At the completion of this chapter, the reader will be able to:*

- ◆ **Identify the constitutional basis for the state regulation of nursing practice and examine the purpose, power, and process of the state board of nursing practice.**
- ◆ **Define the essential elements of a contract and examine the three types of nurse-employer relationships.**
- ◆ **Describe the areas of tort liability that surround nursing practice and examine examples of litigation in each area.**

Law is defined as a social contract designed to assist people in ordering their society, organizing their affairs, and settling their problems; it sets the standard for human conduct and provides an alternative to confusion and force (Cournoyer, 1989). The function of law is to create and interpret legal relationships. It is easier to understand this function if the concept of law is divided into the two broad areas of public law and private law. *Public law* defines and interprets the relationship between the individual and the government. The major categories of public law are constitutional law, administrative law, and criminal law. *Private law* defines and interprets the relationship between individuals. The two major categories of private law are contract law and tort law.

All these areas of law have an effect on the practice of nursing. The clients' and the nurses' constitutional rights and remedies are defined by constitutional law. *Administrative law* determines the licensing and regulation of nursing practice as well as areas such as collective bargaining. *Criminal law* usually involves the nurse as a witness. However, it can also involve the nurse as a defendant who is accused of a criminal offense. *Contract law* identifies the three common types of employer-employee relationships and determines the risks and protections inherent in each type of relationship. *Tort law* is concerned with the reparation of wrongs or injuries inflicted by one person on another. It defines the legal liability for the practice of nursing and identifies the elements that are essential for each tort. The areas of tort liability that affect nursing practice include negligence, assault and battery, invasion of privacy, false imprisonment, and libel and slander.

Legal concepts, legal expectations, and legal consequences surround the practice of nursing. An examination of all these areas is be-yond the scope of this chapter. However, it is possible to identify and discuss the fundamental legal relationships that underlie the practice of nursing. This chapter will examine the nurse/state relationship, the nurse/employer relationship, and the nurse/patient relationship.

### ❖ NURSE/STATE RELATIONSHIP

The relationship between the nurse and the state originates in constitutional law. The Tenth Amendment to the U.S. Constitution permits states to enact legislation in any area that is not prohibited by the U.S. Constitution or pre-empted by federal law (U.S. Constitution). Each state constitution contains a Health and Welfare Clause that allows the legislature to enact leg-islation to protect the health and welfare of its citizens. In 1889, the Supreme Court ruled that occupational licensing was a valid exercise of the state's police power to protect the general welfare of its citizens.* Nursing practice acts that regulate the practice of nursing have been enacted in all states, the District of Columbia, and in the U.S. territories (Snyder and LeBar, 1984). Because the regulation of nursing is

---

*Dent v. West Virginia, 129 U.S. 114 (1989).*

based on state constitutional law, there is no national legal definition of nursing and no na-tional nursing practice act. The regulation of nursing practice is a state right. Therefore, the law, the definition of nursing practice, and the rules that control nursing are always promul-gated in accordance with the specific intent and in the particular terminology of the state legis-lature that enacts the law (Fig. 8-1) and the board of nursing that enforces it. For this rea-son, nurses must know the laws that govern the practice of nursing in the state in which they practice their profession.

Professional nursing organizations, such as the American Nurses' Association, assist states in arriving at some common understanding by promulgating a definition and standards for nursing education and nursing practice that the state legislatures and the state boards of nursing practice can adopt or adapt when enacting their laws and regulations. In 1981, the American Nurses' Association published a revised model definition of nursing practice which states that:

The practice of professional nursing means the per-formance for compensation of professional services requiring substantial specialized knowledge of the biological, physical, behavioral, psychological, and sociological sciences and of nursing theory as a basis for assessment, diagnosis, planning, intervention, and

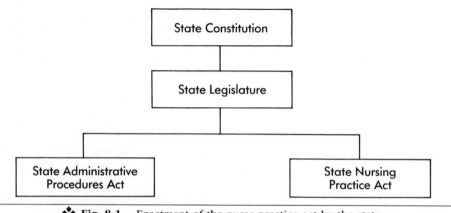

❖ **Fig. 8-1**   Enactment of the nurse practice act by the state.

evaluation in the promotion and maintenance of health; the casefinding and management of illness, injury, or infirmity; the restoration of optimum function; or the achievement of a dignified death. Nursing practice includes, but is not limited to, administration, counseling, supervision, delegation, and evaluation of practice and execution of the medical regimen, including the administration of medications and treatments prescribed by any person authorized by the state to prescribe. Each registered nurse is directly accountable and responsible to the consumer for the quality of nursing care rendered (American Nurses' Association, 1981).

A survey of 51 nursing practice acts conducted in 1983 by the American Nurses' Association revealed that a combination of the four following components were used in formatting the state statutory definition of nursing practice (Snyder and LeBar, 1984).

1. The nursing functions or acts performed that are clearly nursing practice
2. The teaching, supervision, and delegation of nursing practice
3. The execution of the medical regimen
4. The performance of additional acts by specialty-trained nurses

The regulation of advanced practice is an issue involving some disagreement. The first advanced practice or "additional acts" clause was enacted in 1971 in Idaho. Since then, 24 states have included such language in their statutory definition of nursing, and four states have added the language to the definition of the advanced practitioner (Snyder and LeBar, 1984). The American Nurses' Association has opposed the expansion of state regulation into the areas of advanced and specialized nursing practice. They take the position that:

The nursing practice act should provide for the legal regulation of nursing without reference to a specialized area of practice. It is the function of the professional association to establish the scope and desirable qualifications required of each area of practice, and to certify a person as competent to engage in specific areas of nursing practice. It is also the func-

tion of the professional association to upgrade practice above the minimum standards set by the law. The law should not provide for identifying clinical specialists in nursing or require certification or other recognition for practice beyond the minimum qualifications established for the legal regulation of nursing (American Nurses' Association, 1981).

The removal of advanced or specialty nursing requirements from the state's nursing practice act would require nurses to convince their state legislatures that private certification, totally free of state regulation, would not jeopardize the public safety or obstruct the board of nursing's power to suspend or revoke licenses of nurses who have been held incompetent to practice in the advanced or clinically specialized role (Cournoyer, 1989).

Nurses should be familiar with the nurse practice act under which they practice. The structure and function of a particular nursing practice act and the board or agency that enforces it can be more easily understood by examining its purpose, power, and process.

## Purpose

Nursing practice acts usually contain broad statements of purpose that include the protection of life, the promotion of health, and the prevention of illness (N.H. R.S.A. 326-B:1). These statements are the foundation for the power and process of the act. The power must be wielded for the benefit of the public, and the rules and regulations must address public safety and welfare. This is why nursing groups that approach the legislature must be aware that their requests for a new definition of nursing or an expansion of the law or regulations will be carefully scrutinized to ensure that they will protect and benefit the public and not just the nursing profession. For example, nurses attempting to convince a legislature that a nursing practice act should not be amended to allow lay persons to administer medication to clients in nursing homes, may not be successful if they cannot prove that the practice is unsafe and would jeopardize client welfare.

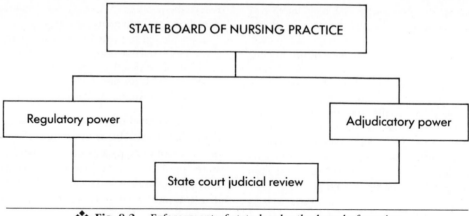

❖ **Fig. 8-2**  Enforcement of state law by the board of nursing.

## Power

Nursing practice acts usually authorize a board or agency to interpret and enforce the act. The regulation of nursing practice is delegated to a board of nursing in all jurisdictions except New York, Connecticut, and Illinois. The majority of jurisdictions have a board that regulates both professional and practical nursing. California, Colorado, Louisiana, Puerto Rico, Texas, Washington, and West Virginia have separate boards for professional and practical nursing. Board composition varies from state to state. Persons who may be authorized by statute to serve on a board of nursing practice include registered nurses, practical nurses, physicians, hospital administrators, hospital trustees, psychiatric technicians, and members of the public (Bullough, 1980).

A board of nursing practice usually has both regulatory and adjudicatory power (Fig. 8-2). The *regulatory power* authorizes the board to develop rules and regulations for nursing licensure, nursing education, and nursing practice. The *adjudicatory power* authorizes the board to investigate, hear, and decide complaints that involve violations of the act or the rules and regulations promulgated by the board. In most jurisdictions the board of nursing practice is responsible for (Snyder and LeBar, 1984):

♦ Determining the eligibility of applicants for licensure
♦ Administering examinations to applicants for licensure
♦ Issuing licenses to qualified applicants
♦ Establishing relicensure procedures
♦ Establishing minimum standards for approving educational programs that prepare a person for licensure
♦ Overseeing mandatory continuing education programs if continuing education is mandated by the act
♦ Investigating complaints against licensees and taking disciplinary action when appropriate
♦ Promulgating rules that regulate nursing practice

In exercising its licensing, rule making, and adjudicatory power, the board of nursing practice must follow the process required by state law.

## Process

Process refers to the manner in which a government agency carries out its regulatory and adjudicatory functions. The procedures used by state agencies can vary significantly from state to state. In addition, there can be differences in the way state agencies within a state operate. In order to achieve some conformity as to the way their state agencies function, most states have enacted an administrative procedures act. The states administrative procedure act specifies the process that the state agencies must follow when making rules, publishing rules and opinions, enacting orders, and conducting investigations and hearings (Schwartz, 1976). It may also indicate the scope of judicial review of the agency's decisions. For nurses to fully understand their legal rights and remedies, the nursing practice act must be read in conjunction with the state administrative procedures act.

**Rule making process.** The rule making process determines the procedures that the board of nursing practice must use in adopting, enforcing, amending, and repealing its rules and regulations. In many states the enactment of rules has become an elaborate and lengthy process that requires involvement of legal counsel, review by a legislative committee, and public hearings. Legislative committees required to review proposed rules may require that each new rule be accompanied by an economic impact statement indicating any new or additional costs.*

**Adjudicatory process.** The administrative procedures act also determines the scope of power that the board of nursing has in investigating, hearing, and deciding cases that involve a violation of the nursing practice act. The nursing practice act usually authorizes the board of nursing practice to discipline a nurse by reprimand, or by denial, suspension, or revocation of the nurse's license. The nursing practice act also indicates the grounds for discipline, which may be further defined in the regulations. For example, the regulations generally contain a very specific and detailed definition of unprofessional conduct.

**Due process.** A nurse's license to practice nursing is recognized by the courts as a constitutionally protected property and liberty right. Therefore, a nurse who is charged with a violation of the nursing practice act has a right to due process in the investigation, hearing, and decision of the charge. The state administrative procedure act determines the procedures that must be followed throughout the adjudicatory proceedings. Due process guarantees usually include a:

1. Notice of the time and place of the hearing
2. Hearing before an authorized group or person
3. Definite statement of the charges
4. Right to cross-examine the board's witnesses
5. Right to produce witnesses and documentary evidence
6. Decision based on the facts presented at the hearing as applied to the nursing practice act
7. Right to be represented by counsel
8. Right to a record of the proceedings
9. Right to a judicial review of the board's final decision

**Judicial review.** Many nursing practice statutes require a rehearing before the board of nursing before the nurse can obtain a judicial review of the board's decision. The nursing practice act or the administrative practice act will usually indicate the nature and scope of judicial review to which the nurse is entitled. For example, in some states the nurse who appeals the board's decision to the court will receive a new hearing and may even be entitled to request a jury trial. In other states, the appellate court is only permitted to review the record of the administrative hearing. Their review will consider whether the board of nursing practice acted fairly, and whether they interpreted and applied the law correctly. The appellate court will only overturn the board of nursing's decision in situations in which they find that the board acted arbitrarily, capriciously, or unreasonably; abused its discretion; violated the nurse's constitutional rights; made an error of law; or based its decision on insufficient evidence (Cournoyer, 1989).

## Challenges to Board of Nursing Power

Challenges to a board of nursing's decision can arise in a number of areas. The following cases provide examples of challenges to the board of nursing's jurisdiction, procedures, interpretation of unprofessional conduct, and to the offense with which the nurse was charged.

**Jurisdiction.** The board of nursing must have the power over the parties and over the subject in order to hear and decide a case.

In *Leggett v. State Board of Nursing,* 612 S.W. 2d 476 (1980), the court held that the board of nursing had no jurisdiction over a licensed nurse who had rendered services as a lay midwife. The court found that she had not represented herself as a nurse midwife or performed as a nurse in her role as midwife. Therefore, the board of nursing could not suspend the nurse's license for functioning as a lay midwife.

**Procedures.** The board of nursing must follow the procedures that are required by the statutes or the regulations.

In *Colorado State Board of Nursing v. Hohu,* 268 P.2d 401 (1954), the court ordered the nurse's license reinstated because all of the members of the board were not present at the hearing as was required by the statute.

In *Wildman v. Axelrod,* 475 N.Y.S.2d 743 (1984), the court held that a delay of 5 years before scheduling a hearing substantially prejudiced the nurse's due process rights.

**Interpretation of unprofessional conduct.** The board of nursing must interpret the meaning of unprofessional conduct according to the definition of unprofessional conduct contained in the statute and in the regulations.

In *Tuma v. Board of Nursing,* 593 P.2d 711 (1979), the court overturned a board of nursing's decision to suspend a nurse license on the basis of her having interfered with the physician-client relationship by having discussed alternative methods of treatment with the client. The court held that the term *unprofessional conduct* was too vague to adequately warn the nurse that the behavior constituted such conduct. The court indicated that the board of nursing should provide a definition of unprofessional conduct in its rules and regulations that would give notice to nurses as to what type of behavior constituted unprofessional conduct.

In *Stevens v. Blake, Alabama Board of Nursing,* 456 So. 2d 795 (1984), the court upheld a finding of unprofessional conduct against a nurse who had self-administered a narcotic while on duty.

**Charge.** The board of nursing must prove the specific offense with which the nurse is charged.

In *Application of Sutton,* 207 N.Y.S. 2d 550 (1960), the court overturned a charge of fraud for making a false statement in the hospital narcotic log because the nurse's entries in the log were correct. She had recorded the right amount of medication in the log, but she had administered a fraction of the dose to the client and self-administered the remainder.

In *Carruthers v. Allen,* 239 N.Y.S. 2d 756 (1963), the court overturned a charge of addiction because the evidence only supported a finding of occasional use rather than evidence that the nurse was addicted, which the board was required to prove.

In *Garrison v. Washington State Nursing Board,* 550 P.2d 7 (1976), the court overturned a charge of distribution because the nurse's actions in taking a drug home did not support a finding of distribution.

In *Hogan v. Mississippi Board of Nursing,* 457 So.2d 931 (1984), the court overturned a charge of misappropriation (taking a drug for one's own use) because the evidence only supported a finding that the nurse could not reasonably account for the wasted narcotics, but did not prove that she actually used them.

In most states, a board of nursing's order to suspend a nurse's license must include a statement of law, which is a specific reference to the section of the nursing practice act or regulations that the nurse has violated and a statement of fact, which indicates the evidence that supports the charge.

The nurse/state relationship is encompassed by the substance and process of administrative law. The complexity and particularity of the requirements surrounding a state board of nursing can be understood by nurses who take the time to read and understand their state's nursing practice act. It is also important for nurses to be aware of the tremendous amount of power that their legislature has delegated to unelected officials who are appointed to serve on licensing boards. They must realize that a government agency is a creature of statute, vulnerable to legal challenges when they exceed their purpose, abuse their power, or disregard their process (Cournoyer, 1989).

### ❖ NURSE/EMPLOYER RELATIONSHIP

The relationship between a nurse and an employer is determined and directed by the requirements of contract law. The nurse must be familiar with the basic elements surrounding contractual and noncontractual agreements in order to recognize the benefits and burdens of an employment relationship.

A contract is defined as a promissory agreement between two or more persons that creates, modifies, or destroys a legal relationship (Prosser, 1971). The four essential elements to a valid contract are mutual assent, consideration, capacity, and a lawful agreement (Schaber and Rohwer, 1975). Mutual assent is the "meeting of the minds," the understanding by the parties that they

have mutually agreed to do something and an agreement on what that something is. Consideration refers to the "bargained for exchange," the service, act, promise, or money that is exchanged between the parties. Capacity means that all the parties to the contract must have the ability to understand the purpose, nature, and effect of the contract. Persons whose capacity to contract may be affected include minors, persons declared legally incompetent, persons who are mentally incapacitated, and prisoners. Lawful agreement requires that the subject matter of the contract be lawful and not against public policy. For example, one could not collect on a gambling debt in a state where gambling is illegal.

### Express and Implied Contracts

A contract can either be express or implied. An *express contract* is one in which the terms are clearly stated in distinct and explicit language either orally or in writing. An *implied contract* is one that is either inferred by the action or conduct of the parties, recognized as a tacit understanding between the parties, or implied by the circumstances surrounding the transaction. For example, clients often enter into an implied contract with their physician by requesting and accepting medical services without first discussing what the physician intends to do or what the charge will be for the service. Once the service is performed, it is the responsibility of the client to pay for it either personally or through third-party reimbursement.

### Oral and Written Contracts

An oral contract is binding and enforceable unless it is precluded by the statute of frauds. Every state has a statute of frauds that identifies the circumstances in which a contract must be in writing in order to be valid. The requirements vary from state to state, but all states require the following transactions to be in writing (Schaber and Rohwer, 1975).

◆ A contract that, by its terms, cannot be performed within 1 year
◆ A promise to pay the debts of another
◆ A contract for the sale of an interest in real estate, including a lease for longer than 1 year
◆ A contract for the sale of goods priced at $500 or more
◆ A contract in consideration of marriage

Although an oral contract may be valid, the person wanting to enforce it may have difficulty proving its terms and conditions.

A written contract can be either a formal document or a written memorandum consisting of a number of notes or writings. A memorandum will be considered a valid contract if the writings are properly connected and identify the (1) names of the parties, (2) subject matter or nature of the transaction, (3) terms or conditions, and the (4) signature or initials of the party to be charged. All written contracts are subject to the parole evidence rule. The parole evidence rule states that any oral or written statements or promises that are made by either of the parties but are not incorporated into the contract will not be enforced by the courts. This means that if these statements or promises were not incorporated into the contract, the court will not allow them to be used to add to, modify, or contradict the written contract. The court, however, may allow the statements or promises to be introduced to show fraud, misrepresentation, duress, mistake, custom, or prior course of dealing (Schaber and Rohwer, 1975).

## Termination of a Contract

A contract can be terminated in five different ways (Schaber and Rohwer, 1975).

1. Performance: when a full, complete, and literal performance of the contract has been obtained
2. Termination: when, under the terms of the contract, the obligation of the parties has ended

3. Accord and Satisfaction: when both the parties agree that the debtor may perform a different promise instead of the one that was owed
4. Impossibility: when an unforeseeable event, such as the death of a person who was to perform a personal service, or the destruction of the subject matter of the contract makes the performance of the contract objectively impossible
5. Rescission: when the parties discharge their respective duties by agreeing to rescind (annul) the contract

## Breach of Contract

A *breach of contract* is an unjustified failure to perform the terms of the contract agreed upon, when the performance is due. Because a contract is a legally enforceable agreement, the breach of such an agreement entitles the nonbreaching party to be compensated for the losses that were incurred as a result of the breach. The three remedies for breach of contract are money damages, specific performance, and an injunction. A demand for money damages requires the breaching party to make good or replace the loss caused by the breach. The nonbreaching party is expected to prove the amount of damages with a reasonable degree of certainty. In addition, the nonbreaching party is expected to mitigate the damages. For example, a nurse who is fired and asking for money damages for unlawful discharge would be expected to seek and obtain comparable employment while waiting for the decision of the court. A request for specific performance would require the person to perform the contract as promised. Specific performance is usually demanded when money damages are inadequate. This can occur when the subject matter of the contract is unique, such as the sale of real estate or an antique or other item that has particular value to the nonbreaching party. A court will not order a person to perform a personal service such as singing or playing football because they would have no control over the manner in which the service was performed. In these situations, it is more appropriate for the nonbreaching party to ask the court to issue an injunction. An *injunction* is a court order requiring a person to do something or refrain from doing something. For example, a court may order a contractor to correct the problems with the work that was covered under the contract. They will not order someone to perform a personal service such as playing football, but they can order the person not to play football for any other team for the duration of the contract.

## Employment Relationships

The employment relationship between a nurse and an employer is controlled and regulated by the requirements of contract law. In order to recognize the benefits and burdens of the employment relationship, the nurse must understand the basic concepts surrounding the various types of contractual and noncontractual agreements. The three types of nursing employment relationships are the collective bargaining agreement, the individual contract, and the employee at will status.

**Collective bargaining agreement.** A collective bargaining agreement is a written agreement between an employer and a union that determines the employees' wages, hours, and working conditions (Henry, 1984). Because the collective bargaining agreement does not guarantee continued employment to the covered employee or create an employer-employee relationship, it is not considered an employment contract (Henry, 1984). A collective bargaining agreement establishes the contractual relationship between the employer and the union and governs the relationship between (1) the employer and the employees and (2) the employees themselves (Henry, 1984).

Three separate areas of the law govern collective bargaining activities. Federal employees such as nurses who work for the Veterans Administration hospitals are covered by the Civil Service Reform Act of 1978, 5 U.S.C. §§ 7101-7135. State employees such as nurses who work in state hospitals or clinics are governed by specific state public employee statutes. Nurses who work for private hospitals or health care agencies are under the jurisdiction of the National Labor Relations Act, 29 U.S.C. §§ 141-187.

**National Labor Relations Act.** The National Labor Relations Act requires that members of a collective bargaining unit have a "community of interest" that is a similar interest in wages, hours, and working conditions. Nurses are included under the definition of professionals and have the right to be included in bargaining units that are made up of professionals. The right of registered nurses to be represented by an "RN only" unit, apart from other health care professionals, is a matter of jurisdiction, entirely dependent on the state in which they are employed. Collective bargaining agreements apply only to employees; therefore, nurses who are considered supervisors are excluded from the agreement.

Every collective bargaining agreement is unique and exists as a result of negotiation and compromise between the employer and the union. Employers and employees are required to meet, furnish information, and attempt to reach an agreement in the areas of hours, wages, and working conditions (Cournoyer, 1989). Collective bargaining agreements usually contain a grievance procedure that must be used to settle disputes arising under the agreement (Peterson, et al, 1981). Collective bargaining agreements generally state that an employer cannot discipline or discharge an employee except for "just cause." Nurses who work in a hospital or agency that is unionized lose the opportunity to personally negotiate their wages, hours, and working conditions. The employer must negotiate with the union, and the union must represent fairly and fully all the employees in the bargaining unit.* The union must also represent nurses who qualify as members of a bargaining unit but have chosen not to join the union.

**Individual express contract.** An express written contract identifies the conditions and terms of employment to which the employer and employee are bound. The nurse negotiates as an individual to create an employment contract that will be interpreted and enforced by the courts if any disagreements arise between the nurse and the employer. Contract law is an unfamiliar area of law for most nurses, and hospitals have been reluctant to encourage nurses to negotiate individual express contracts. Insufficient knowledge and lack of opportunity are two significant factors that can explain why nurses have lagged behind other professionals in recognizing the need to negotiate individual contracts that promote and protect their employment-related interests. Nurses, however, can overcome these impediments. The American Nurses' Association, in conjunction with the Council of Nurse Practitioners in the Nursing of Children has developed guidelines for the individual nursing contract that contain suggested contract language and topics (Potter, 1984). Hospitals have administrative personnel familiar with the intricacies of contract negotiation, while most nurses are generally inexperienced in this area. This unequal bargaining power is a distinct disadvantage that can be remedied by the nurses obtaining legal advice and assistance in negotiating the contract (Cournoyer, 1989). Nurses cannot force a hospital to negotiate individual contracts, but they can remain alert for the situations where such an opportunity might be available. For example, the hospital may have a need for specialized nursing skills or they may want assurances that particular units will be consistently staffed with an adequate number of professional nurses. The greater the hospital's need for nursing services, the greater the chances the nurses will have of negotiating individual contracts.

**Employee at will.** The majority of nurses today do not have the protection of a collective bargaining agreement or an individual express contract and are considered employees at will, a status that is almost entirely weighted toward the employer's interest.

The employee at will doctrine holds that where an employer-employee relationship is not for a definite term, the employee is considered an employee at will. Under the doctrine, the employer has a right to discharge an employee for any reason or for no reason at all. Of course, the employee also has the right to terminate the employment for any reason or for no reason. The majority of nurses employed in the health care industry are hired for an indefinite period of time and are therefore considered employees at will. It is a harsh rule of law that is being undermined in many states by legislative enactments and court decisions that recognize an employee's right to sue an employer for breach of an implied contract or to bring an action in tort for wrongful discharge. The three legal principles that the courts have used to restrict the employer's right to discharge an employee are (1) public policy, (2) implied contract, and (3) promises of good faith and fair dealing (Cournoyer, 1989).

Public policy is defined as that principle of law that holds that no person can lawfully do anything that has a tendency to be injurious to the public or against the public good.* Joining a union, filing a worker's compensation claim, and serving on a jury are the types of activities that are protected by the public policy exemption.† Persons who are considered employees at will should not be fired for taking part in these activities.

---

*Vaca v. Sipes, 386 U.S. 171 (1967).

*Warthen v. Toms River Community Memorial Hospital, 488 A.2d 229 (N.J. Super.AD 1985).
†12 A.L.R. 4th (1982).

A number of courts have limited the employer's right to discharge an employee by recognizing the employee's claim that an implied contract had been created between the employer and the employee (Cournoyer, 1989). Publications and conduct that have been identified as having the potential to establish an implied contractual relationship include the (1) hospital policy and procedure manual, (2) personnel handbooks, (3) oral promises made by supervisory or management personnel, and (4) employer conduct.

One court has held that an employer can create a situation that is "instinct with an obligation" when, presumably in their own interest, the employer creates an environment in which the employee believes that the policies and practices are established and official, purport to be fair, and are to be applied consistently and uniformly to each employee.* In response to this exception, some hospitals have included disclaimers in their personnel manuals that specifically notify the employee that this publication does not constitute a contractual agreement. Courts in jurisdictions that have recognized the implied contract exception have not as yet ruled on the validity of these disclaimers.

Implied promises of good faith and fair dealing have been used by the courts to restrict the employer's right to discharge an employee at will. The employee who files a wrongful discharge suit must be ready to prove that the employer acted unfairly or arbitrarily, or that the employer violated their own policies and procedures. Evidence that a court might consider in determining the nature of the employer-employee relationship includes (1) employment policies; (2) employer assurances, commendations, and promotions; (3) absence of any evidence of direct employee criticism, (4) employee length of service, and (5) the employer's policy of dealing fairly with employees.†

**Litigation.** The employee at will doctrine is being challenged by nurses who feel they have a legitimate claim of wrongful discharge. In some instances there may also be civil rights legislation or state statutes that support their claim. Cases in which the courts have upheld the claim of wrongful discharge include the following:

◆ A nurse anesthetist's claim that she was fired for refusing to participate in a sterilization procedure.*
◆ A nurse's claim that she was fired for reporting patient abuse to an Advocacy Group and for testifying at the patient's hearing.†
◆ A nurse's claim that she was fired for refusing to testify falsely in favor of two doctors at a deposition.‡

On the other hand, the court agreed with the employer and upheld the firing of:

◆ A nurse who had leaked information concerning incidents of patient abuse and improprieties to a newspaper.§
◆ A nurse manager who had been unable to follow staffing patterns and stay within budget.‖
◆ A nurse who had refused to continue to perform dialysis on a client on the basis of her moral and ethical objections, which she claimed was supported by the code of ethics.¶

## ❖ NURSE/PATIENT RELATIONSHIP

The relationship between the nurse and the patient is defined and directed by the principles of tort law. A tort is a private wrong or injury

*Toussaint v. Blue Cross and Blue Shield of Michigan, 882 Mich. Sup. Ct. 1980, 292 N.W. 2d 880 (1980).
†Pugh v. See's Candies, 171 Cal. Rptr. 917 (Cal. App. 1981); Cleary v. American Airlines, 168 Cal. Rptr. 722 (Cal. App. 1980).

*Swanson v. St. John's Lutheran Hospital, 597 P.2d 702 (Mont. 1979).
†Witt v. Forest Hospital, 450 N.E.2d 811 (Ill.1983).
‡Sides v. Duke University Medical Center, 328 S.E.2d 818 (N.C. App. 1985), rev. denied 335 S.E.2d 13 (N.C. 1985).
§Rozier v. St. Mary's Hospital, 411 N.E.2d 50 (Ill.1980).
‖Lampe v. Presbyterian Medical Center, 590 P.2d 513 (Colo. App. 1978).
¶Warthen v. Toms River Community Memorial Hospital, 488 A.2d 229 (N.J. Super.AD 1985).

that results from the breach of a legal duty. Tort liability is founded on the principle that a person who has suffered insult or injury to his or her dignity, health, body, life, or time has the right to be made whole again. Since the law cannot restore these types of losses, the party committing the wrong is made to pay money damages or compensation (Fiscina et al, 1985). The nurse is exposed to tort liability in a number of areas including negligence or malpractice, assault and battery, false imprisonment, invasion of privacy, and libel and slander. The nurse's liability for these torts generally arises in the context of the client's right to (1) receive a reasonable standard of care, (2) consent to care and treatment, and (3) confidentiality concerning the illness.

## Standard of Care

The right to a reasonable standard of care means that the nurse must use the same degree of knowledge and skill as a reasonably prudent nurse would use under the same or similar circumstances. Nurses who fail to provide this standard of care can be held liable for negligence, malpractice, or both. A hospital can be sued directly for failing to provide the patient with a reasonable standard of care. Under the doctrine of *respondeat superior,* they are held liable to pay the damages for the negligent acts of their employees. They can therefore be sued for the nurse's failure to provide a reasonable standard of nursing care to patients.

## Negligence and Malpractice

*Negligence* is the failure to exercise the degree of care that a reasonably prudent person would exercise under the same or similar circumstances. Malpractice or professional negligence refers to negligent acts committed by persons who are acting in their professional capacity. *Malpractice* is defined as any professional misconduct, unreasonable lack of skill, or fidelity in professional or fiduciary duties, evil

practice, or illegal or immoral conduct.* There are some courts that still do not recognize that a nurse's actions are those of a professional; therefore, a nurse can be sued for either negligence or malpractice depending on the nature of the action and the jurisdiction in which it occurs (Cournoyer, 1989). The finding of negligence or malpractice is a jury determination. In order to prevail, the plaintiff must prove that:

1. The nurse had a legal duty to exercise due care.
2. The nurse breached the duty to provide a reasonable standard of care.
3. The plaintiff suffered a physical, emotional, or financial injury.
4. The injury was proximately or directly caused by the nurse's actions.

There are a number of defenses and counterclaims to the charge of negligence or malpractice, the most common of which are the (1) plaintiff's failure to prove negligence, (2) statute of limitations, (3) comparative or contributory negligence of the plaintiff, and the (4) immunity statutes (Cournoyer, 1989).

**Litigation.** "The nursing process is a clinical management system that provides individualized, goal-directed nursing care." (Cournoyer, 1989). It is a four-stage process that consists of the assessment, planning, intervention, and evaluation of care. Although planning and evaluation are an important part of the nursing process, it is in the areas of assessment and intervention that most of the litigation occurs. Claims of nursing negligence or malpractice often center on the nurse's failure to adequately monitor the client, take appropriate action, communicate the client's condition to the physician, or notify administration of an inadequate physician response to a client's need for care. For example, in the following cases nurses have been found negligent for:

*Napier v. Greenzweig, 256 F. 196 (2dCir. 1919).

◆ Failing to follow hospital policy and leaving the operating room at a critical time, which resulted in the anesthetist being without assistance when the client suffered a cardiac arrest. The court held the nurse had abandoned the client even though she claimed she left because she was "being yelled at by two physicians who had started surgery in another operating room." The hospital was also held liable for failure to provide adequate staff.*

◆ Improperly administering intravenous chemotherapy, which resulted in the infiltration of the medicine into the client's forearm, causing severe necrosis and loss of several muscles and tendons.†

◆ Failing to maintain adequate oxygenation levels in a postoperative client. The jury found that the nurse either failed to respond to the alarm, used malfunctioning equipment, or neglected to provide supplemental oxygen when the respirator could not be properly attached.‡

◆ Failing to monitor the infusion pump on a neonate who subsequently suffered fluid overload, respiratory arrest, and severe brain damage. The parties agreed to a $4 million settlement.§

◆ Failing to recognize that the fetal monitor was indicating fetal distress and failing to notify the physician of the fetal distress. As a result, the infant was totally blind and profoundly retarded. The case ended in a $2.2 million settlement. ‖

◆ Failing to turn on the alarm system on a heart monitoring machine when leaving the room. The 70-year-old client suffered irreversible brain damage. The parties agreed to a $2.75 million settlement.*

◆ Failing to tell the physician or administration that an endotracheal tube had been left in the client for 5 days when the hospital policy was for the tube to remain in the client no longer than 3 days. As a result, the client suffered complications that required successive surgery and left the client with a permanent speaking disability.†

◆ Failing to report to the physician that the laboratory test indicated that the client's serum electrolyte levels revealed severe hypokalemia, hyponatremia, and hypochloremia. The client suffered cardiac arrest and sustained permanent neurological and visual impairments.‡

◆ Failing to notify administration that the physician had not responded to her report that there was a foul-smelling substance draining from under the client's cast, that the client's arm was edematous, and that the client had a high temperature. The physician failed to respond to the information for 48 hours at which time the client was transferred to another hospital for treatment, which proved to be unsuccessful and eventually resulted in an amputation.§

## Consent and Informed Consent

The client's right to consent to treatment is founded on the common law right to be free from unwanted, offensive, or harmful touching by another person. A health care provider can be held liable for failing to obtain consent even if the procedure improves the client's condi-

*Czubinsky v. Doctor's Hospital, 139 Cal. App., 3d 361, 188 Cal. Rptr. 685 (1983).
†Ball v. Rolling Hill Hospital, Pa., Philadelphia County Court of Common Pleas, No. 341, 1983, April 16, 1985; 28 ATLA L. Rep. 467 (December 1985).
‡Lindsay v. Mueller, Wash., Pierce County Superior Court No. 83-2-00271-6(June 9, 1985); 28 ATLA L. Rep. 276 (August 1985).
§Jones v. Samaritan Health Services, Ariz., Maricopa County Superior Court No. C487995 (April 1985); 28 ATLA L.Rep. 421 (November 1985).
‖Dobrzeniecki v. University Hospital of Cleveland, Ohio, Cuyahoga County Court of Common Pleas No.17,843 (May 22, 1984); 27 ATLA Rep. 425 (November 1984).

*Statkin v. Capitol Hill Hospital, No. 84-0443 (D.D.C. Oct. 18, 1984), Medical Liability Reporter (1985).
†Poor Sisters of St. Francis v. Catron, 435 N.E.2d 305 (Ind. Ct. App. 1982).
‡Sinks v. Methodist Medical Center, Ill., Peoria County Circuit Court No. 82L3868 (April 1985); 28 ATLA L. Rep. 446 (December 1985).
§Utter v. United Methodist Hospital Center, 236 S.E.2d 213 (W.Va. 1977).

tion. It is important to distinguish the failure to obtain the client's consent from the failure to obtain the client's informed consent. The absence of a client's consent makes a health care provider liable for the intentional tort of battery. The health care provider has a duty to provide the client with adequate information concerning the risks and alternatives so that the client can make an informed decision. The absence of an informed consent makes the health care provider liable for negligence in that they failed to meet the standard for disclosure of information.

### Assault and Battery

An *assault* is a deliberate threat, coupled with the apparent ability to touch another person. *Battery* is the unconsented touching of another. The plaintiffs must prove that they did not consent. Defenses to the tort of assault and battery include proof that the client consented or the invocation of a qualified privilege. The courts recognize a qualified privilege to touch, restrain, or detain a person if it is done in defense of self or others or to prevent self-inflicted harm. Only reasonable force can be used in these situations. Reasonable force is the amount of force that is reasonably necessary under the circumstances.

**Litigation.** Examples of litigation that centered around the failure to obtain the client's consent include:

◆ The physical examination of a client by medical students several times a day despite the client's protests.*

◆ The administration of a drug used to induce labor.†

◆ The administration of medication to a person who had not been found mentally ill, dangerous, or incompetent and who had refused the medication because of her religious beliefs.*

### False Imprisonment

*False imprisonment* is the unlawful restraint of personal liberty or the unlawful detention of the individual. There must be a direct restraint imposed for a period of time during which the person was required to stay somewhere or go somewhere against his or her will. Because the injury is to the person's right to freedom of movement, it is not necessary to prove that damages occurred as a result of the confinement (Prosser, 1971). The elements that must be proven include physical restraint or restraint by threat or intimidation and the absence of consent (Prosser, 1971).

Defenses to the charge of false imprisonment are similar to those discussed previously for assault and battery. The defendant may claim that the plaintiff consented or that the situation involved a qualified privilege. There is a qualified privilege to detain persons who are mentally ill and dangerous to themselves or others. Only reasonable force should be used in detaining them, and the least restrictive alternative should be selected for their detention. State laws regulating involuntary detention should be invoked, and the person's due process rights should be respected.

**Litigation.** A claim of false imprisonment can be brought by persons who are admitted and detained in mental hospitals or on secure psychiatric units in violation of the state's statutory requirements for involuntary commitment.† For

---

*Inderbitzer v. Lane Hospital, 12 P.2d 744 (Cal. App. 1932), aff'd, 13 P.2d 905 (Cal. 1932).*
†Koboutek v. Hafner, 366 N.W.2d 663 (Minn. App. 1985).*

*Winters v. Miller, 446 F.2d 65 (1971).*
†Maben v. Rankin, 10 Cal. Rptr. 353 (Cal. 1961).*

example, a patient sued his employer, the security guard, and a hospital for false imprisonment. He had sought some medication for anxiety while he was at work, and he was forcibly taken to the hospital by the security guard. At the hospital, he was placed in isolation and was not allowed to call anyone, including his lawyer. He was released the following day.* The refusal to discharge clients who come to the emergency department for treatment and are under the influence of alcohol also poses a risk of charges of false imprisonment. On the other hand, if the person were discharged in this condition, and allowed to drive, the hospital could be held liable for injuries to a third party (Cournoyer, 1989).

## Confidentiality

Clients have a right to expect that information learned about them during the course of administrative or clinical inquiries will be kept confidential (Cournoyer, 1989). Informational privacy encompasses a person's right to be left alone, to be free from unwanted publicity, as well as the right to keep private information inaccessible to others.† Informational privacy is a property interest that can form the basis for a claim of invasion of privacy or defamation, two intentional torts that are recognized in common law and in statutory law in many states. Included in the concept of privacy is the freedom from unwanted disclosure of information, the freedom from actual intrusion into private situations, and the freedom to live as one wishes in respect to certain private activities (Greenawalt, 1974).

## Invasion of Privacy

The tort of invasion of privacy consists of four distinct kinds of invasion of four different interests, each representing an interference with the plaintiff's right to be left alone (Prosser, 1971). The interests invaded are the (1) appropriation of the plaintiff's name or likeness, (2) intrusion on the plaintiff's seclusion, (3) public disclosure of private facts about the plaintiff, and (4) placing the plaintiff in a false light in the public eye.

As a defense to the charge of invasion of privacy, some courts have recognized a qualified privilege to release information for purposes that promote the public welfare. This would include disclosures that are part of a legitimate investigation for insurance or credit purposes and employment referrals (Prosser, 1971). Child and elderly protection statutes, communicable disease reporting laws, and criminal law reporting requirements for rape and gunshot wounds create a legal obligation to reveal what is usually considered private information.

**Litigation.** Areas in which hospitals could be held liable for invasion of privacy include the following (Prosser, 1971):

◆ Releasing patient information to unauthorized parties
◆ Permitting unauthorized parties to view medical or surgical procedures
◆ Failing to control visitors in the hospital
◆ Taking pictures of patients without their consent
◆ Disclosing or discussing patient problems or situations in public places
◆ Permitting access to the medical record by unauthorized persons
◆ Publishing the patient's picture to advertise a product or as part of an article, even for educational purposes, without the patient's permission
◆ Public disclosure of a person's x-ray or public exhibition of films, such as a cesarean section, without the patient's consent

---

*Adler v. Beverly Hills Hospital, 594 S.W.2d 153 (Tex. Civ. App. 1980).
†Olmstead v. United States, 277 U.S. 438 (1972), (Brandeis, L., dissenting).

◆ Publishing a patient's case history in a manner in which the patient is identifiable to the public

## Defamation

*Defamation* consists of slander and libel, the twin torts that comprise the invasion of the interest in a person's reputation and good name (Prosser, 1971). A defamatory communication damages a person's reputation by diminishing the esteem, goodwill, respect, and confidence in which the plaintiff is held in the community (Prosser, 1971). It can also create adverse, derogatory, and unpleasant feelings or opinions against the plaintiff (Prosser, 1971).

*Slander* is an oral defamatory statement that is communicated to a third person. The general rule is that slander is not actionable unless the plaintiff can prove actual damage to his or her reputation (Prosser, 1971). The four exceptions to this rule are (1) accusing someone of a crime, (2) accusing someone of having a loathsome disease, (3) calling a woman unchaste, and (4) using words that affect a person's business or profession (Prosser, 1971). In these cases the plaintiff would not have to prove actual damage to his or her reputation because the communications themselves are considered slanderous.

*Libel* is a defamatory communication that is written; however, it also includes signs, photographs, statues, and motion pictures. Some courts require proof of actual damages, while others assume the existence of damages from the publication of the libel itself, without any specific evidence of damage to the plaintiff's reputation (Prosser, 1971).

Defenses to actions for defamation include truth and privilege. The law presumes that all defamation is false. Therefore, proof that the statement is true is an absolute defense to a charge of defamation. The defense of privilege or immunity is founded on the principle that certain conduct is allowed to escape liability

because it furthers some interest of such social importance that the defendant is entitled to protection, even if it results in uncompensated damages to the plaintiff (Prosser, 1971). Examples of situations in which an absolute privilege applies include judges, lawyers, and witnesses in judicial proceedings and legislators and witnesses at legislative hearings. A qualified privilege is allowed for persons reporting to licensing boards, accreditation agencies, and for persons making legitimate inquiries about employment references and credit information.

**Litigation.** The litigation can involve patients suing health care professionals or health care professionals suing each other. For example, in the following cases:

◆ A nurse sued a physician for defamation because of unsolicited statements that he made to the hospital administrator concerning her character and her professional competence.*
◆ A Registered Nurse (RN) sued a Licensed Practical Nurse (LPN) for defamation claiming that the LPN had told a number of persons on the unit that the RN had ordered her to give a medication that the RN knew was wrong.†
◆ A patient had a condition that resulted in a false-positive result on a Wassermann Test. The nurse told the patient's employer that the patient was being treated for syphilis.‡

## Nursing Documentation

The legal process requires that the plaintiff (person suing) prove the elements of the tort he or she claims the defendant (person being sued) has committed. The quantity and quality of the nursing documentation is an important factor that is considered by the hospital in arriving at a decision to defend the suit or to negotiate a

---

*Farrell v. Kramer, 193 A.2d 560 (Maine, 1963).
†Malone v. Longo, 463 F. Supp. 139 (D.D.N.Y. 1979).
‡Schessler v. Keck, 271 P.2d 588 (Cal. 1954).

settlement. The medical record is considered a business record that can be introduced at trial under the business records exception to the hearsay rule. Under the rules of evidence, all or part of the record is considered admissible as evidence if it is accurate, complete, relevant, and recorded, for professional purposes, at or near the time the event took place. Nurses are aware that in the hospital environment, the medical record chronicles the patient's care and treatment and serves as a means of formal communication between health care professionals. Nurses should also realize that in the legal environment, the medical record is considered evidence that can be introduced at trial and challenged by the plaintiff.

**Proving the standard of care.** In 1979, a California appellate court identified the duty of a professional nurse with respect to the care of clients when it approved jury instructions that stated:

It is the duty of one who undertakes to perform the services of a trained or graduate nurse to have the knowledge and skill ordinarily possessed, and to exercise the care and skill ordinarily used in like situations, by trained and skilled members of the nursing profession practicing their profession in the same or similar circumstances.*

A nurse has a legal duty to provide the client with a reasonable standard of care. This is usually referred to as "what the reasonably prudent nurse would do under the same or similar circumstances."

The plaintiff is required to prove the standard of care and the nurse's failure to meet that standard of care. In order to meet their burden of proof, the plaintiffs generally rely on the testimony of expert witnesses and on the introduction of documentary evidence. The types of documents most often used to prove the standard of care include:

American Nurses' Association Standards of Practice
Standards published by the specialty nursing organizations
Joint Commission of Health Care Organizations
State Nursing Practice Act
State nursing practice regulations
Federal and state hospital licensing laws
Federal and state hospital regulations
Hospital bylaws
Hospital policy and procedure manuals

The judge determines whether the document is admissible and what weight the evidence will carry. The jury instructions may state that (1) the document can be considered along with all the other evidence in determining the standard of care or (2) that the document may be considered as evidence of the standard of care unless the defendant can prove otherwise. For example, a jury could be instructed that a hospital policy, stating that "a patient who has a cast must be checked every 15 minutes for signs of circulatory impairment," is the standard of nursing practice, or they could be instructed that the policy should only be considered as part of the evidence and that they can consider other evidence, such as doctor's orders, that may also have been introduced to prove the standard of care in this case.

**Evaluating the nurse's notes.** The quantity and quality of the nursing documentation determines its vulnerability to legal challenge. Nurses' notes should provide a complete, accurate, and timely account of the patient's involvement in and response to the nursing process (Cournoyer, 1989).

The Joint Commission on the Accreditation of Healthcare Organizations' standards state that "the nursing process (assessment, planning, intervention, and evaluation) shall be documented for each hospitalized client from admission through discharge" (Cournoyer, 1989).

When legal action is anticipated, the plaintiff's attorney will subpoena the medical record

---

*Fraifo v. Hartland Hospital, 160 Cal. Rptr. 246 (1979).*

and use nurse experts and legal professionals to review and evaluate both the content and the form of the nurse's notes. The standards of nursing practice require that the nurse's notes contain accurate and appropriate observations, assessments, interventions, and evaluations. Examples of the kind of information that the reviewers are looking for in the nurse's notes include (Cournoyer, 1989):

◆ Descriptions of the patient's appearance, behavior, and symptoms
◆ Initial and continuing assessments that describe a change in the patient's status indicating that the patient is improving or deteriorating
◆ Descriptions of the interventions made in response to the observations of the patient's change of status
◆ Identification of the test, therapy, or treatment and the patient's condition before and after the procedure
◆ Notations for each time a physician is notified with a description of the information communicated to, and the response received from the physician
◆ Identification of patient and family teaching activities and discharge information and instructions
◆ Notations that reveal an evaluation of the patient for the anticipated effects of interventions such as notations that the patient did obtain relief from pain after the administration of a pain-relieving medication
◆ Notations that indicate when the patient has refused treatment or has withdrawn his consent to treatment

Nurse experts and legal professionals reviewing the nurse's notes in anticipation of litigation will pay particular attention to the form of the notes. Hospital policy determines the type of nursing documentation that is used in the institution. Traditionally, nurse's notes consisted of a chronological description of the nursing care provided during three 8-hour shifts, but some hospitals now use a problem-oriented format that records the patient's (S) subjective and (O) objective symptoms and the (A) assessments and (P) plans of the health care professionals to fur-

ther diagnose, treat, and educate the patient. This method of documentation is frequently referred to by the acronym SOAP, derived from the first letter of each area of the required data. In both systems, hospital policy requires that the nurse's notes be (1) timely, (2) complete, (3) legible, (4) correct, (5) accurate, and (6) attributable. This means that reviewers will evaluate whether the (Cournoyer, 1989):

◆ Information is recorded in proper sequence, avoiding time gaps
◆ Delayed entries are identified by time and date and the notation that it is a delayed entry
◆ Record contains all significant information for the appropriate time period
◆ Record contains empty spaces or lines
◆ Notes have been rewritten and the original kept with the record
◆ Handwriting is legible
◆ Record contains marginal notes or information squeezed between the lines
◆ Errors are clearly identified and explained without obliterating any information on the record
◆ Grammar and spelling are correct
◆ Patient is identified on each page of the record
◆ Record contains the legal signature and title of all personnel who have made notations
◆ Notations are recorded by authorized personnel only

The nurses' notes are a primary source of evidence as to the standard of nursing care that the client received from admission through discharge. They can also serve as evidence that the client understood and consented to the care provided. There is no doubt that the nursing process properly documented can provide a reliable and persuasive defense to the clients' claims of substandard care or other tortious (legally wrongful) conduct.

❖ **SUMMARY**

After reading this chapter, nurses will begin to view the law from a common perspective. The information was specifically selected to assist nurses to arrive at a basic understanding of the legal relationships that are fundamental to the practice of nursing. The nurse-state relationship legitimizes the profession of nursing and serves as a vehicle for its refinement and expansion. The nurse-employer relationship establishes the clinical environment and determines the boundaries of professional and economic advancement. The nurse-client relationship creates the requirement of a reasonable standard of care and identifies, promotes, and protects the client's rights.

The laws that influence nurses and nursing practice form a rich tapestry of legal substance and legal process. This chapter has isolated the most common and colorful threads and examined their place and function in the total fabric of legal expectation and legal liability for the practice of nursing.

## ❖ APPLYING KNOWLEDGE TO PRACTICE:

1. Identify and discuss why there is no legal national definition of nursing.
2. Identify and discuss the due process rights that nurses are entitled to if they are charged with a violation of the nursing practice act. Do you think this procedure protects both the nurse and the public?
3. Identify the three types of nurse employment relationships and discuss the benefits and burdens of each.
4. What is the difference between negligence and malpractice? What must a plaintiff prove in order to win a malpractice suit?
5. What is the difference between the medical and the legal purpose of the medical record? How are nurses' notes vulnerable to legal challenge?

## REFERENCES

*Adler v. Beverly Hills Hospital,* 594 S.W.2d 153 (Tex. Civ. App. 1980).

American Nurses' Association, (1981). *The Nursing Practice Act: Suggested State Legislation.* Kansas City, Mo.: American Nurses' Association.

*Ball v. Rolling Hill Hospital,* Pa., Philadelphia County Court of Common Pleas, No. 341, 1983, April 16, 1985; 28 ATLA L. Rep. 467 (December 1985).

Bullough, B. (1980). *The Law and the Expanding Nursing Role.* New York: Appleton-Century-Crofts.

Cournoyer, C. P. (1989). *The Nurse Manager and The Law.* Rockville, Md.: Aspen Publishers, Inc.

*Czubinsky v. Doctor's Hospital,* 139 Cal. App. 3d 361, 188 Cal. Rptr. 685 (1983).

*Dent v. West Virginia, 129 U.S.114 (1889).*

*Dobrzeniecki v. University Hospital of Cleveland,* Ohio, Cuyahoga County Court of Common Pleas No. 17,843 (May 22, 1984); 27 ATLA Rep. 425 (November 1984).

*Farrell v. Kramer,* 193. A.2d 560 (Maine 1963).

Fiscina, S.F. et al. (1985). *A Sourcebook for Research in Law and Medicine.* Owings Mill, Md.: National Health Publishing.

*Fraifo v. Hartland Hospital,* 160 Cal. Rptr. 246 (1979).

Greenawalt, K. (1974). "Privacy and Its Legal Protections," *Hastings Center Studies:* (3) 45–49.

Henry, K.H. (1984). *The Health Care Supervisor's Legal Guide.* Rockville, Md.: Aspen Publishers, Inc.

*Inderbitzer v. Lane Hospital,* 12 P.2d 744 (Cal. App.1932), aff'd, 13 P.2d 905 (Cal. 1932).

Joint Commission on Accreditation of Health Care Organizations, (1985). *Accreditation Manual for Hospitals.* Chicago: Joint Commission, 98.

*Jones v. Samaritan Health Service,* Ariz., Maricopa County Superior Court No. C487995 (April 1985); 28 ATLA L.Rep. 421 (November 1985).

*Kohoutek v. Hafner,* 366 N.W.2d 663 (Minn. App. 1985).

*Lampe v. Presbyterian Medical Center,* 590 P.2d 513 (Colo. App. 1978).

*Lindsay v. Mueller,* Wash., Pierce County Superior Court No. 83-2-00271-6 (June 9, 1985); 28 ATLA L.Rep. 276 (August 1985).

*Maben v. Rankin,* 10 Cal. Rptr. 353 (Cal. 1961).

*Malone v. Longo,* 463 F. Supp. 139 (D.D.N.Y. 1979).

*Napier v. Greenzweig,* 256 F. 196 (2d Cir. 1919).

N.H. R.S.A. 326-B:1.

*Olmstead v. United States,* 277 U.S. 438 (1972) (Brandeis, L., dissenting).

Peterson, D., Rezlee, J., & Reed, K. (1981). "Grievances: Forerunners to Arbitration," *Arbitration in Health Care*: 23.

*Poor Sisters of St. Francis v. Catron,* 435 N.E.2d 305 (Ind. Ct. App. 1982).

Potter, D.O. (Ed.) (1984). *Practices,* Nursing Reference Library. Springhouse, Pa.: Springhouse Corp.,: 684–691.

Prosser, W.L. (1971). *Law of Torts,* (4th ed.) St. Paul, Minn.: West Publishing Co.

*Pugh v. See's Candies,* 171 Cal. Rptr. 917 (Cal. App. 1981); *Cleary v. American Airlines,* 168 Cal. Rptr. 722 (Cal. App. 1980).

*Rozier v. St. Mary's Hospital,* 411 N.E.2d 50 (Ill. 1980).

Schaber, G.D., & Rohwer, C.D. (1975). *Contracts.* St. Paul, Minn.: West Publishing Co.

*Schessler v. Keck,* 271 P.2d 588 (Cal. 1954).

Schwartz, B. (1976). *Administrative Law* Boston: Little, Brown and Co., 21.

*Sides v. Duke University Medical Center,* 328 S.E.2d 818 (N.C. App. 1985), rev. denied 335 S.E.2d 13 (N.C. 1985).

*Sinks v. Methodist Medical Center,* Ill., Peoria County Circuit Court No. 82L3868 (April 1985); 28 ATLA L. Rep. 466 (December 1985).

Snyder, M.E., & LeBar, C. (1984). "Nursing: Legal Authority for Practice." In *Issues in Professional Nursing Practice.* (pp. 1–20) Kansas City, Mo.,: American Nurses' Association.

*Statkin v. Capitol Hill Hospital,* No. 84-0443 (D.D.C. Oct. 18, 1984), Medical Liability Reporter (1985).

*Swanson v. St. John's Lutheran Hospital,* 597 P.2d 702 (Mont. 1979).

3 V.S.A. Chapter 25, Vermont Administrative Practice Act.

*Toussaint v. Blue Cross and Blue Shield of Michigan,* 882 Mich. Sup. Ct. 1980, 292 N.W. 2d 880 (1980).

12 A.L.R. 4th (1982).

U.S. Constitution, Tenth Amendment; "The power not delegated to the United States by the Constitution, nor prohibited by it to the States is reserved to the States respectively, or to the people."

*Utter v. United Methodist Hospital Center,* 236 S.E.2d 213 (W.Va. 1977).

*Vaca v. Sipes,* 386 U.S. 171 (1967).

*Warthen v. Toms River Community Memorial Hospital,* 488 A.2d 229 (N.J. Super. AD 1985).

*Winters v. Miller,* 446 F.2d 65 (1971).

*Witt v. Forest Hospital,* 450 N.E.2d 811 (Ill.1983).

# 9 ◆ Ethics in Health Care Delivery

Sara T. Fry

## OBJECTIVES

*At the completion of this chapter, the reader will be able to:*

◆ Describe how the subject matters of ethics and methods of ethics are used to investigate morality

◆ Describe a decision-making framework for resolving nursing ethics problems

◆ Comprehend how personal values and beliefs, professional moral standards, moral concepts, and ethical principles are used with a decision-making framework to produce moral decisions and actions for nursing practice

The term *ethics* has several meanings. The term is sometimes used to refer to the practices or beliefs of a particular group of individuals, as in Christian ethics, physician ethics, or nursing ethics. *Ethics* also refers to the expected standards and behavior of a group as described in the group's code of professional conduct. Nurses and physicians are expected to maintain certain standards of ethical conduct as described by their professional codes of ethics (i.e., The American Nurses' Association *Code for Nurses* [1985] and the American Medical Association *Principles of Medical Ethics* [1986]). The term *ethics* is also used to refer to a philosophical mode of inquiry that helps us understand the moral dimensions of human conduct. In this sense, ethics is an activity, a particular method of investigation that one undertakes to respond to particular types of questions about human welfare.

Throughout this chapter, the term *ethics* will be used in all of the senses described above. *Ethics* will refer to the moral practices and beliefs of professionals who work together in the delivery of health care, the particular moral standards of a single group of professionals (nurses, physicians, and others), as well as inquiry about the principles of morality. Ethics is a mode of inquiry that helps us understand the moral dimensions of human conduct. To engage in or to do ethics is to undertake a particular method of investigation into matters of human concern (Fry, 1986).

## Subject Matters of Ethics

Ethics has several subject matters or areas of inquiry. *Descriptive ethics* is an area that investigates the phenomena of morality and then describes and explains the phenomena in order

**149**

to construct a theory of human nature that responds to ethical questions (Frankena, 1973). Those who investigate the moral reasoning patterns and moral judgments of nurse subjects (Crisham, 1981; Ketefian, 1981a, 1981b) are usually engaged in descriptive ethics. Other investigators have described how nurses respect the human dignity of patients (Pokorny, 1989) and how nurses make clinical decisions (Prescott, Dennis, & Jacox, 1987).

*Normative ethics* is an area of inquiry that investigates standards or criteria for right or wrong conduct (Frankena, 1973). It usually begins with the question, "What ought I to do?" and examines various ethical principles, rules, or standards of right or wrong commonly associated with moral behavior. The moral weight of the perceived duties and obligations in human interaction is assessed, and theories for moral human conduct are often used to support one normative rather than another. Common moral theories used in normative ethics are util-

itarianism, natural law, formalism, and pragmatism.

*Metaethics* is a secondary level of inquiry that examines the nature of ethical inquiry itself (Frankena, 1973). It gives us theories about ethics rather than theories for ethical conduct. Typical metaethical investigations consider the connections between human conduct and morality, the connections between ethical beliefs (values) and the facts of the real world, and the relationships among ethical theories, principles, rules, and human conduct. Inquiry about the moral language of nursing (advocacy, accountability, loyalty) falls within the area of metaethics as well.

The subject matters of ethics are closely related. Their interactions also yield a system of applied ethics (Fig. 9-1). For example, one might start by engaging in descriptive ethics to describe moral phenomena (such as the protection of patients from harm), then engage in normative ethics to argue for the moral account-

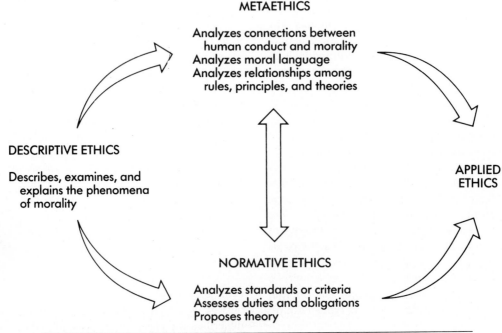

METAETHICS

Analyzes connections between
human conduct and morality
Analyzes moral language
Analyzes relationships among
rules, principles, and theories

DESCRIPTIVE ETHICS

Describes, examines, and
explains the phenomena
of morality

APPLIED
ETHICS

NORMATIVE ETHICS

Analyzes standards or criteria
Assesses duties and obligations
Proposes theory

❖ **Fig. 9-1**    The subject matters of ethics and their relationships.

ability of the nurse in patient care, and then engage in metaethics to explicate the meaning of accountability within nursing practice. The results of this process would then be applied to a particular patient care situation.

Sometimes it is not possible to engage in normative ethics without previous knowledge from metaethics and vice versa. Both normative ethics and metaethics depend on descriptive ethics for the moral phenomena of human conduct. All three subject matters of ethics are particularly helpful in understanding the nature of the increasingly difficult ethical problems experienced by health professionals in the last decade.

## Methods of Ethics

Various methods can be used to investigate morality. Since ethics is a form of philosophical inquiry, one of the most common methods is argumentation. One type of argument often used by ethicists is called "the appeal to authority" (Ladd, 1978). It states that one ought or ought not to do some action because authority tells us so. The authority appealed to may be another person (i.e., mother, father), a group of persons (i.e., the profession of nursing), an institution (i.e., a church or a health agency), or even a hypothetical person (i.e., the patient, members of society). The effectiveness of this method of argumentation is dependent on individual belief and faith in the authority appealed to.

A second type of argument is called "the appeal to consensus" (Ladd, 1978). It cites the supposed agreement of people (or groups of people) on an issue to establish its particular ethical position. Like the first method, it relies on individual belief and faith in the people (or groups of people) who agree on the issue.

A third method of argument is the "appeal to intuition" (Ladd, 1978). This method has a long tradition in ethics and is usually supported by religious conviction. Essentially, this form of argument asserts that self-evidence is a valid form of ethical knowledge. It is meaningful, however, only with persons who likewise rely

on ethical intuitions. It is sometimes regarded as an unreliable method of ethics because individual intuitions often change with time, a change in circumstances, or the conditions that create the intuition. It is always important to know whether an ethical argument is being advanced on the basis of intuition as opposed to other forms of argument.

The fourth and last type of argument is called the "dialectic" or "Socratic" method (Ladd, 1978). It begins by asking questions and then considering answers that are supported by good reasons and logical thought. It enjoys a long and respected tradition in ethics and appeals to reason or rationality for its strength.

It is important to pay attention to the types of arguments used in making ethical judgments. Any ethical judgment must be supported by sound argument. However, results of arguments may differ depending on the type of argument advanced. Since ethical judgments often serve as a basis for moral human actions, one must make sure that the method of argumentation used to reach a judgment is ethically valid and has been correctly followed. This is especially important in normative ethics but may influence metaethical investigations as well.

## ❖ MORAL CONCEPTS IN NURSING PRACTICE

Advocacy, accountability, and loyalty are moral concepts that comprise part of the foundation for nursing ethics. Other concepts considered important are care/caring, compassion, and human dignity. All of these concepts are important, but advocacy, accountability, and loyalty seem to enjoy a special place of honor among nursing standards and statements over the years.

### Advocacy

Advocacy is frequently defined as the active support of an important cause (Fry, 1987a). It is sometimes used in a legal context to refer to the defense of basic human rights on behalf of those who cannot speak for themselves. For example, many institutions employ patient advocates who are expected to defend and speak for patients who cannot, because of hospitalization or diminished autonomy as a result of illness, voice their own concerns and choices or assert their rights. The role of the advocate is to assert the patient's choices or desires on his/her behalf in the same way that a lawyer presents the case of his client, pleads for an interpretation of the case, and defends the client's rights.

There are several interpretations of the advocacy concept (Fry, 1987a). One interpretation (the rights protection model) views the nurse as the defender of patient rights against an impersonal health care system. The nurse informs the patient of his or her rights, makes sure that the patient understands these rights, reports infringements of these rights, and is expected to prevent further violations of rights.

A second interpretation (values-based decision model) views the nurse as the person who helps the patient to discuss his or her needs, interests, and choices consistent with values, life-style, or personal plan of action (Fry, 1987a). The nurse does not impose decisions or values on the patient but helps him or her explore the benefits and disadvantages of available options in order to make decisions most consistent with patient beliefs and values.

A third interpretation (respect-for-persons model) views the patient as possessing certain human characteristics that require our respect (Fry, 1987a). The patient's human dignity is respected and advocated regardless of whether or not the patient is self-determining or autonomous. As advocate, the nurse keeps the basic human values of the patient foremost among his or her considerations and acts to protect the client's human dignity, privacy, and choices (when applicable). When the patient is not self-determining, the nurse advocates the patient's welfare as defined by the patient while he was still self-determining, or as defined by his surrogate decision maker. When no other person

defines the welfare of the patient, the nurse promotes the best interests of the patient to the best of his or her nursing ability. In this role, the nurse assumes responsibility for the manner in which the patient's human dignity and other significant human values have been protected during his or her illness and is accountable to society and other members of the nursing profession for how this important advocate role has been carried out.

This last model of advocacy seems to be consistent with the values in the American Nurses' Association *Code for Nurses* (see the box on p. 153). Indeed, the code describes advocacy as acting so as "to safeguard the client and the public when health care and safety are affected by incompetent, unethical, or illegal practice by any person" (American Nurses' Association, 1985). This means that the advocate role of the nurse has important long-range implications for the quality of care and the role of the nurse in the health care system. It is an important role that cannot be underestimated in today's world.

## Accountability

The concept of accountability seems to have two major attributes: answerability and responsibility (Fry, 1990). Accountability can be defined in terms of either of these attributes, but answerability is preferred in the ANA *Code for Nurses.* The Code defines *accountability* as answerability for how one has promoted, protected, and met the health needs of the client. It means to justify or to "give an account" according to accepted moral standards or norms for choices and actions that the nurse has made and carried out. It involves a relationship between the nurse and other parties and is contractual. The nurse is a professional who enters an agreement to perform services and who can be held accountable for performing them according to agreed-upon terms and standards of practice.

The terms of *legal accountability* are con-

## ❖ AMERICAN NURSES' ASSOCIATION CODE FOR NURSES

1. The nurse provides services with respect for human dignity and the uniqueness of the client, unrestricted by considerations of social of economic status, personal attributes, or the nature of health problems.
2. The nurse safeguards the client's right to privacy by judiciously protecting information of a confidential nature.
3. The nurse acts to safeguard the client and the public when health care and safety are affected by the incompetent, unethical, or illegal practice of any person.
4. The nurse assumes responsibility and accountability for individual nursing judgments and actions.
5. The nurse maintains competence in nursing.
6. The nurse exercises informed judgment and uses individual competence and qualifications as criteria in seeking consultation, accepting responsibilities, and delegating nursing activities to others.
7. The nurse participates in activities that contribute to the ongoing development of the profession's body of knowledge.
8. The nurse participates in the profession's efforts to implement and improve standards of nursing.
9. The nurse participates in the profession's efforts to establish and maintain conditions of employment conducive to high quality nursing care.
10. The nurse participates in the profession's effort to protect the public from misinformation and misrepresentation and to maintain the integrity of nursing.
11. The nurse collaborates with members of the health professions and other citizens in promoting community and national efforts to meet the health needs of the public.

From *Code for Nurses with Interpretive Statements. The American Nurses' Association* (1985). With permission.

tained in licensing procedures and state nurse practice acts. The terms of *moral accountability* are contained in the ANA *Code for Nurses* and other standards of nursing practice in the form of norms set by the members of the profession. In the *Code for Nurses,* it is noted that accountability means "providing an explanation or rationale for what has been done in the nursing role" (ANA, 1985, p. 8). It is a very important concept of professional nursing practice and should be emphasized in the educational process. It is a concept from which important values are derived and principles are frequently formulated. Along with advocacy and loyalty, accountability forms the conceptual framework for the moral dimensions of nursing practice and helps sustain the tradition of nursing by providing both the practice of nursing and the social role of nursing with a necessary historical context.

## Loyalty

Loyalty is a multifaceted concept that includes showing sympathy, care, and reciprocity to those with whom nurses professionally identify. It means to consider the values and goals of those one works with as one's own values and goals. It leads to cooperation and mutual support and flourishes in daily acquaintances and close working relationships. It involves working closely with others toward shared goals, keeping promises, making mutual concerns a priority, and sacrificing personal interests to the maintenance of the professional relationship over time. All these involvements express traditionally valued feelings among human beings (Jameton, 1984).

There are many strong statements of loyalty in nursing's historical documents and professional statements. Isabel Hampton Robb (1900), an early nurse leader and scholar, wrote:

... she must remember that, for the time being, she is a member of a large family and its privacy and internal affairs should be as loyally guarded as those of her own home circle. The individuality of each member of the family should be respected; the shortcomings or mishaps of any nurse should never be made a topic of conversation outside, either to friends in the city or to doctors ... The principle of loyalty must be maintained, irrespective of personal feelings (p. 139).

The obligation of loyalty also gives people the power to work together. The writings of Florence Nightingale (Nutting & Dock, 1907) stress this concept in the following passage:

The health of the unit is the health of the community. Unless you have the health of the unit there is no community health. Competition, or each man for himself, and the devil against us all, may be necessary, we are told, but it is the enemy of health. Combination is the antidote—combined interests, recreation, combination to secure the best air, the best food, and all that makes life useful, healthy, and happy. There is no such thing as independence. As far as we are successful, our success lies in combination (pp. 277–278).

Loyalty seems to be that element that forms human "combination," and that serves to maintain and strengthen the members of a "community" of nurse workers toward a common goal. It does not mean that conflicts will not occur or that the good of patients should be sacrificed for the maintenance of loyalty toward friends or even the employing institution. It does mean, however, that individual goals and interests might need to be compromised in order to achieve organizational and policy changes that will increase the quality of care.

Loyalty is altruistic and expresses the human bonds that grow from working together and spending time together. It can threaten patient care if loyalty to members of the profession or coworkers becomes more important than the quality of patient care. The appropriate role for loyalty, however, is the maintenance of working relationships and conditions that ex-

press obligations toward the patient and that are mutually entered. This is an important concept of contemporary nursing practice and promises to unite nurses in the work environment for important ends related to patient care. Along with advocacy and accountability, loyalty helps form a strong conceptual framework that enables nurses to meet the requirements of professional practice.

## ❖ ETHICAL PRINCIPLES

Ethical principles are action guides to moral decision making and are an important element in the formation of moral judgments in professional practice (Beauchamp & Childress, 1989). They generally assert that actions of a certain kind ought (or ought not) to be performed and serve to justify the rules that are often applied to patient care and the context of professional practice. The ethical principles important in nursing practice are beneficence, justice, autonomy, veracity, fidelity, and avoiding killing (Veatch & Fry, 1987).

### Beneficence

The obligation to do good and to avoid doing harm is understood as the ethical principle of beneficence (Frankena, 1973). Acting on this principle means to help others gain what is of benefit to them, to reduce risks of harm to patients, and to provide positive benefits to clients in terms of goods or assets.

Applying the principle in nursing practice often poses difficult problems for the nurse. For example, it is uncertain whether or not the nurse is obliged to take into consideration all the ways in which the client might benefit. The *Code for Nurses* seems to imply that the nurse should do this when it states that the "nurse's primary commitment is to the health, welfare, and safety of the client" (ANA, 1985, p. 6). This is a substantial obligation and if literally interpreted, would entail multiple obligations toward the patient, some of which may actually lay outside the expertise or competency of the nurse.

A second problem in applying the principle is deciding whether the obligation to provide benefit has greater priority over the obligation to avoid harm. Some ethicists claim that the duty to avoid harm is a stronger obligation in health care relationships than the obligation to benefit (Beauchamp & Childress, 1989; Ross, 1939). If this is the case in nursing practice, nurses could fulfill the obligation to avoid harm by simply doing nothing for patients. Yet, we would hardly call doing nothing for patients acceptable nursing care. The avoidance of harm must be balanced by the provision of benefit, and acceptable ranges of both benefit and risks of harm need to be established.

A third problem in applying this principle in nursing practice concerns the limits of providing benefit to patients. At what point do benefits to other parties (one's own family, the employing institution, coworkers) take priority over the benefits to the patient? Is the nurse obliged to provide benefits rather broadly or simply to the identified patient? Nurses need to be very clear about the boundaries of their obligation to provide benefits and avoid harm in client care.

## Justice

Once the boundaries of the obligation to benefit and avoid harm are determined, nurses should be concerned about how benefits and burdens ought to be distributed among patient populations (Veatch & Fry, 1987). In other words, the nurse must decide what is a just or fair allocation of resources among patients under his or her care.

The formal principle of justice states that equals should be treated equally and that those who are unequal should be treated differently according to their needs (Beauchamp & Childress, 1989). This means that those equal in

health needs should receive the same amount of health care resources. When some people have greater health needs, a principle of justice allows that they should receive a greater amount of health resources. This type of allocation is just, because it distributes health resources according to need in a fair manner. While it is not possible to provide equal amounts of health care goods and resources for everyone in society, it is possible to provide for equal access to health care resources, according to individual need. The focus on need allows for the just distribution of resources among patients and foregoes the distribution of resources outside of need.

## Autonomy

The principle of autonomy ensures that individuals are permitted personal liberty to determine their own actions according to plans they have chosen (Veatch & Fry, 1987). To respect persons as autonomous individuals is to acknowledge their personal choices.

One of the problems that arises in applying a principle of autonomy to nursing care is that persons appear to be autonomous in varying degrees. Patients cannot make choices about their care entirely free from internal and external constraints. Internal constraints on patient autonomy are mental ability, level of consciousness, age, and disease states. External constraints on client autonomy are the hospital environment, nursing resources, information for making informed choices, and financial resources.

The principle of autonomy may also be difficult to apply in patient care when there is a strong conviction on the part of the nurse or other members of the health care team that respecting self-determined choice is not really in the best interest of the patient. In this type of situation, the nurse may need to consider the limits of individual patient autonomy and the criteria for justified paternalism on the part of the nurse. Paternalism is defined as the overriding of patient choices or intentional actions in order to benefit the patient (Beauchamp & Childress, 1989). Although paternalism is seldom justified in the care of patients, there is reason to believe that some situations warrant overriding patient autonomy when the benefits to be realized are great and the harms that will be avoided are significant (Childress, 1982).

## Veracity

The principle of veracity is defined as the obligation to tell the truth and to not lie or deceive others (Veatch & Fry, 1987). Truthfulness has long been regarded as fundamental to the existence of trust among individuals and has special significance in health care relationships.

Truthfulness is expected because it is part of the respect that we owe persons. Individuals have the right to be told the truth and to not be lied to or deceived. Truthfulness also supports the relationship of trust that exists in special relationships. Nurses are obliged to be truthful because to not do so will undermine the effectiveness of the nurse's role with the patient and may, in the long run, bring about undesirable consequences for future relationships with patients.

When patients are seriously ill, nurses may sometimes withhold information from them, thinking that they may not really want to know the truth about their condition. Studies of terminally ill patients, however, have indicated that despite illness, patients want to know the full truth about their conditions (Veatch, 1978). The *Code for Nurses* points out that "truth telling and the process of reaching informed choice underlie the exercise of self-determination, which is basic to respect for persons" (ANA, 1985, p. 2). This means that the nurse is obliged to respect and follow a principle of veracity in providing nursing care.

## Avoiding Killing

The problem of taking life arises in a number of patient care situations and especially in decisions to withhold or withdraw life-sustaining treatments. It can also occur in situations of suicide and whenever clients are suffering from disease or illness. The principle of avoiding killing is defined as the obligation to not infringe on the sacredness of human life, or the obligation to not take human life (Veatch & Fry, 1987).

Killing of patients may be contemplated by the nurse whenever patients are suffering. Someone might consider killing an act of mercy because the patient would be better off dead (or family members would be better off if the client were dead). However, every nurse should consider whether or not the nurse should relieve a patient's misery by hastening his or her death in some manner. Is this a role for the nurse? Are nurses expected to make these types of judgments, especially when the patient is no longer capable of making his or her own decisions or of carrying out such an action alone? Is there a difference between killing a patient for reasons of mercy and withholding or withdrawing treatments knowing that such actions will surely hasten the death of the patient (even though the patient might continue to live a while longer than when the patient is killed outright)?

Some ethicists claim that these questions can be answered by applying the principles already discussed. In other words, the principles of beneficence, justice, and autonomy already provide arguments that will support the avoidance of killing on the part of the nurse. Yet each of these principles has been demonstrated to be insufficient as a justification for the avoidance of killing in client care. A principle of avoiding killing is needed for this reason alone.

The *Code for Nurses* seems to address this issue when it states, "Nursing care is directed toward the prevention and relief of the suffering commonly associated with the dying process. The nurse may provide interventions to relieve symptoms in the dying client even when the interventions entail substantial risks of hastening death" (ANA, 1985, p. 4). Yet the *Code for Nurses* also draws the line against killing patients when it states, "Nurses are morally obligated to respect human existence and ... therefore they must take all reasonable means to protect and preserve human life when there is hope of recovery or reasonable hope of benefit from life-prolonging treatment" (ANA, 1985, p. 2).

Is withholding nutrition and hydration from a patient killing? This question is at the center of some of the most controversial patient care issues confronting nurses today (Fry, 1988). Several philosophers (Lynn & Childress, 1983; Paris & Fletcher, 1983) and some legal cases (In re Conroy, 1983; In re Hier, 1984) have come to the conclusion that nutrition and hydration can be withheld for the same reasons that other treatments are withheld. Others, however, have been reluctant to accept the withholding of nutrition and hydration even when the patient has formally requested this. Some scholars, for example, have expressed concern that the provision of food and fluids are basic caring functions that should always be required in the care of patients (Callahan, 1983). One reason given for this view is that provision of food and fluids is symbolic of our care for the hungry and thirsty among us. If patients in terminally ill states, however, do not experience hunger and thirst, does this mean that food and water should not be administered? The difficult nature of these questions is obvious.

In situations of doubt, the nurse must resort to the weight and importance of the obligation to avoid killing in nursing practice. A principle of avoiding killing is needed because nurses may often be uncertain whether or not their actions will contribute to the patient's death and whether or not such actions are morally

wrong. Killing a patient, under any circumstances, is simply not an option for the nurse.

### Fidelity

This principle is defined as the obligation to remain faithful to one's commitments (Veatch & Fry, 1987). Commitments that usually fall within the scope of fidelity are obligations generic to the trust relationship between patient and nurse. These obligations are keeping promises, maintaining confidentiality, and caring.

Individuals tend to expect that promises will be kept in human relationships. We also expect that promises will not be broken unless there is a good reason. The same expectations concern the obligation of confidentiality, which is one of the most basic ethical requirements of professional health care ethics. However, exceptions to both obligations can sometimes be made. For example, some individuals maintain that it is morally acceptable to break promises when the breaking of the promise produces more good than if the promise is kept. Confidences are often broken for the same reasons.

It is also argued that breaking promises and confidences is morally acceptable when the welfare of a third party is jeopardized by the keeping of the confidence or promise. In the *Code for Nurses,* it is stated that the obligation of confidentiality "is not absolute when innocent parties are in direct jeopardy" (ANA, 1985, p. 4). Some form of this reason is usually given when confidences or promises are broken in order to report child abuse or the laboratory results of a serious communicable disease.

Others, however, argue against the breaking of confidences, in particular, on the basis of benefit to other parties. They claim that keeping information confidential is a right independent of consequences to others. While there may be good moral reasons to break promises to provide benefit to others, it is not morally acceptable to break confidences for the same reason.

One way to understand the conceptual nature of the moral commitments surrounding confidentiality and promise-keeping is to ground these obligations within an independent principle of fidelity. Thus, in order to maintain fidelity with the patient, nurses should carefully consider the information that should be kept confidential and when promise-keeping is a legitimate expectation in the nurse-patient relationship. The duty to keep one's commitments thus becomes the focus of these obligations and not just the keeping of promises or confidentiality.

The duty to care is also included in aspects of the principle of fidelity. In fact, caring is consistently mentioned as one of the most important components of nursing practice, especially in the care of the terminally ill patient (Fleming, Scanlon, & D'Agostino, 1987; Larson, 1986; Mayer, 1987). Individualized caring, affective behaviors, comforting, and nursing competence have all been mentioned by nurses and patients as important to caring and feeling cared for.

In summary, making moral decisions and carrying out moral actions are strongly influenced to the extent to which nurses incorporate ethical principles in their actions and relationships with patients. How do the principles of ethics apply to patient care and how do nurses resolve conflicts of values in patient care?

## ❖ APPLICATION OF ETHICS TO NURSING PRACTICE

No one denies that ethical decision-making ability is a requirement of professional nursing practice (Fry, 1989). Evidence of this ability is generally regarded as a desirable outcome of nursing education. Indeed, the majority of educational programs in nursing in the United States offer some course content in ethics. The goal is to assist the student to integrate his or her personal values and beliefs, the professional code of ethics, moral concepts of nursing practice, and ethical principles into a decision-making framework for making moral decisions and taking moral action (Fig. 9-2).

A recent national study of nursing education, however, has demonstrated that significant numbers of senior nursing students do not feel that they can apply knowledge of ethics to resolve ethical problems in nursing practice (American Association of Colleges of Nursing, 1986). Few of the generic baccalaureate students surveyed (under 40%) consciously used the ANA *Code for Nurses* to guide their actions, and only a minority (23%) reported that they used an ethical framework or model to assist them in the assessment and resolution of an ethical problem (American Association of Colleges of Nursing, 1986). A survey of RN baccalaureate students revealed a perceived increase in their abilities to use ethical frameworks or

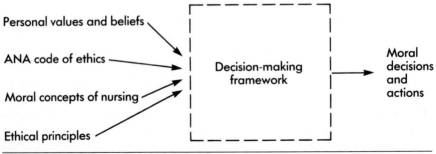

❖ **Fig. 9-2**  Essentials of moral decisions and actions in nursing practice.

models to address ethical problems when the educational process included this type of content (American Association of Colleges of Nursing, 1988).

Are ethical decision-making frameworks really useful in nursing practice? If so, how does one choose such a framework?

## Decision-Making Frameworks

Ethicists recognize that there are many components and variables in decision making. No one decision-making method is appropriate or useful for everyone. However, *ethical* decision making can be enhanced by an orderly process that takes into consideration answers to four questions often called "the fundamental questions of ethics" (Veatch & Fry, 1987). These fundamental questions are:

What makes right acts right?
What types of acts are right?
How do rules apply to specific situations?
What ought to be done in specific situations?

Frameworks for ethical decision making take these questions into consideration and represent the process or approach that one might take in making an ethical decision. They are useful to the extent that they help the decision maker answer the questions needed for an ethical decision. They do not provide a foolproof formula for arriving at the "right" decision. There is no cookbook method for ethical decision making in nursing practice. Each decision maker must supply his or her own values, cognitive ability, moral sensitivity, and rationality to the process to arrive at an ethical decision. Frameworks for ethical decision making simply help the individual use both the questions of ethics and his or her abilities to arrive at an ethical decision for a specific situation.

Since ethical decision making is a moral skill that can be taught in the educational process and that can be learned by anyone with moral conscience, course content in ethics often includes exposure to ethical decision-making frameworks, and the application of such frameworks to patient care situations. When used in conjunction with knowledge of ethics and application of ethics, frameworks promote development of the moral skill needed and required for nursing practice.

A number of ethical decision-making frameworks for nursing practice have been proposed. All of them provide an orderly approach to answering the fundamental questions of ethics, although some seem to be more detailed than others. A number of frameworks proposed by nurses have been derived from physicians' models of ethical decision making (Brody, 1981; Murphy & Murphy, 1976). A few apply contemporary philosophical positions to nursing practice (Benjamin & Curtis, 1986; Aroskar, 1980) while others closely resemble the problem-solving process taught in nursing education (Bergman, 1973; Curtin, 1978; Jameton, 1984; Stanley, 1980; Stenberg, 1979; Thompson & Thompson, 1985). One other framework combines the problem solving process in nursing with a theological perspective (Shelly, 1980). Choice of a framework should be guided by the implicit values of the framework and their importance to the decision maker.

## A Representative Framework for Case Study Analysis

Jameton's Method for Resolving Nursing Ethics Problems is a representative framework that can be used in nursing practice to reach ethical decisions related to patient care. His framework involves six steps:

1. Identify the problem. This means to clarify what is at issue in the situation in terms of values, conflicts, and matters of conscience. The nurse should also examine his or her relation to the problem and assess the time parameters for the decision-making process. This is important because some decisions can (and often should) be delayed, especially if

the decision is not needed at that precise moment. This step of the process will help the nurse answer the first question of ethics: What makes right acts right? Values will be clarified and the nurse's role in the situation will be identified.

2. The nurse should gather additional data. Information that is helpful to this step is deciding the main people involved in the decision, determining what the patient or his surrogate decision maker wants, and constructing the "story" of the conflict as it has developed. This step of the process also helps the nurse answer the first question of ethics by focusing on who is also involved in the decision-making process and who will have final authority for the decision.

3. The nurse should identify all the options open to the decision maker. All possible courses of action should be examined, including the possible outcomes of these actions. Potential impacts of outcomes on individuals affected by the decision should also be discussed. The likelihood of future decisions that might have to be made should also be considered in this step of the process, which addresses the second question of ethics: What types of acts are right? Various theoretical positions in ethics are appealed to in considering the courses of action open to the decision maker and in evaluating their worth.

4. The nurse should "think the ethical problem through" (Jameton, 1984). This means that one should consider the basic human values important to the individuals involved, the basic human values central to the issues, and the ethical principles that can be associated with the situation. Identifying the values and ethical principles is a very important step in the process and enables the nurse to answer the third question of ethics: How do rules apply to specific situations? Answering this question requires rational reflection on the relationships between various rules and principles and how basic values might (or might not) be protected if one course of action is chosen over another.

5. The decision maker should make the decision, meaning that the decision maker chooses the course of action that reflects his or her best judgment of what ought to be done. It is often very individual but is also rational because it reflects a careful process of thought and ethical reflection. In making a decision, the decision maker answers the last question of ethics: What ought to be done in specific situations?

6. The last step is to act and assess the decision or decisions and outcomes. Actual outcomes should be compared with projected outcomes, and the decision maker should ask how the process could be improved in future situations that have similar characteristics. It would also be helpful to consider whether or not the present decision could be generalized to other patient care situations. By completing this step of the process, the decision maker also answers the last question of ethics.

## ❖ RESEARCH ON NURSING ETHICS

Since the 1970s, the results of empirical studies on moral reasoning levels, moral behavior, and moral judgment among nurses have frequently appeared in the nursing literature (Murphy, 1976; Crisham, 1981; Ketefian, 1981a, 1981b). Related studies have focused on the moral reasoning levels of nursing students and nursing faculty (Munhall, 1980), and on client values in relation to treatment choices (Gortner, 1984). More recently, studies have compared nurses' perceptions of moral problems in clinical practice to the perceptions of physicians (Gamelspacher et al, 1986) and have analyzed nurses' beliefs about medical ethical decision making into objective and subjective value dimensions (Self, 1987).

These studies have focused on the ability of the nurse to make moral judgments, the hypothetical moral behavior of the nurse, nurses' perceptions of moral problems, or the value dimensions of nurses' and patients' beliefs about ethical decision making (Fry, 1987b). The measurement tools and the procedures employed have been designed to evaluate the cognitive ability of nurses to perceive value dimensions or to make moral judgments. In most cases, study results have been interpreted according to theoretical structures outside the context of nursing. Kohlberg's stage theory of moral development has been the most frequently cited theoretical structure (Kohlberg, 1981), but bioethical theory (Beauchamp & Childress, 1989) and value theory (Self, 1979) have also been cited.

Observations that can be made about the current "state of the art" in nursing ethics research are the following:

1. Values, value changes, moral judgment, and levels of moral reasoning among nurses or nurse students have not been adequately correlated with formal educational ethics content in nursing curricula. It is also not evident that the formal teaching of ethics affects the development of moral judgment in practicing nurses or that the development of moral judgment and increased levels of moral reasoning among nurses have any effect on the performance of nursing functions or client care outcomes. These are all areas for further study. We tend to think that ethics is an important component in the nursing curriculum and that the ability to recognize values, make moral decisions, and be accountable for decisions are important to the quality of nursing care. Yet we do not really know what type of ethics content is truly effective in the education of nurses. Nor do we know to what extent the effective teaching of ethics influences the ability of the nurse to give more competent client care. Is the morally accountable nurse a more competent nurse?

2. The use of theoretical frameworks to interpret study results should be carefully evaluated. Kohlberg's theory, a structure derived from cognitive psychology and based on studies of male children, has been strongly challenged for its lack of relevance to the concerns and experience of women (Gilligan, 1982; Noddings, 1984). In addition, study tools based on an old interpretation of the ANA *Code for Nurses* or on principles of biomedical ethics need to be reconsidered. Studies from these perspectives have tended to use the *Code for Nurses* and bioethical principles as theoretical structures that may not truly represent the foundations of moral decision making by nurses.

3. The evaluation of nursing research on ethics needs to address the subject matters of ethics rather than typical subject matters of nursing. For example, in a recent review of ethical inquiry in nursing, researchers classified the current state of ethical inquiry in nursing as falling into three units of analysis: the nurse, the client (or family), and the environment (Gortner, 1985). These units of analysis indicate that nurses tend to interpret nursing research in terms of traditional paradigms of nursing inquiry. Unfortunately, they tell us nothing about the discipline of ethics or the state of ethical inquiry in nursing. Ethical inquiry in nursing should be reviewed and evaluated according to the subject matters of ethics: descriptive ethics, normative ethics, and metaethics. We should also be encouraging nurse researchers to pursue research on ethics within these classifications.

## ❖ SUMMARY

The discipline of ethics has different subject matters or areas of inquiry and often uses various methods of argumentation in its investigations of morality. As part of this process, ethical analysis of moral concepts and ethical principles related to the practice of nursing is recommended.

The moral concepts of advocacy, accountability, and loyalty have important moral dimensions and comprise part of the conceptual framework for a theory of nursing ethics. The ethical principles of beneficence, justice, autonomy, veracity, avoiding killing, and fidelity are action guides to moral nurse actions but are often in conflict with one another or with other significant human values. Because of these conflicts, nurses may find that the use of an ethical decision-making framework is useful in patient care situations. Many ethical decision-making frameworks are available in the nursing literature but all seem to answer the fundamental questions of ethics and follow similar steps of reasoning. Jameton's Method for Resolving Nursing Ethics Problems is recommended since it responds to all the questions of ethics in a very clear manner.

As nurses use ethical decision-making frameworks and engage in ethical analysis, the need for additional research on nurses' decision-making patterns and choices will become evident. Descriptive ethics research is at a very early stage of development in nursing, and few good metaethical studies of nursing's moral concepts have been conducted. Normative ethics is also at a very early stage of development as a form of inquiry in nursing.

All nurses should become familiar with the methods of ethics, the use of ethical decision-making frameworks, and the current state of nursing ethics research, so that they can effectively contribute to the growth of ethical inquiry within nursing. If one of the goals of nursing education is to produce a morally accountable individual who can contribute to the quality of client care, then ethics occupies a very important role in nursing education, practice, and research.

## ❖ APPLYING KNOWLEDGE TO PRACTICE

1. To what extent should one's personal code of ethics, integrated with religious beliefs and cultural values, influence moral decision making in nursing practice?

2. If a terminally ill patient under your care asked you to help him or her end his or her life, what would you do? Why?

3. Some ethicists have argued that there is nothing morally unique to nursing practice (i.e., the same moral issues and questions arise in all health professionals' practices). Do you agree or disagree with this statement? Why?

4. The term *applied ethics* means the application of ethical theory, principles, and reasoning to a realm of practice. How would you apply ethics to your own area of nursing practice?

## REFERENCES

American Association of Colleges of Nursing (1986). *Summary Report: Generic Baccalaureate Nursing-Data Project*. Washington, DC: The Association.

American Association of Colleges of Nursing (1988). *RN Baccalaureate Nursing Education: Special Report*. Washington, D.C.: The Association.

American Medical Association Council of Ethical and Judicial Affairs (1986), *Current opinions of the Council of Ethnical and Judicial Affairs of the American Medical Association- 1986*. Chicago: The Association, p. ix.

American Nurses' Association (1985). *Code for Nurses With Interpretive Statements*. Kansas City, MO: The Association.

Aroskar, M. A. (1980). Anatomy of an ethical dilemma: The theory. *American Journal of Nursing, 80(4)*, 658-660.

Beauchamp, T. L., & Childress, J. F. (1989). *Principles of Biomedical Ethics*, 3rd. ed., New York: Oxford University Press.

Benjamin, M., & Curtis, J. (1986). *Ethics in Nursing,* 2nd ed., New York: Oxford University Press.

Bergman, R. (1973). Ethics-concepts and practice. *International Nursing Review, 20,* 140-141.

Brody, H. (1981). *Ethical Decisions in Medicine,* 2nd. ed., Boston: Little, Brown.

Callahan, D. (1983). On feeding the dying. *Hastings Center Report, 13(5),* 22.

Childress, J. F. (1982). *Paternalism in Health Care.* New York: Oxford University Press.

Crisham, P. (1981). Measuring moral judgment in nursing dilemmas. *Nursing Research, 30,* 104-110.

Curtin, L. A. (1978). A proposed model for critical ethical analysis. *Nursing Forum, 17,* 12-17.

Fleming, D., Scanlon, D., & D'Agostino, N. S. (1987). A study of the comfort needs of patients with advanced cancer. *Cancer Nursing 10(5),* 237-243.

Frankena, W. (1973). *Ethics,* 2nd Ed., Englewood Cliffs, NJ: Prentice-Hall.

Fry, S. T. (1986). Ethical inquiry in nursing: The definition and methods of biomedical ethics. *Perioperative Nursing Quarterly, 2,* 1-8.

Fry, S. T. (1987a). Autonomy, advocacy, and accountability: Ethics at the bedside. In M. D. Fowler & J. Levine-Ariff (Eds.), *Ethics at the Bedside,* pp. 39-49. Philadelphia: J. B. Lippincott Company.

Fry, S. T. (1987b). Research on ethics in nursing: The state of the art. *Nursing Outlook, 35(5),* 246.

Fry, S. T. (1988). New ANA *Guidelines* on withdrawing or withdrawing food and fluid from patients. *Nursing Outlook, 36(3),* 122-123, 148-150.

Fry, S. T. (1989). Ethical decision making. Part I: Selecting a framework. *Nursing Outlook, 37(5),* 248.

Fry, S. T. (1990). Measurement of moral answerability in nursing practice. In C. F. Waltz and O. L. Strickland (Eds.). *Measurement of clinical and educational nursing outcomes,* vol IV. New York: Springer Publishing.

Gamelspacher, G. P. et al. (1986). Perceptions of ethical problems by nurses and doctors. *Archives of Internal Medicine, 146,* 577-578.

Gilligan, C. (1982). *In a Different Voice: Psychological Theory and Women's Development.* Cambridge, MA: Harvard University Press.

Gortner, S. R. et al, (1984). Appraisal of values in the choice of treatment. *Nursing Research, 33* (6), 319-324.

Gortner, S. R. (1985). Ethical inquiry. In *Annual Review of Nursing Research,* H. Werley and J. Fitzpatrick, (Eds.)., pp. 193-213. New York: Springer Publishing.

In Re Conroy, No A-108 (N.J. Sup. Ct. Jan. 17, 1985).

In the Matter of Mary Hier, 464 N.E. 2d Series 959, Mass. App. 1984.

Jameton, A. (1984). *Nursing Practice: The Ethical Issues.* Englewood Cliffs, NJ: Prentice-Hall.

Ketefian, S. (1981a). Critical thinking, educational preparation, and development of moral judgment among selected groups of practicing nurses. *Nursing Research, 30,* 104-110.

Ketefian, S. (1981b). Moral reasoning and moral behavior among selected groups of practicing nurses. *Nursing Research, 30,* 171-176.

Kohlberg, L. (1981). *The Philosophy of Moral Development: Essays on Moral Development,* vol 1. New York: Harper & Row.

Ladd, J. (1978). The task of ethics. In W. T. Reich (Ed.) *Encyclopedia of Bioethics,* vol 1 (pp. 401-407). New York: The Free Press.

Larson, P. J. (1986). Cancer nurses perceptions of caring. *Cancer Nursing, 9(2),* 86-91.

Lynn, J., & Childress, J. F. (1983). Must patients always be given food and water? *The Hastings Center Report, 13(5),* 17-21.

Mayer, D. K. (1987). Oncology nurses' versus cancer patients' perceptions of nurse caring behaviors: A replication study. *Oncology Nursing Forum, 14(3),* 48-52.

Munhall, P. (1980). Moral reasoning levels of nursing students and faculty in a baccalaureate nursing program. *Image, 12,* 57-61.

Murphy, C. P. (1976). *Levels of Moral Reasoning in Selected Groups of Nursing Practitioners.* New York: Teachers College, Columbia University (unpublished doctoral dissertation).

Murphy, M. A., & Murphy, J. (1976). Making ethical decisions-systematically. *Nursing 76,* CG 13-14.

Noddings, N. (1984). *Caring: A Feminine Approach to Ethics and Moral Education.* Berkeley, CA: University of California Press.

Nutting, A., & Dock, L. L. (1907). *A History of Nursing,* vol II. New York: G. P. Putnam's Sons.

Paris, J. J., & Fletcher, A. B. (1983). Infant Doe regulations and the absolute requirement to use nourishment and fluids for the dying infant. *Law, Medicine and Health Care, 11(5),* 210-213.

Pokorny, M. E. (1989). Levels of Moral Reasoning in Selected Groups of Nursing Practitioners, University of Virginia (Unpublished dissertation).

Prescott, P. A., Dennis, K. E., & Jacox, A. K. (1987). Clinical decision making of staff nurses. *Image, 19(2),* 56-62.

Robb, I. H. (1900). *Nursing Ethics: For Hospital and Private Use.* Cleveland, E. C. Loeckert.

Ross, W. D. (1939). *The Right and the Good.* London: Oxford University Press.

Self, D. J. (1987). A study of the foundations of ethical decision making of nurses. *Theoretical Medicine, 8,* 86-95.

Self, D. J. (1979). Philosophical foundations of various approaches to medical ethical decision making. *Journal of Medicine & Philosophy, 4,* 20-31.

Shelly, J. A. (1980). *Dilemma: A Nurse's Guide for Making Ethical Decisions.* Downer's Grove, IL: Intervarsity Press.

Stanley, Sr. T. (1980). Ethics as a component of the curriculum. *Nursing and Health Care, 1,* 63-72.

Stenberg, M. (1979). Ethics as a component of nursing education. *Advances in Nursing Science, 1,* 53-61.

Thompson, J. E. & Thompson, N. O. (1985). *Bioethical Decision-Making for Nurses.* Norwalk, CT: Appleton-Century-Crofts.

Veatch, R. M. (1978). Truth-telling attitudes. In W. T. Reich (Ed.) *Encyclopedia of Bioethics,* vol 4, pp. 1677-1682. New York: The Free Press.

Veatch, R. M., & Fry, S. T. (1987). *Case Studies in Nursing Ethics.* Philadelphia: J. B. Lippincott Company.

# UNIT III

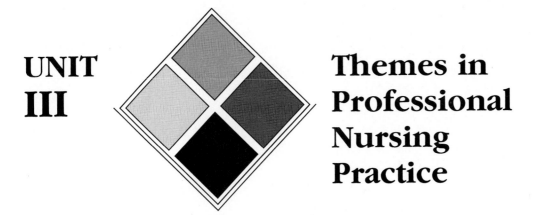

# Themes in Professional Nursing Practice

CONCEPTS common across all areas of professional nursing practice are referred to as themes. Of interest to nurses in a variety of practice settings, these themes serve as unifying threads for nursing practice. For example, as our population becomes more diverse, nurses provide care to clients from varied cultural backgrounds whose value systems may be quite unique. An overview of social and cultural influences and values and beliefs provides the basis upon which to plan and implement individualized nursing care to clients from different cultural backgrounds. Health promotion and wellness is a major thrust in today's health care, and the effect of the environment on individual and community health is of paramount concern at local and national levels. Nurses use interpersonal communication techniques in any nurse-client interaction, and teaching is a fundamental nursing responsibility, whether the client is young or old, ill or well. Finally, the impact of information technology on the planning and delivery of nursing care is a current theme that will become increasingly important in the future. These themes are discussed in this unit.

# Social and Cultural Influences

Kathryn Hopkins Kavanagh

## OBJECTIVES

*At the completion of this chapter, the reader will be able to:*

◆ Understand ways in which cultural differences between a nurse and a client may affect nursing care

◆ Identify communication skills that are useful in intercultural situations

◆ Describe barriers to provision of effective and acceptable transcultural nursing care.

American society is the most diverse in history. It is an intricate fabric of similarities and differences woven from widely varied world views, experiences, histories, and biographies. To provide acceptable and quality care, nurses must understand the design in which those patterned phenomena occur.

There are always reasons for the ways people behave. Those reasons may or may not be understood, and if they are, may or may not be accepted. But within the contexts of social processes, behaviors have function and meaning. The ability to understand interrelationships within society allows informed choices about which aspects of a given society to accept, reject, ignore, or try to change.

## ❖ CULTURE: THE MEDIUM FOR EXPERIENCING REALITY

*Culture* includes shared sets of beliefs, values, ideals and preferences, patterns of environmental adaptation, and rules for socially acceptable behavior that provide normative standards. Every society has at least one culture; some, like ours, are composites of many cultures and subcultures. To realize variation among cultures, one need only venture where life with a different flavor and style predominates.

### Subcultures

Within the vast collage of cultures are far greater numbers of *subcultures*. These smaller composites share cultural values and social norms that, while varying from other subcultures, fit with them under a common umbrella. A generic American culture is difficult to pinpoint, but numerous ethnic, regional, occupational, and other subcultures persist within the rubric of American society.

Nurses and physicians, for example, share systems of norms and values that are somewhat unique among those of society at large, yet also reflect a portion of the generalized system. As distinct occupational groups, however, nurses and physicians also have separate sets of subcultural values and rules for behavior (Leininger, 1976). They may share more in common with each other than either does with members of disciplines not oriented toward health or illness. Yet RNs may find, since care is not cure and society has not learned to value nursing as it has medicine, that they share closer occupational subcultural commonalities with nurses in Asia or Scandinavia than they do with physicians in the next corridor.

### Socialization

One acquires culture through experience. *Socialization* involves lifelong processes of learning the cultural values (that is, patterned ideals, preferences, beliefs, and attitudes) and social norms (the rules that guide behavior in a specific society or part of society) that shape each life stage. International adoptees and migrants, for instance, take on the orientations and behaviors of new homes. Jews spirited out of Nazi Germany and raised in the United Kingdom have British accents, and Asian and Latin immigrants to the United States quickly Americanize, especially if they are young. Genetic constitution notwithstanding, learned, shared culture differentiates humankind from other animals and is the key to functioning in and maintaining society. Shared symbols allow us to communicate with and understand one another. We continue to learn new symbols and meanings as the world in which we live

changes. And we continue to change that world.

### Adaptation and Culture

Culture is both material and nonmaterial. We are surrounded, most of the time, by a physical environment that reflects considerable adaptation on its part and on ours. Look around where you are now. Do you see the natural environment? Or are you encompassed in artifacts produced by a technologically complex and demanding society?

Material culture has an impact on the nonmaterial and vice versa. The relationships that humankind is thought to have with nature shape the handling of physical surroundings. In American society the predominant value allows nature to be mastered, controlled, and exploited. We have, for instance, ready access to foods outside the seasons in which they grow, and we easily control temperature and environment within our homes. We drive nearly everywhere, or save highly valued time by flying. Our physical environment to a large part has been conquered for our use. However, access to these resources depends upon having assets that are valued by society and can be used in trade.

### ❖ SOCIETY: AN ONGOING SYSTEM OF PATTERNED INTERACTION

*Societies* are groups of people who share the same cultural traditions and geographic location. Although it is not always readily apparent, society is organized. There are patterns of interaction that hold it together through structure, organization, and processes that both maintain society and contribute to maintenance of the species. Numerous other animal species also exhibit patterned and organized social behaviors.* However, it is humankind that mea-

---

*See *Cry of the Kalahari* (Owens and Owens, 1988) and Dian Fossey's work with gorillas (e.g., Fossey, 1981) for beautiful descriptions of some of those.

sures experience with such media as the evening news, and who has learned, for better or for worse, to extensively manipulate the environment to its advantage. People have culture, and culture is expressed through social interaction.

## Status and Roles

*Cultural values* shape thinking, preferences, ideals, and therefore, attitudes and goals. Society, the parts that we play in it, and the rules that we learn to get along acceptably provides the medium for behavior, for acting in ways that reflect our values. We become socialized to sets of statuses (social positions) and roles (corresponding social behaviors) (Linton, 1936).

There are numerous positions in society; each of us holds many. A single individual may be, for example, a student, nurse, parent, teacher, child, Catholic, Democrat, Chinese, diabetic, gardener, recycler, licensed driver, health care consumer, and others. Each characteristic carries with it implications for societal position and expectable behaviors. Such socially defined positions may be ascribed and essentially beyond control of the individual (such as being male or female, black or white), or acquired, that is achieved through direct effort, choice, and/or opportunity (such as being an RN, nurse practitioner, prisoner, or president).

Attached to statuses and roles are reciprocal sets of rights and responsibilities, although American society is sometimes characterized as emphasizing privileges over obligations. Nurses who are students, for example, may combine statuses and roles, but they know which sets of behaviors are expected of nurses and which of students, as well as what rights and responsibilities are attached by society to each role and status. Conflicting expectations may lead to role strain: opposing demands built into a single role (see Chapter 5). A nurse, for instance, may be put in a position where he or she is expected to mass produce individualized care.

## Social Norms: Rules for Getting Along in Society

Rules for social behavior are cast in a variety of strengths as folkways, mores, laws, and taboos. All are learned and each is maintained or changed through social sanction (that is, reward or punishment meted out through social interaction). Whatever the scale of the test, from a child's tentative smile to an adult's performance on a career-defining exam, positive responses encourage certain behaviors, and negative responses encourage others.

We learn and are socialized to most of the rules for social interaction without paying close attention to their roles in organizing and perpetuating society. In other words, we typically take societal rules for granted, particularly when the consequences of breaking them are mild.

**Customs and folkways.** *Folkways* and *customs* are aggregates of norms with relatively little social impact. They include the rules that are learned about what to wear to class and to work and to weddings, what to eat for breakfast and for dinner (as if these were not interchangeable), how close to stand to someone when talking with him or her, whom to talk with and whom to avoid, how to behave in a public restroom or in line at the electronic teller, and innumerable other situations. Some are traditions, like eating turkey and cranberries on Thanksgiving, for instance, or ceremonies such as graduation.

Most likely no one sat you down and spelled out those rules; they were learned by observing, interacting, and participating in society. Perhaps expectations for line behavior at bank machines were a thing of the future when you learned the bathroom rules. Standards for behavior change as culture changes. Changes, which occur both within and between cultures, are modified with circumstance (e.g., regional differences, life stage, economic resources, attitude, modeling of others, statements to be made, and types of settings or interactions that are anticipated).

As behavioral patterns are negotiated in everyday life, relatively little happens when minor rules are changed or broken. One might be prohibited from entering an establishment due to unanticipated expectation of a coat and tie, but generally if breakfast and dinner menus are reversed or the dress code is broken, the response is slight. However, if one strays too far outside the boundaries of the norms, wears rags or nothing at all, becomes anorexic, or intrudes too intensely on others' space, social response will be greater. Exactly where those boundaries lay depends on a society's experience with and tolerance for eccentricity and deviance.

**Morals and ethics.** *Morals* and *ethics* are behavioral guidelines that are more heavily weighted in social interaction than are customs or folkways. Condensed extractions from religious and philosophical systems, respectively, they provide a sense of right and wrong and shape judgments, as well as reflect sets of long-standing values held and enforced by specific groups. A divorcing Catholic, for example, may elicit greater social response from his or her fellow parishioners than a divorcing Protestant, for whom marital life might be viewed more as a relationship with legal implications than one with both legal rights and responsibilities and moral implications of permanent commitment.

What is considered a moral or ethical issue reflects broader cultural values and social norms. Some analyses of American society suggest, for example, that unequal distribution of resources demonstrates a throwaway attitude toward some parts of the population. Pro-life and Pro-choice issues are argued at every level of social discourse. Relatively few Americans have accepted, however, the accusation and challenge that the United States' differential infant mortality rates for white and nonwhite babies amount to socially condoned infanticide (Scheper-Hughes, 1987). Nonwhite babies, like babies born to poor families, die at twice the rate at which white babies and those born to nonpoor families die (Boone, 1989), but the problem is not generally examined as an ethical or moral one as are more popular end-of-life and genetic manipulation issues.

**Laws.** *Laws* pose another type of social standard and are distinguished by their reinforcement by the authority of a formal system of government. Such rules do not cover every aspect of life but focus on group-level concern for regulation of behavior. In the United States, an enduring separation of church and state keeps sets of ethical/moral guidelines and of laws relatively separate in reinforcement if not content. However, some topics, such as divorce, may be considered issues of both legal and moral concern, while others, such as the criteria for determining brain death, involve both legal and ethical considerations.

**Taboos.** *Taboos* are the strongest form of behavioral regulator. More conspicuous in traditional cultures than in ours, they include varied interactive prescriptions. Examples of taboos in other cultures include not looking directly at one's mother-in-law, remaining in seclusion during menses, or, depending on specific tradition, ensuring that spirits are either confined or freed at death or burial. In our society, interracial marriage was for a long time treated as a taboo. Breaking these strong social rules can carry severe psychic and/or physical penalties.

Taboos may be strong enough to avoid the need for laws to govern behavior, as is the case with cannabalism in America. On the other hand, incest, against which taboos are common, occurs frequently enough in the United States to warrant establishment and enforcement of laws as well.

## Social Acceptability and Change

The acceptability of any behavior depends upon the cultural context in which it occurs. Expectations vary widely with cultural values and norms, class differences, and time. Few activities can be imagined that are or were not permissible or even rewarded in specific circumstances. Incest, for example, frowned upon in most societies, has also served as the mechanism of resort for continuation of specific, cherished, and often royal bloodlines. What is judged murder in one setting may be viewed as heroic behavior in another. Typically considered unjustifiable by Americans, infanticide has functioned in numerous times and places as an adaptive response to limited resources and one that contributed significantly to maintenance of a society as a whole. Although American society is not disposed at the present to label either of the previously mentioned means of killing as socially acceptable, our current quandaries over preserving life, letting it go, and ending it illustrate the confusion with which we live in a dynamic society influenced by a variety of cultural frameworks and sets of moral and ethical traditions. Science and technology allow things to happen that moral and ethical codes, which reflect cultural and subcultural value orientations, have not been developed to handle. Culture typically changes more slowly than behavior does.

Despite widespread acceptance and the tendency for tradition to endure even when the rationale for behaviors cannot be articulated, societal norms are subject to change. Such norms represent standards of frequency and not necessarily preference or ideals. Behavior that attracts no special notice today may have landed someone in jail or a mental institution a century ago, and may as likely be considered socially inappropriate in future times or other places.

The process of gradual acquisition and the immense complexity of expectations and rules for getting along in a society become acutely evident when one enters an unfamiliar group, that is one for which the social interactive rules are not known. Perhaps if every health care provider experienced at least once the phenomenon of knowing only the "wrong" rules (that is, rules that do not work), our sizable immigrant population would be better understood and served.

## Society: Function and Maintenance

Function and maintenance of society are the outcomes of social action that ranges from the level of the individual to that of society and international relations. Whatever the level, the outcomes are production, reproduction, and defense.

**Production.** What is required to keep a social system going must be produced, whether it be at the level of a solitary person earning a living, adults providing for children and others, or large-scale, interrelated production of goods and services aimed at accommodating the needs (and desires, if it is an affluent society) of the populace.

As members of a technologically dependent, industrialized society, relatively few of us produce goods. Services are the products of our efforts and expertise. The types of services depend on culturally defined values, needs, and priorities. There is no need for a police force where there is no threat to social order or for psychiatrists where there is no concept of mental illness. But where those are not the case, the services will be instituted.

**Reproduction.** In addition to production of goods and services, the perpetuation of society requires biological and social reproduction. Those societies that prohibit reproduction cease to exist. The celibate brothers and sisters of Shaker communities, for instance, formed

America's largest nineteenth-century utopian group. However, as changes in social thought made conversion to the group less appealing, it dwindled gradually to a few individuals.

Despite its undeniable importance, physical reproduction alone cannot sustain a society. If any population duplicated its number, whether by biological reproduction or incorporation of other peoples, but failed to socialize that progeny to the society, the result would be a disorganized aggregate that did not carry on the functions of social life. Social reproduction or socialization (that is, the internalization of cultural values and social norms) is crucial to social interaction and societal continuity.

**Defense.** Defense is the third function of social action. Humankind has always perceived a need to protect itself from its perilous environment. No longer on the lookout for fearsome cave bears or plundering marauders, today's parent cautions instead against specific consequences of the present social conditions, such as traffic, drugs, and strangers. The same adults may actively lobby for better street lighting, schools, or tighter enforcement of laws against drunk driving, all designed to protect the present and future populations of the community. Military systems, symbolizing societal-level defense services, extend the scope of protection beyond national boundaries into international spheres.

## ❖ SOCIETAL RESOURCES AND STRATIFICATION

With the exception of the rare, truly equitable, hunting-and-gathering group, each society distributes its valued resources according to widely accepted social interactive patterns. Although they sometimes overlap and vary greatly among cultures, societal processes distribute the same resources (that is, status, power, and wealth) however these may be manifested in a given society.

### Status

Status, or prestige and the influence that comes with it, comes from ascribed or achieved characteristics. In the traditional caste system of India, for example, one was born into a social position and had no reason to anticipate any alteration of that situation. American slaves experienced the same reality, and, reflecting a lingering post–Civil War caste mentality, Jim Crow laws (which segregated all public resources and were not seriously challenged until the 1960s) demonstrated the slowness with which attitudes change. Despite a common right to voting citizenship and civil freedoms, black and white Americans experienced frankly different social statuses.

### Power

Power, the ability to get people to do things that they otherwise would or might not do, is crucial to accomplishment of many goals and interests. The presence or absence of power is the critical factor in determining majority and minority or subordinate statuses. Blacks in South Africa, for instance, although far outnumbering the more powerful whites, constitute a minority population. Similarly, in the United States, although various religious organizations approximate a system in which no one group dominates the others (despite some groups being larger or smaller than others), *ethnic equality* (that is, equal opportunity to acquire resources) and *ethnic pluralism* (diversity without domination) remain in large part unrealized.

### Wealth

The third resource, wealth, is worth measured in terms of economic and other valued commodities, regardless of the form of exchange. Traditional African Nuer, for example, used cows as their capital, and in South Pacific Yap, acquisition of huge stone discs continues to be valued. Industrialized societies measure economic worth in terms of monetary currency, such as the dollar, rupee, Deutschemark, or yen. Economic worth, or class, is assessed in the United States in terms of income and other assets, the acquisition of which generally depends in part upon status and power. In some instances, however, the resources function independently, as has been the case with black leaders such as Martin Luther King, Jr. and Jesse Jackson. Those men have amassed power and status based not on financial foundations, but on support through community action and common interest, for which black religious organizations served as a vehicle.

### ❖ DISTRIBUTION OF RESOURCES

The distribution of status, power, and wealth involves, in most large societies, variable interrelated factors. Among those, in the United States, are age, sex, education, income, occupation, religion, material possessions, health status, appearance, race, ethnicity, family name, residence, family composition, and landedness. The extent of influence of a given factor differs with time and circumstance, yet, despite civil rights protection against discrimination in many forms, different opportunities are likely to be experienced by a single parent and a two-parent family, a wheelchair-bound worker and his or her able-bodied peer, and a taxpayer who rents a home and another who lives with a mortgage but, by "owning" property, qualifies for a more favorable return.

It is important to recognize that the United States is socially stratified in many ways, despite its traditional idealization as a land of rich opportunity and the realization that it is a place where many people do "get ahead" and effort and accomplishment are correlated, although not always equitably so.

The outcome of social stratification is social inequality. Classifications cannot be made according to criteria that are weighted in importance, worth, or value without some categories

coming out with more positive assessments than others. The experiental consequences of such categorization are unequal life chances and opportunities. Classification of social worth is so much a part of everyday social process that differential distribution of goods and services may evade conscious intent and result from established patterns of interaction and attention. The child who fails fourth grade math in an inner-city school, for example, may be viewed as being unable to handle the work, while his or her suburban counterpart receives supplemental or remedial sessions. The long-term result may be unequal opportunity to achieve status, power, and wealth as productive adults.

Health care settings have long been the subject of study and concern regarding distribution of resources. Since YAVIS populations (that is, those composed of young, attractive, verbal, intelligent, and successful individuals) were distinguished several decades ago as likely to receive preferential treatment at health care facilities, it has also been observed that those persons who are viewed as QUOIDS (quiet, unattractive, old, indigent, dissimilar [perhaps "foreign" or "weird"], and stupid) are likely to receive especially limited attention.

Given American values and norms, and our status as the only industrialized nation without a national health care system, there is limited societal pressure to provide health care (or equitable care) for everyone. One outcome of health care not being a political priority, however, is significant variation in mortality and morbidity rates. American infant mortality rates are higher than those of most other industrialized countries. Similarly, nonwhite male mortality rates to age 65 that exceed white male rates by 40% to 95% exemplify the costs of limited access to health care for large, underserved populations. (*Ethnicity and Health*, edited by Van Horne & Tonnesen [1988], is recommended for further information.)

**Race and ethnicity.** When America was

originally imagined to be on its way to becoming a cultural "melting pot," its immigrants were markedly similar, having come from northern, European, and generally Protestant origins. When members of Southern European and Catholic societies began to arrive in sizable numbers, however, the supposedly amalgamating population experienced some relatively painful, unassimilated lumps. The melting pot idea worked well only for those groups that could and would assume the values of the predominate population, which was white, Anglo-Saxon, and Protestant.

Some groups did not blend in, either because of resistance to giving up cultural values and traditions (that is, adherence to shared cultural traits or ethnicity) or because of inherent "differentness," such as skin color or hair texture, which functioned as disqualification from full integration into society. With time many groups moved toward acculturation and assimilation. A few, such as the Amish and Hutterites, have steadfastly maintained their individuality. For racially distinct groups, meanwhile, there have been many barriers to "melting in," even when the groups are motivated to do so.

Advances in the physical and social sciences have since redefined race as a social rather than a biological phenomenon and have left racist themes of inherent superiority and inferiority untenable. Ethnicity is a more viable tool than race for examination of similarities and differences. In America, the racial die was securely cast, and racist themes continue to influence opportunities to acquire status, power, and wealth. (Van Horne & Tonnesen [1985] and Fee [1983] are recommended for further information.)

The essential fact is that if the earth's more than 5 billion inhabitants were mustered somehow into a single line, starting with the very darkest on one end and ending with the lightest skinned on the other, that vast multitude could not be sorted reliably into races; some are light and some are dark, but the great majority are shades of brown. Skin color does not occur in discrete categories. Nonetheless, access to status, power, and wealth is influenced by such criteria as race, and those resources influence access to health care.

**Sex and gender.** Racism is only one medium for the effect of social inequality on lives. A lengthy list of social stratification criteria implies numerous manipulations of access to resources, including health care. One of the most obvious, and one directly pertinent to nurses, whether male or female, is sexism, with its underlying assumption of the inherent superiority of members of one sex over those of the other. Problems involving sexism cannot, as those involving racism cannot, be resolved within the context of the health care system alone, because they reflect processes that permeate all of society. However, it is important to be aware of gender differences in opportunities to acquire status, power, and wealth because of the influence of those differences on physical and mental health and on access to health care.

In the United States, women earn an average of 60% of men's incomes, even for the same work, and low-income black females are generally the most overrepresented among disadvantaged females. Single parents are typically women (a fact that reflects differences in gender-based rights and responsibilities), and their proportional presence on the welfare rolls has greatly expanded. As more women assume roles as heads of households, socially reinforced ceilings on the worth of women and their work are increasingly apparent in the perpetuation of undervalued feminized occupational patterns such as nursing.

Manipulation of women's roles in society has not left men unaffected. As the process of industrialization moved the locus of economic earning away from the home and farm to the factory and office, men were removed from familial involvement that had traditionally been both their option and a primary source of co-operative labor. While women, like children, were viewed as in need of control and protection, men were deprived of equitable companionship and forced to assume stereotypically paternalistic and patronizing roles. Characteristically stressed by expectations of achievement in the marketplace and estranged from emotional involvement at home, male roles are only now beginning to return comfortably to the family. Society remains a long way from androgynous interchangeability of roles, however, as is made clear by the fact that although nurses constitute an otherwise educationally, ethnically, and experientially heterogeneous aggregate, only a small proportion of nurses are men. Perhaps even more clear is the message communicated by the limited effort to change that.

## ❖ COSTS OF INEQUALITY AND RISKS OF COLOR OR GENDER BLINDNESS

By undermining both personal and organizational integrity, the many costs of social inequality extend to everyone in the social system (Bowser & Hunt, 1981) and in the health care system. It takes energy to believe that racial, ethnic, gender, age, and other issues of inequity are not important or that discrimination does not exist. The consequences include compromised self-respect for the majority population, which must pretend that the problem is the minority's, and the minority population, which may come to question its own worth when made to feel invisible, inferior, and inconsequential. Nurses at times experience that situation.

Social inequality and stratification are cultural traits. Interactions that generate and maintain those phenomena are learned and socially transmitted and are, therefore, subject to change. Phenomena such as "colorblindness" and "genderblindness" (that is, nonrecognition of societal patterns of differential treatment based on race or gender) are nonproductive because they deny variations in life experience that in a stratified society are both real and meaningful.

Effective and acceptable health care involves problem solving on all levels. It is not limited to individual or client-level concerns, but must address higher levels of policy and societal organization. Understanding social processes that underlie the perpetuation of social inequality empowers providers as well as consumers of health care.

Overlooking or ignoring the effects of unequal distribution of resources implies that specific experiences of individuals and groups are not important, and that change is not needed. Since many aspects of racism, sexism, and other systems of unequal opportunity are institutionalized in the social system, failure to recognize and change them serves to perpetuate and condone. For example, unacknowledged diversity among nurses and failure to seriously scrutinize relationships among nurses, as well as between nursing and medical personnel and between health care providers and consumers, are significant because they perpetuate the inequitable status quo.

Two decades ago nursing was at the forefront of the demand for equal rights and recognition. Today there is far less focus on that aspect of social progress. Increased feminism, although undeniably warranted (and perhaps intensifying nursing's association with women), diluted emphasis on relationships rooted in other aspects of power distribution, such as ethnicity, race, and cultural background. Awareness of the function of "blindness" to these and other issues is crucial if nurses are to work together toward common goals, including development of nursing as a unified profession.

## ❖ CULTURE, CARING, AND CURING
### Culture and Perception of Health Status

Since illness and death are part of life, mortal humans have conscious, health-related needs. Systems of beliefs, diagnosis, treatment, and care are required. How illness is defined, however, and what is to be done about it and by whom, are matters of cultural belief systems and social dynamics.

Pinta, a variant of treponematosis that occurs in Central and South America, is named for its white, blue, pink, yellow, or violet skin blotches (McElroy & Townsend, 1989). In some regions pinta is so endemic as to be the norm; the individual without the condition is negatively stigmatized, socially marginal, and decidedly unmarriageable. Given that scenario, who is ill and who is healthy?

Westernized definitions of health and illness are vague. Other ideas may seem, to Western ways of thinking, even more nebulous. Biomedical science deals with disease in terms of deviation from clinical norms or, more broadly, as the result of environmental insult. Illness, on the other hand, is a cultural category based on individual experience, and sickness a manifestation of social behavior.

Mental health and mental illnesses are even more difficult than physical statuses to delineate, due to a lack of readily observable, discrete, and organic phenomena. The consequence is reliance on assessment of behaviors rather than on definitive symptomatology. Diagnoses then involve social competence, which, to be sensitively evaluated, must be assessed against culture-specific criteria. Evaluation of compliance with social rules and expectations requires understanding the rules.

To members of many societies, concepts such as mental health have little or no meaning. One is either ill or not, and that distinction is based on somatic criteria that either allow or impede the ability to perform one's normal roles in society. A physician's diagnosis and prognosis based on unobservable phenomena may seem ludicrous. To many people, impaired function is the only rationale for seeking health care.

The Yanomamo tribesmen with pinta, although diseased by Western standards, may be healthy by those of their society; it is the unafflicted person who is labeled abnormal and assumes a special role outside the social norm.

**Sick role.** Illness, like sickness, varies with cultural definition and social expectation, and is, therefore, subject to change. The classic model of the sick role involved two rights of the patient (that is, the right to exemption from normal social role responsibilities and the right to care until recovery) and two responsibilities (acknowledgment of the sick role as undesirable, which implied an obligation to get well as fast as possible, and utilization of competent help with which the patient cooperated) (Parsons, 1951).

Although Parson's model is still often appropriate, contemporary sick roles are somewhat more complex when applied to chronic, degenerative conditions from which full recovery cannot be expected, and include implications that the failure of the patient to behave in certain ways is responsible for the disease, illness, or both (Alexander, 1982).

### Obstacles to Caring and Curing

Every health care provider has encountered clients who seemed locked within impermeable barriers and remained apparently impervious and unresponsive to all professional ministrations. Responsibility for failure to respond may have been attributed to the "noncompliant" consumer (or potential consumer) who failed to share recognition of the presumed value and benefit of the proferred services.

Given the many ways in which health and illness are perceived, it is not surprising that there is great variety in expectations for appropriate treatment and care. It is increasingly apparent that the ability to communicate interculturally and to understand culture-based care and caring practices are essential to provision of quality, effective, and appropriate illness-alleviating and/or health-promoting care (Leininger, 1985).

**Language and expectations.** There are many cultural phenomena that pose potential barriers in health care. Language, both verbal and nonverbal, is the most obvious obstacle. However, attitudes and expectations that are deeply rooted in class (that is, socioeconomic stratification) and in ethnicity (cultural identity and orientation) also affect health and care. For example, differences in attitudes toward relationships (such as expectations of hierarchy or mutuality, independence or dependence), or toward interacting with others who are perceived as different, may encourage or discourage resource utilization. Expectation of self-care, for instance, may be perceived as inappropriate imposition. Many people view health providers as experts who are expected to provide advice and direction that validate that qualification. Cultural expectations may also be such that illness results in a sick role that is characterized by dependence on others.

**Individuals, groups, and authority.** One of the most taken for granted yet misleading assumptions of Western health care providers is that they are, or should be, dealing with individuals. Despite generalized expectation of highly psychologized and individuated American identities, nurses must face the reality that members of many societies do not perceive themselves first as individuals but as members of groups. As an Asian nurse adroitly explained, she, an individual in Western eyes, is in her view a "small i"; her family is the "large I." Decisions are made by groups or by heads of groups for the good of the group; individuals are first part of the whole and secondly autonomous and separate persons. Therefore, although care may be appropriately individuated for each client, nurses must become more comfortable with perceiving "the client" in collective terms that imply orientation to the common unit and not mere collections of individuals.

It is also unsafe to assume that biological relationships or formal ties such as marriage are the most significant ones. The individual who is culturally expected to make decisions is frequently the dominant male, regardless of who in the group is considered by health care providers to be the focus of care or treatment. For example, no insistence by a community health nurse, that mothers have their children immunized will have the impact that the community leader does after he or she is convinced of the value of disease-preventing inoculations.

**Adaptability.** It is often assumed that health care providers and agencies must find ways to increase compliance of consumers to their policies and procedures. It is equally feasible, however, to examine the possibility of adapting agency policy and protocol to the needs of consumers. This may involve such adaptations as using earth tones in decorating to encourage Native Americans to feel comfortable, or creating flexible schedules for those who do not conform easily to rigid middle class expectations of punctuality and precise appointments.

Another level of agency flexibility is exemplified by clinicians who work toward integration of traditional and folk practices with the biomedical. Clients are experts about their own cultural perspectives. Most can and will provide information, if asked, that allows incorporation of their perspectives into nursing care and medical treatment plans. Clients of Hispanic backgrounds, for example, can be given nutritional information that is congruent with their customs and beliefs about foods that are considered hot or cold (not by temperature, but by theoretical classification), and the relationship between those and health. Diets that are adapted for cultural congruence are more likely to be followed than are those that the client finds unfamiliar and unappealing.

Policy-level accommodation to cultural needs occurs when agency personnel work actively with traditional healers and carers to implement treatment and care plans that are acceptable to clients. Such acknowledgment and integration of alternative practices communicate flexibility, respect, and openness to alternative ways of thinking and caring. When agencies as well as providers make a commitment to provision of culturally congruent care, compliance rates typically increase.

## Intercultural Communication

Meaningful crosscultural, interpersonal interactions quickly lead to the conclusion that empathy alone is not enough. Numerous theories and approaches to intercultural communication exist (Kim & Gudykunst, 1988). One of the approaches most valuable to nursing for its adaptability in clinical situations is Pedersen's. The goal of Pedersen's model is a balance of intercultural awareness, knowledge, and skills conducive to sensitive and acceptable intervention (Pedersen, 1988). This involves articulation of a problem situation from the client's point of view, diminution of resistance and defensiveness that impede goal accomplishment, and the development of recovery skills that allow communication processes to be repaired in the event of interactive problems between the provider and the client.

**Identifying the problem.** Problem identification that is sensitive to cultural needs implies understanding the client's perspective. Pedersen's Triad Model (adapted from Pedersen at al., 1989; Pedersen, 1988) provides a useful tool to that end. It is based on the following ideas:

1. The client has a relationship with the problem as he or she (or they) see(s) it.
2. Effective intervention requires the ability to understand the problem from both the insider's (client's) and outsider's (nurse's) points of view.
3. The influence of the nurse is less than that of the problem, unless the nurse's influence can be combined with that of the client to form a coalition.
4. When the client and provider form a coalition, they can work together toward problem solving.

In conceptualizing a health problem as a three-way interaction with the nurse, client, and problem, relevant questions include (Pedersen et al., 1981):

1. What does the client see as the problem?
2. Who does the client see as responsible for the problem?
3. What does the problem mean to the client?
4. Who has control over the problem?

The triad formed by the nurse, client, and problem is depicted in Fig. 10-1. In this model, *A* represents the client's relationship with the problem as he or she views it. The arrow associated with that relationship depicts the client's

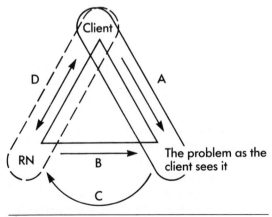

❖ **Fig. 10-1** Pederson's triad model.

efforts to handle the problem. *B* denotes the nurse's relationship with the client's problem and the forces he or she directs toward its resolution. If the nurse does not fully understand the client's perspective of the problem, the nurse's efforts are likely to be less effective than if he or she does understand the client's view. Since perspectives are commonly shaped by cultural orientation, cultural awareness and knowledge are keys to understanding.

*C* represents a shift from the original coalition (*A*) between the client and his or her problem to a coalition between the nurse and the client (*D*). The double-headed arrow (*D*) represents mutual (two-way) interaction between the nurse and client that allows the nurse to accept and understand the client's perspective.

Understanding the client's point of view does not imply that the nurse agrees with or prefers all aspects of it. However, the nurse-client coalition (*D*) allows the nurse and the client to combine efforts (*A* + *B*) to work on problem resolution by setting goals, making plans, and implementing and evaluating them.

**Recognizing resistance and decreasing defensiveness.** Also critical to intercultural communication is recognition of resistance (that is, aspects of the situation that work against meeting the goal) and defensiveness, which is response to the perception of threat. These phenomena can occur in both the client and the provider. Resistance and defensiveness should be understood in specific rather than general terms to avoid vague negativity and to allow productive acknowledgment and change. Understanding, for example, when a female nurse feels defensive because a client has communicated that a man and/or a physician is considered a more appropriate person to handle his or her problem is more valuable than is vague and diffuse defensiveness toward all clients who exhibit similar behaviors or characteristics.

The nondefensive and confident provider can focus on the client's needs, rather than on a personal need to feel more secure in the exchange. Likewise, awareness of why a client may resist specific treatment or care plans allows exploration of alternatives and creation of plans and goals that are acceptable to the client.

Professional camouflage (such as preoccupation with activity and tasks, limitation of interaction due to time pressure, lack of interest, dependence on stereotypes, fear of handling the consequences of communication, and minimizing communication to avoid risk of "hurting someone's feelings") defuses anxiety-arousing situations with defenses that may, in the long run, reinforce rather than reduce interactive barriers. On the other hand, paying close attention to interactive processes and to one's own impact on them, and increasing knowledge about patterns of stress and coping and value conflicts are valuable ways to decrease defensiveness and resistance. Additional tools include the use of questions, confrontation, interpretation, feedback, humor, story telling, self-disclosure, spontaneity, receptivity, apology, and open acknowledgment of resistance and defensiveness (adapted from Pedersen, 1988).

**Recovery skills.** Although the rewards typically more than offset the risks or problems, ventures into unfamiliar interactive situations increase probabilities that mistakes will occur. Never making a communicative mistake implies a failure to take risks, which itself is problematic because even passive behaviors communicate, and lack of activity implies acceptance of the status quo. Since occasional miscommunications are expectable in any active, meaningful exchange, the objective is to be ready with recovery skills to effectively handle the situation when the provider says or does something that arouses a client's anger or suspicion, or finds the client otherwise distanced. Specific skills relevant to communicative recovery processes include refocusing on the topic, changing the topic, challenging the client, using silence, reversing roles with the client, negotiating or arbitrating, role playing, repositioning, providing feedback, using metaphors or examples, apology, termination, and referral (adapted from Pedersen, 1988). Interpersonal communication is discussed in Chapter 14.

Integral to effective intercultural communication is the realization that no one communicates flawlessly; "perfect" communication is not a reasonable goal. It is impossible to know all the interactive rules appropriate to more than 5 billion people who represent thousands of cultures and subcultures, to say nothing of exponential numbers of individualized expectations—virtually any combination of which may present themselves in a given agency. However, learning to be sensitive to, knowledgeable about, and skillful in intercultural situations is rewarding for everyone involved. Since such experience involves occasional mistakes, permission to make mistakes is essential to learning to correct and to live with them.

**Avoidance and coercion.** Fear of uncomfortable situations results in many intercultural situations being handled with either avoidance or coercion, rather than respectful, positive en-counters leading to mutual communication and the maintenance or restoration of integrity. *Avoidance* involves treating situations, and often those persons associated with them, as invisible or unworthy of recognition. However, situations, like feelings, do not go away. A short-term, peacekeeping strategy, avoidance neither prepares for later eruptions of anger and frustration nor fosters mutual effort toward problem resolution or health promotion.

*Coercion* involves the use of status, power, and/or wealth to compel or persuade people to act in specific ways. Neither avoidance nor coercion can be equated with problem resolution or with productive, mutual exchange, although either may result in temporary suppression of the problem. Either can also explain why many "culturally different" clients avoid "complying" with the expectations of Western physicians and nurses. Clients look for, expect, and deserve communication and intervention that recognizes and respects their orientations and experiences.

**Triad model.** Pedersen's Triad Model provides another clinically useful strategy for

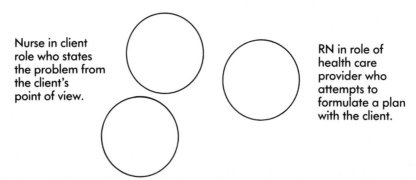

Nurse in client role who states the problem from the client's point of view.

RN in role of health care provider who attempts to formulate a plan with the client.

Nurse in "Challenger" role, who describes barriers to resolving the identified problem as the RN proposes. This individual presents what the client may not feel able to: conflicting beliefs or practices, economic or educational constraints, lack of familiarity with the proposed course of action, and so on.

❖ **Fig. 10-2**  Pedersen's triad model role play.

nurses to work together toward accurate cultural assessment, problem identification, and mutually acceptable intervention and goal formation. Using role play techniques, one nurse represents the client and another the health care provider, who begins a conversation with the client relevant to the problem. A third member of the team functions in a challenger role (that is, he or she represents and articulates obstacles to what the health care provider does and proposes).

Fig. 10-2 depicts the role play's physical arrangement and process. Each circle represents a chair and an actor and is positioned so as to be visible by each other actor. Each role is spoken loudly enough to be heard by all participants.

The challenger role is played, ideally, by someone who is somewhat knowledgeable about the client's culture. It serves as a medium for expression of the client's perspective and allows articulation of aspects of the context that the client may not feel free to express (due, for example, to linguistic barriers, politeness, hesitancy to contradict an authority, fear of rejection, or other reasons).

Used for many years as a crosscultural counseling training technique (Pedersen et al., 1981), the Triad Model Role Play has been found by the author to be equally applicable in clinical nursing situations, in particular team conferences, or staff meetings focused on specific clients' problems. Observations of additional personnel are valuable to help with team analysis of the situation. All involved will increase their awareness and knowledge of the ethnic or cultural perspective that is represented.

## Culturally Congruent Care

The development of caring sciences has emphasized goals of avoiding inappropriate intervention and of providing culturally congruent assessment and intervention. Nurses function as gatekeepers between clients and the health care system, and at times between the client's cultural background and the aspects of American culture that are reflected in health care and/or a client's circumstances. They must, therefore, become comfortable with care meanings, patterns, and processes that allow more flexibility in practice than is sometimes presented in nursing education or modeled by RNs.

Care is the central, dominant, and unifying feature of nursing (Leininger, 1988b). Provision of care that is comprehensive must take into account culture-based factors related to systems of technology, religion and philosophy, kinship and social relations, values and norms, politics and law, economy, and education (Leininger 1988a). Language and environmental contexts are threads throughout those factors and further influence care patterns and expressions of individuals, families, groups, and societies. Fig. 10-3 depicts the interrelationships among sociocultural factors and health care systems (Leininger, 1988a).

Madeleine Leininger, who founded and established transcultural nursing as a distinct subdiscipline with a respectable theoretical and research basis, summarizes the need for effective intercultural nursing care as the following (adapted from Leininger, 1988b):

1. Culturally congruent care is critical for human growth, self and group actualization, human development, and cultural survival.
2. Caring activities, behaviors, and processes link diverse peoples in mutual interdependence and interrelatedness.
3. Caring plays an important role in protecting and maintaining human individuals and groups.
4. Caring behaviors, activities, and processes serve to prevent stress, social disruption and disorganization, and human misery.
5. Culturally sensitive and acceptable caring denotes and sustains human qualities and attributes.
6. Culturally congruent caring facilitates curing and healing.

Culture care

World view

Cultural and social structure dimensions

Cultural values and lifeways

Kinship and social factors

Political and legal factors

Religious and philosophical factors

environment

Economic factors

Language and

Context

Influences care patterns and expressions

Technological factors

Health (well-being)

Educational factors

of

individuals, families, groups, and institutions

Diverse health systems

Folk systems

Nursing

Professional systems

Nursing care decisions and actions

Cultural care preservation/maintenance
Cultural care accommodation/negotiation
Cultural care repatterning/restructuring

Culture congruent care

Code:  — —  Influencers
       ——→  Directional influencers

❖ **Fig. 10-3**    Leininger's model of transcultural nursing.

Within American society, professional biomedical systems, popular medicine (over-the-counter and nonprescription alternatives), and a variety of folk medical systems provide more varied services to consumers than many nurses imagine. Often more than one system is used at a time to deal with a problem. Nurses and nursing, knowingly or unknowingly, may assume a potentially powerful intermediary role in negotiation of the varied options.

**Modes of intervention.** Culturally congruent nursing care decisions and actions have the potential to intervene in one or more of three ways: cultural care preservation, accommodation, or repatterning (Leininger, 1988a). In the first instance, they may serve to preserve or maintain a state of health, aid recovery from illness, or assist with the dying process through reinforcement of traditional cultural values and lifeways that provide familiar, available, and nonthreatening resources.

**Cultural maintenance or preservation.** The need for cultural maintenance or preservation was demonstrated, for example, when a student from New Zealand came to an American university health clinic with complaints of chronic headaches, sleeplessness, inattentiveness, and lack of ability to focus on his school work. He explained that the onset of these symptoms coincided with his father's death, of which he had not learned until it was too late to return to his home for the funeral. Because of his failure to be there when his mother especially needed his support, a relative of his mother had "pointed a bone" at him and that action, he believed, resulted in his present problems.

A thorough assessment failed to produce additional reasons for the young man's somatic complaints, decreased academic achievement, and social unease. Fortunately, a physician was located who had experience with Maori medical beliefs from previous work in New Zealand.

She worked with the university clinic staff and the disturbed student. Together they delineated the problem, worked to understand what it would take to alleviate it, and participated in an adapted ceremony that allowed the client to believe that the effect of the bone-pointing had been neutralized. The student was at peace with the knowledge that it was through no fault of his that he had missed his father's funeral, and knew that further amends for the social transgression could wait until his return to his people after successful completion of his studies, which would allow him to serve more effectively than would premature return as an academic failure.

**Cultural negotiation or adaptation.** The second mode of nursing intervention involves assisting clients in negotiation of or adaptation to new cultural ways (Leininger, 1988a). The need for cultural accommodation was evident when a recently widowed, elderly Japanese man was admitted to a postsurgical unit in a large, urban, American hospital. The client refused to stay in bed, which resulted in a fall, restraints, and a general conviction among the nursing staff that he was "crazy," "uncooperative," and "trying to commit hari-kari." The man's American-born daughter was surprised at her father's sudden "irrational" behavior and pleaded with him not to further embarrass both of them. Fearful that he had permanently lost his ability to reason as well as his limited command of English, she could not explain his "failure to be a good patient." It was not until a Japanese nurse from another part of the hospital talked with the patient that the simple reason for the acute fear underlying the man's behavior became known.

The man demanded to know why he was being laid out to die, that is, why his bed was positioned in the manner that a body would be according to traditional Japanese custom. He was oriented well enough to know the direction of the rising sun, the mountains and the sea, although his anxiety and condition interfered with his ability to communicate his concern, even to his daughter (who did not share that aspect of his knowledge of Japanese tradition).

Despite the apparent potential for quickly relieving the problem by moving the client's bed, the nursing staff soon realized how limited their freedom was to physically reposition people due to structural designs (such as uniform wall hookups) that maximized resources and efficiency by replicating identical facilities throughout each unit. Accommodation of the client's need required moving him to another unit, which, although a physical replica of the first, was located in a wing of the hospital that faced a different direction. In discussions among members of the nursing staff about their reactions to the considerable additional work entailed by working through this problem and move, it became evident that the unit had in the past experienced other patients of Japanese background who had also been characterized as "real bad problems."

**Cultural change or repatterning.** A third approach to intervention involves culturally acceptable and appropriate care that enables changes in lifeways that result in new or different patterns that are meaningful, satisfying, and beneficial (Leininger, 1988a). That type of nursing role is suggested by an incident that occurred when the firstborn child of a young Iranian couple died unexpectedly soon after birth. Several male members of the grieving, extended family, considering the labor room nurse and the obstetrician responsible for their loss, made retaliatory threats against them.

After consultation with a health professional of Iranian background and several members of the family to learn more about their perceptions of and motivations in the situation, the nurse practitioner on the unit was able to work with the family toward understanding the ramifications of carrying out a socially inappropriate action such as physically harming the nurse or physician and to discuss culturally acceptable alternatives to expressing and coping with their grief.

A more common problem in which cultural repatterning was indicated arose when nurses working with pregnant, inner-city, economically disadvantaged teens realized that the young women ate neither nutritionally appropriate foods nor at structured mealtimes. Food intake was often limited to what was immediately available; planning and preparation were minimal. Although awareness of the eating patterns explained underutilization of the nutritional counseling and food plans provided by the nurses, ramifications of the unstructured home environments, which included little sense of time (Taylor, 1989), extended beyond nutritional concerns to poor school performance. By coordinating services of a health department nutritionist (who was familiar with the population's needs and eating patterns) with the school's family life education program, a comprehensive restructuring pattern was developed and implemented.

## ❖ SUMMARY

Contemporary society is a composite of diverse subcultural populations. Despite increasingly homogenized media and technology that permeate the majority of households with standardized versions of event analysis, fast foods, and consumer expectations, significant cultural variation persists and is perpetuated. Nurses are becoming more aware that providing quality care requires awareness and sensitivity, knowledge, and skills that respect and accommodate social and cultural as well as biological, psychological, and spiritual needs. Deep levels of cultural meanings emerge in the quest for health promotion and illness prevention and alleviation. It is in assisting people with personal concerns and losses that nurses encounter patterns of similarities and differences that determine whether the care they give is perceived as acceptable and helpful or as an imposition to be resisted.

Nursing moved decades ago beyond emphasis on physical care into consideration of psychological factors. This provided a more comprehensive perspective for the complex social realities experienced by people, but still limited the focus of attention to individuals and dealt minimally with the multifaceted contexts of actual experience. Humans are social species and many aspects of life are experienced in multiple dimensions. Since nurses and their clientele are members of subcultures and societies with differing histories, worldviews, cultural values, and social norms that influence perceptions of experience, it is important that the potential of these traits and the impact they may have be understood. Effective interventions are founded on informed decisions, not chance happenings.

Nurses are experiencing a need to look more carefully at population-based patterns and needs. In so doing, they realize that familiarity with and willingness to respectfully encounter topics such as race, ethnicity, religion, politics, and belief systems outside the rubric of biomedicine are essential to provision of acceptable and effective care. Overlooking (that is, being blind to) the impact of those aspects of life on actual experience reinforces obstacles to effective health care.

## ❖ APPLYING KNOWLEDGE TO PRACTICE

1. In what ways do cultural differences between a nurse and client affect nursing care?
2. What communication skills are particularly relevant to intercultural situations?
3. What are some barriers to providing effective, acceptable, transcultural nursing care?

### REFERENCES

Alexander, L. (1982). Illness maintenance and the new American sick role. In N. J. Christman & T. W. Maretzki (Eds.), *Clinically applied anthropology: Anthropologists in health science settings* (pp. 351–367). Dordrecht, Holland, The Netherlands: D. Reidel.

Boone, M. S. (1989). *Capital crime: Black infant mortality in America.* Newbury Park, Calif.: SAGE.

Bowser, B. P., & Hunt, R. G., (Eds.). (1981). *Impacts of racism on white Americans.* Beverly Hills, Calif.: SAGE.

Fee, E. (Ed.). (1983). *The politics of sex in medicine.* Farmingdale, New York: Baywood.

Fossey, D. (1981, April). The imperiled mountain gorilla. *National Geographic, 159*(4), 501–522.

Kim, Y. Y., & Gudykunst, W. B. (1988). *Theories in intercultural communication.* Newbury Park, Calif.: SAGE.

Leininger, M. (1976). Two strange health tribes: The gnisrun and enicidem in the United States. *Human Organization, 35*(3), 253–261.

Leininger, M. (1985). Transcultural caring: A different way to help people. In P. Pedersen (Ed.), *Handbook of crosscultural counseling and therapy.* Westport, Conn.: Greenwood.

Leininger, M. (1988a). Leininger's theory of nursing: Cultural care diversity and universality. *Nursing Science Quarterly, 1*(4), 152–160.

Leininger, M. (Ed.). (1988b). Cross-cultural hypothetical functions of caring and nursing care. In *Caring: An essential human need* (pp. 95–102). Detroit, Mich.: Wayne State University Press.

Linton, R. (1936). *The study of man.* New York: Appleton-Century-Crofts.

McElroy, A., & Townsend, P. K. (1989). *Medical anthropology in ecological perspective.* North Scituate, Mass.: Duxbury.

Owens, M., & Owens, D. (1988). *Cry of the Kalahari.* New York: Houghton-Mifflin.

Parsons, T. (1951). *The social system.* Glencoe, Ill.: The Free Press.

Pedersen, P. (Ed.). (1988). The three stages of multicultural development: Awareness, knowledge, and skill. In *A handbook for developing multicultural awareness* (pp. 3–18). Alexandria, Va.: American Association for Counseling and Development.

Pedersen, P. B., Draguns, J. G., Lonner, W. J., & Trimble, J. E. (Eds.). (1981). *Counseling across cultures.* Honolulu, Hawaii: University of Hawaii Press.

Scheper-Hughes, N. (1987). *Child Survival.* Dordrecht, Holland, The Netherlands: D. Reidel.

Taylor, E. (1989). Time is not on their side. *TIME,* 27 February, p. 74.

Van Horne, W. A., & Tonnesen, T. V. (Eds.). (1985). *Ethnicity and the work force.* Milwaukee, Wisc.: The University of Wisconsin System American Ethnic Studies Coordinating Committee, Urban Corridor Consortium.

Van Horne, W. A., & Tonnesen, T. V. (Eds.). (1988). *Ethnicity and health.* Milwaukee, Wisc.: The University of Wisconsin System American Ethnic Studies Coordinating Committee, Urban Corridor Consortium.

# 11 Values and Beliefs

Kathryn Hopkins Kavanagh

## OBJECTIVES

*At the completion of this chapter, the reader will be able to:*

◆ Discuss the roles that values and beliefs play in the identification, expression, and treatment of illness.

◆ Identify universals (similarities) and diversities (differences) among health care and nursing needs of peoples of differing cultural backgrounds.

◆ Describe ways in which American systems of health care interact with the value and belief systems of members of more traditional societies.

◆ Demonstrate an awareness of the impact of cultural influences on nurses, nursing, and the acceptability of nursing care.

A frustrated community health nurse described with disbelief a family with whom she was working. The family had elected against corrective surgery for an infant with severe congenital anomalies. Their rationale, which was reported but obviously not accepted, was that the procedure would be too costly and most likely would not significantly increase the child's chances of becoming a productive adult. The costs, emotional and logistical as well as financial, the nurse could understand. But to deny an individual what might be helpful, she scowled, "How could they do that?"

This real-life example connotes the influence of value differences that underlie attitudes and decisions. When the community health nurse expressed discomfort with a decision

against elective surgery for a child, the response was based on the nurse's own system of values. Certainly acceptable, the response is also quite different from that of the clients. The large extended family, with values focused on the group, believed the decision to be rightly that of the extended family and small community because of its implications for that level of society.

Seldom are we called upon to examine our own values as long as we are with people who share them. But America has a richly diverse population. In routine practice, nurses often interact with people whose world views differ significantly from their own. Many nurses also venture into transcultural and international areas of practice.

## ❖ BASIC CONCEPTS

It may be tempting to avoid close examination of basic values and beliefs because they seem amorphous, complex, or too intimate. However, a grasp of the concepts of normality, abnormality, ethnocentrism, relativism, stereotyping, prejudice, and discrimination as they relate to values and beliefs provides a basis for understanding how society handles differences in attitude and behavior. Social ranking (that is, social stratification) and its consequence, social inequality, affect human experience and opportunity. The interrelationships among values, beliefs, and societal responses to those are important factors in availability, acceptability, and use of health care resources.

Understanding that ideas, values, beliefs, and preferences are culture-, class-, and time-bound empowers providers. Realizing that perspectives are shaped by orientations to specific values and beliefs (which are rooted in specific cultures, classes, or time periods) allows objective assessment of diverse practices that people employ to promote health or cope with illness. Appreciating, for example, that what is to one individual a "superstition" may be to someone else a firmly held and reasonable explanation or belief, allows the sensitive and knowledgeable nurse to objectively consider the practices associated with that belief for their own potential merit, neutrality, or harm. Automatic discrediting of ideas or practices because they are unfamiliar, traditional ("old-fashioned"), not scientific, or otherwise marginal to biomedicine risks alienation of clients as well as loss of potentially useful resources.

### Values and Beliefs

*Values* are composed of ideals and preferences that are specific to a culture, class, or time. They outline general expectations and ideas about such basic phenomena as nature, human interaction, human nature, time, and activity. *Beliefs* are statements or convictions that are held as true and reflect essential values. Values and beliefs function as filters through which reality is experienced. Together they provide keys to understanding those we care for—ourselves as well as others—and for making sense of experience.

Values and beliefs function as screens of interpretation that provide evaluation criteria to use when people interact with the world around them. They also furnish standards for relationships between humankind and essential elements of life. They become embroidered into lush and intricate tapestries through change and interpretation, application, and adaptation. Used in context (that is, to fit the specific circumstances at hand), beliefs and values shape meanings given to traits, behaviors, and events.

Caring behaviors exist in every culture, so nursing is sometimes misconstrued as essentially culture-free. However, specific nursing behaviors, as well as nurses themselves, reflect the cultural contexts in which they occur (Leininger, 1988). It stands to reason, therefore, that there is a need to understand the nursing process from the cultural perspectives of both health care providers and consumers. Care can then be provided by informed practitioners in ways that are perceived as both acceptable and appropriate. The following concepts are germane to examination of values and beliefs as they influence health and health care.

### Normality and Abnormality

*Normality* is both elusive and forthright. It is ambiguous since there is no universally rejected behavior. Even behaviors such as hallucinations, incest, and suicide are considered appropriate and are socially rewarded in some circumstances.

Normality refers simply to statistically normative traits and activities. Most people have, for example, intellectual capacities within a specified "normal" range. However, on either end of that range, some will be found with exceptionally high or low potential. Whether or not any individual has an IQ that represents the precise average or mean for the entire population, the normal range is broad enough to include considerable variation.

"Normal" is something that in the competitive United States everyone and no one wants to be. Garrison Keillor, claiming that in Lake Wobegon "all the children are above average" (Keillor, 1985), endears himself by mocking society's general resistance to being below or even average (that is, "merely ordinary"). At the same time, however, if "everybody" is "above average," average is automatically shifted upward to a new standard. Normality is what is generally expected, based on specific standards ("norms") for a period of time, socioeconomic class, and culture.

In well-baby clinics, for example, the "normal" child is within range of a certain height and weight at a certain age, based on compilations of figures collected from a large and presumably representative sample. The normal Asian child, however, may be smaller in stature than his or her black and white age cohorts and so requires a different standard for measurement, a different "average." Expectations, therefore, must be altered according to context.

*Abnormality,* every bit as difficult to define as normality, is essentially whatever is found at the ends of the Gaussian ("normal") curve. In sociological terms, that becomes the "deviant," the behavior or characteristic that is not typical or expected. In the statistical sense, deviance can represent either more or less of a trait and can be either positive or negative in valuation: the musical genius, the retarded individual, the only boy in his gang who does not use drugs. As with normality, it is the context that determines abnormality. To some adolescents, for instance, deprivation of specific types of clothes threatens abnormality and social rejection, while many adults think it is normal for teens to feel

that way. Observed reality is measured against expectations, not concrete criteria.

## Ethnocentrism and Relativism

We frequently do not realize how thoroughly socialized we are to specific aspects of society, such as ethnic, educational, and occupational background. *Ethnocentrism,* which means being centered in one's culture or people, implies a limited ability or motivation to see beyond that group. Measuring the Asian child, for example, with standards created for non-Asian children, or assuming that the individual who does not speak English clearly is not very intelligent, is ethnocentric behavior. For nurses to work effectively with people from other orientations, considerable flexibility and open-mindedness are needed to avoid imposing biased points of view (for example, those typically determined by white, middle-class, and nursing-based standards). It is essential to view other cultures and societies on their own terms and not as deviations from one's own.

*Relativism* avoids culture-bound ethnocentrism with recognition that various approaches are potentially equally acceptable and applicable. Although blanket relativism (that is, unwillingness to criticize any approach or perspective) is dangerous, errors are more common on the side of rigid, narrow expectations that are unrealistic in a multicultural society.

## Stereotypes

*Stereotypes* are snapshots, images frozen in time. It is healthy to simplify a tremendously complex world by putting observations and experiences into categories, recognizing similarities and differences, and avoiding independent processing of each new bit of information. Knowledge gained through experience is transferred from one setting to another, and similarities perceived between those situations are valuable shortcuts. At times, however, this simplification process leads to dependence on generalized beliefs or impressions that deny actual diversity.

Simplified and standardized conceptions (stereotypes) limit the range of meanings attached to experience. For example, despite their knowledge of American society, German tourists in the United States sometimes return to their homeland disappointed because they did not encounter whooping, painted, and feathered Native Americans. While other Americans may chuckle at that stereotype as antiquated, they may not realize the limitations of its generalizability, even in the past.

An equally invalid, but still widely held stereotype associates poverty with ethnic minority groups in the United States. Opportunity-limiting social processes have resulted in an overrepresentation of members of nonwhite and ethnic minority groups among the economically disadvantaged. However, most members of nonwhite and ethnic minority groups are not poor, and the vast majority of poor people in the United States are white.

## Prejudice and Discrimination

Bias and prejudice signify *prejudgment,* which is reaching a conclusion before the data are all in and before the facts are understood. For example, the biased conviction that everyone who wears glasses must read a lot prejudges data that may provide evidence to the contrary. The negative statement that all people who wear glasses are hiding behind their lenses from direct interpersonal exchange is more than biased; it is prejudicial. Racism, ageism, and sexism are behavioral expressions of pervasive, prejudiced views that some groups are superior or inferior to others.

*Discrimination* puts prejudicial attitudes into action. Individual discrimination occurs when one is denied an opportunity or service because of age, sex, race, national origin, or any

other stratifier, including those such as a particular diagnosis or a need to use spectacles. Institutionalized discrimination involves generally accepted, patterned obstacles that are built into the social organization and limit opportunity to status, power, wealth, and other resources.

The latter type of discrimination is by far the more dangerous, because structural barriers often appear neutral and can be detected only through close observance of their negative consequences. Since discriminatory practices are often part of taken-for-granted societal patterns, it is important to understand this social phenomenon. Limited awareness can result in participation in and perpetuation of inequity by persons who would not do so knowingly.

Looking around where they work, for example, nurses might question what social patterns resulted in roles and statuses being distributed as they are. When a group of health care workers is multicultural or multiracial, nurses tend to be predominantly white, while technicians and auxilary personnel tend to be nonwhite. Likewise, physicians and administrators tend to be male and nurses and subordinate personnel are more likely to be female. The result of institutionalized processes that affect access to opportunity, many such patterns of inequity have not been systematically examined for discrimination and dealt with in the American health care system (Rodwin, 1988).

## ❖ VALUE ORIENTATIONS AND CULTURAL ASSESSMENT

Value systems, which define the merit, worth, or importance of various perspectives, exist in every culture and are expressed through the behavioral norms of each society. Groups have organized and generalized ideas, which are interrelated, learned, and shared. Basic values emphasize ideas about (1) the concept of nature and humankind's relationship with it, (2) the nature of humankind, (3) relationships between and among people, (4) rela-

❖ **Table 11-1**
Kohls' Interpretation of the Kluckholn-Strodtbeck Model

| Orientation | Range | | |
|---|---|---|---|
| **HUMAN NATURE** | Most people can't be trusted | There are both evil people and good people, and you have to check people out to find out which they are. | Most people are basically pretty good at heart. |
| **PERSON-NATURE RELATIONSHIP** | Life is largely determined by external forces, such as God, fate, or genetics. A person can't surpass the conditions life has set. | People should, in every way, live in complete harmony with nature. | Our challenge is to conquer and control nature. Everything from air conditioning to cloning new cells has resulted from having met this challenge. |
| **TIME SENSE** | People should learn from history and attempt to emulate the glorious ages of the past. | The present moment is everything. Let's make the most of it. Don't worry about tomorrow; enjoy today. | Planning and goal-setting make it possible for people to accomplish miracles. A little sacrifice today will bring a better tomorrow. |
| **ACTIVITY** | It's enough to just "be." It's not necessary to accomplish great things in life to feel your life has been worthwhile. | The main purpose for having been placed on this earth is for our own inner development. | If people work hard and apply themselves fully, their efforts will be rewarded. |
| **SOCIAL RELATIONS** | Some people are born to lead others. There are "leaders" and there are "followers" in this world. | Whenever I have a serious problem, I like to get the advice of my family or close friends in how best to solve it. | All people should have equal rights. And all should have complete control over their own destiny. |

From: Pedersen, P. (1988). *A handbook for developing multicultural awareness.* Alexandria, VA. American Association for Counseling and Development, pp. 65-66. Reprinted with permission.

tionships with time, and (5) relationships between people and activity (Kluckhohn, 1953, Kluckhohn & Strodtbeck, 1961). These orientations and the possible range of values associated with each are presented in Table 11-1.

This classic framework continues to function as a major tool in response to a question consistently asked by every nurse and student: "How do I assess for cultural variables?" To be effective, assessment occurs in three areas: the nurse, the client, and the context or setting in which the nurse and the client interact. Self-awareness of values and beliefs is as important as recognition and understanding of values and beliefs of clients. Examination of personal and professional values also empowers decision making in relationships between nurses, with nursing, and with society. Basic questions for the nurse to ask himself or herself and the client include:

Where did my (your) sense of personal and social identity come from?
How was it formed?
What are my (your) values and norms?
Where did they come from?
How and where were they learned?
Are they rooted in a specific ethnic group? Class? Religion? Gender?
What kind of person am I (are you) socialized to be?
How has my (your) social identity changed?
How is it changing?
How do I (you) want it to change?

## Ethnic Diversity and American Cultural Values

American cultural values reflect numerous influences and rich diversity. Nearly one third of the population differs ethnically, racially, or both from the predominant group. There is no single set of American values, and there are apparent conflicts among the many held. However, several value orientations stand out as dominant in generalized American patterns of thinking, decision making, and activity.

**Mastery over nature.** The typical American concept is that humankind is not part of or controlled by nature. This contrasts, for example, with traditional Native American relationships with nature, which emphasize working with or in communion with it, and traditional Arab beliefs that humankind is controlled by nature and so should submit fatalistically to it. Western European and American ideas focus more intently on use and change. Change is associated with progress, which is held in high esteem, and is often dependent upon exploitation of nature. Ideologies based on peacefulness with or submission to nature typically do not promote production of skyscrapers, satellites, superhighways, CAT scanners, or nuclear power plants. Those are constructions of minds and bodies working with the premises that the resources of nature can be harnessed to human advantage, and that it is a human option to orchestrate that transformation.

The ability to control many aspects of nature enables a general standard of living that is unparalleled in the history of the human species. Scientific knowledge, applied through technology, has affected nearly every aspect and scale of life, from arranging plants in aesthetically pleasing or agriculturally productive patterns to preserving lives that would otherwise be lost. The latter example has so modified expectations for human life throughout much of the world that severe pressure from increased population has occurred.

It was not until about 1800 that the human population reached the 1 billion mark. Now, less than two centuries later, there are more than 5 billion people, with a doubling time of only 40 years (Population Reference Bureau, 1988). That increment is not a result of changed fertility, but is due to the ability to decrease death rates. This has occurred primarily through technological development leading to improved sanitation and nutrition. More people live longer and reproduce.

Values tend to change slowly and at times conflict. For example, lowered death rates are highly valued. However, cultural and other factors often interfere with creating a population balance by limiting fertility. Where religious beliefs or ideological values prohibit contraception (in countries such as Mexico or Pakistan, for example) a relatively large proportion of the population is too young to contribute to economic development. Maintenance of disproportionately large populations limits the ability of nations to educate, modernize, industrialize, and increase standards of living that may positively affect health (Popenoe, 1989).

**Acquisition and consumption.** Accumulation of material goods is another prominent American value. This characteristic is an artifact of having more resources than are immediately needed, and of having the ability to preserve or store them. Abundant resources, a sense of personal freedom, and ingenuity encourage high expectations. In American society, attention is focused on providing services. The present age is one of development of increasingly sophisticated communication and informational resources. With long-term and wide-scale mechanization and industrialization, production of goods may be taken for granted and their acquisition more consciously valued.

Americans have the opportunity to learn to be consumers, or potential consumers, from infancy. Only a small minority of American homes do not have televisions, and each button invites an outpouring of occasions to want and acquire both goods and services. As well as being mainstays of American tradition, the lure of free enterprise and consumerism remains among the strongest pulls for immigrants.

In the United States, society has been slower to come to terms with the problems created in the aftermath of consumption than it has been in support of use of resources to improve the standard of living and increase levels of expectation. In addition to environmental concerns related to industrialized patterns of consumerism and materialism, psychosocial problems commonly arise. There is significant confusion between

standard of living, that is, access to and availability of goods and services, and quality of life, which involves congruence between reality and expectations resulting in contentment, sense of fulfillment, and satisfaction.

**Competition.** American values tend to prioritize competition over cooperation. There is greater focus on individual accomplishment than on the good of the group or sharing of resources. Objectives commonly emphasize profit motives, private property, avoidance of unnecessary taxes, and personal achievement.

In some societies, social norms minimize winning and losing. On many of the Pacific Islands, for example, American baseball and British cricket have been adapted to maximize chances of having a good time. No one wins and no one loses. It is almost unimaginable that such an event would be acceptable, let alone appealing, to sportsminded Americans.

Despite the fact that a large part of the world's population does not have equal access to generally abundant resources, most Americans do. Satisfaction and fulfillment of expectations, however, are often not met. Many individuals, as well as sizable groups who feel deprived of access to resources, express need or desire for more. When opportunities to meet expectations are not seen as adequate, escapism becomes commonplace. Popular choices are stimulants (e.g., caffeine), television, and more desperate means (e.g., crime or illegal drugs).

The values of control and competition for resources are taken to the level of aggression and violence in American society. Despite Puritan roots and Victorian influences in many aspects of the culture, children in the United States tend to be heavily exposed to violence and aggression. By their middle teens they have viewed through mass media thousands of killings and deaths, learned that the competitive "rugged individual" is often rewarded, and that personal worth is commonly measured in terms of money. They have associated success with achievement, productivity, speed, and mobility.

**Individualism.** The United States is known throughout the world for its civil rights, personal freedoms, and extreme individualization. Although loneliness and a sense of marginality are common experiences, development of individual identity, independence, and resistance to authority are supported by many American institutions. It is striking to those from other societies to discover, for example, openly advertised radar detectors to foil law enforcers, or the rapidity with which Americans will sue their counterparts.

On the other hand, social conformity remains highly valued. Group ties tend to be weak, but pressure to conform and identification with specific groups affect decision making and other behaviors. Many Americans desire to appear to be parts of groups, while believing that they think independently.

Individuality has not always been highly valued, even in Western society. During the Middle Ages, when religion and spirituality dominated thinking, the idea that persons were responsible for themselves was less developed. Over time, ideas developed that mind and body (psyche and soma) were separate entities, each to be examined more closely. Emphasis on rational and scientific thinking increased. The individual emerged as accountable for himself to his God and society. It took longer for women in patriarchal societies to be acknowledged as truly accountable to society and not merely to an intermediary father, husband, brother, or son. In many ways that expectation of personal accountability remains compromised today.

The conviction that individuals are responsible for themselves allows credit for success or failure to go to persons, rather than to a deity, fate, or the collective. The United States became a symbol of opportunity to take that chance and of the belief that effort and ingenuity would be rewarded. The consequence is that the individual bears the weight of failure as well as of achievement. However, most people believe in a just world (Lerner, 1980) in which there is both the opportunity and a fair chance to succeed.

**Personal achievement.** In America's stratified society (that is, in which groups are ranked by relative worth), the reality is that not everyone has an equal opportunity to achieve. Nonetheless, the myth that they do is central to the presumption that one gets what one deserves. It is widely believed, for example, that a self-perpetuating culture or cycle of poverty, in which many minority groups and individuals are enmeshed, explains the gaps between minority and majority income, education, standard of living, and health status. However, the evidence is strong that the beliefs of poor people about the value of work and education actually mirror those of the rich (*U.S. News & World Report,* 1989). Barriers that are built into the social system (that is, institutionalized discrimination) account for inequitable access to status, power, and wealth. Often there is an underlying assumption that reward comes to the deserving; therefore, the unrewarded must not be deserving. It is quite possible, however, when societal processes work like a deck of cards, that the deck is stacked against the deserving, and that they will go unrewarded.

Many women, for example, are no longer willing to work for grossly inadequate wages. However, relative to men, most women think in terms of jobs rather than careers and involve themselves in a series of jobs. Women are more likely than men to be socialized not to expect careers. Their goals tend not to be set toward long-term upward mobility (that is, increased access to status, power, and wealth) (Tavris & Wade, 1984). Although this is widely accepted (institutionalized) in society, limited goals serve in the long run to limit access by women to socially valued resources. Such practices are perpetuated and their consequences are seldom questioned.

**Time.** Every society has a characteristic notion of time, the meaning of which varies with socioeconomic class and ethnicity. When interviewing nurses about relationships that most influenced them, for instance, I found that only the Asian participants cited persons who were no longer alive as significantly influential in the present. The non-Asian nurses more clearly separated past from present; people who had influenced them in the past were unambiguously relegated to that context.

Youth-oriented and often dissatisfied with the present, Americans tend to focus on the future, on being something other than what they are, and on having more than they have. Associated with the emphasis on becoming and on future options is a restlessness that discourages appreciation of the here and now. This presents a situation not unlike that in the children's story about a bull who was considered bizarre (that is, socially deviant and marginal) because he preferred smelling the flowers to fighting (Leaf, 1936).

The youth who enjoys pumping gas is likely to be advised to take night courses to increase his chances of upward mobility; being a gas station attendant is "not enough" for lifelong work and is often perceived as valuable only as a step to "better things," such as station ownership. Likewise, nurses who return to school sometimes invest in the credential rather than the education. Academic and professional degrees may be viewed as tickets to more status, power, and wealth, usually in the form of autonomy in practice, independence, and income.

The American relationship with time is typically measured in terms of efficiency and productivity, which presents an ongoing problem for nursing, which tends to be time-intensive. Efficiency implies streamlining of activities (that is, routinizing and standardizing them for uniform and business-like delivery). However, it is increasingly evident that one style of care does not accommodate everyone, and quality care must be designed and dispensed with a wide variability of consumer expectations in mind. Therefore, effective care may be very time consuming. It may actually be better measured in time spent than in time saved.

**Activity.** In the American value system, time is closely related to activity. The Protestant ethic, which serves as the capstone of many values and beliefs, provided a framework for a distinct relationship with activity. Long before the rise of Protestantism, idleness was conceived of as evil and its antidote as hard work. Modified precautions against the risks associated with idle hands and the ultimate value of "a good hard day's work" continue to be honored. Work for the sake of work, however, is typically less often treasured, except in the quest for physical fitness. Commensurate compensation is expected for contemporary efforts and expertise. Leisure is also valued, although changes in standard of living devote much of it to interaction with devices that are designed to save time and labor.

Personal identities are in large part oriented toward work, as is often heard expressed in introductions that equate "What do you do?" with "Who are you?" Although work can technically occur anywhere, it is generally viewed as occurring outside the home. As women move into the work force and get paid for their efforts, they often retain the bulk of responsibilities for running homes. Nonetheless, most are more satisfied (albeit exhausted) working outside the home in a status and role that carries greater social value and credibility than homemaking (Tavris & Wade, 1984).

Employment serves as a medium for distribution of resources as well as a mechanism of production. Social categories of work determine economic value in the marketplace and, to a large part, social value (Van Horne, 1985). Numerous institutionalized controls provide different opportunities for different groups.

Nurses, for example, earn better incomes than they did in the past, yet often reach ceilings on earning potential after relatively few years of work. Other groups are similarly affected by societal patterns. Limited child care facilities and support, for instance, make it more feasible for some women to remain at home than to join the general work force and spend disproportionately large parts of their incomes on child care.

**Variation and conflicts.** This brief overview of American values and some of their conflicts is limited to description of broad patterns and does not attend to variations of values among numerous subcultures that interact with the predominant system. Frequently it is those contrasting values that emerge in health care situations, where they may or may not be acknowledged and may or may not be met with tolerance and respect. Understanding the integral role that values play in shaping human behavior, and understanding that people behave in ways that reflect the best of the value-influenced alternatives they perceive at the time, encourages openness and acceptance in provider-consumer interactions.

## Expression of Values in the Health Care System

The values that predominate in a culture are readily apparent in the health care system. For example, American social, political, educational, and legal systems emphasize individual rights and responsibilities. Reflecting that orientation, nurses in the United States tend to value self-expression, self-esteem, self-image, self-control, and self-care, as well as a variety of practices designed to protect personal rights and privacy. While acknowledging the importance of social support systems, it is typically individuals who are cared for, even when they come in groups. What may not be realized, however, is that the level of individualization

that American nurses generally advocate is unusual among the world's cultures. For members of many societies, the good of groups takes precedence over that of individuals. Imposition of expectations oriented toward the self may then be considered inappropriate and unacceptable.

Independence is not a universal goal; interdependence is more widely valued, and in some cultures dependence is the goal. In Japan, for example, the concept of "amae" refers to the relationship between mother and eldest son, who, when he is young and dependent, is prepared for the time when his mother will be old and dependent on him (Doi, 1973). Culturally pervasive, "amae" serves as a model for employer and employee, teacher and student, and provider and consumer relationships within a context in which dependence is viewed as normal and healthy.

**Level of formality.** American values involving relationships between and among people are expressed in nursing through attitudes about and expectations of informality, equality, and mutuality. Clients approach the health care system because they need relief. They go to find expertise (that is, knowledge, skills, training, tools, and experience) that reputation, observation, or desperation leads them to hope exists there. Although formality creates a social distance, extreme informality (manifested, for example, in impersonal casualness, use of first names, or avoidance of names altogether, which often occurs when pronunciations are unfamiliar) may serve to discredit the level of expertise and caring that is available.

**Level of trust.** In addition to being competent, the acceptable health care provider must be viewed as trustworthy. Caring providers have been characterized as those exhibiting the universal attributes of genuineness, love, unconditional acceptance, and positive regard (Sue, 1981). The challenge, however, is in determining how to express those attitudes to clients whose expectations and criteria for caring behaviors vary widely. Trust might be compromised, for example, if mutuality is not valued by someone who has come to a provider expecting to be advised on the expert handling of a problem, but who is met with an expectation of self-care and independence. A trusting relationship is unlikely to develop when a client perceives that a provider does not understand and respect his or her cultural orientation.

**Investment of time.** Time continues to harangue nurses and nursing as it becomes increasingly an entity of accountability. Because efficiency, practicality, and routinization are valued, time is equated with money, and caring with time. Temporal urgency encourages simplification (sometimes oversimplification) of complex situations. For example, assumptions may be made that coping patterns of clients are or should be similar to those of nurses and others socialized to the health care system. Differences may be overlooked in efforts to avoid time-consuming complications. The risk involved in such behavior is that client and provider end up working with different strategies toward dissimilar goals. The nurse, for example, may hurry to include all relevant items in AIDS prevention teaching for high-risk clients, when it is the presence and time spent with them that the clients value, not the information.

Most American health care facilities, reflecting the general social system's preoccupation with time, revolve around fiscal years, hours of productivity, and visits and minutes spent per client. Appointments are levied and meant to be kept; failure to comply is viewed as opportunity lost. However, emphasis on timeliness tends to be far less important to peoples from backgrounds that emphasize history and tradition over the present or future than it is for those from industrialized, clock-bound cultures. Casual time scheduling and tolerance for

lateness or missed appointments may become more pressing issues in the future. The United States' health care facilities will need to adapt to increasing proportions of clientele from Hispanic and other cultures that traditionally devalue punctuality for putting too much pressure on both provider and client.

**Active intervention.** While traditional Chinese are admonished not to do anything when in a situation in which one does not know what to do, the task-oriented American is socialized to act. We have all been cautioned that "He who hesitates is lost" and that "If you don't know what to do, at least do something" (Pedersen, 1988, p. 67). Culturally valued activity is also expressed in the health care setting where there is limited patience with those who are not viewed as adequately motivated toward problem solving and decision making. In a "doing" culture, simply "being" tends to be seen as an inadequate value orientation (Kluckholn & Strodtbeck, 1961; Attneave, 1982; Orque, 1983).

Nursing, reflecting generalized cultural values, also recognizes needs that go beyond those. Being with and caring for sick people is not a highly valued orientation in a youth, health, and fitness-oriented society. Although generally supportive of the biomedical thrust to treat disease, nurses have responded by acknowledging limits to control over nature by helping people to cope with unresolvable situations and to die with dignity. However, that aspect of caring has developed in many cases as a result of observed need, rather than as an expectation introduced in basic nursing education. Nursing theory and practice need to be systematically examined to determine how they reflect population-specific values, and to what extent the potential for flexibility required in work with people with differing values is compromised by adherence to the predominant value system. Provider approaches that reflect an openness to the values and beliefs of others are listed in the box on p. 198.

## ❖ APPROACHES RECOMMENDED FOR ALL CULTURAL GROUPS

1. Provide a feeling of acceptance.
2. Establish open communication.
3. Present yourself with confidence. Introduce yourself. Shake hands if it is appropriate.
4. Strive to gain your client's trust, but don't resent it if you don't get it.
5. Understand what members of the cultural or subcultural group consider "caring," both attitudinally and behaviorally.
6. Understand the relationship between your client and authority.
7. Understand your client's desire to please you and his/her/their motivations to comply or not to comply.
8. Anticipate diversity. Avoid stereotypes by sex, age, ethnicity, socioeconomic status, etc.
9. Don't make assumptions about where people come from. Let them tell you.
10. Understand the client's goals and expectations.
11. Make your goals realistic.
12. Emphasize positive points and strengths of health beliefs and practices.
13. Show respect, especially for males, even if it is females or children you are interested in. Males are often decision makers about follow-up.
14. Be prepared for the fact that children go everywhere with some cultural groups, as well as with poorer families who may have few options. Include them.
15. Know the traditional, health-related practices common to the group you are working with. Don't discredit them unless you *know* they are harmful.
16. Know the folk illnesses and remedies common to the group you are working with.
17. Try to make the clinic setting comfortable. Consider colors, music, atmosphere, scheduling expectations, pace, tone, seating arrangements, and so on.
18. Whenever possible and appropriate, involve the leaders of the local group. Confidentiality is important, but the leaders know the problems and often can suggest acceptable interventions.
19. Respect values, beliefs, rights, and practices. Some may conflict with your own, or with your determination to make changes. But every group and individual wants respect above all else.
20. Learn to appreciate the richness of diversity as an asset rather than a hindrance in your work.

## ❖ CULTURAL INFLUENCE ON BELIEFS ABOUT HEALTH AND ILLNESS

People need to make sense of and understand why and how things happen. There are many ways of doing that, and it is important to realize that individuals may not share identical or even similar explanations for the world they live in and the phenomena they experience. It is possible, and probably quite common in multicultural societies, for health care providers and health care consumers to miss each other like "ships that pass in the night," using different explanations to reach similar or different conclusions.

Many people think and understand in ways and patterns that differ from the patterns generally idealized in Western societies. Western thinking emphasizes linear and measurable relationships between cause and effect and patterns of opposites. Things tend to be viewed as good or bad, right or wrong, either-or, black or white—but not both. Members of other societies, in contrast, may think in more circular than linear patterns, and in less simplified terms. In the United States, for instance, one is typically Christian, Jewish, Muslim, or atheistic. Typically those characteristics and classifications are not combined in the same person. However, there are many ways of knowing and of reasoning. In some societies these may allow, without conflict, allegiance to both Christianity and Buddhism, or any other concurrent ideologies, in the same person.

As members of a discipline committed to logic and reason, as well as to other more humanistic values, nurses frequently assume that problems are and should be defined by frameworks encountered within the boundaries of scientific research and analysis. Science has indeed gone far to elucidate a complex existence. Many problems faced by clients, however, are not inhibited by those artificial boundaries and are perceived and articulated within other frameworks.

## Explanatory Models

Explanatory models are the systems of explanation used to put ideas about the meaning, cause, process, and treatment of illness into workable perspectives (Kleinman, 1980). Conceptual frameworks used to understand health and illness phenomena reflect complex influences such as religion, economic situation, education, language, family composition and other forms of social organization, interactive patterns, ethnic orientation, and general perceptions of the world and self.

## Definition of Illness

In many societies, questions that are related in a medicalized society to health and illness are viewed as related in a more general sense to life or death. Misfortune is seen as a general problem; an illness or injury is a sign of misfortune, rather than a "health" problem. In coping with illness, it is not a malfunctioning body part that is the issue, but an all-encompassing situation

that has an impact on family, friends, and total context (Pedersen, 1988).

Beliefs about illness vary greatly, as do those about determining when one is ill, the meaning of pain and sickness, what to do about them, how to act, to whom to go with specific problems, and when to go. Some health care providers imagine persons who do not share their trust and confidence in biomedicine to be devoid of meaningful beliefs about health and illness. However, rich and complex alternative systems exist with varying degrees of efficacy and potential for congruence with contemporary nursing and medical practices. Ethnomedical (including such subfields as ethnoobstetrics, ethnopediatrics, ethnosurgery, and ethnopharmacology), ethnopsychiatric, and ethnocaring systems have been and continue to be studied by anthropologists, transcultural nurses, and other scientists. Since many systems of beliefs about health and illness exist, it is critical for nursing to be open to their presence and for nurses to communicate openness to clients' sharing of values and beliefs.

## Ideas About Illness Causation

There is probably more variation among etiological beliefs of health care providers within biomedicine than is commonly acknowledged, but a premise of relatively impersonal, natural causation generally prevails. For a variety of reasons or simply by chance, parts and systems malfunction. However, many cultural groups believe illness may also be caused by a supernatural being (a deity or god), a nonhuman being (such as an ancestor, a ghost, or an evil spirit), or another human being (a witch or a sorcerer) (Foster & Anderson, 1978). The sick person in such a case is viewed as a victim (that is, as the object of negative intervention or punishment). Some societies have no concept of accident, so every phenomenon is accounted for as the result of intent by an outside force.

Many other ideas about disease causation also exist, most of them focusing on an equilibrium or balance model. Illness results, for example, when the balance is disturbed, whether the critical components be heat and cold, humors (or "dosha"), yin and yang, or metabolic substances. Indigestible foods, sudden changes in temperature, strong winds, and blood or air "trapped in the body" are other common explanations for illness (Nurge, 1958).

Rooted in Greek ideas about the four elements (earth, water, air, and fire), the theory of humoral pathology has existed for 8000 years. According to that theory, good medical practice involves recognizing the appropriate balance for an individual. This was known traditionally as temperament or complexion. Excesses and deficiencies were controlled through diet, internal medicines, purging, vomiting, bleeding, cupping, and other forms of treatment (Foster & Anderson, 1978).

Early travels and migrations led to widespread acceptance of humoral theory throughout Mediterranean and Asian regions, and its eventual transplantation with the cultural baggage of those who discovered and conquered the New World. Despite dethronement by scientific medicine at the professional level, hot and cold theory and other aspects of humoral origin have been retained, especially in those places influenced by Asian or Spanish cultures. The strongest evidence of this influence remains at the popular (over the counter) level of treatment and in folk systems, where it commonly blended with indigenous (native) healing practices.

## Spanish American Folk Medicine

Spanish American folk medicine, despite some variation with place and group, clearly reflects its humoral antecedents, as well as Catholic ritual and beliefs about supernatural influences. Many illnesses are believed to be "hot" or "cold," so sufferers are treated with medicines and foods of opposite characteristics. These qualities do not refer to temperature but to theoretically subscribed properties. Medically prescribed diets can be adapted accordingly, as an outcome of consultation with clients and awareness and ingenuity on the part of health care providers.

## Folk Illnesses

Many ailments can be translated into English and biomedical equivalents. However, others fall into the category of folk illnesses, which may defy biomedical identification, although they are very real to the persons experiencing them. Examples of Spanish American folk illnesses include "fallen fontanelle" (caida de la mollera), "fallen womb" (caida de la matriz), intestinal clogging (other than constipation) resulting from too much or the wrong types of food (empacho) (Foster & Anderson, 1978), and fright or soul loss (susto) that might occur with a sudden start or sneeze. The evil eye (mal de ojo), unlike witchcraft, is believed to occur unintentionally when, for instance, a careless nurse fails to touch a child he or she has noticed or examined. Herbal remedies and rubbing, massage, or other physical manipulations by curanderos (curanderas, if they are women) are typical treatments. These might be used with less formal home remedies (such as teas) or prayers and trips to religious shrines or charismatic folk healers to alleviate distress.

Along with the predominant allopathic or biomedical approach and the Spanish American system sketched briefly above, other systems of folk beliefs, curing, and caring exist in the United States. These are becoming better known and more often recognized as the visibility of ethnic groups increases.

## African American Folk Medicine

African American folk medicine contains elements of various origins. In the early nineteenth century, Haitian slaves rebelled against their French masters and drove thousands of blacks, mulattoes, and whites to the nearest French port, New Orleans. With them, in the form of voodoo, came a blend of European Catholicism and African tribal religions with modified aspects of humoral pathology. This spread through the Protestant American South and assimilated practices from seventeenth and eighteenth century European occultism (probably due to the insistence of using English rather than African languages) (Foster & Anderson, 1978).

Reflecting its multiple origins, black folk medicine today provides widely varied terms and methods, including, for example, "root" medicine, "rootwork," "mojo," "conjuring," "voodoo," and "hoodoo." Etiologies may be viewed as natural (such as failure to protect the body against inclement weather) or unnatural (for instance, divine punishment for sin) and tend to represent a perspective that holds the world to be a dangerous and hostile place. The individual is viewed as vulnerable to outside attack and as dependent on outside help (Snow, 1977). This perspective was reinforced by nearly three centuries of slavery followed by one of second-class citizenship. The most successful curers were those believed to have occult powers as well as herbal skills, which are renowned. Many writers describe with admiration, for example, the unschooled "granny" midwives who until recently delivered most black infants (and many white ones) and practiced with a wide knowledge of herbal lore.

## Traditional Native American Medicine

Other American groups also share time-honored systems of health beliefs and practices. Native American ideas about health and illness place less emphasis on dysfunction of the body than is typical of biomedicine, and more on relationships within the function of society. For American Indians, health typically denotes a proper relationship between humankind and its physical, relational, and supernatural environment. Illness implies having fallen out of balance with the world.

## The Appeal of Alternative Systems

There are reasons why folk and popular systems of health care continue to appeal to those familiar with them. For example, folk systems, which are available in every large American city as well as many other places, do not require going to unfamiliar places or being seen by people who are strangers. And they are readily understandable to someone socialized to the group.

Only in affluent, service-oriented societies such as the United States do health care providers support themselves solely with those roles. In other social systems, healers are traditionally more a part of society at large, working with the others and practicing healing arts on the side. We might consider how full time occupational roles separate Western health care providers from consumers in thinking and behavior.

Folk systems of medicine are usually readily available, while biomedical facilities may require costly and complicated transportation, as well as long waits. Folk systems are also simply organized, relative to scientific systems, and relatively devoid of intimidating testing, technology, lengthy history taking (which often seems irrelevant to clients and families), and intrusive diagnostic procedures. Interpersonal, social, and kinship relationships are emphasized, rather than the isolated individual. Focus on families and groups minimizes shame and embarrassment of unaccustomed individuated attention. In many cases, care and concern are expressed in essentially public ceremonies that communicate broad-based concern and support. In addition, alternative systems of health care are generally perceived to be humanistic, holistic, and able to inspire confidence.

**Humanism.** Experienced as more humanistic than scientific, folk systems of healing are usually less mechanized, less urbanized, and less intellectualized than biomedicine, which is characteristically bent on fixing body parts, limited in accessibility, and focused on rationality to the extent that emotional needs may be overlooked. The Western health care provider's tendency to use abstract concepts and terms poses an additional barrier in health care situations in which providers and clients do not share common worlds.

**Holism.** A major criticism of biomedicine has been that it tends to dissect a person into mind and body (which may or may not be seen as interdependent, let alone complementary) and then into smaller parts. Somatic responses are sought in some circumstances and psychological responses in others, with relatively little expression of concern for the integrated whole person. The individual is even less likely to be viewed as part of a greater whole (for instance, the family, community, and society). This perspective is uncomfortable for people accustomed to being first and foremost an integral member of a group.

Holistic alternative systems tend to deal with comprehensive contexts in which the person is perceived in his or her entirety and not separate from the environment or nature. Quality of life is likely to be the goal, rather than life for the sake of life or use of highly technical equipment and skills. Use of biomedical health care resources is further discouraged by intolerance for religious and magical orientations and practices, which is common when science and systems of symbolic beliefs and faith are viewed as competitors.

**Confidence.** Confidence and faith in the ability of traditional and folk systems of healing can be very strong. There is virtual consensus among medical and other anthropologists that in its supportive dimension, the psychotherapeutic effect of many alternative systems is remarkably effective (Foster & Anderson, 1978). Popular and folk-healing systems are adaptive cultural institutions that promote the well-being of the societies concerned. They serve, to a far greater extent than is often recognized by health care personnel, to smooth harsh cultural gaps between traditional societies and the predominant American system.

## Folk Systems and Nursing

The variety of popular and folk beliefs and practices currently used far exceeds the limitations of this chapter. It is important, however, that nurses become aware of the existence of those alternatives and recognize that, in addition to numerous traditional, folk remedies that have been incorporated into biomedical pharmacopoeia and practice, there are many others. It is dangerous to assume that all indigenous approaches are innocuous. On the other hand, many observers find most practices to be quite mild and harmless, whether or not they are effective cures. Often such treatments provide valuable psychological support and, because of that contribution, should not be discouraged.

It is essential for clients to feel accepted if they are to share with providers what they believe and practice outside the biomedical system. This will not happen if the client assumes that his or her nonbiomedical beliefs

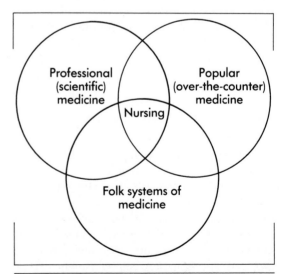

❖ **Fig. 11-1**   Nursing's position in the overlap of professional, popular, and folk health care systems.

and activities are not of interest to health care providers, or will be rejected by them. It is important to know what the client believes and does to facilitate effective progress toward health and to minimize the possibility of harm from treatments or medicines that interact disadvantageously with those of the alternative systems. Nurses are in the position to help effective integration of multiple belief systems toward improved health status and culturally congruent care. These ideas are illustrated in Fig. 11-1.

## ❖ ETHNIC GROUPS IN THE UNITED STATES

Ethnicity is a concept used to classify people who share common cultural traits, a common ancestry, and a perception of being a group that differs from other groups. Ethnicity, more than race, religion, socioeconomic status, or national or geographic origin, describes a sense of commonality (McGoldrick, 1982), and a flavor of difference. A powerful influence in shaping identity, ethnicity in the United States is particularly interesting because a variety of values and identities have been retained for many generations and numerous groups contribute to the composite nation.

### Flexibility in Perspective

Ethnic patterns are strong, but as with "normality" and "abnormality," there is great variation. Rigid expectations that individuals will perform according to general patterns leads to stereotyping that denies the real variation that exists within the patterns. Knowledge of ethnic and cultural patterns is valuable; it provides guidelines for expectations and general areas of concern. But within any ethnic group there will be significant variation as the result of individuals interacting and adapting in a complex world.

Appreciation of ethnic variation is deeply rewarding in its own right, for humans have

created remarkable cultures and societies over time. Such recognition is also integral, however, to understanding beliefs, values, life-styles, needs, and expectations. The key to developing and using sensitivity, knowledge, and skills relevant to ethnic variation is in being flexible. "Cultural encapsulation" (Wrenn, 1985) is the name given to a situation in which stereotypes are allowed to replace real-world data. The unfortunate consequence of disregarding cultural variations among the ways that clients think and feel is that it encourages task- and technique-oriented definitions of the nursing process that may preclude visions of life from the client's point of view.

### Culturally Congruent Care

The importance of understanding cultural backgrounds and value orientations lies in the implications that such characteristics have for nursing care. Population- and culture-specific care represent a significant shift from a largely unicultural approach in human services (Leininger, 1985). In our multicultural world, culturally congruent or acceptable care is not only essential, but also must become explicit. All people value care, and there are some similarities (universals) in care. However, much of its expression (that is, which behaviors are considered caring and which are considered noncaring) varies widely. Differences in meanings, beliefs, practices, characteristics, expectations, and other cultural manifestations of care, as they vary with social structure, cultural values, beliefs, and environmental contexts, have now been studied in several dozen ethnic and cultural groups. Such work continues to be a major area of nursing research (Leininger, 1985, 1988).

### Cultural Values of Predominant Ethnic Groups

Among predominant American groups, white Anglo-Saxon Protestants typically descended from English, Scottish, and Scotch Irish immigrants who came to the United States during colonial or postrevolutionary times. It is that generalized world view that predominates in American institutions today. There is considerable regional variation, however, with Southern, Appalachian, Eastern, Midwestern, and Western Anglo Americans, which reflects somewhat different patterns of coping (McGill & Pearce, 1982).

In health care, sociocultural issues related to minority status (for example, differential opportunities to acquire status, power, and wealth that lead to relative poverty, powerlessness, and other class differences) are frequently confused with ethnic and cultural differences. An important task of nurses and other health providers is to distinguish the consequences of social processes (and discriminatory processes in particular) from cultural or subcultural characteristics.

**Ethnicity among whites.** Despite a common assumption that "whites aren't ethnic," there is a rich diversity of ethnic variation among the many groups that compose much of America. Irish, French, Italian, Polish, Norwegian, and Swedish traditions, as well as many others, brought varied patterns of values and beliefs that have been maintained or modified, but continue to influence individual and group behavior.

Appalachian Americans tend to perceive care as direct help, and caring persons as those who are focused on helping them, trusting them, and understanding their needs (Leininger, 1985). The concept of trust is of vital importance and non-Appalachians, government workers, and strangers require considerable checking over before being trusted. The provider who fails to respect Appalachian lifeways (such as dress and speech) and who cannot be trusted is considered noncaring.

For Jewish Americans, ethnic identity and religious life are often so interwoven as to be indistinguishable. Like members of other groups, they do not present uniform cultural

patterns, but do manifest sets of values (for example, of educational, financial, and social success, of suffering as a basic part of life, and of verbal ability) that influence decision making and other behavior (Herz & Rosen, 1982).

German immigrants have been becoming Americans for three centuries. There are even more Americans of German than of British descent. In German tradition, open display of emotion is minimized, and industriousness and academic achievement are considered appropriate ways of expression and accomplishment. Rationality, patriarchal family structures, and the slow formation of meaningful relationships further characterize German ethnicity (Winawer-Steiner & Wetzel, 1982).

Reflecting the foregoing caricatures of cultural values, white Americans generally favor specific care constructs. For them, care typically implies alleviating stress, discomfort, and anxiety. Providing comfort to self and others is valued, and comfort measures are related both to stress alleviation and nonstress situations. A noncaring person is one who lets another suffer or does not help one to be self-reliant. Education and information are viewed as major instruments of increased self-sufficiency and independence (Leininger, 1985). It is not by accident that these values predominate in nursing.

**African Americans.** There are more than 25 million African or black Americans. Ethnic identities for that large proportion of the population have been influenced by residuals from African cultures, identification with mainstream America, and adaptations and responses to victimization that is the consequence of racism, poverty, and oppression in the United States (Pinderhughes, 1982). Increasingly varied in class, educational background, and coping patterns, it is not possible to classify all black Americans together. It is also important to distinguish American blacks from others who came from the Caribbean Islands (West Indies, etc.) or from Africa (that is, Africans in America, in contrast to African Americans). Values, beliefs, and resources vary widely among various groups, although too often they are thrown together in American thought and policy on the basis of similar physical characteristics.

African Americans are characterized as adaptable and bicultural (that is, able to function in two worlds, one black and one white, which requires considerable effort and energy). They typically value work and education, although they do not always have the opportunity to acquire or use those. Strong family networks tend to extend beyond households to multiple collateral relationships.

Expectations for culturally congruent care among African Americans characteristically include expressions of concern for other blacks ("brothers and sisters") and general concern for one another. "Concern for" is expressed through attention to family needs, food, and coming together to be present and involved in both social and crisis contexts (Leininger, 1985). In a society in which dark skin has rendered people nearly socially invisible for centuries, genuine respect, recognition, and acknowledgment are elements essential to acceptable care.

**Hispanic Americans.** "Hispanic" refers to generally Spanish ethnicity, language skills, and ancestry, but in the United States also implies significant cultural variation. Nearly 16 million American Hispanics come primarily from Cuban, Puerto Rican, or Mexican backgrounds. They vary widely in level of acculturation (that is, integration into the mainstream American system). The average Mexican American, for example, was born in the United States. Although many members of other Hispanic groups are American by birth, many others are immigrants. The amount of Indian and African influence in contemporary Hispanic cultures also varies with historical differences.

Some common themes among Hispanic Americans include Catholicism (although increasing numbers of Hispanics are turning to Protestant and Pentecostal religions), orientation toward extended family systems (which may include godparents [compadres] and other nonbiological kin), distinctly different roles for men and women, high value of respect for self and others, priority of spiritual and humanistic over commercial values, clear hierarchy and patriarchy, and fairly common reliance on folk systems of medicine.

Typical ideas about what constitutes caring behaviors include attention and response to details that are important to family members and others, and succorance, which implies providing specific and direct help both in times of need and in daily activities (Leininger, 1985). Since Hispanic Americans tend to value being listened to and having time spent with them, task-oriented hurrying about is viewed as noncaring. Involvement, loving, and empathy are valued caring behaviors (Leininger, 1985).

**Native Americans.** Native Americans and Alaskan Natives have been referred to as "emigrants in their own homeland" (Attneave, 1982) because of the stresses required to maintain value systems that differ greatly from those of mainstream America. Approximately 2 million American Indians present a rich tapestry of cultural variants. About half live, at least part time, on reservations. Originally representing hundreds of culturally distinct nations, tribes, and bands, Native Americans today tend to get lumped, officially and unofficially, into pan-Indian groups that gloss over tribal identities and those of widely varied Indian nations, as well as distinct traditional beliefs and practices.

In contrast to white, middle-class values, Native American values emphasize harmony with (not control of) nature, a present (not future) orientation, and group (rather than individual) relationships. *Being* is more highly valued than *doing*, and the pervading attitude holds that humankind is essentially good (whereas the U.S. middle class typically views the human species as both good and bad) (Attneave, 1982). The potential for personal confusion is obvious in a situation where mainstream society devalues most of the concepts integral to traditional Native American philosophies and ideologies. The consequence is that those peoples descended from the original inhabitants of this land are among the poorest and most overlooked in society today.

Events in the Indian life cycle are established and rhythmic, and natural phenomena are important. The "real Indian" is one who is in balance as a living being and is growing, becoming, and achieving Indian goals; one continuously becomes and self-development is never completed. Giving is common, and in health care relationships, should be attended to respectfully. In the Indian way of life, noninterference is valued, and behaviors that imply manipulation or control may be offensive. The astute clinician makes sure that the Indian client is aware of the consequences of behavior, but then leaves it to the individual to decide how to proceed. Silence and conservative show of interest (including, for example, minimizing eye contact) are respectful, caring behaviors.

**Asian Americans.** Approximately 6 to 8 million other Americans are of Asian origin or ancestry. These represent diverse cultures from Japan, China, Korea, India, the Philippines and other Pacific islands, and southeast Asia. However, because they are numerically a relatively small proportion of the total U.S. population, they tend to be classified in broad categories that fail to distinguish their cultural differences.

References are sometimes made to Asian immigrants as the most successful newcomers, or as examples that the United States does indeed provide opportunities for success to those who work to take them. The implication is, therefore, that if Asians, who have shorter histories in America than either African or His-

panic Americans, can succeed in traditional American terms in only a few generations, then the non-Asian minorities must have failed to use their opportunities. The problem with that line of thinking is that it does not consider the contexts in which each group has had to struggle to adapt. Asians, far fewer in number than blacks or Hispanics, have been discriminated against. However, they have not been excluded as wholeheartedly (at least since the end of World War II) as have been members of the other groups, for whom racist aspects of American society have undermined values of work and education (Pinderhughes, 1982).

Education and hard work have paid off for many Asian immigrants, and often their transplanted cultural values have fit well with American values. Behavioral patterns tended to be rewarded, even when motivations founded on different values and beliefs prompted them. The other aspect of the "Asian success story" is that it sometimes fails to take into account several important variables. There is, for example, a sizable number of poor Asian Americans despite a low rate of dependence on public assistance and welfare, a continuing discrepancy between education level and income, and a higher percentage of multiple wage earner families among Asians than among other American ethnic groups (Sue, 1981).

Strong Asian values generally involve harmonious interpersonal relationships, webs of obligation, and fear of shame (which is a social concept, in contrast to the Westernized notion of guilt, which is more individualized) (Shon & Ja, 1982). The traditionally extended family is of great importance, and family sharing is a major construct in care. Respect, especially for family, elders, and those in authority, is also seen as vital. Respect is expressed through recognition of family members and in listening to and valuing their input (Leininger, 1985). Reciprocity and generosity are highly valued. Disruptive and conflict situations are viewed as noncaring, and silence is a highly valued caring behavior because it allows one to reflect quietly, rest, and avoid dissonance (Leininger, 1985).

**Middle Eastern cultural groups.** In recent decades the United States has experienced an influx of groups from Middle Eastern and Northern African cultures, such as Iranians, Jordanians, and Arabs. This has increased the American (traditionally Judeo Christian) awareness of the complex cultural beliefs, values, and lifeways of members of predominately Islamic societies.

Despite considerable cultural diversity among Middle Eastern peoples, generally shared value orientations include Moslem (Muslim or Islamic) submission and obedience to God and prescribed rituals of prayer and washing. Strict concepts of what is allowed and forbidden (that is, clean and unclean, good and bad) impose dietary and other rules. Those should be ascertained and accommodated as much as possible in health care situations. Class, status, education, modesty (especially for females), and emotional expression are commonly valued. Patriarchy and the centrality of religion typify Middle Eastern social and familial organizations. Elders are honored, gain in status, and interestingly, tend not to experience the senility common to more youth-oriented cultures (Luna, 1989). Since Middle Easterners are oriented primarily to the present, they may not value making plans because the future is seen as neither uncertain nor preordained, but as something one accepts with fatalistic grace (Jalali, 1982).

## Migration and Culture Shock

A large proportion of health care consumers in America are immigrants; therefore, consideration of problems commonly experienced by migrants is in order. The most obvious response to significant transition is culture shock, which involves reaction to the disparity between what is expected and what actually exists or is experienced (Shon & Ja, 1982). Adjustment is complicated by disappointment, grief over loss and separation, and anger and resentment at the realization that skills and status are often not directly transferable from the old situation or recognized in the new.

Cultural transition can be painful and is strongly influenced by availability of support systems, family constellation and functioning, and degree of fit between the old and new cultures (Landau, 1982). Rates and types of adaptation frequently differ within families, which can be further disrupted as degrees of traditionalism and modernization vary. It is important for nurses to ascertain how long various family members have been in the United States and how the transition process is going for them. Support and referral may be necessary in response to recognition of problems caused as different family subsystems adapt in different ways and at different rates (Landau, 1982).

## ❖ THE CULTURAL ORIENTATION OF NURSING

The above descriptions are brief and do not attempt more than a scant overview of the vastly diverse cultural variations that nurses encounter. It should be noted, however, that the Anglo white description of caring tends to characterize most of nursing. That is, by developing professional nursing as a predominantly white, middle-class discipline, the caring behaviors that are identified, taught, and practiced tend to be those expected by and most appropriate for white, middle-class clients. Nurses deal, however, with peoples from many other groups in addition to white, middle-class Americans of predominately British or German descent. They must learn, therefore, to adapt nursing care to the needs, specifications, and expectations of members of those other groups if they hope to provide care that is both accepted and effective.

*Ethnicity and Family Therapy,* edited by Monica McGoldrick et al. (1982), is highly recommended for its useful information about more than two dozen ethnic groups in the United States. The value of that book extends to all practitioners who work with people of cultural backgrounds other than their own (or who are interested in their own), because it delineates frameworks of historical and value orientations that influence lives in general.

## Values, Beliefs, Nurses, and Nursing: Implications for Professional Development in a Caring Discipline

Nursing as a discipline and subculture needs to examine itself, not because there is anything wrong with it, but to see how to make it better. Realistic expectations for development of nursing as an effective social force require sensitivity to and management of grass roots obstacles. Two major aspects of revised-for-effectiveness nursing might include:

1. Increased attention to diversity among nurses and the impact of social stratification patterns on both nursing and nurses
2. Efforts to increase sensitivity, knowledge, and skills relevant to population-specific and culturally congruent nursing care.

Professional collegiality among nurses is often limited by pressure toward task definition and accomplishment, with relatively low prioritization of staff communication and mutual support. The outcome is inhibited cohesion and generalized perception of powerlessness. There is a hesitancy among nurses to commit to greater collegiality, even in a time of increased awareness of the importance of relationships, support networks, and acquisition of authority and power. There is also little attention to social issues such as:

1. Nursing's continued subordination to other professions and orientations
2. Caring as less distinct and less consciously valued by society than is curing
3. The potential impact of rich ethnic, educational, and experiential heterogeneity among nurses on development of more meaningful patterns of caring.

There is a need to adapt nursing and caring behaviors to the discipline's multicultural clientele (in contrast to focusing on ways to motivate and manipulate consumers and potential consumers to use preset nursing strategies and techniques). That is a logical extension of extensive, research-based evidence that people with varied value and belief systems present diverse, culture-based needs. Values and beliefs shape definitions and expectations of care in more ways than a "single model" discipline can provide. Quality care must be acceptable, and acceptable care necessitates serious consideration of both individual differences and cultural patterns.

## ❖ SUMMARY

Values and beliefs function as filters through which reality is experienced. Systems of health beliefs and practices are adaptive strategies that have developed in diverse cultures and societies to deliberately and as effectively as possible enhance health or relieve discomfort. Throughout history, healing has been a conscious human objective. Networks of supportive action exist in every society. Caring and curing behaviors exist as ritualized attempts to meet the best interests of interdependent, ill individuals and their reference groups. Their goals are transition into new states or restoration of functioning that is as normal as possible. Health and illness are not limited to physical and psychological phenomena but they do have significant social and cultural dimensions.

Nurses play a major part in the promotion of health and alleviation of distress. Given the complexity of that challenge, they must above all be flexible. Homogenized models of nursing, which imply that one style of care fits all people and circumstances, do justice to neither nursing nor society.

## ❖ APPLYING KNOWLEDGE TO PRACTICE

1. Discuss the roles of values and beliefs in the identification, expression, and treatment of illness.
2. What universals (similarities) and diversities (differences) exist among nursing needs of people with differing belief or values systems?
3. What are some ways that American systems of health care might not be congruent with the needs of members of more traditional societies?
4. Identify values and beliefs of nursing in the United States. Discuss how these are congruent or in conflict with the values and beliefs of different cultural groups described in this chapter.

**REFERENCES**

Attneave, C. (1982). American Indians and Alaskan Native families: Emigrants in their own homeland. In M. McGoldrick, J. K. Pearce, & J. Giordano (Eds.), *Ethnicity and family therapy* (pp. 55–83). New York: Guilford Press.

Doi, T. (1973). *The theory of dependence.* Tokyo, Japan: Kodansha.

Foster, G. M., & Anderson, B. G. (1978). *Medical anthropology.* New York: John Wiley and Son.

Herz, F. M., & Rosen, E. J. (1982). Jewish families. In M. McGoldrick, J. K. Pearce, & J. Giordano (Eds.), *Ethnicity and family therapy* (pp. 364–392). New York: Guilford Press.

Jalali, B. (1982). Iranian families. In M. McGoldrick, J. K. Pearce, & J. Giordano (Eds.), *Ethnicity and family therapy* (pp. 289–309). New York: Guilford Press.

Keillor, G. (1985). *Lake Wobegon Days.* New York: Viking Press.

Kleinman, A. M. (1980). *Patients and healers in the context of culture.* Los Angeles, CA: University of California Press.

Kluckholn, F. R. (1953). Dominant and variant value orientations. In C. Kluckholn & H. Murray (Eds.), *Personality in nature, society, and culture* (pp. 342-357). New York: Alfred A. Knopf.

Kluckholn, F. R., & Strodtbeck, F. L. (1961). *Variations in value orientations.* Elmsford, New York: Row, Peterson.

Landau, J. (1982). Therapy with families in cultural transition. In M. McGoldrick, J. K. Pearce, & J. Giordano (Eds.), *Ethnicity and family therapy* (pp. 552–572). New York: Guilford Press.

Leaf, M. (1936). *The story of Ferdinand.* New York: Viking.

Leininger, M. (1985). Transcultural caring: A different way to help people. In P. Pedersen (Ed.), *Handbook of cross-cultural counseling and therapy* (pp. 107–115). Westport, CT: Greenwood Press.

Leininger, M. (1988). Leininger's theory of nursing: Cultural care diversity and universality. *Nursing Science Quarterly, 1*(4), 152–160.

Lerner, M. J. (1980). *The belief in a just world: A fundamental delusion.* New York: Plenum Press.

Luna, L. J. (1989). Transcultural nursing care of Arab Muslims. *Journal of Transcultural Nursing, 1*(1), 22–26.

McGill, D., & Pearce, J. K. (1982). British families. In M. McGoldrick, J. K. Pearce, & J. Giordano (Eds.), *Ethnicity and family therapy* (pp. 457–479). New York: Guilford Press.

McGoldrick, M. (1982). Ethnicity and family therapy. In M. McGoldrick, J. K. Pearce, & J. Giordano (Eds.), *Ethnicity and family therapy* (pp. 3–30). New York: Guilford Press.

McGoldrick, M., Pearce, J. K., & Giordano, J. (Eds.). (1982). *Ethnicity and family therapy.* New York: Guilford Press.

Nurge, E. (1958). Etiology of illness in Guinhangdan. *American Anthropologist, 60,* 1158–1172.

Orque, M. S. (1983). Orque's ethnic/cultural system: A framework for ethnic nursing care. In M. Orque, B. Bloch, & L. Monrroy (Eds.), *Ethnic nursing care: A multicultural approach* (pp. 5–48). St. Louis, MO: C. V. Mosby.

Pedersen, P. (1988). *A handbook for developing multicultural awareness.* Alexandria, VA: American Association for Counseling and Development.

Pinderhughes, E. (1982). Afro-American families and the victim system. In M. McGoldrick, J. K. Pearce, & J. Giordano (Eds.), *Ethnicity and family therapy* (pp. 108–122). New York: Guilford Press.

Popenoe, D. (1989). *Sociology.* Englewood Cliffs, NJ: Prentice-Hall.

Population Reference Bureau. (1988). *1988 World population data sheet.* DC: Population Reference Bureau.

Rodwin, V. G. (1988). Inequalities in private and public health systems: The United States, France, Canada, and Great Britain. In W. A. Van Horne & T. V. Tonnesen (Eds.), *Ethnicity and health.* Milwaukee, WI: The University of Wisconsin System Institute on Race and Ethnicity.

Shon, S. P., & Ja, D. Y. (1982). Asian families. In M. McGoldrick, J. K. Pearce, & J. Giordano (Eds.), *Ethnicity and family therapy* (pp. 208–228). New York: Guilford Press.

Snow, L. F. (1977). Popular medicine in a black neighborhood. In E. H. Spicer (Ed.), *Ethnic medicine in the southwest* (pp. 19–95). Tucson, AZ: University of Arizona Press.

Sue, D. W. (1981). *Counseling the culturally different: Theory and practice.* New York: John Wiley and Sons.

Tavris, C., & Wade, C. (1984). *The longest war: Sex roles in perspective.* New York: Harcourt Brace Jovanovich.

*U.S. News & World Report.* (1989, 7 August). Race relations: An American dilemma revisited, pp. 8–9.

Van Horne, W. A. (1985). Introduction. In W. A. Van Horne & T. V. Tonnesen (Eds.), *Ethnicity and the work force.* Milwaukee, WI: The University of Wisconsin System American Ethnic Studies Coordinating Committee/Urban Corridor Consortium.

Winawer-Steiner, H., & Wetzel, N. A. (1982). German families. In M. McGoldrick, J. K. Pearce, & J. Giordano (Eds.), *Ethnicity and family therapy* (pp. 247–268). New York: Guilford Press.

Wrenn, C. G. (1985). Afterward: The culturally encapsulated counselor revisited. In P. Pedersen (Ed.), *Handbook of cross-cultural counseling and therapy* (pp. 323–329). Westport, CT: Greenwood Press.

# 12 ◆ Health Promotion and Wellness

Rosanne Harkey Pruitt

## OBJECTIVES

*At the completion of this chapter, the reader will be able to:*

- ◆ Define health promotion.
- ◆ Describe the characteristics and benefits of effective exercise.
- ◆ Identify three methods of stress management.
- ◆ Determine the caloric needs of a specific individual.
- ◆ Discuss several ways to evaluate a health promotion intervention.

Health promotion is an interdisciplinary concept that encompasses mental and spiritual health, physical well-being, and social support. Health promotion has always been an important component of nursing practice, particularly in the area of community health. Pender (1987) notes that there is general support for the statement that the goal of nursing is the promotion of health among individuals, families, and communities. Nurses are using aspects of health promotion with groups and individuals in virtually every practice role of the profession. Health promotion includes efforts to assist individuals in taking control of and responsibility for their health to minimize health risks and ultimately improve the quality of life.

### ❖ DEFINING HEALTH PROMOTION

The term *health promotion* comes out of the differentiation of the three levels of preven-

tion by Leavell and Clark (1953) that is widely used in public health and community health nursing. *Tertiary prevention* is health care that focuses on chronic disease and rehabilitation. *Secondary prevention* includes specific screening programs and illness care. *Primary prevention* is usually equated with health promotion in which a specific disease is not the focus of increasing one's level of well-being. Several nursing theorists differentiate even further between health promotion and primary prevention. Health promotion activities are those directed toward sustaining or increasing well-being and self-actualization (Pender, 1987; Shamansky & Clausen, 1980). Primary prevention is defined as activities that decrease the probability of specific diseases. Most frequently, health promotion includes the areas of nutrition, exercise, and stress management. Other areas related to alcohol and drug use and the use of safety belts are included by some, while

**211**

others classify these latter categories as "health protection."

### ❖ WELLNESS

Wellness is often used interchangeably with health promotion. *Wellness* is the state of being healthy or well, while health promotion refers to the activities undertaken to improve one's state of health. The focus of wellness is the improvement of the physical, mental, and spiritual well-being of individuals who are already free of any known diseases. Health promotion encompasses activities to improve the health of those who are not initially healthy as well as healthy individuals.

### ❖ THEORETICAL ASPECTS
### Dunn's High Level Wellness

Some of the earliest work in the area of health promotion was that of Halbert Dunn (1959, 1971). His continuum demonstrates the dynamic interaction of health and environment as one moves toward *high-level wellness.* Health is dynamic with a continuous need for

health-promoting activity to maintain and improve one's health (Fig. 12-1).

While all nursing models address health in some way, several models address health promotion more specifically.

### Neuman's Systems Model

Nursing theorist Betty Neuman (1989) uses a systems format and includes the levels of prevention and the multiple dimensions of health promotion (physical, psychological, spiritual, and social) as well as lines of defense. Health promotion efforts are used to strengthen these line barriers of defense. Activities undertaken to increase stress resistance discussed later in the chapter provide an example of the application of this model. A more detailed discussion regarding other aspects of this model can be found in Chapter 1 and in the book, the *Neuman Systems Model* (1989).

### Pender's Health Promotion Model

Nola Pender's (1987) model is more specifically focused on health promotion (Fig. 12-2).

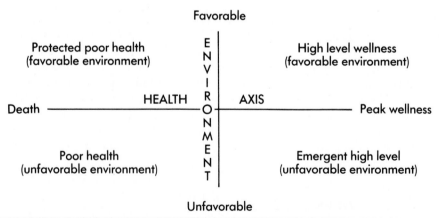

Favorable

| Protected poor health (favorable environment) | E N V I R O N M E N T | High level wellness (favorable environment) |

Death ———————— HEALTH ⟷ AXIS ———————— Peak wellness

| Poor health (unfavorable environment) | | Emergent high level (unfavorable environment) |

Unfavorable

❖ **Fig. 12-1**   Continuum of high level wellness. *From Dunn, H.L. (1959). High level wellness for man and society. American Journal of Public Health 49, p. 88.*

Pender includes the multiple factors that determine how an individual thinks about or perceives participation in health-promoting behaviors, factors that modify initial thoughts and perceptions, and influences that are cues to action, such as the mass media, conversations with others, or feeling better after exercising. The model demonstrates the complexity of whether or not an individual is likely to participate in health-promoting activities. This model is helpful in assessing an individual client as well as including factors to consider in providing a supportive environment for health improvement.

## Green's Health Promotion Model

Lawrence Green, a health educator, developed a model that can be useful in planning and evaluating health promotion activities. He includes the need to consider environmental modifications as well as programs that target individuals. Green's (1986) model demon-

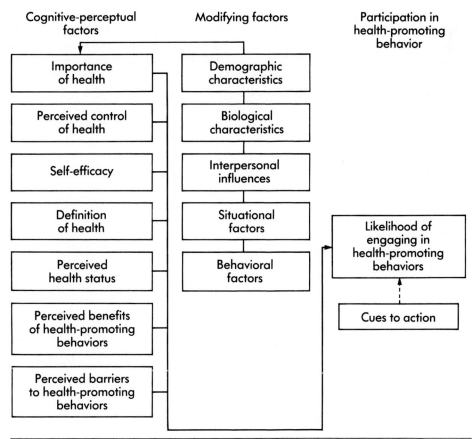

❖ **Fig. 12-2**   Health promotion model. *From Pender, N.J. (1987). Health Promotion in Nursing (2nd ed.), Norwalk, CT: Appleton & Lange, p. 58.* Reprinted with permission.

❖ **Table 12-1**
Green's health promotion model

| Interventions | Process of change | Immediate outcomes | Intermediate outcomes | Ultimate outcomes |
|---|---|---|---|---|
| Health promotion | Economic resources<br>Organization<br>    services | Reduced risk factors<br>Enhanced<br>    well-being | Increases in<br>    productivity<br>Self-esteem | Reduced illness<br>Improved quality<br>    of life |

From A framework for the design of rigorous evaluation of efforts in health promotion by Green, L. W. (1986). *Journal of Health Promotion* 1, (1), 77–78 with permission.

strates the time differences of various outcomes by dividing the complex outcomes into three components: immediate, intermediate, and ultimate outcomes. Effective health promotion efforts have immediate benefits as well as benefits that occur over much longer periods of time. When evaluating the benefits of a health promotion intervention, it is important to include the potential long-term and short-term benefits (Table 12-1).

### ❖ PRACTICE DIMENSIONS

This section focuses on the assessment and counseling in three primary areas of health promotion: fitness, nutrition, and stress management. Other books, such as Pender's (1987) *Health Promotion in Nursing Practice,* can be used if additional detail is needed.

### Fitness

It has been estimated that almost half of adult Americans engage in some form of regular exercise, but many have little or no knowledge of what constitutes a safe and effective fitness program (Dunn, 1987). Unrealistic expectations lead to exhaustion, pain, injury, and a high rate of cessation of fitness activities.

**Effective exercise.** There are several characteristics of effective exercise. The exercise should be integrated into the individual's life-style

at least on alternate days and should be enjoyable for the participant. The activity should produce rhythmic movement with alternating relaxation and contraction, should be vigorous enough to use at least 400 calories, and should sustain the heart rate in the training heart range 20 to 30 minutes (Pender, 1987; Kirkendall, 1986). The training heart range, which is 60% to 90% of the individual's estimated maximum heart rate, is usually estimated by subtracting the individual's age from 220 and then multiplying that number by 0.6 and 0.9. For example, the training heart rate for a 20-year-old is calculated as follows:

$$220 - 20 = 200;$$
$$200 \times 0.6 = 120;$$
$$200 \times 0.9 = 180$$

and would give a training heart range of 120 to 180. Although 20 to 30 minutes is recommended, improvements have been demonstrated in individuals with low initial fitness in sessions as short as 5 to 10 minutes (Kirkendall, 1986).

**Exercise benefits.** Benefits of exercise are psychological and physical. Psychological benefits include increased alertness, general well-being, and lowered stress. Physical benefits include endurance, strength, flexibility and skill, improved aerobic capacity, cardiovascular efficiency, and weight loss (Pender, 1987).

**Components of an exercise plan.** An exercise plan should include warm-up, stretching, and cool-down periods in addition to the endurance exercise. The warm-up increases blood flow to the heart and skeletal muscles and loosens and strengthens muscles, and may include a brisk walk and deep breathing. Stretching is included to maintain and increase flexibility. Stretching is done slowly, holding the position several seconds to the point of tightness, not pain. The cool-down allows body temperature and heart rate to decrease slowly and prevents pooling of blood in the extremities. An example is walking and deep breathing while loosely shaking one's extremities. A variety of different endurance exercises can condition one's heart and lungs. The criteria for evaluation include briskness (raising heart and respiratory rates) and sustained (without interruption) (American Heart Association, 1979). Varying the types of exercise is recommended to prevent boredom.

Starting slowly and then gradually increasing the intensity and duration is the key to a healthy exercise program. A complete history and physical and an exercise stress test (bicycle ergometer or treadmill) is recommended for individuals who are over 35 or who are under 35 but have any existing health conditions or strong family history of cardiovascular or respiratory condition (The American College of Sports Medicine, 1980). If jogging is preferred, one should begin walking and gradually replace it with jogging once he or she is able to briskly walk 3 miles in 45 minutes. The gradual build up should also be employed after any absence from exercise of a week or more.

**Exercise counseling.** Counseling should include coverage of exercise self-care and a tolerance barometer. Exercise self-care includes guidelines for clothing, time of day to exercise, and food and fluid intake. Appropriate footwear for the sport and snug-fitting socks will reduce injury potential. Endurance exercises should not be performed during weather extremes. Guidelines vary slightly depending on the intensity of the exercise regarding food and fluid

intake; however, an increase in fluid intake and a delay after meals is generally recommended. Small amounts of carbohydrates 1 or 2 hours before endurance exercises will help supplement normal reserves.

**Tolerance barometer.** The tolerance barometer refers to potentially dangerous physical symptoms. These include breathlessness, excessive fatigue, and other uncomfortable signs. An individual should be able to talk while exercising. Excessive fatigue refers to feelings of fatigue more than 1 hour after exercising. Uncomfortable symptoms include any chest discomfort, dizziness, faintness, exertional dyspnea, nausea or vomiting, and muscle or joint problems (Oberman, 1984). The pulse rate should be monitored every 5 minutes at any pulse site (except the carotids) as soon as the individual starts breathing hard and until the heart rate resumes normal levels after exercise (Dunn, 1987). The 6-second pulse (multiplied by 10) will minimize disruption of exercise. An individual should slow down if levels exceed the training heart range.

### Stress Management

Stress management comprises efforts to move from distress or overload to eustress. *Eustress* or "good stress" consists of levels of stress low enough to motivate without overwhelming an individual. Distress levels that are too high result in confusion and poor functioning for the individual with resultant physical and psychological complaints. Chapter 17 provides further discussion of the concept of stress.

In order to intervene and assist an individual in managing stress, one must assess the level of existing stress, assess the source of the stress, and determine the appropriate point for intervention to achieve stress reduction. The methods and applications of stress management are diverse and date back to the early part of this century (Goldberg & Comstock, 1976). The techniques used fall into essentially three categories, which reflect the multidimensional nature of the stress response.

**Stress reduction.** The first technique is predominantly cognitive and involves reduction of stress-inducing situations or ways to avoid excessive stress. *Time management* involves determining goals and priorities, organizing one's time to accomplish one's priorities, and learning to say "no" to activities that do not relate to those goals. *Time blocking* is setting aside time to adapt to a change and incorporate it into one's daily routine. This is helpful for a new diabetic, for example, who is learning to adjust to diet, medication, and other life-style changes. *Change avoidance,* employed during periods of high life change, is the avoidance of unnecessary alterations to prevent the need to make multiple major adjustments simultaneously. For example, if an elderly individual can remain in the same home for a period of time after the loss of a spouse, simultaneous multiple readjustments can be lessened. A component of change avoidance is *habituation,* when one attempts to make routine as many aspects of the day as possible during a high-risk period. This can be as simple as parking in the same area or floor of a parking deck to avoid the frustration of looking for one's car. *Environmental modification* involves identifying experiences or personalities that are abrasive or stress-producing and minimizing contact to the extent possible. A helpful alternative for many individuals may be doing something for others or getting involved in helping with activities that interest them to decrease the focus on oneself.

**Stress resistance.** The second point of intervention focuses on behavioral aspects of increasing stress resistance or ways to build resistance to stress. One method to increase stress resistance is enhancing self-esteem by focusing on one's strengths and attributes. This may be accomplished by the individual or may include support groups. Assertiveness training focuses on substituting positive assertive behavior for negative passive behavior. Developing goal alternatives involves helping an individual determine what was important about an initially unachievable goal and how the important aspects can still be achieved. For example, the high school senior who is not accepted in the college of his or her choice often has the option of attending another school and transferring later.

**Lower stress response.** The third stress management technique involves counter conditioning to lower physiological response or ways to alter physiological response to stress. Many methods are included in this category, which encompasses the broad range from self-hypnosis, yoga, and meditation to various breathing and exercise regimens (Pender, 1987; Stoyva & Anderson, 1982). Multiple studies focusing on relaxation activities have documented a decrease of stress-related symptoms in cases of chronic anxiety, tension and migraine headaches, temporomandibular joint (TMJ) syndrome, and localized muscular tension and cramping (Goldberger & Breznitz, 1982). Relaxation exercise includes progressive tension-relaxation exercise, where the individual tenses and then relaxes muscles. This exercise usually begins with individual muscles and combines groups as the individual advances. The disadvantage is that tensing large muscle groups significantly raises blood pressure and is therefore not recommended for individuals with hypertension. Relaxation without tensing is often achieved by progressively moving from head to toe, relaxing various muscles or progressively becoming more relaxed as one counts from ten to one. The use of imagery involves recalling pleasant scenery or experiences from the past to help one relax. Exercise and physical activity are also helpful stress buffers.

**Biofeedback.** Biofeedback assists individuals to become more aware and to ultimately develop more control over responses not ordinarily under voluntary control. The two most prevalent methods are electromyography and skin temperature feedback. Studies have demonstrated successful results with biofeedback in conjunction with one or more of the relaxation methods (Fehring, 1983).

## Nutrition and Weight Control

Guidelines for a healthy diet have changed most in relation to attention paid to the amount of fat and cholesterol over the past few decades. A diet with a fat content of 30% or less is recommended with less than 10% coming from saturated fat. It is estimated that most American diets contain 40% fat (Joint Nutrition Monitoring Evaluation Committee, 1986). The emphasis on fiber has been a part of nutritional advice in relation to digestion and has also gained popularity in relation to its role in lowering low-density cholesterol. The recommendation for a balanced diet with a variety from the basic four food groups to supply the essential vitamins and minerals and an adequate amount of fluid has withstood the test of time as sound nutritional advice.

Nationally, 14% of adult men and 24% of adult women are 20% over their ideal body weight (Vital Health Statistics, 1988). Excessive weight has harmful medical consequences on physical and psychological health as well as longevity (Burton & Foster, 1985).

**Assessment for weight loss.** Before beginning a weight loss program, a history and physical exam must be completed. This is particularly important to identify underlying pathology that is associated with or aggravated by excessive weight and requires medical supervision in conjunction with weight loss efforts. These include diabetes, arthritis, cardiovascular disease, hypertension, hypothyroidism, and renal disease. Weight loss efforts are usually not recommended during chemotherapy due to the already compromised nutritional status and potential impact on therapy (Tait & Aisner, 1989). Lab work that is usually recommended includes an ECG, blood lipids, and glucose.

**Predictors of weight loss success.** The success of a weight loss program depends on a variety of factors:

1. Stability of present weight. If the individual has used starvation diets in the past, he or she may have a more difficult time losing weight because of a resultant lower basal metabolic rate (Ernsberger, 1985). Exercise facilitates weight loss, particularly fat loss, and raises the basal metabolic rate.
2. Realistic expectations. Up to 3 pounds a week is realistic for a healthy weight loss regimen. Gradual declines with a focus on modifying eating habits have been found to have the best long-term success.
3. Motivation to change. Success is more likely to occur when conditions make the weight loss a high priority. A medical diagnosis that makes weight loss imperative has been found to be the most motivating.

**Determining caloric needs.** When working with individuals who wish to lose or gain weight, determinations need to be made regarding ideal body weight and weekly objectives to determine caloric intake. The most reliable source for anthropometric data in order to determine ideal body weight is the 1959 Metropolitan Life Desirable Weight Table. The more recent guidelines have been rejected by many scientists (Semipoulos & Van Itallie, 1984). The American Diabetes Association and the American Dietetic Association have published guidelines, which can be used to estimate caloric needs according to activity level. The midpoint of the ideal weight range (the ideal body weight or IBW) can be used to estimate caloric needs.

1. To determine the number of calories needed to support vital body functions, multiply the ideal body weight by 10.
2. Add activity calories according to the type of activity in which the individual participates during the majority of the day. Sedentary: IBW × 3. Moderate: IBW × 5. Strenuous: IBW × 10.
3. To lose 1 pound per week, subtract 500 calories per day. Note: (500 × 7 = 3500 calories = 1 pound).

To lose 2 pounds per week subtract 1000 calories per day. Calories are added to gain weight (500/day to gain 1 pound/week).

Example: Jim's IBW is 180 and he wishes to lose 2 pounds/week
1. 180 × 10 = 1800 base calories
2. Add 180 × 5 = 900 for a moderate activity level
3. Subtract 1000 calories for a 2 pound loss per week
[1800 + 900 = 2700 − 1000 = 1700 calories per day]

**Behavioral approaches to weight control.** Behavioral approaches to weight control are an important aspect of counseling. These include self-monitoring, conditioning, and stimulus control in addition to exercise (White, 1986). *Self-monitoring* consists of diaries, graphs, or menus that are used to assist an individual in monitoring eating activity. *Conditioning* may be positive, negative, or both. *Positive conditioning* consists of a nonfood reward when short-term goals are achieved. These may be weight-related or may be associated with behavior changes. *Negative conditioning* or aversion therapy is the association of eating and unpleasant things. Most often, this is just a reminder on the refrigerator or pantry door. *Stimulus control* is the reduction of cues that trigger eating. An example is not shopping for groceries when one is hungry.

## Contracting for Health Promotion

*Contracting* is the process of establishing mutual goals as well as strategies for accomplishing them. Contracts between nurses and clients are generally one of two types: contingency or treatment. A *contingency contract* is used for learning or changing behavior with positive reinforcement based on principles of behavior modification. *Treatment contracts* are less common and specify details of therapy: goals, methods, time limits, and responsibilities of the client and the provider (Boehm, 1989). Client involvement in establishing an achievable goal and the selection of an appropriate reward enhances the success of the contract. Contracts can be long-term, but short-term, weekly contracts are recommended for behavior change (White, 1986). Generally, goals are set with progressive, short-term objectives. The nurse can reinforce positive behavior with verbal praise. Self-reinforcement with tangible rewards is helpful for long-term behavioral change. The use of contracts with appropriate positive reinforcement can greatly enhance the success of a behavior change program.

## Motivation

Many factors are responsible for motivating individuals toward making behavioral changes. Pender's model on p. 213 presents factors that include the importance or value of health to an individual and perception of one's own health. Other elements include whether an individual perceives control over his or her own health.

**Self-efficacy.** Self-efficacy is the perceived ability to execute necessary behavior change. Studies have demonstrated a strong relationship between self-efficacy and behavior change and maintenance (Strecher, DeVellis, Becker & Rosenstock, 1987). In an analysis of several studies, Strecher and his colleagues (1987) found that efficacy expectations reflect perceived rather than actual capabilities and that it was the perceptions and not the true ability that influenced behavior change. They recommend that self-efficacy be incorporated into behavioral change programs by breaking down target behaviors into manageable components beginning with the simpler tasks in order to build on success as the individual moves to more difficult tasks.

**Additional motivators.** Still other studies have found different motivators for behavior change. A recent survey of Americans who participate regularly in fitness activities indicated that personal appearance was a top motivator for exercise (Harris, 1986). Convenience of the health care provider and exercise facility, as well as family and peer support, are important in the maintenance and continuation of activities (White, 1987).

## Implementation Methods

Intervention modes are diverse and depend on the audience. Educative roles include group lectures, individual teaching sessions, and sharing or development of printed material. Training lay instructors can expand and extend programs for larger numbers of individuals. Nurses are becoming more involved in the development and dissemination of health education by the media. Newspapers as well as radio and television stations frequently welcome the professional contributions of nurses. Wellness fairs provide another mode of reaching a large number of individuals. Counseling roles may be with individuals or families or may include efforts to develop support groups for individuals with similar needs and objectives. Sometimes policies inhibit efforts for safety and wellness. Nurses can be instrumental in working through bureaucratic restraints. One recent example involved a day care center that was denied access to a residential street. Parents were forced to use a busy street or receive a ticket if they used the safer alternative. Following the health assessment of this school, a registered nurse student worked with the parents to repeal this ordinance. The production quotas and time constraints within many industries also inhibit health promotion efforts. Many industries have been convinced of the need to promote the health of their workers, their most valuable resource. Others still need to be persuaded.

## Interventions with Ill Individuals

Interventions are not limited to essentially healthy individuals. Aspects of health promotion can be incorporated into nursing care for existing health needs. Assistance with nutrition, exercise, and stress management can be approached initially in relation to the improvement of an existing health problem with movement toward a healthier life-style. A recent illness can serve as a very real motivator in the individual's attempt to regain health. This period of changing health status can be used to raise the individual to a higher level of functioning. Research with chronic diseases has consistently shown improved outcomes over time in individuals with lower risk factors. Examples include improved lung function over time by individuals who quit smoking and fewer complications among diabetics who minimize blood sugar fluctuations through diet, exercise, and medication (Tuck, 1988).

## ❖ POLICY DIMENSIONS

Two different political strategies have been used to increase healthy behaviors. The first strategy involves regulation, such as banning certain products, legislating and taxing their use, and restricting sales (McGuire, 1984). State legislation related to alcohol use, speed limits, and safety belts are examples of this type of health protection. Another example is the move of many corporations to restrict smoking by employees. The second strategy attempts to alter health behavior by convincing individuals to exercise personal responsibility. The latter includes media education as well as programs that attempt to motivate risk reduction and skills to adopt more healthy life-styles. In the areas of health promotion, where the risks and costs to others are often unclear, action is more typical of the second strategy, which is education to inform and motivate healthy behavior. Several landmark documents have been published over the past decade. *Healthy People* (1979) by the Surgeon General and the companion document *Promoting Health/Preventing Disease: The Objectives for the Nation* (1980) have been referred to as "the closest thing to a national policy that we have in the United States" (Green, 1986, p. 2). The *Objectives for the Nation* cover 15 areas, five of which specifically address health promotion: exercise and fitness, stress control, smoking, alcohol and drugs, and nutrition. Recent federal legislative proposals have aimed at incentives, such as Medicare discounts for nonsmokers, and special projects and grants, to demonstrate cost savings of preventive efforts in medical care costs. Block grants to states, such as those for maternal child care and health care for the elderly, mandate a certain amount of health education. Enabling legislation for Health Maintenance Organizations (HMOs) mandates inclusion of health promotion activities.

## Economic Dimensions: Costs and Benefits

The economic dimension of health promotion is concerned with costs. Cost considerations included early in the planning stage assist in development decisions as well as the evaluation of programs. Cost estimations include personnel time for planning and conducting the program, materials, promotional costs, transportation, and any fees for rooms. Benefits depend on the program offered. Green's model (Table 12-1) may be helpful in specifying benefits. Dollar amounts are not available for most of the psychological and physical benefits gained by participants. However, expected benefits should be listed for decision makers, including the potential for positive publicity for the organization.

Several different economic methods are available to compare costs and benefits of proposed action. *Cost benefit analysis* (CBA) calculates all benefits and outcomes, including health effects, in monetary terms and determines whether the program or intervention has a positive payoff. *Cost effectiveness analysis* (CEA) assumes the objective is worth achieving and seeks to determine which program, technique, or intervention is the most effective and the least costly (Rogers, Eaton, & Bruin, 1981). CEA is preferred by health-care researchers because of "either the impossibility or undesirability of valuing important outcomes in dollars and cents" (Banta & Luce, 1983, p. 148). *Cost efficiency* compares the costs and benefits of a single program. Economic aspects are an important consideration in supporting the development, continuation, and expansion of health promotion interventions.

## Evaluation of Effectiveness

In addition to the analysis of the costs and benefits of a health promotion program, evaluation of program effectiveness is also critical. *Effectiveness* evaluation focuses on the extent to which a program or activity achieves the intended objectives. Objectives should include should include tangible criteria and be evaluated on a regular basis. These criteria should include behavioral changes of participants, as well as the frequency and duration of participation. Too often, evaluations include only numbers participating and whether or not they enjoyed a program. A variety of methods can be used for evaluation, including record reviews and logs kept by participants and providers. Information on individual progress can include objectives achieved, with group progress monitored by attendance frequency and attrition rate. The evaluation of a weight loss program is much more meaningful, for example, if the number of original participants is reported as well as those who were successful and remained with the program.

## ❖ CLINICAL APPLICATION

The following case study demonstrates the application of health promotion strategies and benefits:

Sam Jones is a 56-year-old man with hypertension that is now regulated with diet changes and medication. On assessment during a follow-up visit, Mr. Jones indicates that he is feeling overwhelmed with occasional headaches and feelings of anxiety. He is unable to determine any specific stressors.

Assuming for this case only that these symptoms are not related to his medication, an intervention is planned with Mr. Jones to lower his stress response through relaxation and exercise. Mr. Jones is taught to use deep breathing and imagery to relax during a 10-minute break in the middle of the afternoon. An exercise plan is developed with small progressive steps. A contingency contract is mutually established between Mr. Jones and the nurse specifying the daily relaxation and progressive exercise,

weekly follow-up, and an appropriate reward. Mr. Jones' primary objectives relate to lower anxiety and feeling better about himself. Potential benefits for Mr. Jones include feeling better, lower anxiety, lower blood pressure, improved self-esteem, and improved cardiovascular efficiency and muscle strength. Achievement of the terms of the contract and these benefits can be used to evaluate the intervention. Cost efficiency of the intervention can be estimated by determining the cost of the visits to Mr. Jones or by specifying the value of nurse's time, room space, and any materials used. Dividing the costs per benefit achieved is one way to deal with values that are difficult to quantify. Demonstrating the cost efficiency of the intervention is particularly helpful in evaluating the intervention to support replication with others and may be useful information for the party paying the bill (if appropriate). The benefits listed above are immediate and intermediate. Potential long-term benefits for Mr. Jones include a decreased need for medication, less illness, and improved quality of life.

## ❖ SUMMARY

This chapter discussed the theoretical aspects of health promotion. Health promotion consists of efforts or activities to sustain or improve well-being. Guidelines for the assessment and counseling for the areas of fitness, nutrition, and stress management were presented. The use of contracts and factors that motivate change were discussed. Implementation methods included educative, counseling, and health policy roles. Health promotion is appropriate for healthy as well as ill individuals. The political and economic dimensions of health promotion were discussed as well as the importance of evaluation.

## ❖ APPLYING KNOWLEDGE TO PRACTICE

1. Select a client for whom you recently provided care in the area of secondary prevention, tertiary prevention, or both. How could you incorporate aspects of health promotion in the care of this individual? Suggest ways that you might involve the family or others in implementation.

2. Determine the ideal body weight range of an individual using an anthropometric chart. Use the midpoint of the range to estimate the caloric needs of this individual. Adjust the caloric intake to assist in a 2 pound per week loss or gain as appropriate to move the individual into the ideal body weight range.

3. Design an effective exercise plan for an individual who has not been exercising regularly and wants to start. Select an endurance exercise and activities for each of the four exercise stages. Be sure to include plans to build the activity level and monitor the exercise tolerance. Include a list of appropriate clothing, shoes, and equipment. Evaluate your selection of endurance exercise according to the characteristics of effective exercise.

4. You have been asked to develop and provide a stress management program for a group in your community. Develop a plan which includes objectives, plans for evaluation, and cost estimations for the proposed program.

## REFERENCES

American College of Sports Medicine (1980). *Guidelines for graded exercise testing and exercise prescription.* 2nd ed. Philadelphia: Lea and Febiger.

American Heart Association (1979). *The exercise standards book.* New York: American Heart Association.

Ardell, D. B. (1986). The history and future of the wellness movement. *Wellness promotion strategies,* J. P. Opatz (ed.). Dubuque, IA: Kendall/Hunt.

Banta, D. H. & Luce, B. R. (1983). Assessing the cost effectiveness of prevention. *Journal of Community Health, 9*(2), 145–164.

Boehm, S. (1989). Patient contracting. *Annual Review of Nursing Research. 8,* 143–153.

Burton, B. T. & Foster, W. R. (1985). Health Implications of Obesity, Consensus Development Conference. *Journal of the American Dietetic Association. 85*(9), 1117–1121.

Dunn, H. L. (1959). High level wellness for man and society. *American Journal of Public Health. 49,* 788.

Dunn, H. L. (1971). *High level wellness.* Arlington, VA: Beatty.

Dunn, M. M. (1987). Guidelines for an effective personal fitness prescription. *Nurse Practitioner. 12*(9), 9–24.

Ernsberger, P. (1985). The death of dieting. *American Health: Fitness of Body and Mind,* 230–235.

Fehring, R. H. (1983). Effects of biofeedback aided relaxation on the psychological stress symptoms of college students. *Nursing Research. 32*(6), 362–366.

Goldberg, E. L. & Comstock, G. W. (1976). Life events and subsequent illness. *American Journal of Epidemiology 104*(2).

Goldberger, L. & Breznitz, S. (1982). *Handbook of stress research: Theoretical and clinical aspects.* New York: The Free Press.

Green, L. W. (1986). Evaluation model: A framework for the design of rigorous evaluation of efforts in health promotion. *American Journal of Health Promotion, 1*(1), 77–78.

Harris, G. T. (1986). Why do people exercise? *American Health. 85*(3), 44–47.

*Healthy People.* the Surgeon General's report on health promotion and disease prevention (1979). Washington, D.C., U.S. Department of Health, Education, and Welfare.

Joint Nutrition Monitoring Evaluation Committee (1986). *Nutrition Monitoring in the United States.* Bethesda:

U.S. Dept. of Health and Human Services. DHHS Pub. (PHS) 86, 1255.

Kirkendall, D. T. (1984). Exercise prescription for the healthy adult. *Primary Care. 11*(1). 22–31.

Leavell, H. R. & Clark, E. G. (1953). *Preventive Medicine,* Toronto: McGraw-Hill.

McGuire, W. J. (1984). Public communication as a strategy for inducing health promotion behavioral change. *Preventive Medicine, 13,* 299–319.

Metropolitan Life Insurance Co. (1959). New weight standards for men and women. *Statistical Bulletin.* Metropolitan Life Insurance Company.

Neuman, B. (1989). *The Neuman systems model* (2nd ed.). Norwalk, CT: Appleton & Lange.

Oberman, A. (1984). Healthy exercise. *The Western Journal of Medicine. 141*(6), 864–871.

Pender, N. H. (1987). *Health promotion in nursing practice.* (2nd ed.). Norwalk, CT: Appleton & Lange.

Pruitt, R. H. (1987). Economics of health promotion. *Nursing Economics.* 5(3), 118–123, 141.

Rogers, B. J., Eaton, E. K. & Bruin, J. (1981). Is health promotion cost effective? *Preventive Medicine. 10,* 324–339.

Semipoulos, A. P. & Van Itallie, T. B. (1984). Body weight, health, and longevity. *Annals of Internal Medicine. 100*(2), 185–195.

Shamansky, S. L. & Clausen, C. L. (1980). Levels of prevention: Examination of the concept. *Nursing Outlook, 28,* 104–108.

Strecher, V. J., DeVellis, B. M., Becker, M. H., Rosenstock, I. M. (1987). The role of self-efficacy in achieving health behavior change. *Health Education Quarterly. 13*(1), 73-92.

Stoyva, J. & Anderson, C. (1982). A coping-rest model of relaxation and stress management. In L. Goldberger & S. Breznitz (Eds.). *Handbook of stress: Theoretical and clinical aspects,* New York: The Free Press.

Tait, N. & Aisner, J. (1989). Nutritional concerns in cancer patients. *Seminars in Oncology Nursing. 5*(2), 58–62.

Tuck. M. L. (1988). Diabetes and hypertension. *Postgraduate Medicine.* 64 (Suppl. 3), 76–83, 90–92.

U. S. Department of Health and Human Services (1988). Health Promotion and Disease Prevention. *Vital and Health Statistics. 10*(16). DHHS. Pub. (PHS) 88–1591.

White, J. H. (1986). Behavioral intervention for the obese client. *Nurse Practitioner. 11*(1), 27–34.

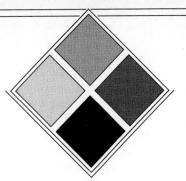

# 13

# Environmental Influences on Health

Lorraine M. Smith ◆ Joan L. Creasia
Barbara Parker

## OBJECTIVES

*At the completion of this chapter, the reader will be able to:*

◆ Identify major environmental health hazards.

◆ Describe the potential health effects of various forms of environmental pollution.

◆ Identify environmental issues of concern at the international, national, and local levels.

◆ Describe the various roles of the nurse in enhancing environmental health and the health of client systems.

We live in a world that is becoming increasingly at risk for environmental disaster. Individuals, community groups, and government officials are now recognizing and documenting environmental abuse. How does environmental abuse affect the health of the world population? As health professionals, we know that health and survival are contingent, in large part, on the integrity of the environment in which people and other forms of life coexist. Today, life is being threatened by a wide range of abuses against basic environmental elements such as air, land, and water. Will these abuses ultimately lead to the destruction of our entire planet? This question has been a major issue for over two decades as levels of air and water pollution continue to soar, land is destroyed, and the population continues to increase. Nadakavukaren predicts that if present trends continue, the "world in 2000 will be more crowded, more

polluted, less stable ecologically, and more vulnerable to disruption than the world we live in now" (1990, pp. 4-5).

Concerns about the relationship between human beings and the environment are not recent phenomena. In Biblical times, the Israelites observed strict laws regarding food preparation and waste disposal. In the Middle Ages, communities reacted to plagues and infectious diseases by quarantining people with signs of disease, isolating community newcomers, and fleeing populated cities during epidemics. Florence Nightingale's writings reflect her awareness of the impact of the environment and the need for sanitation and ventilation.

Whose responsibility is it to attain and maintain a healthy environment? Certainly the complexity of environmental issues requires that solutions come from both public and private sectors at international, national, state, and

225

local levels. However, health professionals have an opportunity and, indeed, a responsibility to address environmental issues that influence the health of client systems. As noted by Gordon (1990) "It is no longer a question of *whether* our environment will be managed, but rather *how* and *by whom*." This chapter focuses on the relationship between health and the environment, with special emphasis on specific environmental hazards that have the potential to adversely affect health. Nursing responsibilities in the areas of assessment, intervention, education, and advocacy are identified.

## ❖ HEALTH AND THE ENVIRONMENT

To establish a common frame of reference, it is important to define key terms related to health and the environment. The World Health Organization (1971) defines health as a state of complete physical, mental, and social well-being and not merely the absence of disease or infirmity. Health status may be either enhanced or impaired by the environment, which Neuman (1989) describes as factors affecting and affected by a client system, including both internal and external forces. Balance and harmony within the individual is the result of successful integration of the body, mind, and spirit combined with a compatible relationship with the environment. The health of the individual as an integrated system within the context of the environment is termed *holistic health*. It follows, then, that the health of individuals is influenced by the condition or health of the environment.

*Environmental health* refers to the state of all substances, forces, and conditions in an individual's surroundings that may exert an influence on health and well-being (Purdom, 1980). When environmental conditions are favorable, health status is enhanced. However, adverse biological, chemical, physical, and sociological forces in the environment, separately or in combination, may disrupt a healthy life-style and impede a person's ability to cope with environmental stimuli.

*Ecology*, the study of living organisms in interaction with the environment, takes into account the effects and influences of a dynamic environment. Broadly conceptualized, ecology is concerned with interrelationships between living and nonliving things, neither of which can be viewed in isolation from the other. The relationship between individuals and the environment is a reciprocal one—that is, individuals affect the environment and the environment affects individuals. The ecological perspective provides a framework for assessing environmental influences on health, the scope of which is reflected in Commoner's (1971) informal laws of ecology:

1. Everything is connected to everything else (i.e., sunlight, oxygen, carbon dioxide, organic compounds, and all organisms are interrelated).
2. Everything must go somewhere (i.e., one organism's waste is another organism's food).
3. Nature knows best (i.e., human interference with nature may be detrimental to its integrity).
4. There is no free lunch (i.e., everything removed from the environment must be replaced).

Commoner's laws describe the interrelationship between living things and the environment in maintaining ecological balance and supporting the need to assess environmental and human health from an ecological perspective. The health status of both humans and the environmment is determined, in large part, by the extent to which these laws are followed or violated.

## ❖ ECOLOGICAL BALANCE

Within the biosphere or world of living things, there are numerous *ecosystems*, each composed of living and nonliving subsystems that support a "circle of life." Four categories of components supply the conditions necessary to support the plant and animal life of an ecosystem:

1. Sunlight, water, oxygen, carbon dioxide, organic compounds, and other nutrients to support plant growth.
2. Plants that produce carbohydrates from carbon dioxide and water through the process of photosynthesis.
3. Consumers of plants and plant products (i.e., humans and animals).
4. Decomposed and other organisms such as fungi and bacteria (Stanhope & Lancaster, 1988).

Often overlooked is the fact that multiple interactions between living and nonliving things are required to maintain a stable environment. A change in one part of the ecosystem necessarily produces a change in another part of the system, and organisms must constantly adapt to stressors or disturbances in the ecosystem to survive. Adaptation is usually not an immediate process, requiring time to respond and adjust to emerging events. Since the interrelationships between parts of the ecosystem are dynamic, there is a constant interchange of demands to adapt.

When studying environmental influences on health, it is important to keep in mind that people are an integral part of the ecosystem composed of the atmosphere, water, soil, plants, and animals that ideally function in harmony to keep the system viable. An individual's attitudes, values, and perceptions about the environment can influence behavior and in part determine the extent to which the ecosystem remains in a state of equilibrium. Threats to the ecosystem may occur naturally or be artificially induced environmental hazards such as those described in the following section.

## ❖ ENVIRONMENTAL HEALTH HAZARDS

Environmental hazards fall into four general categories: biological, chemical, physical, and psychosocial. These hazards will be briefly discussed.

### Biological Hazards

Disease-producing infectious agents in the environment that are capable of entering the human body, such as viruses, bacteria, or other microorganisms, are environmental hazards of a biological nature. Some infectious agents are transmitted by direct or close contact with an infected person, while others are transmitted through contaminated water used for drinking or food preparation. Still others are transmitted by vectors (e.g., rodents and arthropods such as flies, mosquitoes, fleas, ticks, mites, and cockroaches) to other animals or people. As ecological balance is disturbed, human health is threatened by the emergence of new pathogens (e.g., human immunodeficiency virus) as well as mutagenic (e.g., influenza virus) and resistant (e.g., gonococcus) strains of known pathogens.

The use of disinfectant agents and sterilizing methods can prevent many infections. Additionally, control of some vectors can be accomplished through environmental manipulation and regulation to prevent propagation. Good sanitation is also a major concern, and programs must be designed to provide conditions that safeguard the health of individuals, families, and communities. These include a safe and adequate water supply, effective sewage systems, proper waste disposal, and readily available handwashing facilities.

### Chemical Hazards

By far the largest category of environmental hazards is chemical hazards. These include toxic agents such as polychlorinated biphenyls

(PCBs), dioxin (TCDD), asbestos, lead and pesticides such as insecticides (inorganic botanicals, chlorinated hydrocarbons, DDT, kepone, chlordane) herbicides, and rodenticides. Among the major sources of chemical hazards present in our environment are industrial wastes, the use of pesticides in agriculture, and emissions from motor vehicles. Because of modern technology, the number of chemical hazards continues to rise at an alarming rate. Many chemicals being produced are known to be highly toxic, and adverse short-term and long-term effects have been documented. With many other chemicals, however, the relative toxicity is unknown. Human reaction to various chemicals depends on the toxicity and concentration of the chemical, duration of exposure, and susceptibility of the individual. The effect may also be related to body weight and the form (solid, liquid, or gas) of the chemical at the time of exposure.

People are often unaware that they are being exposed to toxic chemicals, but their potential presence may produce adverse physiological and psychological effects (Vyner, 1988). For example, radon, an odorless, colorless gas, can seep into buildings and contaminate indoor air. As it decays, it forms radioactive products, which attach to dust particles and are inhaled, placing individuals at risk for lung cancer. Radon is a naturally occurring chemical that is a product of normal decay of radioactive materials in the soil that are released and normally dispersed in very low concentrations. The recent phenomenon of weatherizing homes and offices for energy efficiency, however, reduces airflow and causes accumulation of radon within modern buildings. The full extent of the radon problem is unknown, but people are generally concerned about their personal risk and the risk to their families. Radon exposure has been identified as a serious problem in the Western United States where homes were built from materials contaminated with waste from uranium mines. More recently, high radon levels have been found in Pennsylvania and New

Jersey as a result of natural conditions in the soil (Edwards & Dees, 1990).

Many liquid chemicals, such as polychlorinated biphenyls (PCB) or dioxin (TCDD), seep into water supplies and contaminate natural waterways and lakes, thus posing hidden threats to health by contaminating drinking water and fish supplies. Results of experimental studies with animals indicate that these chemicals cause severe chronic health problems, thus posing a serious threat to human health (Nadakavukaren, 1990).

## Physical Hazards

Natural disasters such as hurricanes, earthquakes, and volcanoes, and accidents, noise, heat, vibration, radiation, insects, rodents, and certain types of equipment fall into the category of physical hazards. While natural disasters are difficult, if not impossible to control, other physical hazards can be successfully controlled or eliminated. Laws mandating the use of seat belts and airbags, product design which promotes safety, and animal control are some of the ways to address physical environmental hazards.

Depending on the type of industry, physical hazards may be abundantly present in the workplace. Much national attention has been given to providing a safe work environment by enacting legislation to protect workers from adverse environmental conditions. As the result of the *Occupational Safety and Health Act* of 1970 (PL 91-596), the National Institute for Occupational Safety and Health (NIOSH), and the Occupational Safety and Health Administration (OSHA) were created. OSHA's purpose and policy is to ensure as far as possible safe and healthful working conditions for every working man and woman in the nation, thus preserving our human resources (Green & Anderson, 1986).

However, continuous exposure to physical hazards occurs in certain types of work environments. These conditions should be carefully monitored and corrected before irreversible health problems develop. For example, air temperature and humidity may be adversely affected in industries that use blast furnaces, kilns, and laundry equipment, contributing to health problems such as respiratory disorders, dermatitis, gastrointestinal disturbances, and eye inflammation. In addition, an individual's metabolic rate, oxygen consumption, respiration, heart rate, and blood pressure are influenced by temperature. Ventilation systems should be designed to provide physical comfort and safety by controlling the temperature, humidity, and movement of air.

## Sociological and Psychological Hazards

Psychosocial health hazards are not as well delineated as biological, chemical, and physical factors. However, it is recognized that the environment does influence mental health and when conditions are unfavorable, psychological or physiological distress is experienced. Many of the stressors mentioned elsewhere in this book such as violence, stress, and substance abuse and dependence are known threats to the health of individuals, families, and communities. Additionally, feelings of well-being may be altered by factors such as high levels of noise, overcrowding or isolation, lack of adequate resources or opportunities for economic advancement, and rapid societal changes such as those that occur with the increased use of technology. Psychological stress may also be related to biological, physical, or chemical environmental hazards if the individual feels powerless to eliminate the hazard when interacting with a resistant company, industry, or governmental agency.

In the area of environmental health hazards, nursing responsibilities include identifying at-risk individuals and groups and associated environmental conditions that have the potential to exert unfavorable influences on health. Interventions may then be directed toward individuals, aggregates, communities, or political groups as the situation warrants and can be in the form of prevention or treatment modalities, educational programs, or lobbying for a safe environment. For example, occupational health nurses are in the forefront of primary prevention and "must observe (1) how people work, (2) with what they work, and (3) what happens next" (Solomon, 1984, p. 265). Appropriate interventions can then be designed.

## ❖ ENVIRONMENTAL INFLUENCES ON HEALTH

Environmental hazards previously discussed greatly influence the health of client systems. However, there are specific environmental influences on health which, because of their potentially serious nature, warrant further discussion. Since it is not within the scope of this chapter to present a comprehensive review of all major environmental hazards, selected environmental influences on health of paramount concern to health professionals are examined.

### Toxic Agents

With advances in science and technology, many environmental and other types of health hazards have been eliminated. As the ecological perspective suggests, however, solving one problem often produces unintended effects, thereby creating new problems. Toxic agents are present in our environment in ever-increasing numbers, and their effects can be life-threatening as the following discussion illustrates.

**Asbestos.** A chemical hazard when in the form of a dust, asbestos has been used extensively worldwide in building materials and other commercial products. Over the years, asbestos has been linked to diseases such as lung and gastrointestinal cancer and mesothelioma (a rare form of cancer of the membranes surrounding the lungs and the stomach lining). Previously, health concerns focused primarily on construction workers, but there is now evidence that the general public who work in commercial or residential buildings containing friable (crumbles when dried) asbestos is at risk for lung cancer. In addition, asbestos fibers from the workplace may be picked up and carried home on clothing, thus also exposing family members. To protect school-aged children, the *Asbestos Hazard Emergency Responses Act (AHERA)* was enacted. This law requires that all elementary and secondary schools be inspected to determine whether asbestos is present and if so, the school must initiate an abatement program. Nurses, especially school nurses, can be actively involved by being aware of the status of abatement programs and advocating early asbestos removal.

**Lead.** Metal toxicity is one of the lesser publicized environmental hazards. Exposure to small quantities of some metals such as zinc, cadmium, or copper seems to be relatively harmless. However, exposure to larger amounts of heavy metals can have detrimental effects, with lead being a major concern since "it is produced in larger quantities than any other toxic heavy metal ... and is found throughout the worldwide environment" (Nadakavukaren, 1990, p. 194). Sources of lead include old paint, emissions from automobiles that burn leaded gasoline, and solder used on pipes to carry drinking water. Lead biologically interferes with blood formation, often resulting in anemia. It can also cause kidney damage, birth defects, injury to the central nervous system, poor memory, hearing loss, hypertension, mental retardation, convulsions, coma, and death (Healthy People 2000, 1990). In 1971, The Lead Prevention Act was passed, which allocated funds to establish lead screening facilities and to remove old lead paint from buildings. It also banned the use of lead as a paint additive.

The U.S. government is taking the initiative to inform the public about lead exposure and its effects, with The Year 2000 Health Objectives providing direction to target special populations at risk. As noted in this document "Childhood lead poisoning is totally preventable" (Healthy People 2000, p. 317, 1990).

The treatment of lead poisoning involves a three-step plan, which consists of reducing lead in the body through the use of chelating agents, minimizing the sources of lead intake, and improving nutritional status to lessen the vulnerability to lead poisoning (Bullough & Bullough, 1990). Nurses in the community should encourage parents to have their children's blood lead levels measured, assist them with a treatment program if needed, and provide educational programs for community organizations about the sources of lead and risks of lead poisoning.

**Pesticides.** Pesticides such as insecticides, herbicides, fungicides, and rodenticides are used worldwide and result in contamination of the biosphere with pesticide residues, especially those of the chlorinated hydrocarbons (e.g., DDT, kepone, chlordane). These residues are contact poisons and tend to accumulate in fatty tissues in living organisms and remain in the body indefinitely (Nadakavukaren, 1990). Pesticide residues are found throughout the world in all types of animals, fish, and birds and pose a major threat to health. Farm workers are particularly at risk for developing pesticide poisoning due to accidental spraying with pesticides while they are working in the fields. An alternative to chemical pest control is integrated pest management (IPM). This type of management uses various methods such as food deprivation, predators, and other natural controls that are believed to be safer and more ecologically sound than using pesticides.

By conducting a thorough assessment, the nurse can gain an awareness of the extent to which chemical pesticides are in use in the client's home and community. If it is determined that pesticides are used, nursing interventions include teaching about the dangers of pesticides, directions for proper use, signs and symptoms of toxicity, and emergency treatment of pesticide poisoning. As a preventive measure, the nurse must emphasize the importance of keeping pesticides and insect traps out of the reach of children.

## Air Pollution

An environmental hazard of great magnitude, air pollution is an international problem that affects human health, property, animals, and plants. The major sources of air pollution are the products of fossil fuel combustion and motor vehicle emissions. Air pollutants are also generated by volcanic eruptions, forest fires, dust storms, and industrial waste. "At present, in the U.S., the sources of air pollution in order of importance are: transportation, primarily automobiles and trucks; electric power plants which burn coal or oil; industry, the major offenders being steel mills, metal smelters, oil refineries, pulp and paper mills" (Nadakavukaren, 1990, p. 324). The major air pollutants are total suspended particulates (TSP), sulfur dioxide ($SO_2$), carbon monoxide (CO), nitrogen dioxide ($NO_2$), ozone ($O_3$), hydrocarbons (HC) and lead (Pb). These pollutants and their effects are presented in Table 13-1.

The effects of air pollution on the health of individuals depends on the chemical properties of the pollutant and the size of the particle, which in turn affects the site of deposition in the respiratory tract. Adverse health effects from air pollution may range from mild to severe. For example, mild irritation of the respiratory tract can occur when larger particles are entrapped in the upper respiratory tree. On the other hand, severe respiratory problems or even asphyxiation may occur as a result of direct absorption of a pollutant, such as carbon monoxide, from the alveoli into the blood. The risk of developing cancer or a chronic pulmonary disease increases with prolonged exposure to air pollutants.

One solution for decreasing local pollution caused by industrial emissions has been to increase the height of smoke stacks to carry industrial wastes higher into the atmosphere. Unfortunately, solving one problem often leads to creating a new one. The dispersion of particles in the upper atmosphere, when combined with oxygen in the presence of atmospheric moisture, produces sulfuric and nitric acids that fall as acid rain, contaminating soil and rivers. By eating fish or produce contaminated with acid rain, pollutants are ingested through the gastrointestinal tract and may exert a systemic effect on target organs.

Since the problem of air pollution is such a universal one, it is necessary to address it on a number of levels. On the national level, several positive steps have been taken to improve air quality including the enactment of the *Clean Air Act* of 1963, the *Air Quality Act* of 1967, and the *Clean Air Act* of 1970 amended in 1977, which established standards for national air quality. Significant support was demonstrated in the legislative arena to pass a new clean air act in 1990, although, as in the past, some opposition came from various business and political groups. On the international level, another positive step toward improving air quality is collaboration by the federal government with other countries to solve the problems related to air pollution.

Nurses and other health professionals can be involved in informing clients about various pollutants and their influences on health and assessing respiratory function. Assisting clients with proper ventilation of their homes or helping them eliminate certain pollutants in the environment are interventions aimed at alleviating the potentially toxic effects of air pollution. In addition to working with family systems, educational programs can be developed for schools and other community groups to in-

❖ **Table 13-1**
Major air pollutants and their sources and effects

| Pollutant | Form | Major source | Effects |
|---|---|---|---|
| Total suspended particulates (TSP) | Solid or liquid | Combustion, industrial processes | ◆ Acts synergistically with $SO_2$ as respiratory irritant<br>◆ Grime deposits<br>◆ Obscures visibility<br>◆ Corrodes metals |
| Sulfur dioxide ($SO_2$) | Gas | Coal-burning power plants, metal smelters, industrial boilers, oil refineries | ◆ Respiratory irritant<br>◆ Corrodes metal and stone<br>◆ Damages textiles<br>◆ Toxic to plants<br>◆ Precursor of acid rain |
| Carbon monoxide (CO) | Gas | Motor vehicles | ◆ Aggravates cardiovascular disease<br>◆ Impairs perception and mental processes<br>◆ Fatal at high concentrations |
| Nitrogen dioxide ($NO_2$) | Gas | Motor vehicles<br>Power plants | ◆ Respiratory irritant<br>◆ Toxic to plants<br>◆ Reduces visibility<br>◆ Precursor of ozone<br>◆ Precursor of acid rain |
| Ozone ($O_3$) | Gas | Motor vehicles (indirectly) | ◆ Respiratory irritant<br>◆ Toxic to plants<br>◆ Corrodes rubber, paint |
| Hydrocarbons (HC) | Gas | Motor vehicles, evaporation from gas stations, etc. | ◆ Precursor to $O_3$<br>◆ Some types are carcinogens |
| Lead (Pb) | Metal aerosol | Motor vehicles | ◆ Damage to nervous system, blood, kidneys |

From *Man and environment: A health perspective* by Nadakavukaren, A., ed 3, 1990, Prospect Heights, Ill. Waveland Press, Inc. Reprinted with permission, p. 327.

crease awareness about the dangers of air pollution and to propose measures to improve air quality.

## Water Pollution

Population growth and industrial output have created a decline in the quality of water in the world's waterways, lakes, and ground water. In general, underground water supplies are thought to be less subject to contamination than surface sources since they are protected from runoff, which often carries contaminants from pesticides or industrial wastes. However, contamination of underground wells and springs can occur if a hazardous waste dump is located nearby or if the underground water source is close enough to the surface so that contaminants can seep in.

In Third World countries, the most pressing health problems related to water quality involve contamination of waterways with the microbial pathogen found in human body wastes, a problem directly related to lack of or faulty sewage disposal facilities (Nadakavukaren, 1990). While this is usually not a problem in industrialized countries, outbreaks of gastroenteritis caused by pathogenic contamination of drinking water do occasionally occur. A recent example of this problem in the United States is Mexico's sewage infiltrating the water near San Diego.

Swimming facilities, such as swimming pools, wading pools, spas and hot tubs, and natural bathing areas like lakes, rivers, and ponds are sometimes dangerously polluted and provide a medium for vectors to flourish (Green & Anderson, 1986). There is increased attention paid to pollution of natural waterways and, as a result, national, state, and local governments, as well as private and professional sectors, are merging resources to "clean up" the lakes, rivers, and ponds.

There is concern about the presence of organic and inorganic chemicals in municipal water systems because some are toxic, carcinogenic, or mutagenic. But there is not conclusive evidence to determine whether many of these chemicals present long-range threats to health. While most contaminants can be removed by current water treatment processes, nitrites and inorganic phosphates are not effectively removed. Adverse health effects due to these chemicals are thought to be minimal at present, but action is being taken to monitor the level of the chemicals and determine their long-range effects. Contaminants that pose major problems for water sources include fertilizers, pesticides, detergents, radioactive wastes, heavy metals, and salts.

To attain and maintain high quality water supplies, it is critical for communities to plan and build effective water treatment systems, design adequate and more efficient sewage treatment processes (i.e., sludge disposal), and develop alternative technologies for flood and pollution control and construction of wetlands. Legislation such as the *Water Pollution Control Act* of 1965, *Clean Water Restoration Act* of 1966, the *Clean Water Act* of 1972, and the *Safe Drinking Water Act* of 1974, which give the Environmental Protection Agency (EPA) authority to set water standards and to ensure that these standards are upheld, provide the direction for improving the quality of water in the United States. A shortcoming of the latter legislation, however, is that smaller water sources are not monitored by water quality agencies, placing people who live in rural areas, for example, at risk for health problems associated with water contamination.

Nursing measures include assessment of the immediate environment for possible sources of water contamination, examining samples of drinking water for the existence of particles, a strange odor or color, and identifying public health agencies who will test water samples if there is any question about water purity. The nurse can also provide instructions to clients about preventive measures such as boiling water for at least 10 minutes before drinking or cooking, or purchasing bottled spring water for these purposes. If there is evidence of a community-wide problem such as a high incidence of a particular disease or death, further collaboration with other health professionals may be necessary to identify causes and possible solutions. This valuable information can then be turned over to environmental health officials whose responsibility it is to maintain environmental standards.

## Noise Pollution

Noise pollution can be defined as any unwanted or undesirable sound in the environment. Its effects can range from mildly annoying to psychologically and physically debilitating.

The extent to which noise becomes a serious environmental health hazard depends on the level, frequency, and length of exposure as well as the receiver's subjective interpretation of the noise. Some of the negative health consequences of noise pollution include psychological or physical disturbances, such as interference with normal activity and hearing loss.

Noise pollution in the immediate environment may be a result of sounds from airplanes, automobiles, trucks, motorcycles, home appliances, motorized yard equipment, or construction activities. The most severe health problem resulting from noise pollution is temporary or permanent hearing loss. The danger level for hearing loss is thought to be 80 decibels (dB), although the maximum level allowed in the workplace is 90 dB. Loud or continuous noise not only affects hearing but can also affect an individual's psychological and physical health because it disrupts communication, sleep, leisure, and work activities. There is also evidence that noise affects children's language development and ability to read. "High noise levels interfere with the capacity to distinguish certain sounds such as b and v, for example, and can foster a tendency to drop the endings of words, thereby distorting speech" (Nadakavukaren, 1990, p. 384).

Some actions have been taken to reduce noise pollution in the workplace through regulations and standards established by OSHA. Since the *Noise Control Act* of 1972 failed to reduce noise levels in communities, Congress passed a set of amendments called the *Quiet Communities Act* in 1978. This act authorizes the EPA to collaborate with state and local governments in developing programs to reduce noise pollution in their communities.

Nurses working with families can assist them in assessing noise levels within their homes by identifying sources of loud noise such as that from refrigerators, fans, food disposals, lawn mowers, and other devices, and taking measures to reduce or muffle the sound. Families living near an airport or busy highway are at an additional risk for the adverse effects of noise pollution, and the need for sound barriers or other solutions must be communicated to local officials. Once problem areas are identified, nurses can offer suggestions to help families reduce noise levels such as those presented in Fig. 13-1.

## Accidents

Unintentional injuries kill more than 100,000 people each year and incapacitate millions of others, with many incurring lifelong disabilities. Of these, approximately 46,000 deaths are motor vehicle-related as are 3.5 million injuries (Healthy People 2000, 1990). Falls, drownings, and fires are other major causes of unintentional injury.

The physical design of some equipment such as machinery and automobiles can increase the probability of accidents, as can the design of highways, homes, and recreational facilities. It should be noted that "alcohol use is intimately associated with the causes and severity of many unintentional injuries" (Healthy People 2000, 1990, p. 270). Efforts to reduce accident rates must be combined with efforts to reduce drug and alcohol abuse. Providing safety education that emphasizes proper use of equipment, monitoring equipment design, and supervising people who work with high-risk equipment are additional ways to promote safety and prevent accidents. Education programs for school-aged children are recommended to provide safety information aimed at reducing unintentional injuries associated with fires, falls, and motor vehicles.

## Solid and Hazardous Wastes

Wastes are being generated at an alarming rate. The amount of solid waste continues to soar, partly as a result of today's "throwaway" attitude where many products are used once and then discarded. Multiple packaging also creates more waste. "It is estimated that U.S.

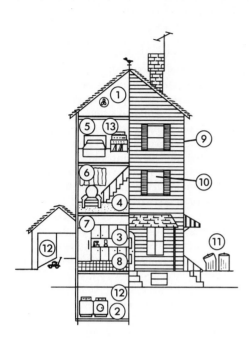

## Inside

1. Install exhaust fan on rubber mounts.
2. Use vibration mounts under electrical appliances like washer, dryer, and dishwasher.
3. Put foam pads under blenders, mixers, and other small appliances (also your typewriter!)
4. Use wall to wall and stair carpeting with felt or rubber padding to dampen noise.
5. Use acoustical tile, spaced below ceiling.
6. Install drapes to absorb sound.
7. Buy quiet appliances.
8. Install floor vinyl or thick linoleum to dampen sound.

## Outside

9. Eliminate noise leaks in walls by sealing holes or cracks.
10. Caulk windows and install storm windows to cut down outside noise.
11. Replace metal garbage cans with plastic ones.

## Protecting your ears

12. Wear ear protectors when you are using very noisy equipment or tools.
13. Keep the stereo volume down.

❖ **Fig. 13-1**    What you can do to quiet your home and yourself from noise. *From the National Bureau of Standards Handbook 119, "Quieting—a practical guide to noise control," 1976.*

cities today collect and dispose of somewhere between 150-180 million tons of wastes annually, representing an average of about 4 pounds of refuse per person per day" (Nadakavukaren, 1990, p. 450). Where to dispose of this waste is a serious problem facing many communities and efforts are being made to recycle reusable materials.

In addition to solid wastes, the disposal of hazardous waste is a critical issue facing the federal government. *Hazardous waste* is defined as any discarded material that may pose a threat to human health or the environment when improperly handled. The EPA has established a two-tiered system for determining whether a specific waste is subject to regulation under current hazardous waste management laws. There are approximately 400 wastes listed

in the federal code. Any waste exhibiting the following characteristics is subject to regulation: toxic, ignitable, corrosive, and reactive. There are two additional categories of wastes (radioactive and infectious) from hospitals and clinics exempt from the above regulations. Instead, they are regulated under the Nuclear Regulatory Commission under the *Atomic Energy Act* and biomedical waste disposal laws that vary from state to state.

Chemical and allied product industries generate most of the hazardous wastes, followed by metal-related, petroleum, and coal product industries. Federal legislation to regulate hazardous waste has been enacted. The *Resource Conservation and Recovery Act* (1976) mandated that the EPA be responsible for monitoring hazardous wastes from the place they are generated to the disposal site. The enactment of the 1980 *Comprehensive Environmental Response, Compensation and Liability Act* (CERCLA) led to the development of a National Priorities List of waste sites (Healthy People 2000, 1990) and the establishment of a "superfund" to provide emergency cleanup of these sites. Nursing actions include assessing hazardous waste disposal practices of clients, if applicable, and being actively involved on the community level to identify any practices that pose a threat to health and well-being. Nurses can also lobby for regulatory legislation.

### ❖ EMERGING ENVIRONMENTAL ISSUES

Many major environmental concerns from the past, such as infectious biological contamination of drinking water, have been eliminated in industrialized countries. At the same time, however, improved technology and scientific advances have created new and more complex hazards. For example, while the spread of infectious diseases through drinking water and hospital wastes has been controlled, chemicals used to accomplish this goal have introduced unintended and unknown effects on the environment. Thus, nurses must not only be aware of health problems within the environment but also the problems resulting from attempted solutions.

As mentioned earlier, environmental issues are complex, and solutions must come from both public and private sectors. Because of the universality of many environmental problems, involvement must occur at the international, national, and local levels.

### International Perspectives

*World Resources 1988-1989* (Paden and staff, 1988) analyzes conditions and trends in the world's natural resources, including global systems, economic policies, and natural resource management. Seven major environmental changes, which will directly or indirectly affect health have been identified:

1. POPULATION: There will be little change in population growth rates by the year 2000. The estimated world population by the end of the century will be 6.3 billion. This means about 100 million people will be added each year. Ninety percent of this growth will occur in the poorest countries.
2. FOOD PRODUCTION: Worldwide, food production is projected to increase by 90% between 1970 and 2000. However, the largest increase of food will occur in the richer countries and the countries of the Middle East. Africa and Southern Asia will continue to have inadequate amounts of food for their people.
3. NATURAL RESOURCES: Nonfuel resources appear sufficient to meet demands through the year 2000, but discoveries and investments will be needed to maintain reserves.
4. WATER: Shortages will become more severe; overpumping of ground water, poor land use practices that increase runoff, and pollution of existing water supplies will reduce the availability of water at a time of rising need.
5. FORESTS: Loss of forests will continue over the next 20 years. Most of the losses will occur in the forests of Asia, Africa, and South America.
6. WILDLIFE: Rates of extinction will increase sharply, resulting in loss of hundreds of thousands of species, especially in the tropical forest regions.
7. POLLUTION: "Increased emissions of carbon dioxide and chlorofluorocarbons in the atmosphere are threatening to alter the world's climate and upper atmosphere significantly by 2050. Acid rain from the burning of fossil fuels is affecting increasingly wider areas with damage to lakes, soil, and crops. Toxic and radioactive wastes continue to be spewn into the air, dumped into waterways, or carelessly buried, presenting health and safety problems in a growing number of countries" (Nadakavukaren, 1990, p. 5).

The trends indicate that the scope of most environmental problems such as air and water contamination do not respect national boundaries. In addition, the trends demonstrate the widening disparity between the health status of developed and developing countries. Maternal mortality and child mortality are much higher in developing countries, and the prevalence of low birth weight infants and children suffering from malnutrition speaks to a tragic ongoing international problem (Paden and staff, 1988). Many health problems in developing nations are directly or indirectly related to poverty. "The poorest countries average less than $5 per capita for annual health expenditures compared to an average of $400 per person in the developed countries of the world" (Shannon, 1990, p. 909). Additional international concerns are those that affect the planet as a whole, regardless of the level of industrial development of the country. Consider, for example, global warming and acid rain.

**Global warming.** As a result of increased burning of fossil fuels, deforestation, and the production of certain synthetic chemicals, there is a dramatic increase in heat-trapping gases in the atmosphere (Begley, 1990). Carbon dioxide ($CO_2$) is the major offender, allowing energy from the sun to pass through, while absorbing radiation from the earth and creating a planetary hothouse.

Data collected from the United States National Aeronautics and Space Administration (NASA) and other sources indicate that there are definite warming trends in global temperature recordings consistent with the greenhouse effect, with the four warmest years on record occurring in the 1980s. NASA has reported that the atmospheric ozone layer, which protects life from harmful ultraviolet radiation, has begun to thin globally. As ozone diminishes in the upper atmosphere, the earth receives more ultraviolet radiation, which promotes skin cancers and cataracts and depresses

the human immune system. Also associated with these warmer temperatures are heat waves, drought, reduced crop yields, depleted marine fisheries, and increased smog. The United Nations is mobilizing an intense international effort to reduce greenhouse producing emissions, a move that is being resisted by a number of industrialized nations (Nitze, 1990). The problem of global warming will affect the health of every person in the world (Brown, 1990) and has profound implications for nursing in the future.

**Acid rain.** Acid rain is caused by emissions of sulfur dioxide and nitrogen oxides. Nitrogen oxides, formed when fuel is burned at high temperatures, come principally from motor vehicle exhaust, electric utilities, and industrial boilers that burn coal or oil. Once released into the atmosphere, these compounds can be carried long distances by prevailing winds until they return to the earth as acidic rain, snow, fog, or dust. Fish and wildlife suffer harm, lakes are contaminated, buildings and statues deteriorate, and people experience health problems such as respiratory impairment.

At the governmental level, countries must work together to prevent global environmental disaster. Since 1972, when the United Nations General Assembly created the U.N. Environmental Program with a mission to safeguard and enhance the environment, collaboration on an international level has continued. During the 1970s, the United Nations convened conferences on environmental topics such as population, food, human settlements, water, and new and renewable sources of energy. Currently, cooperative efforts by the United States with Canada and Mexico to improve environmental conditions along the borders are underway.

The World Health Organization (WHO) has specific responsibilities for international health: to act as the directing and coordinating authority on world health and develop, establish, and promote international standards for food, biological, pharmaceutical, and similar products (Green & Anderson, 1986). When an international, natural, or man-made disaster occurs, WHO, as the authority organization, becomes involved directly or indirectly as an advisory system.

## National Perspectives

As a nation, the United States has identified potential environmental health hazards. The U.S. Surgeon General's Report *Healthy People* (Public Health Service, 1979) identified five areas of environmental health needing improve-

❖ **Table 13-2**
Environmental concerns of the American public and the EPA

| EPA's top 11 (not in rank order) | Public concerns (in rank order) |
|---|---|
| **ECOLOGICAL RISKS** | 1. Active hazardous waste sites (67%) |
| Global climate change | 2. Abandoned hazardous waste sites (65%) |
| Stratospheric ozone depletion | 3. Water pollution from industrial wastes (63%) |
| Habitat alteration | **4. Occupational exposure to toxic chemicals (63%)** |
| Species extinction and biodiversity loss | 5. Oil spills (60%) |
| | **6. Destruction of the ozone layer (60%)** |
| **HEALTH RISKS** | 7. Nuclear power plant accidents (60%) |
| Criteria air pollutants (e.g. smog) | 8. Industrial accidents releasing pollutants (58%) |
| Toxic air pollutants (e.g. benzene) | 9. Radiation from radioactive wastes (58%) |
| Radon | **10. Air pollution from factories (56%)** |
| Indoor air pollution | 11. Leaking underground storage tanks (55%) |
| Drinking water contamination | 12. Coastal water contamination (54%) |
| Occupational exposure to chemicals | 13. Solid waste and litter (53%) |
| Application of pesticides | **14. Pesticide risks to farm workers (52%)** |
| Stratospheric ozone depletion | 15. Water pollution from agricultural runoff (51%) |
| | 16. Water pollution from sewage plants (50%) |
| | **17. Air pollution from vehicles (50%)** |
| | 18. Pesticide residues in foods (49%) |
| | **19. Greenhouse effect (48%)** |
| | **20. Drinking water contamination (46%)** |
| | 21. Destruction of wetlands (42%) |
| Scientists and the public draw different conclusions about the seriousness of various environmental problems. Above: the worst environmental problems, as identified by EPA's Scientific Advisory Board. Right: the public's top concerns, as reflected in a March 1990 Roper Poll. (Figures in parentheses are the percentages that rated each problem "very serious"; boldfaced items also appear on EPA's list.) | 22. Acid rain (40%) |
| | 23. Water pollution from city runoff (35%) |
| | 24. Nonhazardous waste sites (31%) |
| | 25. Biotechnology (30%) |
| | 26. Indoor air pollution (22%) |
| | 27. Radiation from x-rays (21%) |
| | **28. Radon in homes (17%)** |
| | 29. Radiation from microwave ovens (13%) |

From Roberts, L. (1990). Counting on science at EPA. *Science, 249* (4969), p. 616.

ment to ensure health and quality of life: toxic agent control, occupational safety and health, accidental injury control, fluoridation of community water supplies, and infectious agent control. The *Nation's 1990 Objectives* were developed to address these concerns. Many hazards were identified in each of the five areas, along with recommendations for detection, control, and health protective measures. A midcourse review (Public Health Service, 1986) found that significant progress had been made in some areas (e.g., accidental injury control) while there was little improvement in others (e.g., toxic agent control).

*The Year 2000 Objectives* were developed following a series of hearings around the country and meetings with professionals from a number of disciplines, including nursing. The objectives focus on improving environmental health in the areas of "childhood lead poisoning, ozone and respiratory disease, recently recognized hazards like radon, the need to develop ongoing mechanisms for exposure and disease surveillance, and environmental hazards in the home environment" (e.g., lead and radon) (Public Health Service, 1989, 8-1). The objectives are listed according to the focus on health status, risk reduction, services, protection, and personnel surveillance and data needs. These objectives are being directed toward special populations who are more vulnerable or at risk than other population groups.

To gain some sense of the opinions of the general public regarding environmental concerns, a public opinion poll was conducted in 1990. Concerns identified in this poll are ranked and listed in Table 13-2 along with the EPA's top 11 environmental concerns. Although the EPA's concerns are more global in nature, several concerns common to both groups were identified.

Education at all levels, including legislators, policy makers, business leaders, professionals, and the general public is a critical component in attaining and maintaining a healthy environment. Nurses can increase their involvement in addressing environmental concerns by developing community educational programs on topics such as lead poisoning, household toxic substances, and the health effects of air and water pollution.

**The Environmental Protection Agency.** Legislation establishing regulations and policy occurs at the national level. The EPA is an independent agency formed to coordinate environmental programs related to air and water pollution, solid and hazardous waste management, noise, public water supplies, pesticides, and radiation. The agency also administers the municipal sewage treatment construction grant program authorized by Congress in the 1972 *Clean Water Act.*

The administrator of the EPA is appointed by the President. There are five assistant administrators for each major division within the Agency: (1) Office of Planning and Management, (2) Office of Enforcement, (3) Office of Air and Waste Management, (4) Office of Water and Hazardous Substances, and (5) Office of Research and Development. The EPA's functions are based on the following legislative acts:

1. AIR QUALITY CONTROL ACT, 1970, AMENDED: This act establishes national air quality standards and assists states in revising plans if they do not meet the standards.
2. WATER POLLUTION CONTROL ACT, AMENDMENTS, 1972: This act provides authority for restoring and maintaining the integrity of the country's natural waters.
3. MARINE PROTECTION RESEARCH & SANCTUARIES ACT, 1973: This act establishes a dumping permit program and sites for dumping in the oceans.
4. NOISE CONTROL ACT, AMENDED, 1978: This act establishes standards and regulations concerning major sources of noise.

5. SOLID WASTE DISPOSAL ACT, 1965: RESOURCE CONSERVATION AND RECOVERY ACT, 1976: These acts establish regulations and devise EPA programs to ensure safe disposal of wastes (i.e., toxic substances, pesticides, and explosives), and review states' existing waste disposal sites.

6. TOXIC SUBSTANCES CONTROL ACT, 1976: This act compels industry to develop adequate data on the effect of chemical substances on health and the environment, and to regulate and ban substances when necessary.

7. SURFACE MINING CONTROL AND RECLAMATION ACT, 1977: This act requires mining companies to restore the land, remove wastes, replace topsoil, and replant grass and trees.

8. COMPREHENSIVE ENVIRONMENTAL RESPONSE, COMPENSATION AND LIABILITY CONTROL ACT, 1980: This "superfund" legislation created a 1.6 billion dollar fund to be used for emergency cleanup of abandoned hazardous waste dumps.

Other environmental issues are delegated to several federal agencies and cabinet level departments. These agencies and departments are responsible for making national policies related to the environment. In addition to the EPA, governmental agencies include the Centers for Disease Control, Public Health Service, Consumer Product Safety Commission, Nuclear Office of Science and Technology Policy, Office of Technology Assistance, Food and Drug Administration, Occupational Safety and Health Administration, Fish and Wildlife Service, Office of Surface Mining Reclamation and Enforcement, Bureau of Land Management, and the Soil Conservation Service. As nurses increase their knowledge of environmental hazards and environmental effects on the health of communities, a clear understanding of which federal agency will provide assistance and supervision is required to expedite solutions to acute problems.

## Local Community Involvement

Nurses in the community function in the roles of advocate, counselor, educator, and community planner. Working with clients in the community fosters an awareness of the influence of the environment on the health of individuals and families. For example, occupational health nurses may identify a cluster of symptoms within a particular unit of an industry and need to determine potential sources of contamination or exposure to other environmental stressors. One aspect of occupational health and safety of particular concern in many industries is environmental effects on pregnant workers. Since questions have been raised regarding employers discriminating against women of childbearing age in an attempt to reduce administrative costs, two occupational health nurses conducted a study to determine the consequences of work adjustments necessitated by pregnancies of female employees (Mahone & Wilkinson, 1985). The nurses interviewed managers at a large pharmaceutical company chosen because of the potential need to temporarily reassign pregnant employees because of their work with chemical and biological hazards. The managers described positive and negative effects of the pregnancy reassignments and leaves of absence. Positive effects included cross-training skills of other employees, increasing departmental flexibility for other leaves, and the identification of exceptional potential employees hired as temporaries who were later offered permanent positions. Burdens included the temporary loss of experienced workers through pregnancy leave and the forfeiture of some work. Since some of the women delayed their return to work because of the lack of child care, the occupational health nurses also identified the need for an industrial-based child care facility.

In working with families in the home, sources of pollution from noise, chemicals, contagious diseases, contaminated water, or other pollutants may be identified as an actual or potential nursing problem. Nurses in rural areas need to be especially alert to a family's water supply if well water is consumed. The nurse's knowledge regarding the appropriate local or state authority to contact for assistance is frequently the family's only source of information.

All nurses need to be informed of the national goals and priorities developed by the Department of Health and Human Services. Nurses can continue to be involved in the development of these objectives through association with professional organizations. In addition, interventions at the local level to educate the public are an important component of disease prevention and health promotion. Public Health Service publications may be useful for nurses to assess environmental issues facing their communities.

Local nursing involvement may also include joining one of the many organizations devoted to environmental concerns. These organizations inform members of local issues, publish newsletters, lobby for environmentally sensitive legislation, and provide an opportunity for networking with other concerned citizens.

## ❖ SUMMARY

This chapter addresses some of the major environmental concerns affecting the health of individuals, families, and communities. Health hazards of a biological, chemical, physical and sociological/psychological nature were briefly described, and emerging environmental issues were identified. Environmental concerns were addressed at the international, national, and local levels. Nursing actions and responsibilities were highlighted throughout. In general, they include assessment, intervention, education, and advocacy.

## ❖ APPLYING KNOWLEDGE TO PRACTICE

1. What kind of environmental hazards are present at your place of employment? (i.e., infectious wastes, radioactive materials). Who is responsible for the safe disposal of these materials? Do you think that nurses should be concerned about these issues or are they the responsibility of another department?

2. What environmental issues are of concern to the home health nurse? Discuss how a home health nurse could appropriately dispose of infected medical supplies.

3. Identify major sources of pollution (air, water, chemical, physical) in your community. Identify at least one government agency and volunteer organization who are concerned with each of these hazards.

4. This chapter identifies Nightingale and Neuman as nursing theorists who have recognized the relationship between the individual and the environment. Describe how other nursing theorists conceptualize this relationship (review Chapter 1).

## REFERENCES

Begley, S. (1990). Pollution knows no boundaries. *National Wildlife, 28,* 34-44.

Bullough, B. & Bullough, V. (1990). *Nursing in the community.* St Louis: C. V. Mosby.

Brown, R. (1990). *State of the world.* New York: W. W. Norton & Co.

Commoner, B. (1971). *The closing circle: Nature, man and technology.* New York: Alfred A. Knopf, Inc.

Edwards, L., & Dees, R. (1990). Environmental health: The effects of life-style on the world around us. In S. J. Wold (Ed.). *Community Health Nursing: Issues and Topics.* Norwalk: Appleton & Lange.

Gordon, L. (1990). Who will manage the environment? *American Journal of Public Health.* 80(8), 904-905.

Green, L. & Anderson, C. (1986). *Community health.* St. Louis: Times Mirror/Mosby.

Mahone, M., & Wilkinson, W. (1985). Women, work and pregnancy: Implications for occupational health nursing. *Occupational Health Nursing.* 33, 343-348.

Nadakavukaren, A. (1990). *Man and environment: A health perspective* (3rd ed.). Prospect Heights, Ill.: Waveland Press, Inc.

Neuman, B. (1989). *The Newman systems model* (2nd ed.). Norwalk: Appleton and Lange.

Nitze, W. A. (1990). A proposed structure for an international convention on climate change. *Science, 249*(4969), 607-608.

Paden, M. E., Managing Editor & Staff (1988). *World resources 1988-89: An assessment of the resource base that supports the global economy with data tables for 146 countries.* New York: Basic Books, Inc.

Public Health Service (1979). *Healthy people: The Surgeon General's report on health promotion and disease prevention.* Washington, DC: U.S. Government Printing Office.

Public Health Service (1986). *The 1990 Health Objectives for the nation: A midcourse review.* Washington, DC: U.S. Government Printing Office.

Public Health Service (1989). *Promoting health/preventing disease: Year 2000 health objectives for the nation.* Washington, DC: U.S. Government Printing Office, Department of Health and Human Services.

Public Health Service (1990). *Healthy people 2000: National Health Promotion and Disease Prevention Objectives,* Conference Edition. Washington, DC: U.S. Government Printing Office.

Roberts, L. (1990). Counting on science at EPA. *Science, 249*(4969), 616-618.

Shannon, I. (1990). Public health's promise for the future: The 1989 presidential address. *American Journal of Public Health, 80*(8), 909-912.

Solomon, C. (1984). Occupational health problems in high tech industries. *Occupational Health Nursing,* 32, 261-265.

Stanhope, M. & Lancaster, J. (1988). *Community health nursing: Process and practice for promoting health* (2nd ed.). St. Louis: C. V. Mosby.

Vyner, H. M. (1988). The psychological dimensions of health care for patients exposed to radiation and other invisible environmental contaminants. *Social Science and Medicine, 27*(10), 1097-1103.

World Health Organization (1971). *Constitution: World health organization.* Geneva: World Health Organization.

# 14

# Interpersonal Communication

Sandra J. Sundeen

## OBJECTIVES

*At the completion of this chapter, the reader will be able to:*

◆ Identify and describe the components of the communication process.

◆ Discuss the characteristics of each of the four phases of the nurse-client relationship.

◆ Analyze interpersonal relationships by applying theories of communication.

From birth until death, the ability to communicate enables humans to acquire sustenance, support, and survival techniques for the many challenges of life. The growth of skill in communication is a lifelong process. Its culmination is reflected in the wisdom that is associated with advanced age. People interact with others at many levels: one-to-one, with their families, various groups, and on an international level. The outcome of an effort to communicate may be positive or negative; it may be expected or a total surprise. It is certain, however, that constant involvement in communication is inevitable. One cannot *not* communicate (Watzlawick, 1967).

The potential for communication rests in one's biological heritage. This is a capacity that is shared with many other species. Human beings are different from other species in their ability to understand and send complex messages. People also have the ability to develop backup systems for communicating if the primary channel breaks down. For instance, although hearing is considered to be very important for accurate communication, hearing-impaired individuals can learn to compensate for their disability by focusing on other senses, such as vision.

The ways that people communicate have evolved throughout recorded history and continue to change and develop today. Ancient cave paintings and hieroglyphics are studied by scientists so that we may understand the thoughts and feelings of our ancestors; other scientists are busy inventing new ways to transmit messages. Just in the last century, we have witnessed the invention of the radio, television, computer, and communication satellites. Consider how quickly we can receive messages from people on the other side of the world or even the moon. The accomplishments that allow us to do this were motivated by a desire to communicate.

Communication is also essential for successful nursing practice. Florence Nightingale (1859) recognized this when she wrote, "He (the patient) feels what a convenience it would be, if there were any single person to whom he could speak simply and openly; . . . to whom he could express his wishes and directions without that person persisting in saying 'I hope that it will please God yet to give you twenty years,' or, 'You have a long life of activity before you' " (p. 55). She went on to advise that platitudes and empty advice were not needed by the sick. Rather, the nurse should focus on listening to the concerns of the patient and on keeping him apprised of current events.

Contemporary nursing theorists are equally concerned that nurses be aware of the importance of the interpersonal nature of patient care. The caring nature of nursing is known through the experience of a gentle touch or an understanding word. This chapter will explore the various ways in which communication skills may be used to enhance nursing practice.

## ❖ DEFINITIONS

A general definition of communication is found in Webster's New Collegiate Dictionary: "A process by which information is exchanged between individuals through a common system of symbols, signs, or behavior." Theorists who have studied communication have developed their own definitions. Ruesch (1972) has described it as "all those processes by which people influence one another." An additional observation has been made by Watzlawick and his colleagues (1967). They state that all behavior is communication, and conversely, all communication is a form of behavior. The emphasis on behavior and influence is important to the consideration of communication within the context of nursing. Through the conscious use of communication skills, nurses can have an influence on the health-related behavior of their clients.

## ❖ LEVELS OF COMMUNICATION

The levels of communication include verbal, nonverbal, and metacommunication. Verbal communication includes all aspects of communication that depend on speech. All other communications are nonverbal. In general, much more information is communicated nonverbally than verbally. Nonverbal communication includes the study of body language or kinesics, territoriality, and personal space. Written language relies on the use of words but is considered to be nonverbal, since it does not involve speech.

### Types of Nonverbal Communication

Ruesch and Kees (1956) identified three types of nonverbal communication. These are action, object, and sign. *Action nonverbal* refers to sending a message through the use of body activity. It does not include the use of signs or symbols. Examples of action nonverbal messages might include jumping or hitting. *Sign nonverbal* is the use of symbolism. For instance, the exchanging of "high fives" at a sporting event symbolically communicates shared excitement. *Object nonverbal* communication relates to the messages that are given by personal possessions. An example of this is the message that is given by the car a person drives.

### Metacommunication

*Metacommunication* refers to the covert messages that are transmitted directing how to interpret or decode an overt message. For instance, a parent may scold a child in the presence of an adult friend, simultaneously winking his eye. The child receives the message, "What you did is wrong, but not serious. I'm doing this for the benefit of this outsider." The parent may then say, "Let's have some ice cream," which is a verbal metacommunication that reinforces the message given by the wink. Metacommunication depends on the relationship between the participants for success. The better they know each other, the more successful the metacommunication. Cultural similarity also helps in decoding metacommunications.

## ❖ CHARACTERISTICS OF A HELPING RELATIONSHIP

Peplau (1952) has described nursing as "a significant, therapeutic, interpersonal process." By using good communication skills, the nurse establishes and maintains a helping nurse-client relationship. Carl Rogers, a psychologist who based his helping theory on the interpersonal relationship, asked questions designed to describe the characteristics of the helping relationship. They are:

1. Can I *be* in some way that will be perceived by the other person as trustworthy, as dependable, or consistent in some deep sense?
2. Can I be expressive enough as a person that what I am will be communicated unambiguously?
3. Can I let myself experience positive attitudes toward this other person—attitudes of warmth, caring, liking, interest, and respect?
4. Can I be strong enough as a person to be separate from the other?
5. Am I secure enough within myself to permit that person separateness?
6. Can I let myself enter fully into the world of his or her feelings and personal meaning and see these as he or she does?
7. Can I be acceptant of each facet that clients present to me? Can I receive them as they are? Can I communicate this attitude? Or can I only receive them conditionally, acceptant of some aspects and silently or openly disapproving of others?
8. Can I act with sufficient sensitivity in the relationship that my behavior will not be perceived as a threat?
9. Can I free them from the threat of external evaluation?
10. Can I meet this other individual as a person who is in the process of becoming, or will I be bound by his past and by my past? (Rogers, 1961).

A nurse who can give a positive response to each question should be able to establish nurse-client relationships that enhance nursing care. A negative or uncertain response indicates an area that the nurse needs to address through exploration of personal attitudes and beliefs or with the help of a nurse-mentor.

## ❖ THE COMMUNICATION PROCESS

The process of human communication has been examined by theorists from many fields, including psychology, sociology, anthropology, linguistics, and cybernetics. Study of these theories can help the nurse clarify a personal conceptual model of communication applied to nursing practice.

### Structural Components of Communication

The structural components of communication include the sender, receiver, message, feedback, and the context. A structural model of communication is illustrated in Fig. 14-1. The *sender* is the person who initiates communication by transmitting a message, verbal or nonverbal, to the receiver. *Feedback* refers both to the verbal or nonverbal response from the receiver and the internal evaluation of the communication that occurs within the sender. The

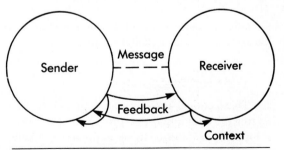

❖ **Fig. 14-1**   Components of the communication process. *(From Sundeen S, et al: Nurse-client interaction, ed 4, St Louis, 1989, The CV Mosby Co.)*

effective communicator constantly monitors how accurately the message was perceived by observing nonverbal responses and listening to verbal ones. The context in which communication takes place also affects the process. For instance, an intimate conversation is awkward in a crowd. A noisy classroom interferes with the student's ability to concentrate (Sundeen, 1989).

## Communication Processes

Three processes of communication have been identified by Ruesch (1972). These are perception, evaluation, and transmission. *Perception* refers to the use of the senses to recognize the presence of a message. Perception usually takes place through auditory, visual, or tactile channels. It is affected by many factors. These may include the person's past experiences, emotional state, the setting in which communication takes place, and the relationship between the people involved. *Evaluation* is the internal assessment of the message. This includes recognition of the overt message, comparison of the message to past experiences, and the emotional reaction to the message. *Transmission* is the conscious and unconscious, verbal and nonverbal, response to the message. This is then perceived by the original sender as a new message, and the cycle continues.

## ❖ COMMUNICATION THEORIES

Selected theories of communication further illustrate the communication process.

### Transactional Analysis

Transactional analysis is an approach to analyzing the communication process that was developed by Eric Berne. It was popularized when he published "Games People Play" (1964) and "What Do You Say After You Say Hello?" (1970). Berne viewed communication as a series of transactions between people. Transactions may be open and clear, but they are often clouded because the participants are playing interpersonal games. These games are related to roles that are learned as a result of life experiences. As people go through life, they learn to assume roles in various situations. In other words, they live out life scripts. The role that a person assumes in a particular transaction represents an ego state. If the person is authoritarian and directive, the ego state is that of "parent." ($P$). If the response is submissive or playful, the "child" ($C$) ego state is operational. The "adult" ($A$) ego state is characterized by being objective and rational. No ego state is considered to be the "best" one. Each may be functional, depending on the situation. For instance, the child allows a person to have fun and to see the humor in life; the adult is helpful when there is a need to be productive at work; the parent is effective when a crisis must be handled quickly and efficiently. The well balanced person is able to move among ego states as needed. It should also be noted that the ego states are not usually entered consciously. They occur spontaneously in response to the situation. However, it is possible, with training, to analyze the ego states that are present in personal interactions and to work to change these patterns. This is the purpose of therapy based on transactional analysis.

Berne (1964) has classified transactions according to the combination of ego states that are operating in a particular interaction. A *complementary* transaction is one in which the response corresponds with the sender's expectation. For instance, a parent message receives a child's response:

P: Pick up your clothes.
C: Do I have to?
P: Yes, you have to.
C: Okay, if I have to.

Adult to adult transactions are also complementary. These transactions encourage the continuation of communication. *Crossed* transactions take place when the response is not congruent with the sender's expectation. Examples of crossed transactions would be a parent to child or a child to parent response to an adult to adult message. For example:

A: We need to leave soon or we'll be late.
C: Why is it always my fault when we're late?

Crossed transactions tend to cut off communication and cause frustration. The third type of transaction is called *ulterior.* In this case, the message is directed toward more than one ego state. The response may be in terms of one or both of the ego states addressed in the message. Paradoxical communications are examples of ulterior transactions. An example of such a transaction follows:

A/P: You probably shouldn't come home for the holidays. The weather could be bad.
C: Why are you saying that? You know I always come home.

Ulterior transactions are at the core of interpersonal games. In families, members may rely on games so much that it is very difficult for an outsider to understand their communication. It can even be hard for a family member to be sure that the real message is understood. Transactional analysis often takes place in groups. When group members interact, they tend to use the same patterns of communication they use in their families. Games can then be identified and ulterior transactions replaced with complementary ones. Sometimes when a nurse is confused by a client's communication, it can help to review the interaction in terms of transactional analysis theory. Ulterior transactions may be taking place; the nurse may be trying to respond to the verbal message while unconsciously recognizing the conflicting nonverbal one.

## Erickson's Theories

Milton Erickson is another communication theorist whose work can be helpful to nurses. He is known best for his work as a hypnother-

apist, but actually bases his theories of hypnosis on communications concepts. Lankton (1985) has described the elements of Erickson's approach to interpersonal interaction, several of which are particularly pertinent to nursing practice. *Communication should be positive and individualistic.* Erickson believed that people who are given encouragement and support will usually choose the best course of action available to them. Their options may be limited based on past learning. The caregiver's role is to help the person learn new options for behavior and to use problem-solving resources that are already available. *Interventions should be active and goal-oriented.* A thorough understanding of human needs and development is more important than labeling behavior. The helping relationship is based on working together with the client to promote goal accomplishment by changing behavior. *Approaches need to be systems oriented.* Any change that is undertaken must occur within the context of the social system in order to mobilize support for the client.

Applications of Erickson's theories can be very complex and require specialized training. Some aspects of neurolinguistic programming, an interpersonal approach that is based on Erickson's theories, may be applied in nurse-client situations and will be addressed later in this chapter.

## ❖ SELF-AWARENESS AND COMMUNICATION

Since communication is interactive in nature, the nurse must function as a participant-observer. This can be difficult. It requires the nurse to be aware of personal responses, feelings, preferences, prejudices, and attitudes that might influence interactions with clients. Consider the following clinical vignette:

Ms. E. was a 45-year-old nurse who worked for a community health agency. One of her responsibilities was to teach a health education course at the local high school. While she was teaching the unit on substance abuse, one of the students challenged her statement that the use of illicit drugs is not a healthy behavior. She became extremely defensive and was aware that her credibility with the students was compromised. After class, she examined her response and realized that it was related to her fear that her own adolescent son would experiment with drugs.

Awareness of the underlying reason for a response can help a person put it into perspective. Varied life experiences can facilitate successful communication with clients if the nurse is in touch with the effect of the past on the present.

## The Influence of Feelings on Communication

Self-awareness also helps the nurse to be sensitive to subtle messages that are received from clients. Feelings, in particular, may be transmitted nonverbally. Nurses who pay attention to their own feelings in response to the client may receive clues about the feelings of the client.

**Anxiety.** Anxiety is known to be contagious. It spreads from one person to another because it is communicated nonverbally. Those who are near an anxious person will perceive clues about his or her state. For instance, he or she may be fidgety, tense, flushed, perspiring, with loud and rapid speech. This person does not need to verbalize anxiety. It is apparent to anyone.

A nurse who feels anxious while caring for a client needs to analyze the origin of the feeling. It could be that the nurse is anxious because of something about the clinical situation or a personal matter unrelated to work. It is important for the nurse to recognize that he or she is anxious because this will be communicated to the patient. If the nurse cannot identify a personal reason for feeling anxious, it is likely that the feeling is being communicated by the client. This perception needs to be validated by

assessing the client's feelings verbally and through observation.

**Anger.** Another feeling communicated interpersonally is anger. Anger that is unconsciously perceived in another person will not necessarily make the receiver angry; it might result in anxiety. This is why it is important to validate the client's emotional state when one becomes aware that feelings are having an impact on the relationship. It is also useful to be aware of one's own usual reaction to anger. A defensive or rejecting response will not allow the client to feel secure enough to express anger or to describe its perceived cause. Invalidation of anger usually makes the feeling more intense. A fearful response may complicate the anger with anxiety that the situation could get out of control. Most people will respond positively to an opportunity to talk about their anger if they are reassured that they have a right to their feelings. This can be followed with a discussion of ways to express angry feelings in a healthy way. It should also be noted that a nurse who is angry at work will communicate this feeling to others. If the anger is related to the work situation, it should be dealt with before interacting with clients if this is at all possible. If the anger is unrelated to work or if it cannot be overcome, it is best to explain that the nurse may seem preoccupied because of personal issues unrelated to the client. This avoids having the client assume that the nurse is angry at him or her. Of course, the nurse still takes care not to take the anger out on the client or to use the client as a counselor.

**Caring.** The profession of nursing is built around the fact that caring is also communicated interpersonally. Human caring is first experienced in the parent-child relationship. A loving environment in infancy and childhood leads to the capacity to be a loving adult. Many of the clients who are in need of nursing care were deprived of a caring childhood. Nurses have an opportunity to mend some of the damage that this causes. When nurses speak of "caring for" someone, they are usually thinking of the totality of nursing interventions. An important part of "caring for" is "caring about." This refers to the emotional aspect of caring, or becoming involved with the client as one person to another. This is the type of caring that Rogers (1961) described as characteristic of the helping relationship. Some nurses are hesitant to care about clients, because they fear "overinvolvement." Self-awareness is again the key to caring about the client while retaining a professional relationship. Caring in the nurse-client relationship is for the purpose of meeting the needs of the client for human relatedness. The nurse correctly seeks to meet personal needs for caring in other contexts. However, when the nurse is cared about as a person outside of the nurse-client context, a capacity is developed to relate to clients in an unconditionally caring way.

## ❖ APPLICATIONS TO CLINICAL PRACTICE

The principles of communication are applied to nursing practice through the establishment of the helping nurse-client relationship.

### The Nurse-Client Relationship

The nurse-client relationship has four phases: preorientation, orientation, maintenance, and termination. The phases of the relationship may be aligned with the stages of the nursing process. Preorientation and orientation are related to assessment. Planning is the bridge between the orientation and maintenance phases. Implementation and maintenance occur simultaneously. Evaluation occurs throughout the relationship, but is particularly prominent during termination.

In many settings, the course of the relationship may be abbreviated because of short hospital stays or brief episodes of outpatient care. However, it is important to understand the characteristics of the relationship so that the nurse may plan realistically for the interpersonal aspects of patient care. In general, the maintenance phase of the relationship will be most affected by short-term contacts.

Forchuk and Brown (1989) developed an instrument to help community mental health nurses measure the progress of nurse-client relationships by describing the behaviors of the nurse and the client during each phase of the relationship (Fig. 14-2). They based their work on Peplau's (1952) model of the nurse-client relationship. In this model, the maintenance phase is called the working phase and is subdivided into two parts—identification and exploitation. The resolution phase is the same as the termination phase.

**The preorientation phase.** The *preorientation* phase begins before there is an encounter between the nurse and the client. During this phase, the nurse reviews available information about the client and plans for the first meeting. In particular, the nurse looks for information about the client's response to earlier contacts with the health care system, as well as identifying the circumstances that have led to the current contact. Information may be limited and should be used as background. Any impressions that are formed at this stage need to be validated with the client later. Care should be given to planning for the first contact with the client. If at all possible, a private area should be found. Distractions should be kept to a minimum. Anything that can be done to create a relaxed environment is very helpful. Most people are anxious when they encounter a health care provider, and this can inhibit communication.

**The orientation phase.** The first phase of the relationship that involves both the nurse and the client is the *orientation* phase. This

❖ **Table 14-1** Community mental-health-promotion program phases of nurse-client relationship*

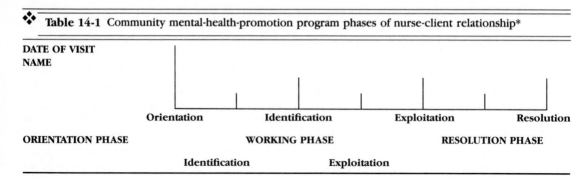

| ORIENTATION PHASE | WORKING PHASE | | RESOLUTION PHASE |
|---|---|---|---|
| | Identification | Exploitation | |
| **Client** | | | |
| Seeks assistance. | Participates in identifying problems. | Makes full use of services. | Abandons old needs. |
| Conveys educative needs. | Begins to be aware of time. | Identifies new goals. | Aspires to new goals. |
| Asks questions. | Responds to help. | Attempts to attain new goals. | Becomes independent of helping person. |
| Tests parameters. | Identifies with nurse. | Rapid shifts in behavior; dependent—independent. | Applies new problem-solving skills. |
| Shares preconceptions and expectations of nurse due to past experience. | Recognizes nurse as a person. | Exploitative behavior. | Maintains changes in style of communication and interaction. |
| | Explores feelings. | Realistic exploitation. | Positive changes in view of self. |
| | Fluctuates dependence, independence and interdependence in relationship with nurse. | Self-directing. | Integrates illness. |
| | Increases focal attention. | Develops skills in interpersonal relationships and problem-solving. | Exhibits ability to stand alone. |
| | Changes appearance (for better or worse). | Displays changes in manner of communication (more open, flexible). | |
| | Understands purpose of meeting. | | |
| | Maintains continuity between sessions (process and content). | | |

❖  **Table 14-1 (cont.)**

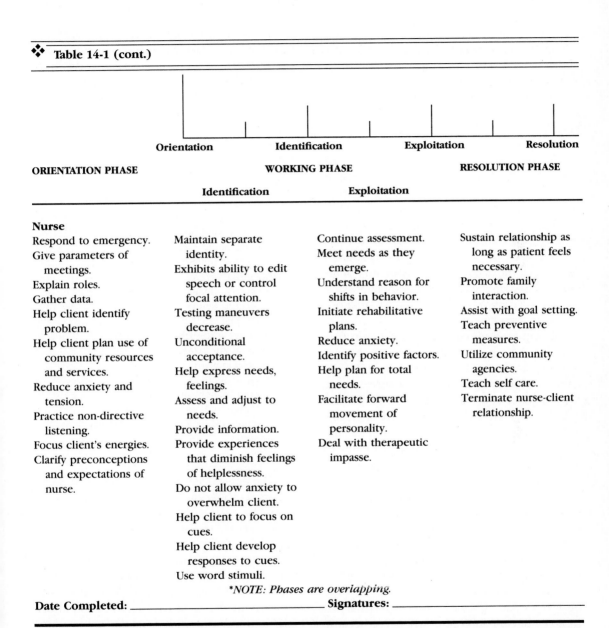

| Orientation | Identification | Exploitation | Resolution |

**ORIENTATION PHASE**          **WORKING PHASE**          **RESOLUTION PHASE**

                 Identification          Exploitation

| **Nurse** | | | |
|---|---|---|---|
| Respond to emergency. | Maintain separate identity. | Continue assessment. | Sustain relationship as long as patient feels necessary. |
| Give parameters of meetings. | Exhibits ability to edit speech or control focal attention. | Meet needs as they emerge. | Promote family interaction. |
| Explain roles. | | Understand reason for shifts in behavior. | Assist with goal setting. |
| Gather data. | Testing maneuvers decrease. | Initiate rehabilitative plans. | Teach preventive measures. |
| Help client identify problem. | Unconditional acceptance. | Reduce anxiety. | Utilize community agencies. |
| Help client plan use of community resources and services. | Help express needs, feelings. | Identify positive factors. | Teach self care. |
| Reduce anxiety and tension. | Assess and adjust to needs. | Help plan for total needs. | Terminate nurse-client relationship. |
| Practice non-directive listening. | Provide information. | Facilitate forward movement of personality. | |
| Focus client's energies. | Provide experiences that diminish feelings of helplessness. | Deal with therapeutic impasse. | |
| Clarify preconceptions and expectations of nurse. | Do not allow anxiety to overwhelm client. | | |
| | Help client to focus on cues. | | |
| | Help client develop responses to cues. | | |
| | Use word stimuli. | | |

*NOTE: Phases are overlapping.*

**Date Completed:** _____  **Signatures:** _____

From Forchuk, C. & Brown, B. (1989). Establishing a Nurse-Client Relationship. J. Psychosocial Nursing and Mental Health Services. (*27*)(2), p. 32.

begins with introductions.

*Introductions.* The nurse's introduction should include name, title, and function. For example, "I am Mary Smith. I'm a staff nurse on this floor and I will be your primary nurse. That means that we will plan your nursing care together and I will provide your care whenever I am working." A wealth of information has been given. Since the client may be anxious, this may need to be repeated at the beginning of the next contact. The nurse should then inquire about how the client would like to be addressed. Following the client's preference in this regard helps establish a helping relationship. The preferred mode of address should be recorded in the nursing care plan. It is extremely important to identify oneself to every client at each encounter unless it is absolutely certain that the client knows the identity of the nurse. Most identification badges are impossible to read and cannot be relied upon for orienting clients to their care providers.

*Interpersonal contract.* Following introductions, the nurse needs to orient the client to the parameters of the relationship. This includes the purpose of the nurse-client contact, the frequency of meetings, the duration of each meeting, and the duration of the relationship. This will vary a great deal. Some nurses may encounter clients for a brief time in a clinic or an emergency room; others may engage in long-term relationships in nursing homes or home care settings. However, in each case, the basic types of information described above should be communicated. The client may need an opportunity to react to the nurse's description of their relationship. For instance, the nurse may describe a long-term series of meetings when the client expects only a brief contact with the health care setting. Clarification is necessary or a barrier to communication will occur because of conflicting goals. Agreement on the purpose, frequency, and duration of the relationship constitutes the interpersonal contract. The information about the nature of the relationship

should be repeated at the end of the first contact and as often as necessary to be sure that the client understands it.

*Data collection and goal setting.* Following the establishment of the contract, the nurse and client are ready to move forward to data collection and goal setting. Data collection will lead to the formulation of a nursing diagnosis. Some NANDA diagnoses that may be applied to the communication process or the interpersonal relationship include:

Impaired verbal communication
Impaired social interaction
Social isolation
Altered role performance
Altered parenting
Altered family processes
Ineffective individual coping
Defensive coping
Ineffective denial
Ineffective family coping
Decisional conflict
Self-esteem disturbance
Chronic low self-esteem
Hopelessness
Powerlessness
Altered thought processes
Dysfunctional grieving
Potential for violence
Anxiety
Fear

The nurse needs to identify the client's expectations about the episode of care. Feedback should be given about whether or not the client's goals are realistic in relation to what the nurse has to offer. Openness about realistic expectations avoids later disappointment when unrealistic goals are not met. As the nurse proceeds with the nursing assessment, additional information will be provided leading to mutual goal setting. The establishment of mutually agreed upon goals marks the end of the orientation phase of the relationship. As goals are identified, they also become part of the contract between the client and the nurse.

**The maintenance phase.** The maintenance phase of the relationship is sometimes called the working phase, because it is the time during which the nurse and the client work on accomplishing the identified goals of the relationship. The nurse uses the relationship with the client to assist in addressing the identified health care needs by using interpersonal skills. These might include such techniques as interviewing, empathizing, listening, nondirective interventions, and elements of neurolinguistic programming. The particular technique used depends on the needs of the client, the focus of the relationship, and the abilities of the nurse. It is helpful to develop a variety of relationship skills so that they may be adapted to meet the needs of various clients.

*Interviewing.* Interviewing skills are needed during all phases of the relationship. The interview may be structured or nonstructured. In a *structured interview,* the nurse follows a set format to elicit information from the client. An example of this is the use of a standardized assessment tool to collect health data upon admission to a health care program. This is an efficient way to collect information but may be limited depending on the adequacy of the instrument or format that is used. It is also useful for the collection of data for research purposes. A strictly structured interview may lead the nurse to use "tunnel vision," with more attention focused on the completion of the data collection form than on the interpersonal clues that are being communicated by the client.

*Nondirective therapeutic communication techniques.* The *unstructured interview* allows the nurse to use nondirective therapeutic communication techniques to enable the client to explore areas of concern. Skillfully employed nondirective techniques do not hamper the relationship, but indicate to the client that the nurse is interested in clarifying his or her messages. Practice is needed in order to feel comfortable with these approaches. Several common nondirective techniques as described by Sundeen, Stuart, Rankin, and Cohen (1989) will be discussed.

*Establishing guidelines* is a reorientation of the client to the reason for the interaction with the nurse. Even if the relationship is long-term, continuity is maintained by reviewing the overall purpose and goals, as well as the specific objectives to be accomplished during the current meeting. In addition, it is helpful to explore the client's recollection of the last meeting and to bring up any issues that were not resolved. This repetition of the goals and frequent reassessment keeps the relationship from drifting off course and gives the participants a sense of progress as goals are accomplished.

The client is assisted to clarify and explore thoughts and feelings when *broad openings* are offered. The purpose of this technique is to indicate willingness to interact with the client without influencing the content of the discussion. The nurse may use such statements as "Tell me what's been happening to you," or "How are you doing?" This technique should be used discriminately. When the client introduces a topic, the nurse will usually need to be more directive in order to address it in greater depth.

*Restating* is another nondirective approach. In this case, the nurse paraphrases the client's statement or a part of it to encourage continuation and to validate understanding of the meaning of the communication. A related technique is *reflecting.* This requires the nurse to identify the main theme of the thoughts or feelings that are being expressed by the client and to share this perception with the client. If the nurse is on target, the client feels understood. If the nurse has misunderstood the client's message, reflecting allows for correction while indicating to the client that the nurse wants to understand. Neither restating nor reflecting means parroting. Unskilled interviewers sometimes overuse these approaches. The result may be that the interaction resembles a comedy routine.

Client: I have a headache.
Nurse: You have a headache.
Client: I would like an aspirin.
Nurse: You would like an aspirin.
Client: My headache is getting worse.
Nurse: You feel like your headache is worse.

In this rather extreme example, it is easy to see that the nurse is not getting the information needed to help the client. A switch to structured interviewing would have been appropriate.

It is very important to be sure that the client's message is understood, so that appropriate responses can be made. This can be accomplished by using the technique of *clarification*. When a message is unclear to the nurse, the client is asked to explain its meaning. This is not impolite or intrusive. Clients appreciate the nurse's effort to understand their communication. A related technique, *consensual validation*, refers to assuring mutual understanding of words or phrases. It is particularly important to use this approach when interacting with a client from a different age group, culture, or ethnic background.

Each interaction should end with a *summary*. The nurse and client share their perceptions of what happened during the interaction and plan for the next meeting, if there is to be one. This enhances the sense of mutuality between the participants in the relationship.

***Nontherapeutic communication techniques.*** As the nurse conducts the interview, it is also necessary to be careful not to use *nontherapeutic communication techniques*. Sundeen, Stuart, Rankin, and Cohen (1989) have described several of these. They are usually signals that the nurse feels uncomfortable addressing the issues that the client is trying to discuss. Clients may bring up difficult subjects indirectly or with hesitation. Then it is easy for the nurse to avoid confronting these messages, allowing the interaction to shift to more comfortable themes.

The nurse may simply choose not to acknowledge a message. In this case, the nurse may change the subject or may focus on a superficial aspect of the client's statement. For example:

Client: My son is having a hard time now that he's started high school. I'm worried that he'll get into trouble.
Nurse: What grade is he in?

The nurse's response is not really relevant to the client's concern. The message is one of disinterest in exploring the client's worry about her son, thus cutting off the communication. A more therapeutic response would have been, "I can see that you are worried about him. Tell me more about that."

The nurse may be more active in discouraging the client from sharing anxiety-provoking concerns. Conveying *value judgments* about the client's statement closes off communication channels. This includes using phrases such as "that's good," or "that's too bad." "Shoulds" and "should nots" interfere with the client's ability to consider alternative solutions to problems. Therefore, *advice giving* also interferes with the therapeutic relationship. By advising the client about a preferred course of action, the nurse assumes responsibility for the client's behavior. If the advised action is not successful, the client is less likely to learn from the experience because the decision to act was made by someone else. It is more helpful to assist the client to identify alternative courses of action, the positive and negative consequences of each alternative, and to support him in carrying out the selected alternative.

*Reassurance* is often viewed as helpful to someone who is distressed. In reality, it is more helpful to the reassurer. If a nurse tells a client, "Don't worry. Everything will be all right," the real message is "I don't want to talk with you about the concerns you have that things will not be all right." This approach is particularly unhelpful in situations such as grief or terminal illness when both the nurse and the client recognize the emptiness of the reassurance, but tacitly agree to avoid the painful issues that need to be addressed.

A related nontherapeutic intervention is the use of *stereotyped responses*. These are almost automatic and require conscious effort in order to avoid them. For example:

Nurse: Good morning, Mr. Jones. How are you today?
Client: Not so good. How are you?
Nurse: Fine, thank you.

In this case, the nurse responded to the usually expected social greeting ritual, rather than responding to the client's deviation from the ritual.

When people are under stress, they may become very critical of others, particularly those upon whom they must depend. *Defensiveness* is not a therapeutic response in this situation. If a client criticizes the nurse or other staff members, it is important to listen carefully and to use good communication skills to discover the underlying concerns. If the client has a good reason to complain, the nurse should act as an advocate and try to rectify the situation. If the client is responding to anxiety, the nurse can intervene to alleviate his distress, thereby reducing the need to attack others.

*Active listening.* In order to communicate effectively with others, it is essential to engage in *active listening*. This means that the nurse gives full attention to the client. This is communicated verbally and nonverbally. Eye contact conveys interest and involvement (Fig. 14-3). Head nods and facial expressions also indicate understanding. These should be used consciously. Unconscious nodding may indicate unintended agreement.

A particular type of active listening is the use of *neurolinguistic programming*, described by Richard Bandler and John Grinder. This communication technique is based on the work of such experts in the field of communication as Virginia Satir, Fritz Perls, and Milton

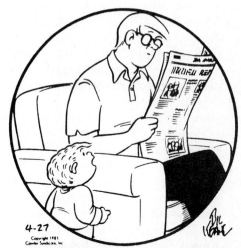

4-27

"You hafta listen to me with your eyes, Daddy. Not just your ears."

❖ **Fig. 14-2**    Communication involves all of the senses.

Erickson. This is a complex approach to communication that requires specialized training. Two concepts that are part of neurolinguistic programming will be discussed here. They may help the nurse to enhance assessment and interaction skills. They are pacing and representational systems.

According to King, Novik, and Citrenbaum (1983), *pacing* involves sending a message to the client that is reflective of his or her current experience. For instance, the nurse might say, "You made a face when I gave you this medicine. I guess it tastes pretty bad." Pacing is used to establish lines of communication with the client. It is then possible to lead the client to a desired behavioral change. In the preceding example, the nurse might go on to say, "This water will take the bad taste away." Of course, this would not work if water was not effective for overcoming the taste of the medicine. The communication is used to enhance the effect of the intervention and to indicate to the client that the nurse is in tune with his or her feelings.

Another approach to pacing is described by

Knowles (1983). She describes a process called *mirroring.* In this case, the nurse imitates the client's body position, gestures, or even breathing patterns. When this is done inconspicuously, it is a powerful way of communicating understanding, thereby facilitating the communication process. Once the nurse has succeeded in pacing the client's current behavior, it may be possible to lead the client toward behavioral change. For instance, if the client is anxious, the body position may be rigid, there may be loud and fast speech, and breathing may be rapid. After synchronizing his or her own body position, speech, and rate of breathing with those of the client, the nurse can gradually relax, speak quietly, and breathe more slowly. If the pacing has been successful, the client is likely to do the same.

One may also gain access to the client by identifying and using congruent *representational systems.* Knowles describes the three sensory modalities that are included: auditory, visual, and kinesthetic. This theory is based on the premise that every person has a preferred sensory channel for communication. It is possible to identify and access the preferred channel in order to communicate in a way that is comfortable for the client. One way to identify the sensory modality that the person uses most frequently is to listen for the predicates in sentences. Individuals tend to use predicates related to one of the three modalities more often than those related to the other two. For instance, in response to the comment, "My husband and I are angry with each other," a person who uses the visual modality might say, "I see what you mean"; one who uses the auditory might say, "I hear what you're saying"; and one who uses the kinesthetic modality, "I feel that I understand what you mean." The box that follows provides lists of predicates related to the three sensory modalities (Knowles, 1983).

---

### ❖ PREFERRED PREDICATES

| AUDITORY | KINESTHETIC | VISUAL |
|---|---|---|
| listen | feel | see |
| hear | knock out | behold |
| gripe | turn | observe |
| hassle | thin-skinned | view |
| attend | tender | witness |
| give ear to | stir | perceive |
| get | excite | discern |
| listen in | arouse | spy |
| eavesdrop | whet | sight |
| hang upon every word | sharpen | discover |
| tip | sore spot | notice |
| take in | itch | distinguish |
| overhear | creeps | recognize |
| register | sting | imagine |
| reach | thrill | catch sight of |
| listening | tingle | take in |
| hearsay | shudder | look |

According to the NLP communication model, most people's speech reflects a preference for one of three sensory categories. The lists above suggest typical word choices in each group.

From Knowles, RD. (1983). Building rapport through neurolinguistic programming AJN, 1011–1014. Reprinted with permission.

*Empathy.* The use of good communication skills, active listening, and the techniques of pacing and using representational systems all help the nurse develop empathy with the client. *Empathy* refers to the ability to relate to another person at a feeling level with a deep understanding of the other's experience, without losing the perspective of one's individuality. Empathy is often differentiated from sympathy in which the individual reacts from the standpoint of past personal experiences, rather than trying to see the situation through the other person's eyes.

Ehmann (1971) has described four steps in the process of empathy. The first is identification. During this stage, the nurse becomes open to the other person's feelings by focusing on the verbal and nonverbal messages that are being received. The second step is incorporation. At this point, the nurse internalizes the feelings of the other person, while not taking ownership of them. At the third step, reverberation, the nurse compares the perceived experience of the client with past personal experiences and the feelings that were associated with them. Detachment is the last step. The nurse moves back from the internal process and is able to share the perception that resulted with the client. Kalisch (1973) has developed an assessment tool that allows the nurse to evaluate the level of empathic response to a client (Table 14-2). Self-evaluation of this skill will help the nurse improve the ability to communicate meaningfully with clients.

*Trust.* Purposeful application of all the techniques of communication will assist the nurse to work productively with the client toward goal achievement. It will also help the nurse establish trust as a solid foundation for the relationship. *Trust* is basic to the success of all human relationships, beginning with the maternal-infant bond. Trust does not happen

❖ **Table 14-2**
The nurse-patient empathic function scale: a schematic presentation

| | Level of patient's feelings | |
|---|---|---|
| **Categories of nurse empathic functioning** | **Conspicuous current feelings** | **Hidden current feelings** |
| 0 | Ignores. | Ignores. |
| 1 | Communicates an awareness that is accurate at times and inaccurate at other times. | Ignores. |
| 2 | Communicates a complete and accurate awareness of the essence and strength of feeling. | Communicates an awareness of the presence of hidden feelings but is not accurate in defining their essence or strength; an effort is being made to understand. |
| 3 | Same as category 2. | Communicates an accurate awareness of the hidden feelings slightly beyond what the client expresses himself. |
| 4 | Same as category 2. | Communicates without uncertainty an accurate awareness of the deepest, most hidden feelings. |

From Kalisch, B: What is empathy? Copyright © 1973, American Journal of Nursing Company. Reproduced with permission from the American Journal of Nursing, September, Vol 73 No 9.

automatically. The nurse needs to work to build trust. An important element of trust is reliability. This refers to carrying out promises, to responding to requests promptly, and to keeping appointments. Another component of trust is honesty. Questions should be answered clearly and completely. If the nurse is unsure of the answer to a client's question, this should be communicated. The nurse then finds the correct information and provides it to the client as soon as possible.

Proper management of confidential information is also important to the maintenance of trust. Any information that is given to the nurse in the context of the professional relationship is confidential. This means that it may not be shared with anyone who is not directly involved in the client's health care. This should be explained to the client. It may also be necessary to tell the client that the nurse is obligated to communicate pertinent information to other members of the health care team. An element of judgment related to confidentiality is required. Clients sometimes give nurses information that is not relevant to the immediate health care problem. The nurse must decide whether it is in the client's best interest to share that information with other team members. For instance, a person who is being treated for stable diabetes may mention marital discord. The nurse may be concerned that the added stress could cause the diabetes to become uncontrolled. In this case, it would be appropriate to inform the client that the nurse plans to share this information with the physician. On the other hand, the nurse could assess that the problem appeared to be transient and not particularly stressful. Then the nurse might decide not to share the information at that time. A good rule is, "When in doubt, communicate." All members of the health care team are bound by rules of confidentiality and a code of ethical behavior. The nurse should be particularly wary of a client's request to keep a secret as a condition for giving information. If the client

shares information that is critical for the provision of safe health care, the nurse must communicate it to colleagues. Examples of such situations are threats of suicide or confessions of failure to take prescribed medications. The nurse should respond to requests for secrecy by explaining the need to be sure that the client receives safe care and that the nurse must be free to take whatever action is needed to ensure safety.

The trusting relationship with a nurse will help the client have a positive experience with the health care system. The maintenance phase of the relationship continues until the goals are accomplished or other conditions require termination. Examples of other conditions include discharge of the client from the health care agency, completion of a student learning experience, and resignation of the nurse from the agency.

As the nurse practices good communication skills, proficiency will increase and interactions with clients will become more rewarding. As health care becomes more technological and people feel more alienated, the need for caring relationships will increase. It is up to nurses to make sure that the health care system continues to be a caring system.

**Termination.** The last phase of the helping relationship is *termination.* Ideally, this occurs when the nurse-client goals have been accomplished and both participants feel satisfied with the outcome. However, the reality of the health care system is that sometimes termination must take place before goal accomplishment is completed. When this is the case, it is important to help the client identify additional resources for continued assistance. *Summarizing* the accomplishments of the relationship helps to identify the work that has been done and what needs to be done. Both the nurse and the client should contribute to the summary. This can also be an excellent learning experience for the nurse in terms of the success or failure of past interventions.

When two people terminate a meaningful relationship, it helps to be able to envision the other person in the future. It can be a time of sharing future plans. For instance, if the relationship is ending because of the end of a student experience, the client may like to know what experience the student will have next; or if graduating, what the student's job plans are. If a client is being discharged from the health care setting, it can be reassuring to know that the familiar staff will still be there if a problem recurs.

Sometimes clients wish to give the nurse a remembrance of the relationship. Most health care agencies prohibit the acceptance of gifts or gratuities from clients. The nurse needs to evaluate these offerings in the context of the relationship. If the client asks the nurse to accept a small token of little monetary value, such as a handmade trinket, it may be thoughtful to accept. It is even better if the nurse has anticipated this event and is prepared to reciprocate. Items of value should never be given or received in a professional relationship. Also, the nurse must be careful not to use the giving of gifts to avoid confronting the feelings associated with termination of a relationship.

The ending of a close relationship can be difficult for both the client and the nurse. Terminations serve as reminders of past losses, and feelings associated with those losses may be reexperienced, especially if they were not resolved at the time. The nurse needs to analyze personal responses to termination in order to prevent interference with the helping relationship. It can be very helpful to clients to assist them to express their feelings in the context of termination and to learn to resolve feelings that may have been troublesome in the past. Anger is a feeling that is expected to accompany termination. It is frequently expressed indirectly by missing appointments or refusing to interact. If the nurse is alert to signs of anger, it can be

acknowledged, accepted, and the nurse and client can move on to sharing the positive feelings they have for each other. Sadness is also typical of partings. The nurse may be able to facilitate the client's expression of sadness by sharing personal feelings. In this case, the nurse's goal is not to receive help from the client in handling feelings, but to demonstrate that the relationship was meaningful and sadness is appropriate. Mutual expression of sadness often leads to sharing of the caring feelings that have developed between the nurse and the client. When a relationship has been terminated successfully, the participants will be left with feelings of warmth for each other and nostalgia for the relationship.

## ❖ PROFESSIONAL COMMUNICATIONS

The professional relationship is unlike other relationships in life. Expectations of the participants are unequal. The client expects that the nurse will assume responsibility for the progress of the relationship. The nurse expects the client to participate in directing the goals of the relationship as much as possible, but realizes that the primary responsibility rests with the nurse. Meetings are planned, formalized, and goal-directed. The relationship itself is time-limited and termination is final. The promise, actual or implied, of continuation of the relationship after termination is unfair to the client because it blocks addressing the experience of loss. Participation is also not equal at the feeling level. Nurses encourage clients to share their most personal feelings and help them to learn to manage personal problems. The nurse, however, must find other resources for dealing with personal difficulties.

Because of the uniqueness of the professional relationship, an ongoing supervisory relationship with an experienced nurse colleague is highly advisable. The supervisor can help the nurse to analyze interactions and to identify the influence of personal needs and feelings on the nurse-client relationship. Peer supervision, with or without a designated group leader, can be very helpful for experienced nurses. The supervisory relationship is based on the same principles of trust and confidentiality as the nurse-client relationship.

## ❖ COMMUNICATIONS RESEARCH

Communications and nurse-client interaction are fertile areas for nursing research. This is also a complex area of research. Descriptive research may assist with identification of the structural components of communication. Examples of this type of study include the work that has been done by Birdwhistell (1970) in kinesics and by Hall (1959) in the use of personal space. Experimental studies in the application of communication theory are much more difficult to design. It is difficult to isolate the effect of a particular intervention when the client is being exposed to multiple health care providers and multiple therapeutic approaches, as well as interactions with relatives and friends. However, it is possible to find examples of research that has been completed and is useful in understanding the characteristics of communication and the helping relationship.

Extensive relationship research has been conducted by Carkhuff, Truax, and their associates (1967, 1969). They identified the core dimensions of the helping relationship. These include accurate empathy, nonpossessive warmth, and genuineness. Aiken and Aiken (1973) built upon this work related to the nurse-client relationship. They identified the dimensions of empathic understanding, positive regard, genuineness, and concreteness or specificity of expression. Nursing research has investigated the characteristics of empathy in the context of the nurse-client relationship. For example, Stotland and Mathews (1978) explored the relationship between ability to empathize and the amount of time spent with clients by nursing students. They found that early in the

semester, the highly empathic students spent less time with clients than the other students did. They hypothesized that this was related to the empathic students' awareness of the disparity between the relationship needs of the clients and their ability to meet those needs. As they grew in confidence, they spent more time with the clients. Other nursing studies have been conducted by Williams (1979) who investigated the relationship between empathic communication and self-concept and by Mansfield (1973) who looked at the verbal and nonverbal communication of empathy. Wheeler (1988) has published a summary of research on the subject of empathy. She emphasizes the need for a unified conceptual model.

Other nurses have investigated other aspects of communication. Topf (1988) provides a model for studying communication characteristics and developing an assessment tool for nurses. Smith and Cantrell (1988) have explored the concept of distance in the nurse-client relationship. They applied the personal space theories developed by Hall and added the concept of "verbal distance," which has to do with the intrusiveness of the interaction. They found that physical distance was only anxiety-provoking when accompanied by verbal intrusiveness. This was the case for all distances. These examples demonstrate the real need for nurses to investigate other aspects of relationships and communication between nurses and clients. Increased knowledge about these elements of nursing practice will assist nurses to base more of their interventions on theory rather than intuition.

## ❖ SUMMARY

This chapter explored the nature of communication as it relates to the therapeutic nurse-client relationship. Levels of communication were discussed and the structure of communication was described. Characteristics of a helping relationship as listed by Rogers were presented. Samples of theories of communication included transactional analysis and the work of Milton Erickson. The concepts of anxiety, anger, and caring were discussed as they relate to the nurse-client relationship.

The phases of the nurse-client relationship were explored and characteristics of the professional relationship were examined. Supervision was recommended as a way to identify areas of personal conflict that may interfere with interaction with clients. Some examples of research related to communication and the helping relationship were presented, and the need for more nursing research on nurse-client communication was identified.

## ❖ APPLYING KNOWLEDGE TO PRACTICE

1. Compare and contrast the similarities and differences between your relationships with a close relative, a close friend, a casual acquaintance, a colleague at work or school, and a client. Consider the parameters of interpersonal closeness, openness, equality, responsibility, and anticipated duration.

2. Describe the nursing actions that you initiated in your last client contact that would support the development of trust. Did you do anything that would inhibit the development of trust?

3. It might be said that some therapeutic communication techniques, such as reflecting, restating, mirroring, and pacing, are contrived and manipulative. Do you agree or disagree? Support your opinion with examples.

4. Using theories of communication presented in this chapter, analyze the following interaction. If you think that the nurse has made a response that is nontherapeutic, substitute a therapeutic one.

   Situation: The client has come to the emergency room complaining of "pain in my head." The emergency room is very busy, with recent admissions of four victims of a serious automobile accident and two people with gunshot wounds. Two staff members called in sick. One was replaced with a nurse who had never worked in the E.R. The other was not replaced.

   Nurse (looking at the admission sheet): "I see you have a headache."
   Client: (softly) "I feel awful."
   Nurse: "How long have you had this headache?"
   Client: "I can't stand this feeling any longer."
   Nurse: (sounding impatient) "I can't help you if you don't tell me about your headache."
   Client: "What?"
   Nurse: (loudly) "You have to tell me about your headache."
   Client: (looks puzzled) "What headache?"
   Nurse: "It says here that you have a pain in your head."
   Client: "I guess you could call it that. I said my head was bothering me. I was dizzy and I fell down and hit my head on a table. It *does* hurt where I hit it."
   Nurse: "I think we need to start over. Tell me how you're feeling."

*Continued.*

❖ **APPLYING KNOWLEDGE TO PRACTICE—cont'd**

**5.** Analyze the following interaction using concepts of transactional analysis and neurolinguistic programming.

Client: "My foot feels funny."
Nurse: "It looks all right to me."
Client: "Why do you nurses always brush me off?"

Nurse: "I'm not sure I see what your problem is."
Client: "You're supposed to make me feel good. I don't feel good. Make me feel better."
Nurse: "You have to help us help you."

## REFERENCES

Aiken, L., & Aiken, J. (1973). A systematic approach to evaluation of interpersonal relationships. *American Journal of Nursing*; 73, 863.

Berne, E. (1964). *Games People Play*. New York: Grove Press, Inc.

Berne, E. (1970). *What Do You Say After You Say Hello?* New York: Grove Press, Inc.

Birdwhistell, R. (1970). *Kinesics and Context*. Philadelphia: University of Pennsylvania Press.

Carkhuff, R. (1969). *Helping and Human Relations, Volumes I and II*. New York: Holt, Rinehart and Winston.

Carkhuff, R. & Truax, C. (1967). *Toward Effective Counseling and Psychotherapy*. Chicago: Aldine Publishing Co.

Ehmann, V. (1971). Empathy: Its origin, characteristics, and process. *Perspectives in Psychiatric Care*; 9(2), 77.

Forchuk, C. & Brown, B. (1989). Establishing a nurse-client relationship. *Journal of Psychosocial Nursing and Mental Health Services* 27(2),30.

Hall, E. (1959). *The Silent Language*. Garden City, New York: Doubleday & Co.

Kalisch, B. (1973). What is empathy? *American Journal of Nursing* 73, 1548.

King, M., Novik, L., & Citrenbaum, C. (1983). *Irresistible Communication: Creative Skills for the Health Professional*. Philadelphia: W. B. Saunders Company.

Knowles, R. D. (1983). Building rapport through neurolinguistic programming. *American Journal of Nursing* 83(7), 1011–1014.

Lankton, C. H. (1985). Elements of an Ericksonian approach. In S. R. Lankton (Ed.), *Elements and Dimensions of an Ericksonian Approach*. New York: Brunner/Mazel Publishers.

Mansfield, E. (1973). Empathy: Concept and identified psy-

chiatric nursing behavior. *Nursing Research*, 22, 525.

Nightingale, F. (1859). *Notes on Nursing*. London: Harrison and Sons.

Peplau, H. (1952). *Interpersonal Relations in Nursing*. New York: G. P. Putnam's Sons.

Rogers, C. R. (1961). *On Becoming A Person*. Boston: Houghton Mifflin Co.

Ruesch, J. (1972). *Disturbed Communication*. New York: W. W. Norton & Co., Inc.

Ruesch, J. and Kees, W. (1956). *Nonverbal Communication*. Los Angeles: University of California Press.

Smith, B. J. & Cantrell, P. J. (1988). Distance in nurse-patient encounters. *Journal of Psychosocial Nursing and Mental Health Services* 26(2), 22.

Stotland, E., Mathews, K. E. Jr., Sherman, S. E., Hansson, R. O., & Richardson, B. Z. (1978). *Empathy, Fantasy, and Helping*. Beverly Hills, California: Sage Publications.

Sundeen, S. J., Stuart, G. W., Rankin, E. D., & Cohen, S. P. (1989). *Nurse-Client Interaction: Implementing the Nursing Process*, (4th ed.) St. Louis: The C. V. Mosby Co.

Topf, M. (1988). Verbal interpersonal responsiveness. *Journal of Psychosocial Nursing and Mental Health Services* 26(7), 8.

Watzlawick, P., Beavin, J., & Jackson, D. (1967). *Pragmatics of Human Communication; A Study of Interactional Patterns, Pathologies, and Paradoxes*. New York: W. W. Norton & Co., Inc.

Williams, C. (1979). Empathic communication and its effect on client outcome. *Issues in Mental Health Nursing* 2(1), 16.

Wheeler, K. (1988). A nursing science approach to understanding empathy. *Archives of Psychiatric Nursing*. 2, 95.

# 15 Teaching and Learning

**Mary Ann Gniady Wilkinson**

## OBJECTIVES

*At the completion of this chapter, the reader will be able to:*

◆ Compare and contrast different frameworks for learning.

◆ Identify characteristics of learners across the life span and develop appropriate teaching strategies for each group.

◆ Formulate a list of behaviors and activities necessary for successful teaching.

Teaching is an essential part of professional nursing practice. Not only is teaching mandated by nurse practice acts and professional competencies (DeBack, 1987), but it is also recognized by nurses themselves as an important aspect of nursing practice (Honan, Krsnak, Peterson, & Torkelson, 1988). Nurses may believe they know how to teach, but research indicates that both new and experienced nurses perform poorly in this area (McClosky, 1983; McClosky & McCain, 1984, 1987, 1988). One factor influencing the nurse's ability to teach is a lack of knowledge of teaching and learning techniques (Murdaugh, 1980; Faulkner, 1983). Although most nursing programs include teaching and learning content in their curricula, it is often delegated to a few hours of lecture and assigned readings. Unless additional courses are taken or graduate study is pursued, the nurse becomes a self-taught teacher. When they are offered the opportunity, however, registered nurses readily participate in research that includes training in teaching techniques (Wilkinson, 1988).

This chapter is designed to enhance the existing skills of experienced practitioners by exploring teaching and learning principles and applying them to practical situations.

## ❖ THEORETICAL FRAMEWORKS FOR LEARNING

Any attempt to discuss teaching must also explore learning. Learning is the expected outcome of teaching, the change that results from gaining new knowledge, skills, or attitudes. Each of the three major classifications of learning theories (behaviorist, cognitive, and humanistic) identifies change as a critical outcome of the learning process, but each has different explanations regarding why or how the change occurs.

### Behaviorist Theory

Behaviorists explain that change results from conditioning and is closely linked to physical response. Given a stimulus (which is external and environmental), the individual responds in a manner that can be seen and measured. Thus the learner reaches the correct response through trial and error. Reinforcement is used to increase the frequency and consistency of the correct response. This stimulus-response sequence is referred to as *conditioning*.

Both positive and negative reinforcement result in a physical response. Positive reinforcement influences learning and can be adjusted until the learner performs as desired. This changing learner response is known as *shaping*. The amount, timing, and frequency of the positive reward are important for changing behavior in the desired direction. Conversely,

negative behavior can be extinguished by withholding reinforcement or substituting a positive response for the negative behavior through *counterconditioning*. Learning can be measured by the resulting observable behavioral change.

Modeling theory is an application of these behaviorist principles. In *modeling*, the learner observes the new behavior and the resulting consequences. The learner then models the behavior to gain the same reward. The result, attained through repeated practice, is the internalization and personalization of the behavior. Table 15-1 summarizes the learning principles and teaching applications relative to behaviorist theory.

 **Table 15-1**
Behaviorism

### MAJOR THEORIES AND THEORISTS

| | |
|---|---|
| Connectionism | E. L. Thorndike |
| Stimulus-response | I. Pavlov |
| Operant conditioning | B. F. Skinner |
| Stimulus substitution | J. Wolpe |
| Modeling | A. Bandura |

| Learning principle | Teaching application |
|---|---|
| Humans learn through trial and error. | Provide opportunity for problem solving. |
| Learning develops over time. | Provide adequate practice time. Plan retesting or repeat demonstrations both immediately and at later intervals. |
| Given a stimulus, the learner responds. | Plan teaching strategies to trigger the desired response. Avoid unnecessary information that may detract from the desired response. |
| Positive and negative feedback influence learning; positive feedback is remembered longer. | Reward the learner for all correct behavior; praising positive behavior is better than punishing mistakes. |
| Learning is strengthened each time a positive response is received or a negative consequence is avoided. | Continue praise and positive reinforcement throughout the teaching transaction. |
| Learning occurs through linking the behavior with the associated response. | Proceed from simple to complex; provide information to show that learning is occurring. |
| Learning remains until other learning interferes with the original learned response. | Assess prior experience with the subject; some "unlearning" may be needed before new learning can take place. |

## Cognitive Theory

While behaviorist theory is based on observed change to validate learning, cognitive theory relates learning to an internal change in perception, which is not as obvious or measurable. A basic tenet of cognitive theorists is that learning relates to the information processing ability of the individual who receives information from the environment in different ways.

Early cognitive research demonstrated that children are motivated to learn in order to make sense of what they see in their environment. Children progress through predictable stages of cognitive development. Piaget (1954) identified stages of cognitive development that reflect a child's qualitative ability to relate to the world and thus organize information for learning. Children take in information through *assimilation,* modify the information to fit their individual understanding by *accommodation,* seek an intellectual balance or *equilibrium,* and finally merge reflex and cognitive pro-

cesses. Mastering words and their meaning are the most important cognitive tasks of children from birth to 2 years in the *sensorimotor stage* of development. Sensory impressions and motor actions are most involved in the learning process for children between the ages of 2 and 7, the *preoperational stage.* Higher learning, including the ability to reason and distinguish reality, occurs between the ages of 7 and 11 years during the *concrete operation stage.* Adolescents, ages 11 to 14 years, develop the ability to become logical as well as abstract thinkers capable of forming their own values during the *formal operational stage.* Gagne (1974) developed principles for teaching children based on the cognitive principles of building simple and complex skills. Determining meaning from perceptions is the basis for cognitive theory.

*Gestalt,* a type of affective learning, is categorized as cognitive learning. Affective learning deals with the personal, social, or emotional patterns of adjustment. Feelings, emotions, in-

---

   **Table 15-2**
Cognitive

### MAJOR THEORIES AND THEORISTS

| | |
|---|---|
| Cognitive discovery | J. Piaget |
| Field theory | K. Lewin |
| Information processing theory | R. Gagne |
| Hierarchal structure | B. Bloom |

| Learning principle | Teaching application |
|---|---|
| Learning is based on a change of perception. | All learning cannot be readily observed; information must be internalized. |
| Perception is influenced by the senses. | Use multisensory teaching strategies. Adjust environment to minimize distractions. |
| Perception is dependent upon learning and is influenced by both internal and external variables. | Assess attitude toward learning, past experiences with similar situations, culture, maturity, developmental level, and physical ability before designing teaching plan. |
| Personal characteristics have an impact on how a cue is perceived. | Identify learning style and target it in the teaching process; develop a flexible approach. |
| Perceptions are selectively chosen to be focused on by the individual. | Focus the learner on what is to be learned; provide support and guidance. |

terests, and attitudes are part of the affective domain. Cognitive behaviors are generally accompanied by affective behaviors. Gestalt, from the German word for *organization,* relates to analyzing learning as a whole, not looking at individual parts. Gestaltists assert that an individual's perceptions are influenced by a number of positive and negative factors in the past and present. Individuals strive for balance and equilibrium. When something is unknown, a state of disequilibrium results. An individual's motivation to learn is the result of an attempt to restore order and balance to his or her perceptual field.

Bloom (1956) divided cognitive learning into six levels: knowledge, comprehension, application, analysis, synthesis, and evaluation. His work further identified specific language to use when writing behavioral objectives for each category. Table 15-2 summarizes cognitive theory.

## Humanistic Theory

The humanist sees learning as an integrated process involving both cognitive and affective areas. The individual is believed to be self-motivated toward achieving full potential and seeking experiences toward that goal: learning is self-motivated, self-directed, and self-evaluated. Each person is viewed as a unique composite of biological, psychological, social, cultural, and spiritual factors.

Learning focuses on self-development and achieving full potential. The teacher provides information to assist in the process of increasing cognitive and affective functioning. The learner is supported during the interaction to not only gain skills and knowledge, but also to enjoy the process. The goal of teaching is to produce individuals who reach their full potential and develop a positive self-concept from the learning process. Table 15-3 lists humanist theorists, basic principles, and teaching applications.

All three theoretical approaches can be used to guide the teaching and learning process. For example, in teaching a manual skill,

**Table 15-3**
Humanistic

### MAJOR THEORIES AND THEORISTS

| | |
|---|---|
| Self-directed learning | C. Rogers |
| Hierarchy of needs | A. Maslow |
| Perceptual-existential theory | A. Combs |
| Values clarification | J. Dewey |
| Reality theory | W. Glasser |
| Andragogy | M. Knowles |

| Learning principle | Teaching application |
|---|---|
| Learning is self-initiated. | Promote self-directed learning. |
| The learner is an active participant in the teaching-learning transaction. | Serve as a facilitator, mentor, and resource for the learner to encourage active learning. |
| Learning should promote the development of insight, judgment, values, and self-concept. | Avoid imposing own values and views on the learner; support development of learner's self-concept. |
| Learning proceeds best if it is relevant to the learner. | Expose the learner to new, necessary information; pose relevant questions to encourage the learner to seek answers. |

such as how to change a dressing, all three approaches might be necessary. The behaviorist approach would be useful in teaching the psychomotor skills necessary to perform the task and to correctly repeat the demonstration. The cognitive approach would be useful if the learner recalled past injuries or infections as a way to understand the concept of asepsis. Humanistic learning might be involved if the experience is used to build curiosity about health care and healing. Nurses can facilitate learning by understanding the different approaches and applying the principles in planning and directing learning.

The following section illustrates teaching techniques for learners of different ages and abilities who have varying health needs.

## ❖ TEACHING

Teaching is a set of planned, purposeful activities that assists the learner. Teaching success is measured by the change demonstrated by the learner, such as acquisition of new knowledge, attitudes, or skills. Thus, teaching activities will change according to the needs of the learner. Supporting, guiding, directing, demonstrating, facilitating, correcting, communicating, caring, evaluating, and praising are among the many terms that can be used to describe teaching activities. As described in the following sections, selecting the appropriate teaching technique is dependent in part on the characteristics of the learner.

### Pedagogy

The art and science of teaching children is called *pedagogy*. When teaching children, methods, implementation, and evaluation are generally initiated by the teacher. Planning appropriate educational programs for children requires the nurse's understanding of growth and development and age-appropriate expectations. As a general rule, the younger the child, the

simpler the teaching technique should be. Since children have a short attention span, teaching should be creatively planned to hold their interest. Because children learn primarily through their senses, successful teaching is directed toward the psychomotor and cognitive domains.

Since learning involves change, some children may be fearful. This may be a special concern if the child has no previous experience with which to link the new information. Thus it is important for the teacher to provide security so the child feels comfortable enough to learn.

### Nursing applications: strategies for teaching children

**Infants and very young children.** The age and developmental stage of the child influences the selection of teaching techniques. It is most difficult for health professionals to teach infants and very young children who have not yet developed language skills. Nonverbal communication can be a most effective teaching strategy for this age group. The use of touch and a soothing tone of voice are examples of techniques that can convey the meaning of safety and security to very young children. Frequent reinforcement is a critical and effective technique for this age group.

**Toddlers and preschoolers.** Some additional techniques are available for use with toddlers and preschool children. This age group most often learns through play, exploration, and observation. The following example describes the use of these techniques:

Puppets were used to prepare a preschool class for the arrival of a handicapped student. With the goal of teaching to allay anxiety and fear of the unknown, simple puppets were constructed to represent the teacher, class members, and the handicapped child. The handicapped puppet was equipped with glasses, leg braces, and a wheelchair. A ten-minute puppet show was presented to illustrate common fears and misconceptions about the handicapped. Simple language was used, and new terms were defined. The script included a question and answer session between the children puppets and the handicapped puppet. Following the puppet show, the children were invited to play with the puppets and were encouraged to ask questions of their own. The next day, the handicapped child came to school and was readily accepted by the group.

Analysis of this teaching-learning situation illustrates Gagne's (1974) eight component functions of the instructional situation:

1. Presenting the stimulus: puppets were used to provide a multisensory approach.
2. Directing attention and other learner activities: the puppets provided sudden, vivid stimulation and the children's attention was focused using verbal directions.
3. Providing a model for terminal performance: puppets served as models, illustrating how to touch, talk to, and play with the handicapped child.
4. Furnishing external prompts: puppets provided information about the handicapped child.
5. Guiding the direction of thinking: the script included questions and answers to guide the children's thoughts, presenting accurate information, and correcting false beliefs.
6. Inducing the transfer of knowledge: the class asked questions of the puppets and transferred this information to their interaction with the handicapped child.
7. Assessing learning attainment: this was accomplished by observing the students' interaction with their handicapped classmate and assessing their behavior.
8. Providing feedback: the question and answer session provided immediate feedback.

**School-aged children.** School-aged children have a larger vocabulary and greater repertoire of skills and abilities than do preschoolers. Children advance from the intuitive cognitive process of 6- to 7-year-olds to the ability to reason, see another's point of view, and solve problems by age 10 (Piaget, 1954). They can learn through formal teaching inter-

actions and through play. Attention span, while still short, increases as the child gets older. Younger, school-aged children enjoy coloring, creating, handling objects, and asking questions. Older children can understand more abstract ideas, have begun to develop value systems, and benefit in both formal and informal situations from selective behavioristic, cognitive, and humanistic teaching strategies. The following example illustrates a nutrition lesson plan, integrated across subject areas, with appropriate modifications based on the age of the child.

The class' knowledge of nutrition can be assessed by administering a simple nutrition quiz on the five basic food groups. Compensate for different reading levels by putting the test in different forms. Younger children can answer verbal questions by circling pictures on an answer sheet, and older children can use the multiple choice or a fill-in-the-blank format. Interest in the topic can be stimulated by having the children keep a diary of all food eaten during a 24-hour period. Parental involvement is needed to help younger children with this activity, while older children can work independently. The teacher can analyze the individual food diaries and provide relevant feedback. For instance, pictures or written descriptions can be used to illustrate the long-term implications of continuing the nutritional pattern shown in the diary into adulthood. Choosing appropriate slang can be humorous yet effective with older children.

Once individuals have been given feedback, group learning can be reinforced across various subject areas of the curriculum. For example, teaching about nutrition can be integrated with mathematics. Using a small scale and pictures of food attached to washers of different weights can illustrate what foods need to be chosen to balance the scale for a normal size child. Too many choices would tip the scale for an overweight child, too few for an underweight child. Nutrition can be incorporated into science by showing, for example, the mineral composition of healthy bones or by analyzing the fat content of foods.

**Adolescents.** Adolescents present further challenges to health care professionals. They are struggling for their identity and are strongly influenced by their peers. Teenagers, bolstered by their feeling of immortality, are falsely self-confident and tend to depersonalize threats. Often resistant to traditional teaching techniques, they demand of the teacher both creativity and respect for their growing intelligence. Consider the following example of teaching about sexually transmitted diseases to a group of adolescents in a job training facility.

A series of posters was developed on common sexually transmitted diseases, which included lists of symptoms, long-term effects, treatment, and prevention. Simple, straightforward language and colorful pictures were used. The posters were displayed in the hallway outside the cafeteria where students waited for their meals. Students were encouraged to seek further information from the health nurse during their routine health maintenance visits. As a result, students began to report their symptoms earlier, and many referred their sexual partners for health screening. Condoms, birth control pills, and information were freely available, and an increased demand for them was observed.

The previous example illustrates an effective teaching technique that allows adolescents to determine the timing and relevance of teaching to their own situation. Learning was facilitated through continuous reinforcement, since the adolescents passed the posters each day on their way to meals. The invitation to seek further information during individual health maintenance visits provided the opportunity for privacy and individual discussion of unique needs and concerns.

## Andragogy

Malcolm Knowles is recognized as the father of adult education theory—*andragogy*. According to Knowles (1984), the adult learner is motivated by the desire for self-growth and self-direction. Five characteristics of adult learners are identified:

1. Adults are motivated to learn as they experience needs they want to satisfy and interests they want to pursue. These needs become the basis for teaching adults.
2. An adult's orientation to learning is life-centered. This means that learning must be perceived as relevant and practical.
3. Experience is a rich resource for adults. Effective education of adults, therefore, builds on the individual's past experience.
4. Adults are self-directing. The teacher role is one of facilitator, encouraging mutual inquiry.
5. With age, individual characteristics emerge that require special consideration. Thus, the effective teacher provides for differences in style, time, place, and rate of learning.

Given these characteristics, consider the following principles for effective teaching of adults:

1. Involve learners in planning, carrying out, and evaluating their own learning.
2. Build new knowledge on the base of the learner's past experience.
3. Center learning experiences around real-life situations.
4. Treat mistakes as occasions for learning.
5. Help individuals identify their own needs for self-improvement.
6. Build self-satisfaction by providing immediate opportunities to practice new learning.

### Nursing applications: strategies for teaching adults

Teaching begins with establishing a therapeutic relationship through the process of gaining trust and acceptance and establishing rapport. Part of the trust a client feels toward the nurse is based on the belief that the nurse is a competent professional. Using the personal approach when communicating with the client builds further trust. Rapport can be quickly established and maintained by focusing verbal and nonverbal behavior on the client. This may be accomplished by formulating responses of empathy in a language and manner that is most easily understood by the client. Specific techniques that are useful include the following: using a tone of voice, rate, and volume of speech similar to the client's; mirroring the client's posture; and using his or her significant gestures when responding (Knowles, 1983).

Since adults learn in different ways, it is important to identify the client's preferred sensory channel (i.e., auditory, kinesthetic, or visual) for receiving and retaining information. Sensory channel preference can be determined by simple questioning and listening to the client's choice of words when he or she is discussing past learning experiences. Spoken language is the clue to identifying the preferred sensory channel. Listen for language that indicates whether the client is using the visual, auditory, or kinesthetic sense. Identifying and using the client's preferred sensory channel individualizes instruction and may increase learning (Van Hoozier, 1987). Teachers also have their own preference and tend to teach accordingly (Jonassen, 1981). However, selected teaching techniques, such as verbal instruction, can be individualized by choosing words directed toward the client's preferred sensory channel. Examples of sensory-based vocabulary that can be used to determine a client's preferred sense and to present information to different types of learners are listed in Chapter 14.

Personalized communication and use of the client's preferred sensory channel is illustrated in the following example.

In this situation, the goal was to teach simple, stress-reduction techniques to a busy, young, professional woman. The interview was conducted with the nurse sitting opposite the client. The nurse observed the client's posture and slowly adjusted her own so that they were in mirror positions. During assessment questioning, the nurse matched the client's voice tone, tempo, and volume. In addition, the nurse used the client's key words with the same tone, emphasis, and gestures when restating information.

After identifying that a major source of stress was the client's troubled relationship with her employer, the nurse attempted to assess and validate the client's preferred sensory channel. This was accomplished by asking: "Can you describe a work situation that was stressful?" The word "describe" was selected to prompt the client to provide cues to the preferred sense. The italicized words in the client's response show that this person is most influenced by the kinesthetic or feeling sense.

"Yesterday, I was very busy *sitting* at my desk *working* on a project that I *felt* was really important. My boss *walks* up and starts to interrupt me. He wants me to *go* to a meeting for him. He *thinks it will be good for me.* I *think* he's just trying to *weasel* out of it and knows he can *pressure* me into *going.* Then I *feel rushed,* I *can't concentrate,* my chest *feels tight,* I get a *headache.* I wish I could *wring his neck,* instead I just *smile and go.*"

When the client said "wring his neck," the nurse noticed that she used a hand gesture to exemplify wringing out something. This significant gesture and phrase then was used in summary when the nurse related her understanding of the relationship. She restated her conclusions using kinesthetic words:

I get the *feeling* that you may be *frustrated* by not being able to do your *work* because your boss *interferes.* This makes you *feel bad.* Instead of *"wringing his neck,"* there are several things you can *do* to help you control that stress and *feel better.*

When the nurse repeated this information, the client listened intently and nodded in agreement when the conclusion was made, thus validating that the nurse's opinions were congruent with the learner's. Teaching then progressed using kinesthetic or feeling terminology whenever possible. Verbal instructions were given simultaneously with demonstrations and return demonstrations of the relaxation techniques. In this situation, the client was taught exercises, including deep breathing and progressive muscle relaxation rather than imaging techniques that are more helpful for visual learners. In contrast, the person who is auditory might respond better to stress reduction involving listening to soothing music or relaxation tapes.

## Teaching special groups

***Culturally diverse groups.*** Immigrants to the United States present special teaching challenges because of language and cultural differences. As the United States' population becomes more diverse, it is important to learn more about the beliefs and behaviors of specific cultural groups to help assess teaching and learning needs and the level of understanding. For example, in some cultures, personal disclosure may be difficult, and members may not comfortably answer sensitive questions such as those on marital problems or sexual functioning. In other cultural groups where it is important to "save face," clients may not admit a lack of understanding. Clients from some cultural groups may be reluctant to ask questions in fear that they may appear to challenge authority. Finally, it is important to remember that people's ability to speak the language does not necessarily correlate with their intellectual ability or with the amount of information they understand.

Several strategies may be adopted to facilitate the teaching and learning process with clients who have a limited ability to speak or understand English (see the box that follows).

Instructions should be given by speaking slowly and clearly, using normal volume. Inflection and tone of voice should at first be calm and relaxed; later, inflection and tone can be varied for particular emphasis. Simple, concrete words, combined skillfully with gestures and pictures, will also assist the learner. Important information should be repeated several times and in different ways, while avoiding slang expressions and jargon. In addition, nurses working with clients who have a language barrier need to ensure that written materials and pamphlets are available in whatever languages their clients speak and read. Ongoing evaluation of teaching and learning effectiveness may be accomplished by frequently validating the learner's understanding.

***Low literacy adults.*** An additional consideration in planning teaching activities is the client's ability to read written materials. It is estimated that many American citizens are at a tenth grade literacy level, and 20% of the population are estimated to read at the fifth grade level (Bartlett, 1984). Pamphlets and educational materials are useful only if they are understood by the learner. Rorden (1987) and Redman (1988) offer several formulas to assess

❖ **TEACHING STRATEGIES FOR CLIENTS WITH A LANGUAGE BARRIER**

**WHEN SPEAKING**
1. Use simple, concrete language; use pauses for emphasis. Consider the language level of the client. Attempt to keep all words below three syllables.

**ON VISUAL AIDS**
2. Keep sentences short using simple, concrete, laymen's terminology. This limits the amount of information the learner has to focus on at one time and makes passages easier to read.
3. Use a sequential organization layout. Beginning with simple concepts and progressing to more complex ideas allows the learner time to assimilate and build on previous knowledge. Spacing and numbering may help focus the reader.
4. Include pictures to illustrate and help hold interest. Figures such as the simple international sign symbols are easy to draw and can be used effectively to illustrate health teaching. A simple picture vocabulary can be created to show signs and symptoms, do's, and don'ts. Clocks can show times for medication dosages.

the reading level of printed materials. In addition, there are several strategies to determine the reading ability of a particular client. Before making this assessment, however, it is important to recognize that reading difficulty might be a sensitive topic, and the client may be ashamed to admit his or her inability to read. Many people have successfully hidden this limitation by memorizing signs and symbols or stating that their reading glasses are elsewhere. Some indicators of reading ability can be determined by obtaining information regarding the client's education and employment. However, at times it may be appropriate for the nurse to ask the client to read and then explain a short passage to confirm reading ability and comprehension. When problems are identified, the nurse can adapt teaching strategies to include materials specifically developed for low literacy.

***Hearing or visually impaired individuals.*** Hearing-impaired clients benefit from printed materials and other forms of visual communication. The same visual aid strategies described in the box on p. 271 also may be effective when working with this group. Since many hearing-impaired clients are proficient at lip reading, the nurse should position himself or herself in front of the person and establish eye contact before beginning to talk. Lip reading is facilitated if the nurse does not stand in front of a bright window or in a shadow. Gestures and pictures are useful for reinforcing the spoken message. If the person understands sign language, an interpreter should be used.

Teaching plans for visually impaired clients require different strategies. Along with traditional teaching methods, an additional strategy is the use of audiotapes with step-by-step instructions. When developed with a pause at the end of each step, clients can pace and individualize their learning. Depending on the amount and type of visual impairment, some clients may be able to use pamphlets if the print is large,

and color contrast is added for emphasis. For blind clients who know braille, teaching materials in braille may be used.

## ❖ DESIGNING THE TEACHING AND LEARNING EXPERIENCE

The nursing process may be used as a prototype for designing the teaching and learning experience. Initial assessment of the client is followed by development of an individualized teaching and learning experience, including conditions for implementation of the teaching plan and evaluation of its effectiveness. During this process, appropriate goals and objectives should be identified, and effective teaching strategies and evaluation procedures should be selected.

### Assessing the Learner

First and foremost, the level of knowledge of the learner must be ascertained so that relevant teaching and learning experiences can be designed. As discussed earlier, it is also critical that certain characteristics of the individual be taken into account, such as age, preferred sensory channel, and ability to read and understand English. A thorough assessment can identify not only knowledge deficits but also special circumstances that require individualized attention.

Characteristics of the learner can serve as facilitators or barriers to learning and influence the outcome of the teaching and learning experience. One significant characteristic that facilitates learning is *motivation,* the inner drive in individuals that causes them to seek out new knowledge. Assessing the learner's level of interest in a topic can provide some insight into the motivation to learn. Factors that influence motivation are internal and external. For instance, motivation to learn about a specific illness may include internal factors such as the individual's degree of susceptibility or likelihood of contracting the illness, the perceived seriousness of the illness, and the belief that actions being taught would prevent the illness and that preventive actions are easier to perform than dealing with the disease itself (Becker, 1974). External factors include the degree of difficulty of the suggested activity, trust in the teacher and external constraints (such as a demanding job or caring for family members), expense, availability of equipment, and other environmental considerations. An additional issue related to motivation is the physical condition of the client at the time of the teaching activity. For example, pain, physical discomfort, and fatigue serve as barriers to learning because they adversely affect motivation and decrease readiness to learn.

Anxiety may be either a facilitator or a barrier to learning. A large amount of anxiety tends to interfere with the learning process; however, a mild to moderate amount of anxiety may increase a person's motivation to learn. For example, people who deny their diagnosis or are immobilized by anxiety over it may be unwilling or unable to learn about their condition. On the other hand, mild anxiety about the diagnosis often motivates people to seek information about the condition.

## Developing the Teaching Plan

Following the assessment, the needs of the client are identified and prioritized. Then a specific teaching plan is developed that includes the following:

1. A realistic goal
2. Objectives that are measurable and are constructed in a format that includes the subject, an action verb (behavior), a condition, and a criterion
3. Content outlines to correspond with each objective
4. Teaching methods to be employed
5. Expected learner activities

6. Evaluation plans, including expected progress toward goal achievement
7. Alternative plans and revisions if needed

An example of a teaching plan is presented in the nursing care plan on pp. 274-276.

## Selecting the Teaching Mode

An integral part of developing the teaching plan includes determining the most appropriate mode or modes of teaching. Modes to consider include group instruction, demonstration/return demonstration, role playing, and one-to-one discussion.

Traditionally, client teaching has been regarded as a one-to-one endeavor. However, group instruction is a time-saving option that is appropriate when there are several people with the same learning needs. Group instruction may also be augmented by having members share experiences or successful strategies for problem solving.

Some types of learning (for example, motor skills) are facilitated by using a demonstration/return demonstration model. A good demonstration provides the learner with a clear mental image of what is to be learned. Nurses can reduce the client's perception of artificiality by choosing the type of materials the client will actually be using. For example, it would be inappropriate to teach a mother how to read a glass mercury thermometer by demonstrating with an electronic thermometer.

Role play can be effectively incorporated into a teaching plan to rehearse new behaviors or illustrate the feelings of others in a nonthreatening format. Role play is especially effective in teaching communication skills (such as assertiveness) or teaching school-aged children. Once a new skill has been learned, the client can gain confidence and proficiency by practicing the behavior in a situation where the new skill could be used. Teacher involve-

# ❖ NURSING CARE PLAN

## AIDS PREVENTION TEACHING PLAN

**ASSESSMENT OF THE LEARNER**
18-year-old female who denies sexual activity but has boyfriend who wants to have a sexual relationship. Boyfriend has a history of IV drug use. Unable to answer questions on basic knowledge of AIDS. Expresses interest in staying healthy.

**NURSING DIAGNOSIS**
Lack of sufficient knowledge about acquired immune deficiency syndrome to maintain health when sexually active.

**LONG-TERM GOAL**
Client will remain free from AIDS.

**INTERMEDIATE GOAL**
Client will practice safe sex with partner 100% of the time.

**SHORT-TERM GOAL**
Client will gain sufficient knowledge necessary to protect self from HIV infection as measured by correct answers and demonstrations after instruction.

*By the end of the teaching and learning session, the client will:*

| BEHAVIORAL OBJECTIVES | CONTENT OUTLINE | TEACHING METHODS |
|---|---|---|
| 1. Correctly identify the human immundeficiency virus (HIV) as the cause of AIDS. | 1. Review AIDS and potential bodily effects (flulike symptoms, destruction of helper T cells in blood, depression of the immune system, Kaposi's sarcoma, pneumocystis pneumonia, diarrhea, yeast and other opportunistic infections, death). | 1. Determine and use appropriate sensory based language according to individual needs. |

**NURSING CARE PLAN—cont'd**

### AIDS PREVENTION TEACHING PLAN—cont'd

| BEHAVIORAL OBJECTIVES | CONTENT OUTLINE | TEACHING METHODS |
|---|---|---|
| 2. State four ways AIDS can be transmitted. | 2. Discuss modes of transmission (direct contract with AIDS-infected blood or body fluids), methods of spread (sexual intercourse with infected partner, sharing contaminated needles during intravenous drug use, from infected mother to developing fetus, from infected mother to breast feeding infant, from infected blood transfusions given before screening for AIDS had begun, any direct blood contact with AIDS virus). | 2. Review content using visual aids. |
| 3. Identify two rules to prevent the transmission of AIDS. | 3. Warn against taking any body fluids during any kind of sexual intercourse and don't share needles. | 3. Discussion of sexual intercourse, IV drug use, past blood transfusions, and infected mother to unborn or nursing child as methods of transmission. |
| 4. Demonstrate, on an anatomical model, the correct way to wear and remove a condom. | 4. Assemble all supplies: model of penis, different types of condoms, AIDS-effective spermicidal foam/jelly, written directions and drawings of steps. Demonstrate, have client return demonstration. | 4. Pamphlets about AIDS and condoms. |

*Continued.*

## ❖ NURSING CARE PLAN—cont'd

### AIDS PREVENTION TEACHING PLAN—cont'd

| BEHAVIORAL OBJECTIVES | CONTENT OUTLINE | TEACHING METHODS |
|---|---|---|
| 5. List five safe, intimate activities. | 5. Review safe activities that do not transmit AIDS, including safe kissing (no french kissing or kissing if lesions on mouth or bleeding gums), giving blood, hugging, shaking hands, using toilets, eating and drinking with someone who has AIDS. | 5. Role play dialogue convincing partner to wear condom. 6. Demonstration of correct application and removal of a condom.<br><br>7. REVIEW KEY POINTS. |

**EXPECTED LEARNER ACTIVITIES**

Ask questions, add comments, discuss feelings and fears, participate in role play, return demonstration on how to apply a condom; apply learning to real situations 100% of the time.

**EVALUATION**

Ask questions to determine the success of teaching; reteach as necessary. Arrange telephone contact for follow-up evaluation and support.

ment in one of the roles reduces emotional distance and may facilitate role modeling. Instructions should be easy and informal so participants can enjoy the activity and experience success.

Individual discussion is probably the most common teaching mode used by nurses. Individual discussion includes taking time to explore the individual's feelings and particular concerns regarding the teaching activity. An interview before and after the instruction will en-

courage participation and facilitate evaluation. At the conclusion of the instruction, some insight relative to the expected level of compliance can be gained by asking the client specifically what he or she plans to do after returning home.

## Implementing the Plan

The best plan of instruction can fail if the environment is not conducive to learning. Al-

❖ **Table 15-4**
Choosing and using audiovisuals

Assessment questions:
| | |
|---|---|
| 1. Is the material accurate and current? | 6. Is it worth the time and money? |
| 2. Is the age/learning level appropriate? | 7. Is the appearance and quality satisfactory? |
| 3. Is it interesting? | 8. Is it appropriate for the size audience? |
| 4. Is it the best available in the price range? | 9. Is the equipment available; can I operate it? |
| 5. Is it an acceptable time length? | 10. Is a different medium a better choice? |

| Media | Advantages | Considerations |
|---|---|---|
| Audiotapes | ◆ Useful for individuals and groups, involves auditory learners<br>◆ Economical, easy to prepare<br><br>◆ Can be used independently | ◆ Assess hearing with individuals, room size with groups<br>◆ Make backups or use good quality tapes<br>◆ Review mechanics, check batteries or power |
| Books/pamphlets | ◆ Useful for individuals, involves visual sense<br>◆ Easy to use<br><br>◆ Allows client to self pace | ◆ Assess reading ability and level of material<br>◆ Cost, must obtain permission to copy<br>◆ Texts go out of date rapidly |
| Computer programs | ◆ Allows self-pacing, multisensory involvement<br>◆ Sequential programs can be used by all learner levels<br>◆ Entertaining | ◆ Requires added time to learn computer use<br>◆ Equipment expensive<br><br>◆ Professional programming required |
| Films | ◆ Suitable for groups, involves sight, hearing<br>◆ Can stimulate emotions, build attitudes<br>◆ May be available from a public library<br>◆ Useful for compression of time and space | ◆ Does not permit self-pacing<br><br>◆ Difficult to produce<br><br>◆ Expensive to buy, allow time for order<br>◆ Requires darkness, special equipment |
| Flipchart/chalkboard | ◆ Suitable for groups, involves sight<br>◆ Allows step by step buildup<br>◆ Inexpensive | ◆ Bulky to transport<br>◆ Back to audience while writing<br>◆ Not reusable |
| Models/real objects | ◆ Useful for individuals/small groups<br>◆ Multisensory involvement<br>◆ Permits demonstration and practice | ◆ May not be easy to obtain<br>◆ Models costly<br>◆ Models often easily damaged |
| Posters/overheads | ◆ Useful for individuals/small groups, involves sight<br>◆ Easy to produce, inexpensive<br><br>◆ May be reused, easy to store | ◆ Requires viewing space and/or equipment<br>◆ Avoid crowding; consider color, size, and space<br>◆ For best appearance, have professionally done |
| Slides | ◆ Suitable for large groups<br>◆ Inexpensive, easy to produce/duplicate<br>◆ Easy to add/subtract material accordingly | ◆ Need partial darkness<br>◆ Test equipment, have extra light bulb<br>◆ Duplication of color slides expensive |

though some environmental aspects (such as the condition and location of a classroom) may be difficult to control, certain steps can be taken to minimize their negative impact on learning.

Facilitating learning begins with setting the climate for instruction by first advertising for the class with posters, fliers, and announcements to spark interest and explain the content. The room environment may be modified by adjusting the temperature and lighting and by arranging comfortable seating. If discussion is to be used, chairs may be arranged in circles instead of in rows. The nurse must make sure all the supplies are available ahead of time, and that they are arranged to be shown to their best advantage. Audiovisual materials should be tested for viewing from several locations in the room to ensure that all participants can easily see all materials. Audiovisual aids can add interest to presentations but should only be used if they are of good quality and appropriate for the content. Table 15-4 describes factors to consider in selecting audiovisual materials.

The "tone" of the class can range from formal to informal depending on the audience and the materials to be presented. For example, most childbirth education classes are happy events and are presented in a somewhat informal, relaxed manner. On the other hand, teaching newly diagnosed cardiac patients about dietary and activity restrictions might require a more formal, serious presentation. Cultural differences could also influence the level of formality. For example, clients of an Asian background expect an educational experience to be a formal lecture and might feel uncomfortable in a very informal environment. Beginning with the opening activity, learning should progress according to the purpose and objectives delineated in the plan. The length of instruction is determined by the content to be learned and the age and physical comfort of the learner. As a rule of thumb, however, any teaching activity should provide a break at least hourly.

## ❖ EVALUATING TEACHING AND LEARNING EFFECTIVENESS

Comprehensive evaluation of the teaching and learning experience includes identifying changes in the learner as well as measuring teacher effectiveness.

### Evaluating the Learner

Learning in each of the three domains (cognitive, affective, and psychomotor) is evaluated by measuring change in knowledge, attitude, or skill of the learner. Criteria for evaluation are derived from the stated goals and objectives. Conclusions about the level of learning can be drawn by measuring the extent to which goals and objectives are attained. Frequently, the only evaluation methods available to nurses are immediate feedback or return demonstrations.

More comprehensive evaluation mechanisms can offer information on long-term outcomes reflected by internalization of change by the client. Follow-up client evaluations can be done by telephone, mailed survey, or home visit depending on the availability of time and resources. Because of the personal nature of phone calls and home visits, more information will generally be obtained. Evaluation of teaching and learning can be accomplished by simple questions about the client's knowledge of the content, life-style changes that have been implemented, and satisfaction with the teaching and learning experience.

### Evaluating the Skills of the Teacher

Actual observation of the teaching process is a method of evaluation that is particularly enlightening. By using video or audio recording or a peer observer during the presentation, teaching activities and actual client responses can be recorded using a behavior checklist. Feedback should include comments as well as the written checklist results. Beginning with

### ❖ TEACHER EVALUATION FORM

| Behavior | *Satisfactory (S) Improvement Needed (I) | | |
|---|---|---|---|
| | S | I | Comments |
| Establishes environment conducive to learning | | | |
| Appearance is appropriate for teaching | | | |
| Establishes rapport | | | |
| Ensures mutuality | | | |
| Uses appropriate speech tone | | | |
|     tempo | | | |
|     volume | | | |
|     vocabulary | | | |
|     gestures | | | |
| Clarifies unfamiliar terms | | | |
| Avoids needless speech ("you know," "uh," "um") | | | |
| Provides a lesson overview and objectives | | | |
| Organizes presentation from simple to complex | | | |
| Length of instruction is learner-appropriate | | | |
| Enthusiastic presentation style | | | |
| Uses a multisensory approach | | | |
| Actively involves the learner | | | |
| Asks questions | | | |
| Waits for responses | | | |
| Encourages discussion | | | |
| Praises the learner throughout | | | |
| Uses analogies to link new information to old | | | |
| Reinforces key information | | | |
| Uses accurate and appropriate content | | | |
| Summarizes | | | |
| Allows practice time | | | |
| Determines skill development by return demonstration | | | |
| Listens to client questions | | | |
| Provides correct, complete answers | | | |
| Verbally checks client understanding | | | |
| Simplifies or restates as required by client response | | | |
| Observes and responds to nonverbal reaction | | | |
| Appropriately uses audio visual aids | | | |

*Comments should support areas that are satisfactory and areas that need improvement.

❖ **Fig. 15-1**  Checklist to evaluate teacher skills.

positive areas and progressing to areas for improvement will make the evaluation less threatening. The checklist in Fig. 15-1, adapted from information found in Jeffers and Guthrie (1988), provides an example for evaluation of teacher effectiveness, which can be used in both live and taped situations.

Videotaping has the additional advantage of allowing nurses to view their own teaching abilities. Tapes can be repeatedly reviewed, each time with a different focus. Disadvantages of videotaping include the necessity of obtaining written consent from the institution and the participants, expense of equipment, and the necessity of a designated area for the taping. Some technical ability is also necessary to set up and record the interaction. The advantages far outweigh the disadvantages, however, if videotaping can be arranged.

### ❖ SUMMARY

This chapter reviews theories of learning and different teaching techniques and applies them to client populations of varying ages and abilities. Examples for individual and group instruction are included. Contained in the chapter are practical methods for individualizing presentations and for determining success of the instruction. Finally, the role of the nurse and specific behaviors necessary for successful practice as a client educator are reviewed.

### ❖ APPLYING KNOWLEDGE TO PRACTICE

1. Jasmine is a 4-year-old girl who has been recently diagnosed with juvenile diabetes. Using the techniques described in the chapter, develop an age-appropriate teaching plan to help her learn the foods to select and avoid. Include strategies and rationale for cognitive, affective, and psychomotor learning as required.
2. In order to advance up the clinical ladder at your hospital, you are required to provide continuing education for staff on your unit. Outline a plan for content that would best address the needs of the entire staff. Include assessment, behavioral objectives, teaching format (lecture, visual aid, pamphlet, etc.), rationale, and a plan for evaluation.
3. Review the teaching strategies you currently employ with clients in your setting. Based on the knowledge gained from this chapter, decide which are the most and least effective and explain why.

# REFERENCES

Bandura, A. (1971). Analysis of modeling processes. In A. Bandura (Ed.), *Psychological modeling.* Chicago: Aldine.

Becker, M. H. (1974). In M.H. Becker (Ed.) *The health belief model and personal health behavior.* Thoroughfare, NJ: Charles B. Slack.

Bloom, B. S. (1956). *Taxonomy of educational objectives: Handbook I: Cognitive domain.* New York: Longman, Green.

Combs, A. (1965). *The professional education of teachers.* Boston: Allyn Bacon, Inc.

Dewey, J. (1938). *Experience and education.* New York: Macmillan.

Faulkner, A. (1983). Nurses as health educators in relation to smoking. *Nursing Times, 79,* (15), 47-48.

Gagne, R. M. (1974). *Essentials of learning for instruction.* Hinsdale, Ill: Dryden Press.

Glasser, W. (1965). *Reality therapy.* New York: Harper & Row.

Honan, S., Krsnak, G., Peterson, D., & Torkelson, R. (1988). The nurse as patient educator: Perceived responsibilities and factors enhancing role development. *Journal of Continuing Education in Nursing, 19*(1), 33-37.

Jeffers, J. M. & Guthrie, D. W. (1985). Self-assessment via videotaping to maximize teaching effectiveness. *Journal of Continuing Education in Nursing, 19*(5), 223-226.

Jonassen, D. H. (1981). Personality and cognitive style predictors of teaching style preferences: An exploratory study. In M. Simonson, & E. Hooper (Eds.), *Proceedings of selected research paper presentations at the 1981 Convention of the American Association for Educational Communications and Technology.* Ames, Iowa: Iowa State University.

Knowles, M. (1984). *The adult learner: A neglected species* (3rd ed.). Houston: Gulf Publishing.

Knowles, R. D. (1983). Building rapport through neurolinguistic programming. *American Journal of Nursing, 83*(7), 1010-1014.

Lewin, K. (1951). *Field theory in social science.* New York: Harper.

McClosky, J. C. (1983). Nursing education and job effectiveness. *Nursing Research, 32,* 53-58.

McClosky, J. C. & McCain, B. E. (1984). *Commitment, sat-isfaction, performance of hospital nurses.* (DHHS Publication No. NU 01050). Washington, DC: US Government Printing Office.

McClosky, J. C. & McCain, B. (1987). Commitment, satisfaction, performance of newly employed hospital nurses. *Image: The Journal of Nursing Scholarship, 19,* 20-24.

McClosky, J. C. & McCain, B. (1988). Nurse performance: Strengths and weaknesses. *Nursing Research, 37*(5), 308-313.

Maslow, A. H. (1970). *Motivation and personality.* New York: Harper & Row.

Murdaugh, C. (1980). Effects of nurses' knowledge of teaching-learning principles on knowledge of coronary care unit patients. *Heart and Lung, 9,* 1073-1078.

Pavlov, I. P. (1927). *Conditioned reflexes.* (trans. G. V. Anrep). London: Oxford U. Press.

Piaget, J. (1954). *The language and thought of the child (3rd ed).* London: Routledge & Kegan Paul of America, Ltd.

Piaget, J. (1970). *Genetic epistemology.* New York: Columbia U. Press.

Redman, B. K. (1988). *The process of patient education,* (6th ed.). St. Louis: C. V. Mosby.

Rogers, C. R. (1961). *On becoming a person.* Boston: Houghton Mifflin.

Rogers, C. R. (1969). *Freedom to learn.* Columbus, Ohio: Chas. E. Merrill.

Rorden, J. W. (1987). *Nurses as health teachers: A practical guide.* Philadelphia: W. B. Saunders.

Skinner, B. F. (1953). *Science and human behavior.* New York: Macmillan.

Thorndike, E. L. (1913). *The psychology of learning.* New York: Teachers College.

Van Hoozer, H. L., Bratton, B. D., Ostmoe, P. M., Weinholtz, D., Craft, M. J., Gjerde, C. L., & Albanese, M. A. (1987). *The teaching process: Theory and practice in nursing.* Norwalk, Conn.: Appleton, Century, Crofts.

Wilkinson, M. A. (1988). *The impact of NLP rapport skills training for RN's on one-on-one teaching of AIDS prevention.* Unpublished doctoral dissertation. Blacksburg: Virginia Polytechnic Institute and State University.

Wolpe, J. & Lazarus, A. (1966). *Behavior therapy techniques: A guide to the treatment of neurosis.* Oxford: Pergamon Press.

# 16 Information Technology

Lorraine Spranzo Keller

## OBJECTIVES

### At the completion of this chapter, the reader will be able to:

◆ Discuss the conceptual dimensions of information technology in relation to information, automation, technology, and its relation to the profession of nursing.

◆ Describe the societal dimensions of information technology in relation to knowledge, transformation of work and roles, and the issue of privacy and confidentiality.

◆ Outline, with examples, the growth and development of information technology in health care and related nursing implications.

◆ Discuss, with examples, the use of information technology to control and advance nursing as a knowledge-based discipline.

## ❖ INFORMATION TECHNOLOGY: EVOLUTION AND REVOLUTION

Human society is considered to be in the midst of a revolution in the nature of social communication. The information-processing capabilities of computers and the dissemination of information through telecommunications make up the distinctive technological basis for this revolution. Although the exact nature of the revolution and the anticipated transformations are conjectural, the pervasiveness of information technology is undeniable. Because of the rapid evolution of the technology and its recent impact, choices and rules for its use are still being formulated.

Nursing's choices and rules for the exploitation of information technology are emerging.

Nurses are increasingly becoming educated consumers of this technology, providing directions for its use in the advancement of nursing as a knowledge-based practice discipline. This chapter is an exploration of the dimension of information technology in terms of its technical evolution, societal impact, incorporation within the health care system, and implications for nursing.

### Assumptions Related to Nursing

Two premises serve as the organizing ideas for the content of this chapter. First, it will not be our technical skills in the use of this technology that will determine our advancement as a profession. It will be our intellectual skills. An understanding of the nature of the technology and its actual and potential impacts will aid us in applying our intellectual skills to its successful incorporation into practice. Second, this technology provides us the opportunity to examine and then explain the nature of nursing as a cognitively based discipline that uses information in the making of decisions and in the taking of actions to provide humanistic care. In order to effectively use the technology, this process is essential. The process itself is transforming—we learn to define nursing in ways that can be effectively communicated, measured, and applied to improve client care. In the long run, this will be the basis of our advancement as a profession, The technology is simply an advantageous tool to be used in this process.

### ❖ CONCEPTUAL BASES
### Information and Knowledge

A definition of information and its relationship to knowledge and decision making serves as a conceptual basis for understanding the nature of information technology. *Information* is derived from data (basic facts or observations) that are organized to be understood. Hadden (1986) considers information as meaningful data and distinguishes it from *knowledge,* which is an evaluation that can put the information to use. Table 16-1 provides two examples of this distinction using an adaptation of Gordon's (1982) nursing diagnosis formulation exercises.

According to Dowling (1988), information is needed to support action and decision. Analysis of the actions to be taken or decision making leads to an understanding of what information is needed for successful completion of the task at hand. A nursing diagnosis is used to represent a decision, and data are transformed to provide the needed information. Intrinsic to this transformation is the extent and degree of underlying knowledge the person brings to this process.

### Automation of Information

Computer processing enables the transformation of factual data into needed information rapidly, efficiently, and in large amounts. Before computerization, the task must be analyzed, broken down into its smallest parts, and programmed into a computer. This involves a rationalization of the task, whether the task is to automatically spray paint a car or to generate a medication report. The computer program represents the logic of the task that can be interpreted through computer processing, which results in a consistently executed task. To the extent that a human task can be logically analyzed and translated into a computer program, it can be automated. This has served as a driving force for the use of automation as a means to extend our human ability to perform tasks. The proliferation of automatic teller machines and optical scanners in supermarkets are just two of many examples.

❖ **Table 16-1**
Distinguishing information from knowledge

| Information | Knowledge |
| --- | --- |
| Client is unresponsive to stimuli; no voluntary movement of extremities | Total self-care deficit/comatose state |
| Client is comatose, drooling, unresponsive to stimuli, $PO_2$ 78mm | Potential airway obstruction |

## Dual Nature of Automated Information

Zuboff (1988) encourages us to consider information technology as being composed of the dual capacities of automating and "informating" (p. 10). For example, the scanner devices in supermarkets automate the checkout process and simultaneously generate data that can be used for inventory control, warehousing, scheduling of deliveries, and market analysis. By automating a nursing personnel file, data can be generated for the planning of staff development, allocation of nursing resources based on skill mix, payroll increases, and turnover analysis. New streams of information are generated, and the activities and events of an organization become more apparent. According to Zuboff (1988), if the focus is on exploiting the informating capacity of the technology in ways that promote intellectual skill development throughout an organization, then innovative change will occur. If the focus remains solely on its automating capacity, the technology will merely permit a new way to continue the status quo. The technology itself is not revolutionary. It is the choice we make in how to use it that will determine the nature of the predicted revolution.

## Concept of Information Technology

Galbraith (1977) defines *technology* as "...the systematic application of scientific or other organized knowledge to practical tasks" (p. 77). This permits a consideration of the impact of technology beyond its hardware or machinery components. According to Banta (1986), a broader meaning enables a wider consideration of the influence of technology on our organizations, values, and culture. Based on these ideas, *information technology* is defined as a term that represents a combination of technical developments in a number of fields (mathematics, microelectronics, computer science, telecommunications, software engineering, and systems analysis). Developments in the technology itself cause reciprocal interaction and continued growth in these fields. The practical task that information technology performs is the recording, storing, analyzing, and transmission of information in ways that allow flexibility, accuracy, immediacy, volume, and complexity (Zuboff, 1988). Developments in telecommunications (electronic mail, teleconferencing, facsimile systems, electronic bulletin boards, etc.) have permitted geographic independence, or the ability to share sources of information over great distances (Rosenberg, 1986). Evidence of how this feature alone can influence the work culture is the increased movement toward home-based work environments. Essentially, it is the capacity of the technology to distribute information directly to the user that holds the greatest promise for the restructuring of organizations and transformation of work roles.

## Nursing Informatics

Advances in information technology and the fact that health care professionals operate in environments dense with information have influenced the evolution of the term *informatics* to represent the application of computerized information processing and communication to health care processes. *Nursing informatics* is defined as "the use of information technologies in relation to any of the functions which are within the purview of nursing and which are carried out by nurses" (Hannah, 1985, p. 181). This is intended to include the use of this technology in client care activities, client education, nursing education, nursing management, and/or research on information use and decision making in nursing. The definition alone indicates the broad influence of this technology and the information needs of nursing. Graduate programs are evolving that will generate nurse specialists in this practice field (Heller, Damrosch, Romano, & McCarthy, 1989). Competencies and guidelines are being produced to assist nurses to effectively use this technology (Ronald & Skiba, 1987; Zielstorff, McHugh, M, & Clinton, J., 1988; Peterson & Gerdin-Jelger, 1988). The American Nurses' Association and the National League for Nursing have developed councils and task forces to provide expertise and guidance for the incorporation of information technology into practice. Within the past 5 years, new vocabularies, competencies, and organizational thrusts have begun to evolve.

## Societal Pervasiveness

A brief scan of one's environment is convincing enough of the pervasiveness of information technology. It enables new sounds in music, new images on screens, new forms of learning and entertainment for children (and adults), new ways of being placed on unneeded mailing lists, new ways of forecasting weather, fixing cars, and monitoring unpaid bills. Every segment of society is influenced directly or indirectly by computers and the associated technology of linking or networking among computers. At its core is the silicon chip. A brief review of its evolution will partially explain its pervasiveness.

## ❖ COMPUTERIZATION: MINIATURIZATION AND PROLIFERATION
### Computers as Electronic Devices: Technical Evolution

The modern electronic computer is an elaborate counting device composed of a processor (logic unit) and a memory (storage) unit. The processor performs and controls computations and the memory unit stores the programs and data required for the processing. The stages of evolution of the modern computer, referred to as computer generations, represents developments in its electronic components (Saba & McCormick, 1986; Blum, 1986).

The first-generation (1953-1958) modern

computer developed from a mechanical calculator into a huge electronic device that occupied one large room, required constant attention to its 5000 vacuum tubes, and had to be kept well-ventilated. The first commercial computer (UNIVAC I, Sperry Rand Corporation) could add two numbers in 2 millionths of a second. It set the stage for competitive technology development (Blum, 1986).

The technical developments focused on increasing the speed, reliability, and capacity of the storage and processing components. Transistors were developed during the second generation (1958-1964) as replacements for the vacuum tubes. By the third generation (1964-1974), the transistors and their electrical circuits could be etched on a semiconducting material—the silicon wafer. In 1971, Intel Corporation introduced large-scale integrated circuitry. This is a microminiaturization of transistors and circuits chemically etched onto silicon chips (Saba & McCormick, 1986). Hundreds of thousands of transistors can be built on a chip measuring no more than a fraction of an inch. In 1975, the microprocessor on a chip evolved, heralding the fourth generation, and the personal computing market developed into a major industry. Computing power, previously available only to large businesses, industry, and government, was now available to the lay consumer.

According to Porter and Millar (1985), the cost of computer power relative to the cost of manual information processing is at least 8000 times less than the cost during the generation of the UNIVAC I. The reduced cost created increased proliferation during the fourth generation (1975–present) and further refinements in software and hardware architecture created an astonishing market response. Currently, computers are available as embedded devices, parts of the tool we use, and as a networked resource linking us through a telephone system to large, varied, and distant informational data bases (Saba, Oatway, & Rieder, 1989). Local area networking technology enables the linking and sharing of resources among computers within an organizational setting, and the means of access are becoming more simple to operate.

### Fifth-Generation Computers

According to Blum (1986) the fifth-generation (1990 + ) computer (as predicted by the Japanese) will continue with trends of the fourth generation with reduction in costs, size, and increased computing power. The advances in telecommunications and networking (the joining of computer systems) will make invisible the distinctions between where one computer starts and another ends. Parallel processing (the use of more than one processor in parallel) will stimulate growth in advanced programming languages resulting in growth in the field of artificial intelligence including knowledge-based expert systems, robotics, computer vision, and natural language processing. This could result in systems capable of processing voice input; expert consultation; and improved technologies to access data bases for decision making (Rosenberg, 1986).

The rapid growth, proliferation, increased power, flexibility, and usefulness of the personal computer are all factors that are stimulating changes in attitudes toward computerization. Users (constantly increasing in number) are becoming less intimidated, and the computer display terminal is becoming an accepted part of our environment. The following discussion highlights the societal changes that have been forecasted as a result of the permeation of information technology.

### ❖ "INFORMATION SOCIETY:" TRANSFORMATIONS AND IMPLICATIONS
### Information Society Defined

"Information societies" has become a popular term when referring to several Western European nations, Japan, and the United States. Although not specifically defined, scholars generally agree that an *information society* is one where the economic growth is related to technological advances, where knowledge and "know-how" are valued commodities, and where these commodities are applied to improve the production of services and the revitalization of businesses (Williams, 1986). According to Salvaggio (1986), characteristics of an information society include instantaneous transmission of information, intensive knowledge bases, and a trend toward decentralization.

Bell (1973), who preferred the term "post-industrial society," viewed the technology as enabling a competitive society based on the economic resources of information and knowledge. Bell predicted the evolution of a knowledge elite (scientists) who would be egalitarian in applying the knowledge to solve societal problems. Other scholars view the technology as a political or cultural product used to serve the interests of those in power and to create inequities in the distribution of employment ("deskilling of jobs") and domination by large organizations (Rosenberg, 1986). Technological optimists forecast primarily the benefits of the technology and the increased leisure it will allow (Williams, 1986). Increasingly documented is the need for a multidimensional approach to the assessment of impacts with a focus on the contexts in which the technology is incorporated. These contexts have in place a philosophy or culture of socioeconomic organization that will ultimately shape the development, implementation, and use of information technologies (Salvaggio, 1986).

### Implications for Change: Work and Roles

Evidence is accumulating to support the contention that computing is too weak a force in itself to affect organizational structures in significant ways. Rather, the net effect of computing is contingent on the existing management practices, financial resources, and information control structures that will govern how computing will be used and the priorities for its use (Northrup, Kraemer, & King, 1989). While the technology is supportive of either centralizing or decentralizing structures, it is the history and traditions of the organization that will decide which arrangement is followed.

It is generally acknowledged that once employees become familiar with computers, most feel better about their work and perform better. The job displacement effects so far have been offset by expansion of current jobs and the creation of new jobs. This is particularly true in health care organizations. In most cases, hospitals undergoing computerization find it essential to name a single nurse or group of nurses as computer specialists who serve as systems analysts, liaisons with computer companies, and content designers. This has generated a cadre of nurses cross-educated either formally or "on the job" in the information sciences and who have pioneered the forward movement of computers in nursing (McCormick & McQueen, 1988).

Zuboff (1986) states that the optimizing benefits of computerization occur for those individuals who are permitted to and can conceptualize the nature of their work in ways that make known the underlying principles and "whys" of their actions. This requires an explicit understanding of the work process itself (the "know-how") and the logic and structure of the information system (Milholland, 1986). It seems, then, that in order to achieve the best results this technology can provide, contexts promoting inquiry, collective discussion, and participatory problem solving are required. Organizational contexts that perceive nursing as having a fundamental problem-solving role in the management and delivery of client care will incorporate the technology to enhance the nurse's ability to be a productive and effective problem solver. Organizational contexts that perceive nurses as skilled servants will still incorporate the technology, but it will not be one

that facilitates the advancement of nursing practice.

## Privacy and Confidentiality

Scholars generally agree that invasion of privacy is the most serious negative impact possible from incorporation of information technologies. The miniaturization of the technology has enabled compression of vast and varied data bases. Refinement of data base management systems has facilitated ease of use and the capacity to link data bases (enabling a complete profile of an individual's health, financial status, and educational status). Telecommunications permit instantaneous access from great distances. Unauthorized access to data bases and wiretapping has occurred. Sensor technology (electronic tracking) is expected to grow in use (e.g., parents may perceive it as a logical way to keep track of their children). Although laws are in place (*Electronic Communications Privacy Act* of 1986) to federally protect electronic communications from unlawful invasion, the open interpretation of such laws and the rationalized need for information by government and organizations creates an uneasy tension relative to privacy (Salvaggio, 1986). For example, an implantable body sensor enables the monitoring of parolees, and its use is argued from the fact that physical incarceration and prison regimen imposes a larger invasion of privacy (Rosenberg, 1986). According to Salvaggio (1986), privacy is often relinquished for more apparently valued commodities such as profits, safety, health, efficiency, and productivity. Organizations and individuals, then, may continue to vary in their willingness to violate codes of ethics and laws.

## Confidentiality, Technology, and Nursing

Computerization raises both the complexity and importance of the issue of privacy as a personal right. Nurses rely on disclosure by the client of complete health-related data in order to provide comprehensive care. The client, in a sense, relinquishes the control of privacy to the nurse. The nurse's duty is to maintain secrecy about the information. While this duty predates the advent of computers, nurses will need to incorporate this duty into practice in new ways. The incorporation of the technology into health care settings will require nurses to be involved in determining the levels of responsibility for the extent and type of data collection (including sensor technology), rationalizing the need for and the monitoring of the use of data, maintaining correct access to and security of computer systems, and advocating for related procedures that uphold the duty to safeguard the secrecy of information (Romano, 1987).

## Data Security and Data Integrity

Nursing responsibility for the use of the technology in practice settings includes consideration of authorized access, which is one form of data security (Covvey, H., Craven, N., & McAlister, 1985; Romano, 1987). *Data security* involves participation in both the definition and ongoing monitoring of policies and procedures designed to protect access. This control of access may be in the form of passwords, badges, or management of user identification. Another related concern is that of data integrity. *Data integrity* involves mechanisms to ensure the accuracy, reliability, and completeness of the data. Romano (1987) recommends that nurses insist that computer systems include mechanisms for error checking and confirmation of accuracy of data before their incorporation into a permanent data base. This confirmation process provides feedback to the user nurse and allows correction of errors in transcription. Nurses will play a key role in reviewing and recommending software for clinically based practice. To be effective in this role, nurses must insist on software that meets high standards for data security, data integrity, and that operates at a perfect level of accuracy.

## ❖ HEALTH CARE INFORMATION TECHNOLOGY: GROWTH AND DEVELOPMENT
### Nurses' Roles

Nurses will be involved as educators, designers, developers, implementors, users, and evaluators of applications of information technologies within health care settings. What follows is a brief overview of types of computer applications or systems used in health care settings and related nursing implications. The following references offer more detail on software applications pertinent to nursing and health care: Bolwell, E. *Directory for Educational Software in Nursing,* Rowland, H. *Hospital Software: A Sourcebook,* proceedings from the *Symposium of Computer Applications in Medical Care,* and the *International Symposium on Nursing Uses of Computers and Information Science,* and the journal of *Computers in Nursing.*

### The Objects of Processing: Data, Information, Knowledge

According to Blum (1986), computerized applications in health care can be grouped according to the objects they process. The three types of objects are data, information, and knowledge. In reality there can be overlap of these objects in computerized systems. However, the grouping by objects processed is a useful means for understanding the types of applications available to health care settings.

### Data Oriented Systems

Data oriented applications are those that operate on uninterpreted elements (data) such as a client's name, test result, electrical activity of the heart, blood pressure, or a symptom. The mathematical computation of such an application operates only on data. A simple example is computation of body surface area from height and weight (Blum, 1986). Applications that fall into this category are business data processing (financial systems), clinical laboratory systems, client monitoring, diagnostic systems, and imaging applications (CAT scanners).

Client monitoring devices have been in wide use in intensive care, emergency, and operating-recovery units. Computerized monitoring involves the use of a sensor to collect physiological activity and convert it to a signal that can be shaped for further processing or display. This processing may be a simple comparison with a reference signal level, or it may be sophisticated analysis to recognize events such as cardiac arrhythmias and to interpret signals for diagnostic purposes, (e.g., electrocardiogram) (Blum, 1986). The trend is for an increase in both external and implantable microprocessors for diagnostic, monitoring, and therapeutic uses (e.g., cardiac pacemakers, hearing aids, and voice-activated wheelchair controllers).

Although not supportive of the entire nursing process, computerized monitoring has benefited nursing assessments by decreasing errors of observation, streamlining assessment documentation, increasing detection of abnormals, (via alarms) and increasing access to information by means of graphic display. Cardiac arrhythmia monitoring has been shown to increase detection of arrhythmias dramatically, which resulted in a decreased mortality rate in cardiac care unit patients (Saba & McCormick, 1986). However, more evaluation studies are needed to assess the costs and benefits of computerized monitoring devices. Nursing will become increasingly involved in assessing the efficacy of these instruments as they become incorporated into clinical practice (ease of use, degree of false alarms, accuracy, degree of intrusiveness, and changes in physical care requirements). Additionally, the trend is toward integrating the physiologic monitoring systems and client data management systems in such a way as to generate a completely computerized clinical record (Milholland, 1986). This would include the nursing process (nurse care planning) and is a movement to the information-oriented type of application.

## Information Oriented Systems

Information oriented applications organize and join data in ways that allow meaningful interpretation by the user. Information systems commonly refer to the automation of data into information and are built on the concepts of long-term data base, storage, retrieval, and communication. Hospital Information System (HIS), Patient Care System (PCS), Health Care Information System (HCIS), and Clinical Information System (CIS) are systems that automate the flow of information relative to client care within a health care setting. The primary function of such systems is to speed up the communication of information to those who need it, decrease the redundancy of data entry, increase sharing of data among the reports generated, and decrease the errors of transcription (Blum, 1986; Saba & McCormick, 1986; Ball, Hannah, Gerdin-Jelger, & Peterson, 1988).

**Health care information systems.** Although HIS models vary widely, they generally consist of applications centering around services, such as nursing, pharmacy, laboratory, radiology, and admissions. The functions may include the client record (admissions, discharge, transfer), order entry and results reporting, drug profiles, care planning, personnel and staffing, and financial. The functions included depend on the level of HIS development. The lowest level of development is the financial tracking system, which is an automation of the admission, discharge, and billing of clients. The next level of HIS is the recording and retention of the client record and facilitation of interaction between the nursing unit and ancillary services. The highest level of HIS allows for all the mentioned functions plus the use of the computer to analyze trends in client responses, drug use studies, admissions by diagnosis/acuity, and statistics for planning and research (Sauter, 1988).

**Modular development: nursing information system.** As a result of advances in networking technology and reduction in costs for computer equipment, the current trend in HIS development is toward integration of an existing system (Ball, Hannah, Gerdin-Jelger, & Peterson, H., 1988). In this approach each service unit is considered a functional unit or module linked by communications. The units or modules can either share a common database (integrated system) or each module can manage its own data base and coordinate changes to the shared database (integration of independent systems). The concept of integration allows each unit to detail the functional specifications of the computerized system—hence each service can develop applications that best meet its information needs. Modules that become outdated can be replaced with newer, more updated modules at a reduced cost. According to Blum (1986) the major advantages of this approach are the decentralized control of information, low risk of investment in obsolescence, and the increased potential for the accommodation of new clinical tools.

Information-oriented applications in nursing are generally designed to support administrative functions such as patient classification, staffing and scheduling, budgeting, and personnel filing, and to meet documentation needs in nursing care (care-planning, nursing notes, discharge planning). The current emphasis in nursing information applications is the automation of the nursing process. Brennan and Romano (1987) provide a cogent argument for the automation of the nursing process (inclusive of nursing diagnoses) so that it becomes a more visible part of the health record, stimulates the perpetuation of nurse thinking, and contributes to the definition of nursing practice. In order to develop such systems that take advantage of the current level of technology and meet the information needs of practicing nurses, the American Nurses' Association published *Computer Design Criteria: For Systems That Support the Nursing Process*. This serves as a valuable guide for the development of nursing systems that are flexible enough to accommodate the technological enhancements of the future.

**Evaluation of information oriented systems.** Evaluations of HIS to date have demonstrated that the work flow is modified to decrease or reassign the clerical tasks of documentation and that the greatest changes were in the nursing activities associated with information handling (Blum, 1986; Kjerulff, 1988). Consistently documented is the estimate that nurses spend 30% to 40% of their time in communicating and managing information. Clearly, automating the information flow processes can offer considerable benefits to nursing practice. Several HIS systems demonstrate an "access to information at point of care" philosophy of development (Hughes, 1988, p. 139). This places data collection systems at the place of nurse-client interaction (e.g., the bedside). These systems ease the information handling burdens in nursing. However, they vary in the degree to which they provide interaction with the fully functional HIS system. Hence, the nurse may or may not have ready access to retrieval of information for review or decision making. This is one important consideration in judging the effectiveness of bedside systems.

Information-oriented applications assist in decision making by displaying clinical information in an orderly and organized manner and by providing access to a complete and accurate data base conducive to further analysis and inquiry. The design of these systems can include automatic surveillance, while client data that are entered can be compared to a set of predetermined criteria (e.g., drug to drug interaction alerts, risk for falls alerts, etc). Finally, a system can be designed with features that take the form of telling the decision maker what to do (e.g., automatic reminders for medications, careplan update, and barium enema prep) (Blum, 1986). The supply of information in such applications is limited to what is available in the data base and what has been encoded through algorithms and programs. The value of the information to decision making relies on the knowledge the user brings to the system.

## Knowledge Oriented Systems

Knowledge oriented applications are those designed to provide more information than is provided in a computerized clinical data base. Knowledge in the form of rules, facts, and relationships is structured to enable the application of inference or a problem-solving process for the purpose of generating solutions, recommendations, or explanations for complex problems. Bibliographic retrieval systems, decision support systems, and expert systems are types of knowledge oriented applications that augment the user's decision-making effectiveness. Their development and application to the health care field represents a major research frontier (Blum, 1986; Hannah, 1988; Ozbolt, 1988).

**Bibliographic retrieval systems.** Bibliographic retrieval systems organize knowledge for identification and extraction by the user. Once the knowledge is integrated by the user, it can be used to determine a course of action or to arrive at a solution. The National Library of Medicine uses the Medical Subject Heading (MeSH) vocabulary to classify publications in the health care field. The Medical Literature Analysis and Retrieval System (MEDLARS) is searched using the MeSH language, which contains 14,600 headings and subheadings and provides access to citations and abstracts of articles in over 3000 journals, including nursing journals. MeSH incorporates subheadings for nursing ethics, nursing laws, and the nursing profession; however, subheadings for nursing clinical judgment areas such as rehabilitation, health promotion, prevention, cure, and maintenance are not currently indexed using the MeSH vocabulary. McCormick (1988) proposes that further research be directed at correlation of the nursing diagnosis taxonomy to the MeSH vocabulary. Such initiatives would contribute to the

development of a unified nursing language system, which would both improve the efficiency of searching the nursing literature and serve as a unifying framework in computerized nursing applications. This approach facilitates the linking of different kinds of nursing information resources and improving direct access by the practicing nurse to literature pertinent to clinical decision making. Saba, Oatway, and Rieder (1989) provide a comprehensive review on available data bases pertinent to nursing, current access methods, and recommendations for a national nursing information system.

**Research data base for bibliographic retrieval.** Evolving is the concept of on-line access to knowledge (as opposed to citations and abstracts), which requires that the knowledge be extracted from the literature and then structured for retrieval by means of an easy-to-use interface. This provides access to a data base that is tailored to a specific environment (Blum, 1986). Graves and Cocoran (1988) provide several examples of demonstration projects that build on this concept. The Quantitatively Expressed Ideas Database (QEID) stores research variables studied together in the area of oncology with a special focus on childhood cancers. As a result of querying the data base of all variables studied, survival probabilities, treatment strategies, and source reports can be generated. The emphasis of such demonstration projects is to provide the latest research knowledge in support of clinical decision making specific to practice domains.

Improvements in access to data bases will continue with an emphasis on the structure and connection of data bases as knowledge resources, the generation of full text reporting, and the linking of these knowledge resources directly to clinical practice areas. Nursing information systems that do not exploit the current and evolving technologies in providing access to the discipline's research literature are lacking an important element in the advancement of nursing as a knowledge-based discipline.

**Decision support systems.** Decision support systems (DSS) can be considered a bridge between information-oriented and knowledge-oriented applications. The goal of information-oriented systems is to increase clerical efficiency for rather routine and structured decisions. The goal of DSS is to increase decision-making effectiveness in semistructured situations characterized by uncertainty or risk (e.g., choosing among several pain management strategies (Hadden, 1986). A growing number of analytical tools are being developed to support decision making. Brennan (1988) provides a useful review with pertinent applications to nursing. Bayesian analysis (use of probabilities) to predict the outcome for one client based on the outcome from a larger population of similar clients is one area of major research activity in the application of DSS to the health care environment.

*Components of decision support systems.* DSS are composed of three components: (1) a language component or interface that facilitates inquiries, (2) a data base organized for use in decision making, and (3) a problem processing component that contains the analytical models used to generate alternative solutions. It is the problem processing component that distinguishes a DSS from an information-oriented system. According to Brennan (1985), a nurse using an appropriately designed DSS could enter client signs and symptoms (diagnostic cues or defining characteristics), and the computer displays the recommended nursing diagnoses, enabling more accuracy in the selection of a diagnostic label. The recommended diagnoses are based on the computer program, which includes rules (problem solving component) linking the defining characteristics to diagnostic labels. The rules are derived from nursing knowledge and research on the probabilities of linkage between the diagnostic cues and the diagnosis. While such systems for suggesting nursing diagnoses are experimental at present, the growing number of nurses with the technical expertise for such applications holds prom-

ise for further research and developments in the area of decision support in nursing.

*Examples of decision support systems.* The HELP System, developed at the Latter Day Saints Hospital in Salt Lake City, uses decision analysis (Bayesian statistics) and its HIS data base to assist in clinical decision making. The system integrates client data from physiological monitoring and the many other sources of data entry and allows decision making in the form of interpretations, warning alerts, or treatment protocols when abnormal conditions are recognized. Conditions for these alerts are defined in HELP sectors (e.g., likelihood of pleural fluid in a client, hypoxia, renal failure). These sectors are considered knowledge frames that represent the data and logic to formulate a decision. Roughly 2000 such medically oriented knowledge frames are embedded in the HELP system, which is operational on clinical units throughout the hospital (Blum, 1986; Saba & McCormick, 1986). Heriot and colleagues (1988) report on the development and testing of a pain management support system for nursing that can be used as a functioning part of the HELP system. The knowledge frames are based on facts and logic from both literature sources and domain experts. The testing of the logic will be based on real client data recorded during use of the system. Comparisons between the actual nurse decisions and the system-recommended decisions for pain management will be used for further refinement of the system. This research represents one beginning point in the area of modeling clinical decision making in nursing and then embedding the knowledge derived in a computerized system that will provide further dissemination and use of that knowledge.

**Expert systems.** Expert systems generally refer to knowledge-based systems that incorporate artificial intelligence (*AI*) principles. *AI* is a field of study concerned with making a computer emulate human thinking, including learning from experience, justifying its reasoning, and correcting inconsistencies in its knowledge base. *AI* researchers initially hoped to find general laws of reasoning but soon discovered that programs embodying such laws solved specific problems poorly. Through observation of human experts, researchers discovered that people scale problems down to manageable size using heuristics or rules of thumb (common sense reasoning) and that expertise entails both knowledge as well as these problem-solving techniques (Blum, 1986; Hadden, 1986; Hannah, 1988).

*Components of expert systems.* Expert systems built using AI techniques include a representation of domain-specific knowledge, including reasoning rules, a method of interrogating the user logically, a provision for an explanation of the rationale supporting a decision, and the capacity to incorporate into the knowledge base feedback about the outcomes of the decisions generated. The knowledge base could then grow and become cumulative.

*Examples of expert systems.* In medicine, MYCIN was developed to provide consultation on infectious diseases and antimicrobial therapy. INTERNIST has been developed and verified for use in the area of medical diagnosis consultation. PUFF is an expert system that interprets measurements from respiratory tests administered to patients in a pulmonary function lab. Used daily at the Pacific Medical Center in San Francisco, it has interpreted 4000 cases, 85% of which were accepted without modification (Weiss, 1984). Happ (1988) provides a useful review of past and current applications of expert systems in health care with attention to various management and cost issues.

While medicine has been involved in expert system development since 1976, nursing's progress in this area is more recent. In nursing, the current focus is on building expert systems that: (1) focus on narrowly defined problems considered important, (2) require judgement (i.e., solutions are not so obvious), and (3) have gained acceptance in the area of nursing exper-

tise. Chang and Hirsch (1988) cite these criteria for the selection of the problem of self-care deficit as the focus for their expert system project. The current stage of the project is the field testing of an assessment guide used to collect client data related to the problem and the generating of probabilities of both defining characteristics and etiologies that will form the knowledge base for an expert system intended to be used as a diagnostic reasoning aid. Larson (1988) reports on the planning phases of a micro-computer-based expert system to address the nursing care needs of AIDS clients. Petrucci (1989) is currently field testing an expert system designed as an advisory system for the nursing management of urinary incontinence. Ozbolt (1988) is researching the application of conceptual models to define the nursing knowledge base for management of elimination needs in the elderly.

**Benefit of knowledge-oriented systems to nursing.** It is still unknown how these systems could benefit nurse decision making in the practice arena. Considering Benner's (1982) formulation of nursing proficiency as a continuum from novice to expert, it can be conjectured that expert system dissemination could hasten the novice nurse's progress toward becoming an expert. The experienced nurse who bases clinical judgment on an intuitive level that includes the recognition of patterns and a sense of salience (perceived importance of observations) may benefit from using an expert system if it is designed not as a diagnostic aid, but as a generator of alternative or competing hypotheses, interventions, and outcomes based on individualized client situations (Ozbolt, 1988).

Despite conjecture on its eventual use, expert system development offers great insight into what constitutes nursing knowledge and the directions for its further refinement. The knowledge acquisition phase of expert system development requires the location, collection, and refinement of knowledge from nurse experts, relevant literature, personal experiences, and existing data bases. Knowledge engineering, the discipline of expert system development, is a process of defining the knowledge, relevant constructs (rules and reasoning) and then converting it to applicable forms (electronic representation and dissemination). Currently, this is an extremely difficult process given the degree of introspection required of the human expert to express knowledge concisely and completely, the level of interpretation needed by the knowledge engineer (educated in computer science, cognitive science, and artificial intelligence), and the general lack of domain-independent knowledge rules or heuristics. Technological advances such as parallel processing, symbolic programming languages (LISP, PROLOG), and experimental machine learning programs designed to assist in the knowledge engineering process are evolving to loosen the constraints in expert system development. These technical developments, in addition to nursing's growing interest in the research and development of expert systems, are creating a necessary knowledge engineering role for nurse information specialists of the future (Weiss, 1984; Hadden, 1986; Grosso, 1988).

**Knowledge and nursing.** In actuality, all computerized applications apply knowledge; the data-oriented types use knowledge in the form of algorithms, and the information-oriented types embody knowledge in the form of programs. Given that computerization requires a rationalization of the process of knowing, then rational or empirically based patterns of knowing are most amenable to this technology. In nursing, to the extent that we are able to describe, explain, and verify our knowledge, then it can be codified. Yet, according to Carper (1978), this cognitive pattern represents but one of four patterns of knowing demonstrated in nursing clinical practice. The second pattern,

esthetics, blends both cognitive and affective processes and enables the attachment of meaning to a situation. This aspect, often referred to as the art of nursing, defies codification. A third pattern of nursing knowledge is personal knowledge, which centers on the therapeutic use of self in a relationship with another person. Personal knowledge is too idiosyncratic to be computer emulated. Ethical knowing, a fourth pattern characterized by advocating, valuing, and clarifying, can be codified to the extent that its rules are made explicit as in the profession's code of ethics. However, intuitive or emotionally based ethical knowing defies codification (Fitzpatrick, 1988).

Viewing nursing knowledge as a composite of interrelated patterns permits an appreciation of the complexity of nurse thinking and an understanding of the limitations of computerization to advancing nursing knowledge. One may well add that there should be limitations, given the highly humanistic manner of nurse thinking and the crucial role it serves in clinical decision making. The fine tuning of a nurse's critical thinking skills is intimately tied to the human experience of knowing. Yet successful incorporation of information technologies requires careful study and explication of our "know-how." Even if the explication is unidimensional or cognitively focused, the search may result in further understanding of the nature of the remaining dimensions and their influence on the clinical judgment process of nurses.

## ❖ INFORMATION TECHNOLOGY AND NURSING: INTEGRATION AND DIFFERENTIATION
### The Need for Information Technology in Nursing

It is no longer argued whether the integration of clinically oriented information technologies into nurse practice settings is necessary. The volume, complexity, and time involved in information handling by nurses is common knowledge. The current and projected trends of complex care needs of clients requiring timely, accurate data retrieval and documentation are increasingly evident. Public policy directions in health care cost containment and consumer expectations for quality of care challenge health professionals' obligations to maintain productivity and high quality service. Nursing is at the focus of client care decisions and the information flow about those decisions. The success of an information system in meeting the needs for timely and effective decision making is directly related to how involved nursing is in its planning, implementation, and evaluation (Dowling, 1988).

## The Profession of Nursing and Information Control

Rather than its necessity, prevailing arguments are concerned with how best to use this technology to advance the discipline of nursing. Clinton (1988) considers information as a discipline's essential and particular knowledge, which needs to be controlled in order to maintain control of nursing practice. Control of nursing practice is conceptualized as the extent to which the discipline of nursing can define, verify, and communicate the basic nature and benefits of its services. Nursing information is cardinal to all the profession's functions, including its definitions of practice, ethics, standards, and the testing of its knowledge base to evaluate, improve, and explain its services to the public and policy officials. Clinton advocates that use of this technology promotes control of practice because it facilitates control of information.

## Toward a National Nursing Data Base

Consistent with this focus is the national nursing leadership emphasis on the testing and

refinement of the Nursing Minimum Data Set (NMDS) (Werley & Lang, 1988). The NMDS is a standardized base of information concerning a specific aspect of nursing that meets the essential data needs of multiple users. The NMDS is composed of three broad categories: (1) nursing care, (2) client/patient demographics, and (3) service characteristics. Currently, the last two categories contain items that are already included in the Uniform Hospital Discharge Data Set (UHDDS). Essential nursing care data are specific items of information used on a regular basis by the majority of nurses across all settings (nationally and internationally) in the delivery of client care. The nursing process is the frame of reference for the extraction of essential nursing care data, which is categorized into nursing diagnosis, nursing intervention, nursing outcome, and intensity of nursing care. Each data category is defined and is currently undergoing pilot testing for refinement and eventual submission to the Department of Health and Human Services (DHHS) for approval. If approved, the NMDS can then be integrated into DHHS programs requiring minimum core data retrieval.

## Integration of Nursing Data to Differentiate Practice

The purposes of the NMDS are to (1) establish comparability of nursing data across clinical populations/settings, (2) describe nursing care of clients in a variety of settings, (3) demonstrate or project trends on allocation of care and resources according to health problems/nursing diagnoses, and (4) stimulate nursing research through links to the detailed data existing in nursing information systems and other health care information systems (Werley & Lang, 1988). The goal is to integrate nursing data elements into existing methods of national data retrieval systems and consequently enable differentiation of nursing as a well-defined health care service that serves as a vital link between cost and health care quality.

## Application of Integration and Differentiation

Nursing information system (NIS) developments that exploit the informating capacity of the technology and support the concept of control of nursing practice are evident. Halloran and associates (Halloran, Patterson, & Kiley, 1987; Halloran, 1988) designed, developed, and are testing a multidimensional NIS complementary to the medical data system and social service data system. The goal of the system is to demonstrate both the collaborative and discipline-distinguishing data sources that combine to explain the client care resource use and cost. The system is focused on the recording of client needs for nursing based on the clinical judgment of the nurse providing care (using a nursing diagnosis classification scheme), the provision of decision support for clinical management decisions, and the identification of patterns of nursing care and nursing care products. This project exemplifies the application of knowledge and technology to capitalize on the nurse as relevant decision maker in the clinical practice arena.

The successful incorporation of information technology to advance nursing will require active involvement of the nurse in articulating and prioritizing information needs required for effective clinical decision making in client care specific to the practice setting. To maximize the informating capacity of the technology requires the practicing nurse to conceptualize his or her role as a relevant decision maker as opposed to an information coordinator. To achieve this requires organizational contexts that share a belief in nursing as a viable resource in the clinical management of clients and that are able to harness the resources and expertise to incorporate the technology in ways that augment the nurse's clinical judgment process.

## ❖ SUMMARY

The discussion in this chapter focuses on the nature of information technology and the implications of this tool for the advancement of nursing. The nature of the technology was described in relation to data, information, and knowledge. The technical evolution of computers and telecommunications was summarized to emphasize how advancements in the technology permitted the proliferation of computers. Actual and potential societal impacts were presented with an emphasis on the nurse's role in privacy and confidentiality of computerized information.

The current level of information technology in health care was outlined with examples of data-oriented, information-oriented, and knowledge-oriented applications. The level of incorporation of these technologies into nursing was addressed with the related implications. In closing, emphasis was placed on the applications of the technology for the advancement of nursing with examples such as the Nursing Minimum Data Set and the development of an integrated nursing information system. By understanding the nature and potential impacts of information technology, nurses are better able to make conscientious choices about its use.

## ❖ APPLYING KNOWLEDGE TO PRACTICE

1. To what extent is Bell's idea of the evolution of a "knowledge elite" consistent with the professional practice of nursing and its societal influence? In what ways can information technology support the advancement of nursing as a scientifically based discipline? Discuss the pros and cons of conceptualizing nursing as "knowledge elite."

2. Review the nurse's role in privacy and confidentiality of client information. Given the predicted problems in maintaining privacy with the incorporation of information technology, discuss the nurse's responsibility for upholding confidentiality with computer based systems. Can you identify potential problems in your practice setting?

3. Distinguish between the informating and automating capacities of information technology. Describe the incorporation of computers into your practice setting and categorize the application as to informating or automating. Discuss how the informating capacity is used in your setting.

4. Describe your role as relevant decision maker in the clinical management of clients in your practice setting. What are your information needs in maximizing your decision making? Categorize your needs in relation to their source (e.g., the nurse-client encounter, face-to-face contact with colleagues, textbooks/journals, policies/procedures, etc.). Discuss the design of an NIS that would meet your information needs in decision making.

## REFERENCES

Ball, M. J., Hannah, K. J., Gerdin Jelger, U. & Peterson, H. (1988). *Nursing informatics: Where caring and technology meet.* New York: Springer-Verlag.

Banta, H. D. (1986). Technology assessment in health care. In S. Jonas (Ed.), *Health care delivery in the United States:* (3rd ed.) (pp. 465-482). New York: Springer.

Bell, D. (1973). *The coming of post-industrial society.* New York: Basic Books.

Benner, P. (1984). *From novice to expert.* Menlo Park, CA.: Addison-Wesley.

Blum, B. I. (1986). *Clinical information systems.* New York: Springer-Verlag.

Brennan, P. F. (1985). Decision support for nursing practice: The challenge and the promise. In K. J. Hannah, E. J. Guillemin, and D. N. Conklin (Eds.). *Nursing Uses of Computer and Information Science: Proceedings of the IFIP-IMIA International Symposium* (pp. 315-319). North-Holland: Elsevier Science.

Brennan, P. F., & Romano, C. A. (1987). Computers and nursing diagnoses: Issues in implementation. *Nursing Clinics of North America, 22*(4), 935-941.

Brennan, P. F. (1988) Modeling for decision support. In M. Ball, K. Hannah, U. Gerdin Jelger, & H. Peterson (Eds.), *Nursing informatics: Where caring and technology meet* (pp. 267-273). New York: Springer-Verlag.

Carper, B. A. (1978). Fundamental patterns of knowing in nursing. *Advances in Nursing Science, 1,* 13-23.

Chang, B. L., & Hirsch, M. (1988). An expert system for nursing diagnosis: Field testing of phase 1, Assessment. In Irish Nursing Board *Proceedings of the Third International Symposium on Nursing Use of Computers and Information Science* (pp. 152-164). St. Louis, Mo.: C. V. Mosby.

Clinton, J. F. (1988). The relationship between control of nursing information and control of nursing practice. In H. Werley, & N. Lang (Eds.), *Identification of the nursing minimum data set* (pp. 339-346). New York: Springer.

Covvey, H., Craven, N., & McAlister, N. (1985). *Concepts and issues in health care computing.* St. Louis, Mo.: C. V. Mosby.

Dowling, Jr., A. F. (1988). Considerations for data set development: Planning for future needs and the nature of information. In H. Werley, & N. Lang (Eds.), *Identification of the nursing minimum data set.* New York: Springer.

Fitzpatrick, J. J. (1988). Nursing knowledge and practice. In Irish Nursing Board *Proceedings of the Third International Symposium on Nursing Use of Computers and Information Science* (pp. 58-65). St. Louis, Mo.: C. V. Mosby.

Galbraith, J. (1977). *The new industrial state*. New York: New American Library.

Gordon, M. (1982). *Nursing diagnosis: Process and application*. New York: McGraw-Hill.

Graves, J., & Cocoran, S. (1988). Design of nursing information systems: Conceptual and practice elements. *Journal of Professional Nursing, 4*(3), 168-177.

Grosso, C. (1988). Knowledge acquisition for development of expert systems for nursing. In Irish Nursing Board *Proceedings of the Third International Symposium on Nursing Use of Computers and Information Science* (pp. 152-164). St. Louis, Mo.: C. V. Mosby.

Hadden, S. G. (1986). Intelligent advisory systems for managing and disseminating information. In B. Bozeman & S. Bretschneider (Eds.), *Public Administration Review, 46*(Special Issue), 572-578.

Halloran, E. J. (1988). Conceptual considerations, decision criteria, and guidelines for the nursing minimum data set from an administrative perspective. In H. Werley, & N. Lang (Eds.), *Identification of the nursing minimum data set* (pp. 48-66). New York: Springer.

Halloran, E. J., Patterson, C., & Kiley, M. L. (1987). Casemix: Matching patient need with nursing resource. *Nursing Management, 18*(3), 27-42.

Hannah, K. J. (1985). Current trends in nursing informatics: Implications for curriculum planning. In K. J. Hannah, E. J. Guillemin, and D. N. Conklin (Eds.) *Nursing Uses of Computer and Information Science: Proceedings of the IFIP-IMIA International Symposium* (pp. 181-187). North-Holland: Elsevier Science Publishers.

Hannah, K. J. (1988). Classification of decision-support systems. In M. Ball, K. Hannah, U. Gerdin Jelger, & H. Peterson (Eds.), *Nursing informatics: Where caring and technology meet* (pp. 260-266). New York: Springer-Verlag.

Happ, B. (1988). The management of artificial intelligence/expert systems in nursing and health care. In Irish Nursing Board *Proceedings of the Third International Symposium on Nursing Use of Computers and Information Science* (pp. 506-518). St. Louis, Mo.: C. V. Mosby.

Heller, B. R., Damrosch, S. P., Romano, C. A., & McCarthy, M. R. (1989). Graduate specialization in nursing informatics. *Computers in Nursing, 7*(2), 68-77.

Heriot, C., Graves, J., Bouhaddou, O., Armstrong, M., Wigertz, G., & Ben Said, M. (1988). A pain management decision support system for nurses. In Irish Nursing Board *Proceedings of the Twelfth Annual Symposium on Computer Applications in Medical Care* (pp. 63-68). Washington, D.C.: IEEE Computer Society.

Hughes, S. (1988). Bedside information systems: State of the art. In M. Ball, K. Hannah, U. Gerdin Jelger, & H. Peterson (Eds.), *Nursing informatics: Where caring and technology meet* (pp. 138-145). New York: Springer-Verlag.

Kjerulff, K. H. (1988). The integration of hospital information systems into nursing practice: A literature review. In M. Ball, K. Hannah, U. Gerdin Jelger, & H. Peterson (Eds.), *Nursing informatics: Where caring and technology meet* (pp. 243-249). New York: Springer-Verlag.

Larson, D. (1988). Development of a microcomputer-based expert system to provide support for nurses caring for AIDS patients. In Irish Nursing Board *Proceedings of the Third International Symposium on Nursing Use of Computers and Information Science* (pp. 682-690). St. Louis, Mo.: C. V. Mosby.

McCormick, K. A. (1988). A unified nursing language system. In M. Ball, K. Hannah, U. Gerdin Jelger, & H. Peterson (Eds.), *Nursing informatics: Where caring and technology meet* (pp. 168-178). New York: Springer-Verlag.

McCormick, K. A., & McQueen, L. (1988). New computer technology. In M. Johnson & J. McCloskey (Eds.), *Series on nursing administration* (Vol. I, pp. 58-69). Menlo Park, CA.: Addison-Wesley.

Milholland, K. (1986). Assessing the impact on nursing practice of CDMS. *International Journal of Clinical Monitoring and Computing, 3,* 191-197.

Northrup, A., Kraemer, K., & King, J. (1989). What every public manager should know about computing. In R. Cleary, N. Henry, & Associates (Eds.), *Managing public programs: Balancing politics, administration, and public needs* (pp. 167-192). San Francisco, CA: Jossey-Bass.

Ozbolt, J. G. (1988). Knowledge-based systems for supporting clinical nursing decisions. In M. Ball, K. Hannah, U. Gerdin Jelger, & H. Peterson (Eds.), *Nursing informatics: Where caring and technology meet* (pp. 274-285). New York: Springer-Verlag.

Peterson, H. E., & Gerdin-Jelger, U. (1988). *Preparing nurses for using information systems*. New York: National League for Nursing.

Porter, M., & Millar, V. (1985). How information gives you competitive advantage. *Harvard Business Review,* July/August, 152.

Romano, C. A. (1987). Privacy, confidentiality, and security of computerized systems: The nursing responsibility. *Computers in Nursing, 5*(3), 99-104.

Ronald, J. S., & Skiba, D. J. (1987). *Guidelines of basic computer education in nursing*. New York: National League for Nursing.

Rosenberg, R. S. (1986). *Computers and the information society*. New York: John Wiley & Sons.

Saba, V. K., & McCormick, K. A. (1986). *Essentials of computers for nurses.* Philadelphia, PA: J. B. Lippincott.

Saba, V. K., Oatway, D. M., & Rieder, K. A. (1989). How to use nursing information resources. *Nursing Outlook, 37*(4), 189-195.

Salvaggio, J. L. (1989). *The information society: Economic, social, and structural issues.* Hillsdale, NJ: Lawrence Erlbaum.

Sauter, V. (1988). Using computers in health care. In E. Sullivan & P. Decker (Eds.), *Effective management in nursing* (2nd. ed., pp. 463-494). Menlo Park, CA: Addison-Wesley.

Weiss, S. M. (1984). Expert problem-solving and consultation. In S. Weiss & C. Kulikowski (Eds.), *A practical guide to designing expert systems* (pp. 1-15). Totowa, NJ: Rowman and Allanheld.

Werley, H. H., & Lang, N. M. (1988). *Identification of the nursing minimum data set.* New York: Springer.

Williams, F. (1988). *Measuring the information society.* Newbury Park, CA: Sage.

Zielstorff, R. D., McHugh, M. L., & Clinton, J. (1988). *Computer design criteria: For systems that support the nursing process.* Kansas City, Mo.: American Nurses' Association.

Zuboff, S. (1988). *In the age of the smart machine: The future of work and power.* New York: Basic Books.

# PART 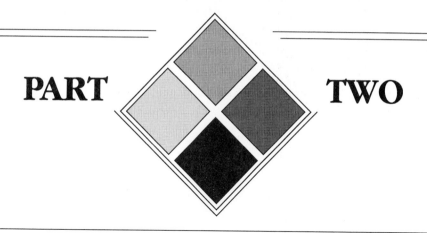 TWO

# CONCEPTS RELATED TO CLIENT CARE

Concepts related to client care are issues found in all clinical settings. A number of concepts are identified and described to assist the nurse in assessing the presence or absence of a particular phenomenon, identifying strategies to increase or decrease the behavior or its impact, and implementing and evaluating the success or failure of these strategies.

Client care concepts are divided into three overall categories: client stressors, client strengths, and major life themes. This classification scheme is somewhat different from other approaches since it recognizes that nursing interventions should not only be designed to relieve problems or stressors, but also to build on individual and family strengths. While this approach is unique, we believe it is an important conceptualization of professional nursing care.

Most registered nurses' previous education will, by necessity, have focused on problem identification, pathology, and technical skills. An appropriate objective in higher education is the provision of comprehensive care in the hospital and the community. This involves the use of creative strategies for long-term coping and adaptation. The identification and support of individual and family strengths will facilitate this process.

Most episodes of nursing care will incorporate aspects of both stressors and strengths. There may be times, however, when the focus of care will be devoted primarily to either one or the other. This will most often occur in times of crisis or urgent situations with stressors such as violence or acute pain. In general, interventions geared toward building on strengths have a more long-term focus and are designed to promote permanent, lasting changes in behavior.

Certain concepts related to client care defied categorization as either stressors or strengths but were too important to ignore. These concepts are described as major life themes as they occur throughout the life span.

In this section each concept is described followed by definitions of key terms, an in-depth discussion of the concept, and application of the concept to clinical practice. Sample nursing care plans are incorporated to assist in the clinical application of the concept. Research on each concept is integrated throughout the chapter, and discussion questions are provided to assist in further application of the concept to clinical practice.

# UNIT IV

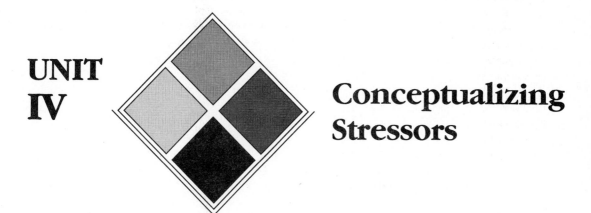

# Conceptualizing Stressors

CLIENT stressors are problems faced by individuals and families amenable to nursing interventions. The concepts are broad in scope and affect clients of all ages and in most clinical practice areas. Some concepts such as stress, disease, and pain will be encountered in most client interactions. Others such as sensory alterations, crisis, addiction, and violence might be seen less frequently and yet are phenomena that all nurses will encounter regardless of the practice setting.

The chapters in this unit describe the concept, incorporate nursing research relevant to the topic, and provide a sample nursing care plan specific to the topic. The care plans incorporate a sample medical diagnosis, nursing diagnoses or clinical description, goals, intervention, and evaluation as a model for nursing intervention. The care plans provide a beginning model for the use of the concepts in practice.

# 17 Stress

Joyce K. Engel

## OBJECTIVES

*At the completion of this chapter, the reader will be able to:*

◆ Describe three different sets of theories related to stress.

◆ Describe the effects of stress.

◆ Discuss Roy's adaptation model and stress.

◆ Identify factors to be considered in caring for clients and families experiencing stress.

Stress. Rarely has any one topic created so much fascination among both lay and professional sectors. This fascination has been present since the 1930s when Hans Selye, a Canadian endocrinologist and the most widely recognized stress researcher, first articulated a relationship between environmental stimuli and physiological reactions. His early postulations described phenomena that were common to the human experience and condition and thus began a search for further articulations of this shared experience.

Concern with the stress experience spans many disciplines; medicine, psychiatry, anthropology, sociology, and psychology are all represented in stress theory and research. Nurses, too, have been sensitive to the relevancy of theories and concepts of stress, change, coping, and adaptation and have recognized the potential of these concepts in the delivery of nursing care. This recognition is evident in the works of theorists such as Roy and Neuman, who have been heavily influenced by stress theory.

The purpose of this chapter is to provide an overview of the terms and concepts related to stress and to discuss the relevance of stress to nursing. This discussion includes delineation of major trends in stress theory and research as well as an overview of nursing theory and research that is directly related to the concept and to nursing practice.

## ❖ THE HUMAN SYSTEM AND STRESS

The stress response involves specific physiological and psychological processes. The primary effects of this disruption are experienced in the immune and endocrine systems.

When the individual senses disruption, the sensory motor receptors are activated. The signals are transmitted to the reticular activating system, which screens and selects incoming stimuli. The limbic system, which is concerned with emotions, and the thalamic and hypothalamic centers, which are responsible for autonomic and endocrine responses, work together to regulate the stress response through a series of feedback loops.

Physiological responses occur primarily as a result of the hypothalamic stimulation of the autonomic and endocrine systems. In response to stimulation, the sympathetic nervous system activates the mass-discharge phenomenon of fight or flight. This degree of arousal increases the body's capacity for energy above that needed for everyday function. Cardiac output and heart rate increase, and blood is diverted from peripheral vessels and gastrointestinal organs toward the head and trunk. Stimulation of the posterior pituitary results in secretion of vasopressin, which functions to increase circulating fluids and increase blood pressure. As changes in cardiac functioning and circulation occur, the individual may subjectively experience a pounding heart, racing pulse, and a knot in the stomach.

As the fight or flight response progresses, epinephrine is released and a number of hormones [gonadotropic hormone, thyrotropic hormone, and adrenocorticotropic hormone (ACTH)] are also released. The gonadotropic hormone causes increased secretion of glucagon and the initiation of lipolysis and glycogenolysis. Thyrotropic hormone stimulates secretion of thyroxine from the thyroid, which increases the basal metabolic rate and increases the rate of absorption of food and secretion of digestive enzymes. ACTH, together with stimulation by the sympathetic nervous system, increases production of mineralocorticoids and glucocorticoids by the adrenal gland. The mineralocorticoids influence the functioning of the kidneys, leading to the enhanced fluid retention that increases circulating blood volume. The glucocorticoids stimulate glycogenesis, which further increases serum glucose, and also promotes protein catabolism and lipolysis. Break-

down of proteins and fats provides the free amino acids necessary for metabolic functions and increases the serum levels of circulating free fatty acids, triglycerides, and cholesterol. These increased levels are essential in the provision of energy for fight or flight.

The adrenal cortex secretes the antiinflammatory glucocorticosteroids, cortisol and cortisone. Cortisol and cortisone are influential in decreasing the activity of the thymus gland, and so affect immunological functioning. In response to stress, there is often generalized decrease in leukocytes, eosinophils, and helper T-cells.

During sympathetic stimulation, norepinephrine and epinephrine are released. These substances constrict arterioles, resulting in increased blood pressure, increased serum glucose levels, and free fatty acid levels. Gastrointestinal and urinary sphincters constrict, and respiratory functioning is affected.

## The Physiology of Stress and Illness

Overall, the individual under short-term stress experiences increases in blood pressure, temperature, pulse, and respirations. Palms are sweaty and pupils are dilated. Gastrointestinal activity is increased and large skeletal muscles are tensed for action. Triglyceride, cholesterol, cortisol levels, and serum glucose levels are all increased. Over time, the chronically stressed individual may experience weight loss, wasting of muscles, and decreased resistance to infection. The relationship of these long-term effects to diseases such as hypertension, arteriosclerosis, and immune disorders seems evident. These relationships are being investigated from both the prevention and treatment aspects of disease control. Dixon and colleagues (1989) and Hyman and associates (1989), report relationships between stress and hypertension, nausea, vomiting, and the onset of rheumatoid arthritis. Caution must be exercised, however, in envisioning a simple causal relationship between specific stressors and illness. The possible cumulative effects of stress as well as several factors related to stress make the relationship between stress and illness consistent but weak.

## ❖ OVERVIEW OF CONCEPTS

Despite widespread familiarity with stress theory, there are no agreed upon conventions regarding either terminology or the domains of stress (Lazarus, 1966). Stress, for example, has been used synonymously with anxiety, frustration, and stimulus. In a review of nursing literature, Knapp (1988) found strain, stress, and stressor to be used interchangeably, and suggested the need to be more precise in our use of key terms. Knapp points out that even Selye contributed to the confusion by failing to adequately differentiate between *stress* (the cause of wear and tear) and the *strain* (the wear and tear itself). While attempts to achieve conceptual clarity are essential, one senses that the task becomes increasingly complex as the term becomes more diffuse. Mirskey (1964) referred to the diversity and complexity inherent in defining stress by commenting "I have heard a word used frequently ... which bothers me a good deal and that is the word 'stress.' If one examines the literature dealing with 'stress', it becomes apparent that almost every energy transformation can be interpreted as stressful phenomenon" (pp. 533-534).

Lazarus (1966) suggested that stress be considered an area of study and abandoned efforts to operationally define stress. In his opinion, stress is not a stimulus, a response, or an intervening variable, but a collective term that includes physiological, psychological, and sociological phenomena within a field of study (Zegans, 1982). Furthermore, Lazarus noted that there were three main variations in the concept of stress. The most common approach has been to view stress as a *stimulus* or condition that evokes disequilibrium or turbulence. Other writers have conceptualized stress as the "*reaction* of the body to any threat or change in equilibrium and is therefore a direct result or adaptation of events in the social, physical and emotional environment" (Rawlings, 1988, p. 552). Such a variation is consistent with the viewpoint Knapp presented earlier in this discussion. Still others have viewed stress as a *transaction* involving mediated interchange between the individual and the environment.

## ❖ STRESS AS A RESPONSE
### Selye and Stress

The classic definition of stress as a nonspecific response of the body to any demand placed upon it (Selye, 1974) well illustrates the conceptualization of stress as a response. Selye's definition is derived from his General Adaptation Syndrome (GAS) in which stress is considered a physiological response to stressors. Selye coined the term *stressor* to refer to the cause of stress. A *stimulus* is a stressor only if it produces a stress response, which is objective and observable.

Selye first elucidated his GAS theory of stress following an attempt to discover a new sex hormone. During his experimentation with rats, Selye discovered that rats developed anomalies of the endocrine and gastrointestinal systems following injections of crude ovarian extract. Crude extracts from other organs and from stimuli such as heat, cold, epinephrine, and pain produced similar results (Elliott and Eisdorfer, 1982). On the basis of these findings, Selye suggested that stimuli produce a typical nonspecific response of the hypothalamic–pituitary–adrenal axis. Selye insisted that regardless of the type or intensity of body assault, the hypothalamic–pituitary–adrenal axis organizes and expresses the defensive reactions. The response is considered nonspecific because the body does not selectively respond to particular stressors.

Selye ascribes the notion of internal regulation as a response to body assault to even earlier researchers and theorists. During the 1920s, noted American physiologist Walter B. Cannon suggested the term *homeostasis* for the coordinated physiologic processes which maintain most of the steady states in the organism (Cannon, 1939). Cannon further established the presence of many mechanisms that protected the body against disruption. He particularly emphasized the stimulation of the nervous system and the resulting response of the endocrine system, which occurs during crisis situations. This response is clearly linked to Selye's later theory of stress.

## The General Adaptation Syndrome

Selye (1982) divided the nonspecific response of the organism to threat into three phases. Selye (1982) believes that even very early humans must have been intuitively aware of this triphasic response to hardship.

... prehistoric man must have recognized a common element in the sense of exhaustion that overcame him in conjunction with hard labor, agonizing fear, lengthy exposure to cold or heat, starvation, loss of blood, or any kind of disease. He probably also soon discovered that his response to prolonged and strenuous exertion passed through three stages: first the task was experienced as hardship; then he grew used to it; and finally he could stand it no longer. The vague outlines of this intuitive scheme eventually were brought into precise scientific terms that could be appraised by intellect and translated into precise scientific terms (p. 8).

Using a more precise scheme, Selye labeled and described the phases of the General Adaptation Syndrome.

1. *Alarm reaction* is the fight or flight response. During the alarm reaction the individual is mobilized for defense. Tissue catabolism and hemoconcentration occur, which is characteristic of the early phases of burn injury. Because of its intensity, the alarm reaction can-

not be maintained continuously and indefinitely without death ensuing.
2. *The stage of resistance* reflects the adaptation of the individual to stress and a return to homeostasis, survival. Adaptation refers specifically to positive alterations that individuals make in their pattern of interaction with stimuli. These alterations perpetuate and increase survival, satisfaction, and utility. Selye outlined physiological changes that occur during the stage of resistance (adrenal enlargement, thymolymphatic involution, hemodilution, and anabolism) that represent the body's nonspecific response to demand. If the individual is overwhelmed by the amount, duration, or intensity of stress, or if the individual's adaptive mechanisms are ineffective, a state of exhaustion ensues.
3. *The stage of exhaustion* occurs when all energy stores are depleted. Unless this stage can be controlled, death may result. Selye believed that with most stresses, individuals experience only the first two stages of the GAS, or General Adaptation Syndrome. Encounters with stress, which Selye believed were continuously present, enhance the abilities of individuals to adapt. The most positive outcome of stress is adaptation. A common maladaptive response to stress may be illness. Even though the causal link between stress and illness may be less impressive than it initially was (Dixon, Dixon, & Spinner, 1989), much research into the links between stress and disease was initiated by Selye's work and continues at this time. More current research favors the concept that stimuli alone may not produce illness but rather that illness may result from the perception and mediation of the stimuli.

According to Selye, it was immaterial whether the situation produced *eustress* (good stress) or *distress* (bad stress). What mattered was the intensity of the demand for readjustment that was created (Selye, 1976). Selye suggested that all situations regardless of whether they were perceived as pleasurable or disturbing in outcome were stressful, and this stress response was primarily physiological. Although

Selye acknowledged the importance of perception in the stress experience, he did not modify his theoretical explanations. He did not explicitly acknowledge cognitive processes in his model and thereby did not allow for individualized responses to stress.

## Stress as a Response: Further Refinement

John Mason, among others, raised serious questions about the all-or-none nature of Selye's physiological response theory and whether it could occur in the absence of cognitive and psychological factors. The inflexibility and simplicity of the model seemed unable to completely explain the complexity of stress. Mason and his colleagues, in experiments with primates, demonstrated that different patterns of hormone excretion occurred in response to heat, cold, hunger, and exercise. Stressors were found to be function-specific or organ-specific (Mason, 1975). This finding has been supported by more recent experiments with human subjects.

In her experiments with human subjects, Frankenhaeser (1986) delineated two important components of stress and demonstrated the specificity of the sympathetic-adrenal and pituitary-adrenal activity to these two components. *Effort* is associated with engagement, involvement, and active efforts to gain and maintain control. *Distress* is associated with boredom, uncertainty, anxiety, and feelings of helplessness. In situations where distress and effort were both present (a state typical of daily hassles), Frankenhaeser found that catecholamine and cortisol levels rose. In effort without distress, characterized by joyous and high involvement, only catecholamine levels increased. The state of distress without effort, characterized by depressed clients, resulted in increases in cortisol secretion and possible increases in the release of catecholamines. This study suggests that epinephrine release is a non-specific response since increases are present in both pleasurable and distressing situations, which is somewhat consistent with Selye's work. Of perhaps greater significance is the fact that the endocrine profile varies specifically with the psychological impact of the situation, a finding that is consistent with Mason's work. These findings suggest the possibility of mediating between the initial stimulus and the ensuing response. As Frankenhaeser suggests, the key concern is how to facilitate effort without distress.

## ❖ STRESS AS A STIMULUS
### Stress and Major Life Events

When stress is regarded as a stimulus, it is viewed as disruptive. Stressful stimuli include situations that are new, changing, or intense. Stressful stimuli may include overstimulation, joy, boredom, fatigue, isolation, failure, rapid social change, loss of function, or failure of social feedback mechanisms. The stress-as-stimulus concept was also responsible for very active research into the links between stress and illness. The major disadvantage of stress-as-stimulus research was again a tendency to ignore highly individualized responses. No account was made of the individual's coping abilities, understanding of the event, or social network. Each individual was perceived as responding to stressful stimuli in the same manner, and the interpretive meaning of the event was ignored. Assumptions critical to the stimulus model of stress include: (1) life changes are experienced similarly across time and individuals, (2) perceptions of the event as positive or negative are irrelevant, and (3) there is a threshold beyond which disruption and potentially, illness may result (Beare & Myers, 1990).

Holmes and Rahe, perhaps the most widely known of the life events researchers, conducted studies with a massive number of patients and concluded that major illnesses were briefly preceded by significant life events. On the basis of this research, Holmes and Rahe (1967) developed the Social Readjustment Rating Scale (SRRS) to measure and to predict the impact of stressful events on health (Table 17-1). By adding the values for recent life events, one could determine the risk for major illness within the next 2 years. The model depicts the individual as receiving stress without effort and does not account for individual interpretations of the event. Stress can indeed

trigger a functional or organic disease, but it can also produce joy, stimulate creativity, and contribute to health. The model views stress as a consequence of adaptive challenge and not as a consequence of adaptive failure (Zegans, 1982). Many felt that such a view, which has now been supplanted by later theories, ignores the positive potential of stress as well as the multiple variables that influence the development of illness.

❖ **Table 17-1**
The social readjustment rating scale

| Life event | Mean value | Life event | Mean value |
|---|---|---|---|
| 1. Death of spouse | 100 | 23. Son or daughter leaving home | 29 |
| 2. Divorce | 73 | 24. Trouble with in-laws | 29 |
| 3. Marital separation | 65 | 25. Outstanding personal achievement | 28 |
| 4. Jail term | 63 | 26. Wife begins or stops work | 26 |
| 5. Death of close family member | 63 | 27. Begin or end school | 26 |
| 6. Personal injury or illness | 53 | 28. Change in living conditions | 25 |
| 7. Marriage | 50 | 29. Revision of personal habits | 24 |
| 8. Fired at work | 47 | 30. Trouble with boss | 23 |
| 9. Marital reconciliation | 45 | 31. Change in work hours or conditions | 20 |
| 10. Retirement | 45 | 32. Change in residence | 20 |
| 11. Change in health of family member | 44 | 33. Change in schools | 20 |
| 12. Pregnancy | 40 | 34. Change in recreation | 19 |
| 13. Sex difficulties | 39 | 35. Change in church activities | 18 |
| 14. Gain of new family member | 39 | 36. Change in social activities | 17 |
| 15. Business readjustment | 39 | 37. Mortgage or loan less than $10,000 | 16 |
| 16. Change in financial state | 38 | 38. Change in sleeping habits | 15 |
| 17. Death of a close friend | 37 | 39. Change in number of family get-togethers | 15 |
| 18. Change to different line of work | 36 | 40. Change in eating habits | 13 |
| 19. Change in number of arguments with spouse | 35 | 41. Change in schedule (vacation) | 12 |
| 20. Mortgage | 31 | 42. Christmas | 12 |
| 21. Foreclosure of mortgage or loan | 30 | 43. Minor violations of the law | 11 |
| 22. Change in responsibilities at work | 29 | | |

Scores of 150–199 indicate a 37% chance of physical illness
Scores of 200–299 indicate a 51% chance of physical illness
Scores of 300 indicate a 90% chance of physical illness

From T. Holmes and R. Rahe, J (1967). Psychosom Res *2*(4), p. 214. With permission.

## Stress and Minor Life Events

Still others believe that minor life events experienced on a daily basis are as troublesome as those of greater magnitude. Minor life events have been characterized by daily hassles and are defined as irritating and bothersome demands that have greater significance than major events because of their frequency and proximity (Kanner, Coyne, Schayer, & Lazarus, 1981; Delongis, Coyne & Dokob, 1982). Later research is supportive of the premise that daily hassles are more likely to produce a stressful life experience. In a study of women, Woods, Most, & Longenecker (1985) found that a generally stressful life experience and in particular, daily stressors, had more impact on premenstrual symptoms than episodic, major life events. In another study by Hall and Farel (1988), maternal everyday stressors were more strongly associated with mothers' reports of disruptive child behavior responses than with major life events, although maternal life events and everyday stressors considered simultaneously provided the best prediction of child behavior problems. Furthermore, maternal everyday stressors were strongly associated with maternal depression while life events were not. The implications of theories and research related to life events is the necessity to assess the stressful life experiences of individuals and their perceptions and adaptation related to that experience, rather than to assume a linear relationship between stress and disease or maladaptation. A major advantage of the work in life events was the expansion of stress into a broader context, which demanded a clearer and more in-depth understanding of stress and adaptation.

## ❖ STRESS AS A TRANSACTION
## Individualized Responses to Stress

Stress as transaction is a concept that encompasses the notion of the individual and the environment in constant interchange with each other. This concept of stress recognizes that stress is a complex phenomena that encompasses cognitive, affective, and adaptational or coping strategies (Beare & Myers, 1990) and is useful in explaining individualized responses to stimuli.

When an event or situation occurs, it is essentially neutral in orientation. Once the stimulus is identified, the individual appraises the situation, attaching meaning to what is perceived. In the Lazarus model of stress, *primary appraisal* includes judgment about the event and whether it is likely to cause threat, produce challenge, or result in harm or loss. *Threat* refers to the anticipation of harm or loss to a judgment that damage has already occurred. *Challenge* includes the judgment that the individual can influence or control the outcome as well as appraisal of what is at stake (Holroyd & Lazarus, 1982). This initial appraisal involves recognition of what is at stake and answers questions related to the jeopardy inherent in the situation. Appraisal is completed within seconds and is mediated by self-concept, beliefs, motivation, and other variables. During *secondary appraisal,* the individual evaluates the resources and options available for managing the potential or actual harm. While discussed separately here, primary and secondary appraisal are highly interdependent and may be difficult to delineate individually in many contexts.

## Individualized Responses to Stress and Coping

Once appraisal has taken place, the individual engages in the process of *coping* or self-regulation. Like stress, coping is a commonly used but ambiguous term. Lazarus views coping as behavioral and cognitive efforts to minimize stress and to master conditions that cause threat, harm, loss, or challenge. Coping may be *problem-focused* and includes information seeking and problem solving. Coping that attempts to regulate emotion is *emotion-focused.* Emotion-focused efforts include affective regulation (getting away, exercise) and emotional discharge (taking feelings out on others, letting feelings out, and substance abuse). Emotions will vary with an individual's assessment of the situation; there is no one emotion that characterizes a stress response. Coping tends to be a dynamic combination of both emotion-focused and problem-focused activities. Coping activities can serve to either aggravate or to ameliorate the stressful event, depending on the success of coping strategies. (See Chapter 26.)

## Coping and Relevance to Nursing Practice

Johnson and Lauver (1989) suggest that the ability of clients to regulate emotions will be reflected in their distress level. Regulation of problems will be reflected in the ability of clients to solve problems relative to reaching goals. Furthermore, in their study of preparatory teaching for clients, Johnson and Lauver found that concrete, objective, and unambiguous information assisted clients in problem-focused coping efforts. Fear-producing information was not seen as motivating to the client. Instead, the study suggested that fear-arousing information that focused on the emotional or reactive portions of an experience was ineffective and potentially harmful.

In another study of the impact of information on client coping, LaMontagne (1987) suggests that the flow of information between parents and doctors is of key importance to the coping of children who are hospitalized for surgery. Furthermore, coping is an age-related activity. Children are more likely to use active methods of coping as they grow older. This progression is likely related to increasing abilities in abstract thinking and therefore increasing abilities to consider alternative methods and preventive strategies as a child matures. LaMontagne found that children tended to become more active as they received greater amounts of information, and the more active they were in

coping, the more likely they were to receive information. This study emphasizes the impact of information on client coping during illness, but suggests that other variables may affect coping as well.

Chronicity may have an impact on coping. (See Chapter 21.) Gurklis and Menke (1988) suggest that physiological stressors rather than psychosocial stressors may have greater impact among chronically ill clients. In a study of 68 clients who had been on dialysis anywhere from 3 to 200 months, the researchers found that these clients were problem-focused rather than emotion-focused in their coping. Over time, these clients may have had the opportunity to focus on physical rather than emotional needs and so were more concerned with the practicalities of adjusting to fatigue, pain, repeated dialysis, and altered sleep and rest patterns.

The various aspects of coping delineated in nursing research illustrate Lazarus' premise that coping should not be viewed simplistically. Attempts to cope will be mediated by the situation and by factors such as age and previous exposure to the situation. Coping may contribute to adaptation, which is considered a positive outcome of a stressful experience.

## ❖ ADAPTATION

Although used synonymously with coping by many writers, some conceptualize coping and adaptation as being quite different. Some writers conceptualize *adaptation* as positive alterations that a person must make to improve his or her existence and perpetuate survival. Sundeen, Stuart, Rankin, and Cohen (1989) subsume coping under the term adaptation by stating that adaptation includes all reflexes, instincts, behaviors, and coping efforts needed to meet the demands of the task during a difficult situation. Adaptation includes changes in a number of responses: physiological, sociocultural, physiochemical, and behavioral. Failure to respond or change may effectively result in *maladaptation.* Maladaptation can result in illness or disharmony for the individual and the environment. Examples of maladaptation can be seen in individuals who are unable to adapt positively to chemical emissions from various plants and subsequently develop respiratory illnesses. Examples of adaptation are found in children from families where marital discord or mental illness are present, and they are still able to lead well-balanced and productive lives. Attempts to define adaptation in terms of success or failure, however, must be made cautiously. The woman who remains passive and disinterested in self-care following a mastectomy may not be maladaptive. She may instead be allowing her husband the satisfaction of "doing for" her in a positive and mutually satisfying manner. Adaptation, like stress and coping, must be considered within the complexity of context in which it occurs.

## ❖ STRESS AND NURSING

Nursing research and care delivery models suggest that nurses can alter the stress experience by enhancing the client's ability to cope with stress, either directly or indirectly.

### Roy's Adaptation Model of Nursing and Stress

Roy's Adaptation Model of nursing relies heavily on stress theory, the concept of adaptation, and the ability of the nurse to facilitate adaptation to stress. The term *adaptive* appears frequently throughout the model and is used to describe that which promotes the integrity of the person in terms of survival, growth, reproduction, and mastery.

Roy states that the individual is a biopsychosocial being who exists within an environment. The individual and the environment are sources of stimuli. The constant interaction between the individual and the environment produces change, and change necessitates efforts

to maintain integrity or to adapt. The individual is regarded as an adaptive system (see Chapter 1).

In describing the interchange between this adaptive system and the various stimuli from the environment and itself, Roy appears to adopt the view of stress as a response. Stimuli or input occur and humans respond through the use of two control mechanisms (Fig. 17-1). The *regulator* control mechanism parallels very closely Selye's conceptualization of the body's neuroendocrine response to stressors, while the *cognator* control system reflects the ability of the system to process the stimuli through intellectual and emotional methods. In her model, Roy postulates that the regulator and cognator subsystems frequently work together to facilitate adaptation in four different modes.

The four different channels for adaptation include physiological function, self-concept, role function, and interdependence. Physiological function has been further subdivided into oxygenation, nutrition, elimination, activity and rest, skin integrity, the senses, fluid and electrolyte balance, neurological function, and endocrine function (Roy, 1984). Behaviors in each of these modes may be affected by focal, residual, and contextual factors. Adaptation may occur predominantly in one mode or simultaneously in several modes. Adaptive problems such as the effects of stress occur when excesses or deficits exist in the modes (see the box on p. 315). The client who has recently suffered a myocardial infarction may deny changes or the need for alterations in self-concept, role function, and interdependence and yet, his physical self is adjusting to the insult of an infarction. Adaptation is conceptualized as multidimensional and was developed in response to Roy's concern as to how people respond to change.

The output of an adaptive system is either adaptation or an ineffective response. Obviously, the role of the nurse is to promote adaptive responses. Roy, however, expands the

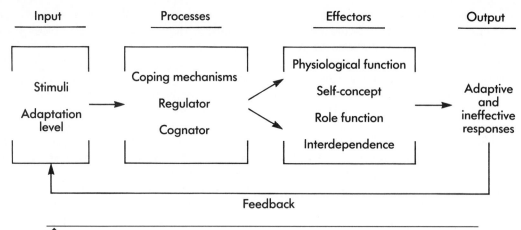

| Input | Processes | Effectors | Output |
|---|---|---|---|

Feedback

❖ **Fig. 17-1**    The person as an adaptive system. *From Roy, C. (1984). Introduction to nursing: An adaptation model (2nd ed.) Englewood Cliffs, New Jersey: Prentice Hall, p. 30, with permission.*

nursing role even further. The nurse must also act to expand the individual's coping abilities so that a wider range of stimuli is tolerated. According to Roy's model, each individual has limits to adaptation that are affected by the condition of the person or the individual's state of coping. This introduces the idea of control into stress, which goes beyond earlier theories of stress in which the individual was considered a passive recipient of stimuli. It also reflects a more optimistic view of the human capability and provides an arena in which nursing activities can occur.

### Nursing Care and Stress

Like Roy, other researchers and writers in nursing suggest that nurses can promote the adaptation of clients to stress. A number of strategies such as problem-solving, assessment of social supports, life-style modification, relaxation training, therapeutic touch, biofeedback, massage, meditation, and imagery have been identified as potentially useful in the management of stress (Clarke, 1985). Clarke states that nurses can and should assist in strengthening a client's

resistance to stressors and teach indirect coping strategies of therapeutic relaxation or guided imagery. However, the effectiveness of techniques needs to be evaluated carefully since research findings in this area are controversial. For example, Crowther (1983) found that progressive muscle relaxation and imagery was effective in reducing blood pressure in hypertensive patients but Hyman and associates (1989) and Mast (1986) caution that the effects of indirect techniques may have more limited value and generalizability.

Before attempting to enhance the coping skill of clients, nurses must exercise discretion in the assessment of stress. Studies related to the evaluation of stress (Biley, 1989, Carr & Powers, 1986) found differences between nurse and patient perceptions as to the stress experience of being a patient. This research is significant in that it demonstrates the differences that occur in perceptions, depending on the perspective from which the experience is viewed. Nurses may view the patient's experience normatively while the patient views it from a totally individualized and personalized perspective. The differences in perception can

## ❖ EFFECTS OF STRESS ORGANIZED BY ROY'S ADAPTIVE MODES

**BASIC PHYSIOLOGIC NEEDS**
◆ Exercise and rest
Little or no exercise, little or no recreation, poor time management, fatigue, sleep difficulties, difficulties relaxing, reliance on drugs/medications/alcohol for relaxation.
◆ Nutrition
Weight loss/gain, muscle wasting, ulcers, skin lesions, indigestion, nausea, vomiting, changes in appetite, elevated triglyceride and cholesterol levels.
◆ Elimination
Diarrhea, constipation, urinary frequency.
◆ Fluid and electrolytes
Inadequate nutrition, excessive perspiration.
◆ Oxygen
Increased respiratory rate.
◆ Circulation
Rapid pulse, elevated blood pressure, palpitations, cardiovascular disease.
◆ Regulation
Increased temperature, dilated pupils, elevated cortisol and serum glucose levels, decreased resistance to infection, impotence, decreased pain tolerance.

**SELF-CONCEPT**
◆ Physical self
Ineffective health protection behaviors, changes in health behaviors.
◆ Personal self
Difficulty making decisions, confusion, negative thinking, difficulties learning, poor self-esteem, decreased self-confidence, unrealistic expectations of self, depression, anxiety, anger, feeling overwhelmed, spiritual distress, confusion about beliefs and values.
◆ Interpersonal self
Increased isolation, loneliness, dysfunctional relationships, dissatisfaction with relationships.

**ROLE MASTERY**
Unrealistic expectations of self and others, ineffective functioning in roles, increased conflict with others, inability to handle stressful situations.

**INTERDEPENDENCE**
Isolation, loneliness, aggression, anger.

From Roy, C. (1980). Conceptual models for nursing practice. In Riehl, J. P. and Roy, Sr. C. (editors). Norwalk, CT: Appleton-Century-Crofts.

## ❖ NURSING CARE PLAN

| | |
|---|---|
| **CLIENT:** | John P. |
| | 48-year-old businessman. Impending divorce. |
| **MEDICAL DIAGNOSIS:** | Myocardial infarction. |
| **NURSING DIAGNOSIS:** | Anxiety: related to loss of physiological health, role failure, loneliness. |
| | Cardiac output decreased: related to physiological alterations. |
| | Noncompliance: related to hostility, powerlessness. |

| GOALS | INTERVENTIONS |
|---|---|
| John will experience decreased anxiety. | ◆ With client, identify stressors in illness experience and prehospitalization experience. |
| | ◆ With client, identify emotional, cognitive, and physiological responses to stressors (especially impending divorce, and perceived impact of a medical diagnosis upon work performance). |
| | ◆ Assist client to identify past effective coping strategies, resources, and support systems that have been effective in coping with stress. |
| | ◆ Assess motivation to learn alternative methods for coping with stress. |
| | ◆ If client is motivated, develop a contract with client related to present and future stress management strategies. |
| | ◆ Provide (or arrange with other disciplines) for appropriate teaching related to the stress management contract. |
| | ◆ Facilitate visits and involvement with significant support persons. |
| John will experience increased cardiac output. | ◆ Monitor cardiac functioning. |
| | ◆ Ambulate progressively. |
| | ◆ Encourage client to relax, using relaxation techniques (if specified in client contract). |

**NURSING CARE PLAN—cont'd**

| GOALS | INTERVENTIONS |
|---|---|
| John will comply with treatment regimens and stress management strategies. | ◆ Encourage expression of feelings.<br>◆ Identify learning needs related to treatment regimens and stress management programs.<br>◆ Provide teaching appropriate for the learning needs assessment (start with client's priorities).<br>◆ Reinforce the client's attempts to positively control his treatment regimen and stress responses. |

**EVALUATION**

John reports reduced anxiety as a result of identifying stressors and previous effective coping strategies. The stress management contract includes specific stress management strategies such as the use of support systems or relaxation techniques. John's ability to walk progressively longer distances is one indication of increased cardiac output. Over time, John continues to adhere to his treatment protocol and effectively uses stress management techniques.

only be understood through assessment and appreciation of the true complexity of the stress experience.

From the perspective of nursing care, the nurse and client together must identify the stressors from the client's perspective, and then identify effects (affective, cognitive, and physiological) of the stressors upon the client. Since identification of stressors can further accentuate feelings of being overwhelmed, the nurse must, together with the client, identify coping skills and life-style patterns that have positively and negatively influenced the stress response. With this as a basis, nursing actions will emphasize protection of the client against further stress as a result of the health care experience, mobilize positive behaviors and resources, and facilitate alternative methods of dealing with stress. Ongoing and final evaluation of the cli-

ent's level of stress and abilities to cope with stress are essential to the determination of whether nursing interventions have been sufficiently individualized and effective to promote stress management. A sample care plan is shown on pp. 316 and 317.

### Families and Stress

Finally, any consideration of the individual's stress experience must also take into account the stress experienced by the family. The stress of illness and disability and of the individual's experience also produces stress and disequilibrium in the family, which is a network of interconnected and interdependent relationships. Hayes and Knox (1984), in a study of parents of children hospitalized for long-term disabilities, found that the distance between the parental and professional understanding of the hospital experience contributed greatly to family disequilibrium and parental stress. Oberst and Scott (1988) found that the stress of spouses of nonterminal surgical clients with cancer was remarkably similar, although the sequence in which it occurred during the care of the client was different. Families experience a high need for information about their loved ones. Nurses, as readily available contact persons, are in a position to offer information and education. The need for information and involvement, however, varies markedly with each family and must be individually assessed. Too much involvement in care may increase the stress of family members.

Assessment of the family's coping skills, problem solving abilities, and needs is an essential step to understanding the stress of the family and to their inclusion in care (Alcock & Mahoney, 1990; Logan, 1988). Involvement in the actual care of clients varies with the needs of each family (Alcock, 1990; Nielson, 1990) and can only be determined through ongoing assessment of the family. Families generally need accurate current information, physical proximity to the ill or disabled relative, and support and empathy for the feelings of family members (Alcock & Mahoney, 1990; Hull, 1989; Nielson, 1990). Finally, families need to be considered as an integral part of any treatment constellation that directs its efforts toward alleviation of stress caused by and contributing to the experience of illness.

## ❖ SUMMARY

The concepts of stress are complex. To attempt definition of terms or clarification of concepts demands acknowledgment of the diversity of thinking and theories in the field.

The psychological response of the body to stress is complex and primarily affects neuroendocrinal and immunological functioning. Long-term stress may have a link with disease because of the alterations in body functioning that are produced by stress.

Stress may be variously defined as a response, stimulus, or transaction. These definitions are derived from the works of eminent researchers and theorists in the field of stress.

Adaptation is a concept central to stress theory and related intimately to coping. Perceptions of adaptation, in terms of success or failure, may vary with the individual who perceives the adaptation.

Stress theories and stress research are relevant for nursing. Research suggests that professional nurses can use knowledge of stress to alter the stress experience positively for clients and their families. Roy's model of adaptation provides an excellent example of how a nursing theorist has adapted stress theory to the care of clients. Her model delineates both the responses of clients to stress and the role of the nurse in assisting the client to reach adaptation. Interventions must acknowledge the complexity of stress by recognizing the interaction of the individual and his or her environment and the differing perceptions of individuals in relation to the same stimuli. In this way, nurses can use stress theory to enhance nursing care and to assist the client in minimizing stress.

## ❖ APPLYING KNOWLEDGE TO PRACTICE.

1. Find at least two research studies that deal with stress related to nurses. Outline key elements in these studies that could be applied to your setting to either aid in understanding stress or relieving stress.
2. Discuss the relationship between stress and burnout.
3. Discuss the difficulties inherent in defining stress. Define stress according to your understanding of the phenomenon.
4. Describe a client for whom you have cared whose response to stress was maladaptive. What nursing interventions did you use to promote adaptation?

## REFERENCES

Alcock, D., & Mahoney, W. (1990). Parents of long-stay children. *Canadian Nurse, 86*(1), 20-23.

Appley, M. H., & Trumbull, R. (1986). *Dynamics of stress. Physiological, psychological, and social perspectives.* New York: Plenum Press.

Beare, P., & Myers, J. (1990). *Principles and practice of adult health nursing.* St. Louis: C. V. Mosby.

Biley, F. C. (1989). Nurses' perception of stress in preoperative surgical patients. *Journal of Advanced Nursing, 14*(7), 575-581.

Cannon, W. B. (1939). The Wisdom of the Body. New York: W. W. Norton, Inc.

Crowther, J. H. (1983). Stress management. Training and relaxation imagery in the treatment of essential hypertension. *Journal of Behavioral Medicine, 6*(2), 169-187.

Carr, J. A., & Powers, M. J. (1986). Stressors associated with coronary bypass surgery. *Nursing Research, 35*(4), 243-246.

Clarke, M. (1986). Stress and coping. Constructs for nursing. *Journal of Advanced Nursing, 9*(2), 90-95.

Delongis, A., Conyne, J., & Dokof, G. (1982). Relationship of daily hassles, uplifts, and major life events to health status, *Health Psychology, 1*(2), 119-136.

Dixon, J. P., Dixon, J. K., & Spinner, J. (1989). Perceptions of life-pattern disintegrity as a link in the relationship between stress and illness, *Adv. Nurs. Sc., 11*(2), 1-11.

Elliott, G. R., & Eisdorfer, C. (1982). *Stress and human health. Analysis and implications of research.* New York: Springer Publishing Company.

Frankenhaeser, M. (1986). *A psychobiological framework for research on human stress and coping.* In M. H. Appley, & R. Trumbull, (eds.), Dynamics of stress. Physiological, psychological, and social perspectives, (pp. 106–107), New York: Plenum Press.

Gurklis, J. A., & Menke, E. M. (1988). Identification of stressors and use of coping methods in chronic hemodialysis patients. *Nursing Research. 37*(4), 236–241.

Hall, L. A., & Farel, A. M. (1988). Maternal stresses and depressive symptoms: Correlates of behavior problems in young children. *Nursing Research, 37*(3), 156-161.

Hayes, V. E., & Knox J. E. (1984). The experience of stress in parents of children hospitalized with long-term disabilities. *Journal of Advanced Nursing, 9,* 333-341.

Holmes, T. H., & Rahe, R. H. (1967). The social readjustment rating scale. *Journal of Psychosomatic Research, 11,* 213-218.

Holroyd, K. A., & Lazarus, R. S. (1982). *Stress, coping, and somatic adaptation.* In L. Goldberger, & S. Bretznitz (eds.), S. Handbook of stress. Theoretical and clinical aspects. New York: The Free Press.

Hull, M. M. (1989). Family needs and supportive nursing behaviors during terminal cancer: A review. *Oncology Nursing Forum, 16*(6), 787-792.

Hyman, R. B., Feldman, H. R., Harris, R. B., Levin, R. F., & Malloy, G. B. (1989). The effects of relaxation training on clinical symptoms. A clinical analysis. *Nursing Research, 38*(4), 216-220.

Johnson, J. E., & Lauver, D. R. (1989). Alternative explanations of coping with stressful experience associated with physical illness. *Advances in Nursing Science, 11*(2), 29-59.

Kanner, A., Conyne, J., Schaefer, C., & Lazarus, R. (1981). Comparisons of two modes of stress management: Daily hassles and uplifts versus major life events. *Journal of Behavioral Medicine, 4*(1), 1-39.

Lazarus, R. (1966). *Psychological stress and the coping process.* New York: McGraw Hill.

LaMontagne, L. L. (1987). Children's preoperative coping. Replication and extension. *Nursing Research, 36*(3), 163-167.

Logan, M. (1988). Care of the terminally ill includes the family. *Canadian Nurse. 84*(5), 30–32.

Knapp, T. R. (1989). Stress vs strain: A methodological critique, *Nursing Research, 37*(3), 181-184.

Mason, J. W. (1975). A historical view of the stress field. Part II, *Journal of Human Stress, p. 22.*

Mast, D. E. (1986). Effects of imagery. *Image, 18*(3), 118-120.

Mirsky, I. A. (1964). Discussion in the Timberline conference on psychophysiologic aspects of cardiovascular disease. Part II, *Psychosomatic Medicine, 26,* 533-534.

Nielson, D. (1990). One parent's perspective. *Canadian Nurse, 86*(1), 18-19.

Oberst, M. T., & Scott, D. M. (1988). Post discharge distress in surgically treated cancer patients and their spouses. *Research in Nursing and Health. 11*(4), 223–230.

Rawlings, M. (1988). *Anxiety, fear, and stress.* In J. B. Flynn, & P. Heffron, (eds.): Nursing. From concept to practice. (pp 543–558) Norwalk, Appleton and Lange.

Roy Sr. C. (1980). *The Roy adaptation model.* In Riehl J. P., & Roy, C. (eds.), conceptual models of nursing practice. (2nd ed.) (pp. 179-188). Norwalk, CT: Appleton-Century-Crofts.

Roy, Sr. C. (1984). *Introduction to nursing: An adaptation model.* Englewood Cliffs, Prentice-Hall Inc.

Selye, H. (1974). *Stress without distress.* Philadelphia: JB Lippincott.

Selye, H. (1982). *History and the present status of the stress concept.* In L. A. Goldberger, & S. Breznitz, (eds.), Handbook of stress. Theoretical and clinical aspects. New York: The Free Press.

Sundeen, S. J., Stuart, G. W., Rankin, E. A., & Cohen, S. A. (1989). *Nurse-client interaction. Implementing the nursing process.* (208-244). St. Louis: C. V. Mosby.

Woods, N. F., Most, A., & Longenecker, G. D. (1985). Major life events, daily stressors, and premenstrual symptoms, *Nursing Research, 34*(5), 263-267.

Zegans, L. S. (1982). *Stress and the development of somatic disorders.* In L. A. Goldberger, & S. Breztnitz, (eds.), Handbook of stress. Theoretical and clinical aspects. New York: The Free Press.

# 18 Disease

Joyce K. Engel

## OBJECTIVES

*At the completion of this chapter, the reader will be able to:*

◆ Describe the links between health, disease, and stress.

◆ Describe disease and stress as personal constructs.

◆ Relate the impact of disease and stress to nursing care and to the ecological model of disease.

◆ Describe Neuman's model in relation to health, disease, stress, and nursing care.

Traditionally, the link between stress and disease has been conceptualized as causal and linear, which has been consistent with the medical model of cause, disease, and treatment. The work of Hans Selye, who pioneered the idea of a nonspecific physiological response to stressors or stress-inducing stimuli, provided a basis for considering stress as a causal agent for disease. While this link has been upheld consistently but weakly in more contemporary research studies, newer theories have necessitated consideration of a new relationship: disease as a stressor.

The focus of this chapter will be on consideration of health, disease, and stress as part of the entire life process. The relationship of each construct to the other is a function of how the individual appraises stimuli interrelationships among body, mind, spirit, and environment. Subsequently, stress may be conceptualized as an antecedent to disease, a consequence of disease, or as a component of health. In caring for individuals who experience disease, the nurse must be alert to the personal and evolving meaning of disease, stress, and health for the client, and assume a broader ecological stance that acknowledges the impact of mind, body spirit, and environment.

## ❖ OVERVIEW OF CONCEPTS, THEORIES, AND RESEARCH

*Stress* is a multidimensional concept and has been subjected to a variety of definitions. The definitional dilemma is one of defining the parameters of stress. Selye (1974) defined stress in physiological terms as the nonspecific response of the body to any demand placed upon it. Holmes and Rahe (1967) perceived stress as a stimulus to major life disruptions, particularily disease. While these two schools of thought seem basically polarized, some see the concepts as part of a sequence from stressor through reaction to consequence (Crosby,

1988; Elliott & Eisdorfer, 1982). When presented with stressful stimuli or stressors, a feedback loop occurs that effectively translates cognitive, emotional, and behavioral assaults into the familiar response of Selye's General Adaptation Syndrome (GAS). When faced with stressors, the individual initiates coping strategies that may result in complete or partial *adaptation,* which is defined as positive, purposeful alternations that maintain stability and perpetuate survival. Partial adaptation may result in a state of residual stress that is transmitted to the sympathetic-adrenal-medullary system. The sympathetic nervous system provides for activation of the neural system and prepares the individual to confront the stress by dilating the pupils, shunting blood away from the periphery of the body, and increasing the circulatory rate (Crosby, 1988). The endocrine system responds with numerous secretory changes that involve growth hormone, ACTH, cortisol, thyroid stimulating hormone, thryoxine, vasopressin, follicle-stimulating hormones, epinephrine, norepinephrine, and insulin. Excessive stress on a longer term basis has been implicated with changes in the immunological system, hypertrophy of the adrenal cortex, gastrointestinal ulcers, loss of body weight, and irregularities in body temperature. These changes have been further implicated in pathophysiologies such as rheumatoid arthritis, infections, allergic diseases, hypertension, cancer, and cardiovascular diseases.

## Disease as a Stressor

Disease as a consequence of stress may in turn produce stress, which then completes the sequence of stressor, reaction, and consequence. In research with patients with rheumatoid arthritis, Crosby (1988) found that emotional stress and physical symptoms were directly related. As emotional stress levels increased, the symptoms of rheumatoid arthritis intensified. As the symptoms of rheumatoid arthritis intensified, emotional stress levels increased. On this basis, Crosby suggested that nurses need to consider both psychological and physiological manifestations when caring for clients with this disease.

While Crosby's study recognizes links between stress as a cause of disease and disease as a cause of stress, other writers such as Lazarus indicate that stress may be even more complex. In an attempt to explain why responses to a stressor are so individualized, Lazarus (1966) theorized that stress was a transaction and an adaptive commerce between the organism and the environment.

## The Impact of Appraisal Upon Disease and Stress

Consideration of the interaction between the individual and environment reflects movement towards a more contemporary, holistic view of health that recognizes the complexity of any experience, including that of disease and stress. Parse (1981), a recent nursing theorist, views this relationship between man and environment as dynamic and freely interchanging. Humans are inseparable from their environment and ascribe meaning to this coexistence with environment through languaging, imaging, and valuing. Humans thus language, image, and create their own health, which is continuously changing and transcending what is possible. The concepts of languaging, imaging, and valuing in relation to health and environment fit closely with contemporary theories of stress in which the individual ascribes personal meaning to stimuli. The process of appraising stimuli is the process of interpreting the stimuli in terms of their potential for stress. This process may explain why some individuals are devastated by illness and disabilities while others react to similar situations with less evidence of stress.

According to Lazarus, stress is mediated by cognitive, affective, and coping strategies. Any stimulus, including disease or disability, is neutral until interpreted and filtered through a perceptual screen. Since the perceptual screen of each individual is affected by factors such as experience, cognition, and emotion, perceptions and responses to similar stimuli will vary. Lazarus uses the term *appraisal* to refer to the process of assessing stimuli and resources for coping with the stimuli. This process is integral to understanding why certain individuals are exposed to apparently noxious stimuli without experiencing illness or other symptoms of distress while others are exposed to fewer noxious stimuli with greater negative effects. The possibility of individual susceptibility to stress necessitates some caution in attributing a direct, causal relationship between stress and disease and disease and stress.

The difficulty in singling out specific stress-related causes for disease is further complicated by the residual impact of stress. Over time, these residual effects may accumulate, making it difficult to determine which stressful factors produced the pathophysiology. This is particularly relevant since some stress-related disorders may take up to 20 years to develop. Time, accumulation of stress, and individual susceptibilities complicate the view that stress is a perfect prediction of illness (Holmes & Rahe, 1967). Stress cannot be considered a singular cause of disease (Jasmin & Trygstad, 1979) and any consideration of stress as a causal agent must recognize the interaction of cognition, resources, and environment.

## The Impact of Disease: Constructing Patterns and Interrelationships

The complexity of perception and appraisal in stress, disease, and health is recognized in the *ecological model* of disease. In this model, disease is a construct inferred from interactive processes within a naturally occurring system (Hughes & Kennedy, 1983). Disease is a disharmony or failure of adaptation within the larger phenomenon of life. Like health, which is also part of that phenomenon, disease is constructed out of the interrelationships among mind, body, spirit, and environment. The impact of disease is also a construct of these interrelationships and is dynamic and personal.

Dubos (1959), an earlier writer, envisioned health broadly as the condition of the total or whole person engaged in effective interaction with the environment. This definition differs remarkably from any view of health in which the individual passively engages in an absence of disease or infirmity, or as in the response approach to stress, where the individual responds to stimuli. It implies a dynamic, personal perception of health that is determined through interaction with the environment. This perception of health is much like that of Dunn (1961), who defined health as an emergent process, characteristic of an entire life span. Like Parse, Dunn believed that health was a continuously unfolding process, created and enacted by the individual. Within this process, stress could be conceptualized as either part of health or as part of disease. Stress, disease, and health are all part of the entire life process and reflect adaptations to the environment.

Concern with the personal nature of health and disease, as well as with the broad, multidimensional nature of environment may be reflective of a shift of perspective in relation to health and disease (Allan & Hall, 1988). Traditionally, the emphasis was on establishing the cause of disease and fixing it. Disease was treated as a self-contained unit, separate from the individual who housed it. The primary thrust was that of establishing a single cause for each disease (Allan & Hall, 1988). Much emphasis was placed on the care of the disease, and little attention was focused on impact. This approach ignores the multidimensional nature of health and disease, which involves biology, environment, life-style, and health care (La-

Londe, 1974). The monocausal, technocratic medical model ignored environment and factors that could not be understood through a simple, causal relationship. The movement towards an ecological model of health and away from the technocratic medical model has been necessitated by pressing environmental problems, recognition of the value of disease prevention, and failure of the medical model to adequately deal with chronic illness and mental health problems, which have replaced communicable diseases as predominant health concerns (Epp, 1986). As well as the inability to establish single causes and cure in several instances of these health concerns, the medical model fails to consider the impact of these conditions upon the life-style of the client.

## The Impact of Disease Upon Environment

Consideration of an ecological model of health, in which the emphasis is upon identification of patterns and person-environment interactions (Newman, 1986) necessitates movement away from the medically oriented search for causality of disease. In the medical model, stress is considered relevant primarily because it may act as a precipitating factor in the development of disease and because of its impact upon already established disease. The client who has experienced a myocardial infarction is told to reduce a life-style of stressors because the rigors of his life contribute to continuing pathology. While this approach has merit and has certainly been supported by the "stress as a response" and "stress as a stimulus" framework, it largely ignores the impact of disease on the individual and his environment, of which the family is an important component. Out of the latter viewpoint arises concern with how a myocardial infarction will affect function and lifestyle. Will the client and family be immobilized because of fear of recurrent pain? Or will the client reach for a level of health superior to that experienced before the myocardial infarction? "The focus of nursing on function and on care defines the phenomena of illness and health more broadly than a focus on disease, cause, cure, emotional response, or reaction to stress" (Visintainer, 1986) and is consistent with a broader view of health and disease. This viewpoint facilitates consideration of disease and stress from a multifactorial perspective. It also recognizes the need to focus on the consequences rather than the cause of disease, which is integral to any discussion of disease as a stressor.

## ❖ NEUMAN, DISEASE, AND STRESS

The value of Neuman's model to a discussion of disease as a stressor is the emphasis that the model places upon both the antecedents and the consequences of disease. While the model may not totally embrace a holistic view, Neuman embraces the need to consider health from a multidimensional viewpoint.

Neuman (1989) views the person as a composite of physiological, psychological, sociocultural, and developmental factors who responds to stimuli with a normal range of responses. Each person is surrounded by three hypothetical boundaries: lines of resistance, normal lines of defense, and flexible lines of response. The lines of resistance represent the individual's final and most intimate defenses. When this is overcome, the very core of the individual becomes vulnerable. The normal lines of defense represent patterns of coping and problem-solving behaviors that the individual usually evokes when confronted with environmental demands. Because this line of defense is influenced by physical and genetic factors, it is easy to envision that normal coping mechanisms may be altered by the experience of illness or fatigue. The flexible line of defense has the most potential for change, since it can be strengthened by the acquisition and learning of new behavior and can perhaps be most influenced by interventions designed to optimize the individual's state of health.

Unlike theorists such as Parse, Neuman views health as a state. This state is one of balance and harmony between the individual and environment and is influenced at any one time through interaction and adjustment with the environment. The emphasis on adjustment rather than creation of change (Thibodeau, 1983) suggests that the individual tends to be controlled by, rather than in control of, the environment.

The concept of health is closely linked to the boundaries that surround the core of the individual. The normal line of defense represents a steady state or state of illness that is specific for each individual. Illness occurs when the line of defense is overwhelmed by stressors. Factors such as time of occurrence, past coping mechanisms, intensity, and perception influence how an individual responds to stressors. Nursing is a "unique profession in that it is concerned with all of the variables affecting an individual's response to stressors" (Neuman, 1974, p. 102). The emphasis on strengthening and maximizing coping as well as on the effects of multiple variables in mediating stress is particularly consistent with current thinking related to stress. This aspect of the model together with the various levels of prevention establishes a useful basis for dealing with the stressful consequences of disease.

## Levels of Nursing Intervention

Nursing intervention, which involves the cooperation of the client, can occur at primary, secondary, and tertiary levels. *Primary prevention* is carried out before a response or disease occurs. The goal of primary prevention is strengthening the normal lines of defense through prevention of invasion by stressors, provision of information to strengthen and maintain existing client strengths, and support

of positive coping (Neuman, 1989). *Secondary prevention* focuses on early detection of symptoms once a reaction has occurred and includes maximization of the client's own resources, negotiation with the client for change, and support of a positive reaction to illness. *Tertiary prevention* follows active treatment and is directed at assisting the client to achieve a new level of stability through negotiation of change, education, support of client-directed efforts, and coordination of health resources. These levels of intervention are illustrated in the nursing care plan on pp. 326 and 327.

While Neuman's model may conceptualize the client as more passive than active in relation to the environment, the model is valuable in that it provides direction for illness-oriented activities through the concept of primary prevention, as well as direction for reconstitution of the client during and following illness. The recognition of the need for reconstitution is an important aspect in dealing with a client who is experiencing or has experienced disease and acknowledges that disease has an impact on the stability of the human system.

## ❖ THE IMPACT OF DISEASE UPON THE INDIVIDUAL

The need to strengthen and maximize coping is particularly applicable to the adjustment of clients to acute and chronic illness. Disease provides a disequilibrium that challenges coping abilities and the boundaries of these individuals. In a study of clients with chronic coronary artery disease, Riegel (1989) delineated the profound emotional response of clients to physical crisis and limitations. Clients with chronic coronary artery disease experience fears of recurrence, depression, fatigue, anxiety, and changes in self-esteem that persist for years. Denial and invalidism, which occur in response to disease, can affect adjustment and contribute to an ongoing cycle of disease-response-disease.

# ❖ NURSING CARE PLAN

| | |
|---|---|
| **CLIENT:** | Mary M. |
| | 35 years old |
| | Housewife/Mother |
| **MEDICAL DIAGNOSIS:** | Rheumatoid arthritis |
| **NURSING DIAGNOSIS:** | Activity intolerance |
| | Mobility, impaired physical |
| | Comfort, alteration in: pain |

| GOALS | NURSING INTERVENTIONS |
|---|---|
| **PRIMARY PREVENTION**<br>Mary will reduce factors that may precipitate fatigue. | ◆ Encourage 8 to 10 hours of uninterrupted sleep.<br>◆ Encourage Mary to alternate activities with rest periods.<br>◆ Assess for home arrangements that will prevent fatigue (e.g., assistance of husband with instrumental activities).<br>◆ Provide education related to positive management of stress. |
| Mary will maintain areas of health. | ◆ Teach client nutritional practices that will avoid obesity.<br>◆ Have client sleep on a firm mattress to prevent back deformities. |
| Mary will retain current mobility status. | ◆ Teach ROM exercises to prevent stiffening. |
| **SECONDARY PREVENTION**<br>Mary will maintain physical and emotional strength. | ◆ Encourage verbalization of feelings and identification of specific stressors and coping skills.<br>◆ Encourage Mary to carry out responsibilities and activities when pain relief is experienced. |
| Mary will experience minimal pain and stiffness. | ◆ Administer medications as ordered to relieve pain.<br>◆ Encourage expression of thoughts and feelings related to pain and disease.<br>◆ Encourage active participation in treatment regimens. |
| Mary will minimize limitations in mobility. | ◆ Encourage repositioning every 2 to 4 hours.<br>◆ Encourage full participation in care planning and treatment regimens. |

**NURSING CARE PLAN—cont'd**

| GOALS | NURSING INTERVENTIONS |
|---|---|

**TERTIARY PREVENTION**

Mary will achieve maximal relaxation and rest.

♦ Teach imagery, relaxation techniques.
♦ Encourage family problem solving around Mary's need to rest.

Mary will achieve pain relief.

♦ Assess efficacy of pain relief measures.
♦ Encourage Mary to identify factors that increase pain.
♦ Provide back massage to ease pressure.

Mary will experience relief of deformity and mobility restrictions.

♦ Provide ambulatory aids.

**EVALUATION**

Mary engages in primary prevention activities such as alternating activity with rest periods during the day and obtaining several hours of uninterrupted sleep. In addition, she reports nutritional intake that limits obesity and performs ROM exercises daily. Mary undertakes secondary prevention activities when she controls her pain, verbalizes the use of specific coping skills and changes position at least every two hours. Success of tertiary prevention measures include reports of pain relief, the use of imagery and relaxation techniques, and the use of aids to reduce deformity.

## Disintegrity as a Stressor

The experience of *disintegrity* or being unable to live one's life as one should (Dixon, Dixon, & Spinner, 1989) appears as a major stressor in disease. Studies of clients with acute and chronic illness have demonstrated that clients are particularly concerned about the limitations that the disease imposes on life-style (Crosby, 1989; Dixon, Dixon, & Spinner, 1989; Gurklis & Menke, 1988; Lambert, 1985). Clients on renal dialysis and with rheumatoid arthritis worry about mobility; the ostomy client is faced with physical symptoms and alterations in function that are more severe than expected; and the client with cancer struggles to redefine life. All concerns represent a response to disequilibrium, a disequilibrium that has been brought about by disease and that cannot be easily solved with a specific cure or solution.

## Managing Defenses Against the Effects of Disease

The need to support and strengthen physical responses to demands placed on the human organism is familiar to nurses and is operationalized through appropriate management of hydration, mobility, and other needs. Neuman's model implies, however, that the support of the client goes beyond management of physical needs and must include education, mobilization of resources, and enhancement of the client's own efforts to cope. Dimond (1980) and Clarke (1985) specifically outline methods for enhancing the client's own abilities to cope such as giving information, assisting with problem solving, and teaching the client techniques such as guided imagery and relaxation. While research into the effectiveness of guided imagery and relaxation techniques (Hyman, Feldman, Harris, Levin, & Malloy, 1989; Mast, 1986; Crowther, 1983; Hughes, Brown, & Lawlis, 1983) is inconclusive, there is sufficient evidence to suggest that such techniques may serve to augment a client's coping abilities in some instances.

The importance of social support in buffering and mediating the stress experience is well documented (Riegel, 1989; Mercer & Ferketich, 1988; Roberts, 1988). Social support, however, may not be useful unless it is perceived as support. Riegel (1989) suggested that perceived support was congruent with the needs of the client in relation to timing, source, and structure. Furthermore, Riegel found that the needs of spouses of clients with coronary artery disease interfered with their ability to provide perceived support. Spouses were caught between a need to support and a need to be supported, which was often expressed in behavior that was overprotecting and solicitous.

## ❖ THE IMPACT OF DISEASE UPON THE FAMILY

The response of spouses to disease processes is an essential factor in the provision of support and the positive adjustment (Neuman, 1989) of the client to disease. Studies have demonstrated that spouses and family members also experience disequilibrium as a result of illness, even though their experience may not parallel that of the client in relation to time of occurrence. In a study of clients who are surgically treated for cancer, Oberst and Scott (1988) found that the intensity of distress experienced by clients and spouses was remarkably similar, whereas the temporal occurrence was significantly different. Spouses tended to be more distressed immediately before the discharge of the client and considerably less so after the client had been at home for 10 days. Clients tended to be the most distressed 10 days after discharge, having confronted unexpected or unexpectably severe physical symptoms.

The need to support spouses and family members is particularly evident both during crisis and in the long-term course of progressive or chronic illness. As Robinson (1989) points out, the family caregivers of dementia victims experience particularly low support at a time when their own needs are highest, because they sacrifice their own relationships and because the ill person may have been their main source of support. This lack of support occurs at a time when family members are required to make changes in their own functioning and roles.

Strengthening the coping skills and social support of the family can be accomplished through a number of different interventions. Communication is likely the main intervention in relation to all levels of prevention. Communication is essential in educating, supporting, and in encouraging the use of social networks that will enhance the family's coping and maintain normal lines of defense. Hayes and Knox (1984) suggest that the space that exists between a parent and a nurse in relation to a hospitalized child can be lessened through effective communication of differing perceptions. Furthermore, communication can be used to lessen the space that exists between the perceptions of the nurse and those of the client or a significant other person in relation to the disease and treatment experience.

### ❖ THE IMPACT OF DISEASE UPON THE NURSE

The nurse, as part of the client's external environment, influences and is influenced by the client's adaptation to disease. Studies suggest that the disease experience is perceived differently by the nurse and client and validate earlier suggestions that perception mediates the stress experience. Studies by Biley (1989) and Carr and Powers (1986) both suggest that nurses rate the distress of the hospital experience higher than the clients themselves rated the experience. The greatest significance of these studies is that they suggest that a space exists between the experience of the nurse and the client in relation to the experience of disease and disease-related experiences. Interventions must address the gap in perceptions to facilitate a nurse-client relationship that does not further contribute to the impact of disease as a stressor.

### ❖ SUMMARY

The concept of disease as a stressor is multifaceted and involves analysis of ideas related to stress, disease, and health. Disease as a stressor must be conceptualized as an interaction that occurs within a broader arena of health and disease than that envisioned by the medical model. A variety of nursing theorists contribute to a perspective of disease and health that involves clients and their interactions with the environment. Knowledge of these patterns and interactions facilitate responses to the disease experience of the individual and family that enhance their coping and facilitate a positive adjustment to disease.

### ❖ APPLYING KNOWLEDGE TO PRACTICE

1. Apply the concept of stressor-reaction-consequence to a client situation from your own experience.
2. What factors contribute to the gap between nurses' and clients' perceptions in relation to illness-based stressors? Discuss particular examples from your experience.
3. Select a medical diagnosis that is mediated by stress and provide specific examples of primary, secondary, and tertiary prevention in relation to stress.

### REFERENCES

Allan, J. D. & Hall, B. A. (1988). Challenging the focus on technology: A critique of the medical model in a changing health care system. *Advances in Nursing Sciences, 10*(3), 22-34.

Biley, F. C. (1989). Nurses' perceptions of stress in perioperative surgical patients. *Journal of Advanced Nursing, 14*(7), 575-581.

Carr, J. A., & Powers, M. J. (1986). Stressors associated with coronary bypass surgery. *Nursing Research, 35*(4), 243-246.

Clarke, M. (1985). Stress and coping: constructs for nursing. *Journal of Advanced Nursing, 9*(1), 3-13.

Crosby, L. J. (1988). Stress factors, emotional stress and rheumatoid arthritis disease activity. *Journal of Advanced Nursing, 13,* 452-461.

Crowther, J. H. (1983). Stress management training and relaxation imagery in the treatment of essential hypertension. *Journal of Behavioral Medicine, 6*(2), 169-187.

Dimond, M. (1980). Patient strategies for managing maintenance hemodialysis. *Western Journal of Nursing Research, 2*(3), 255-268.

Dixon, J. P., Dixon, J. K., & Spinner, J. (1989). Perceptions of life-pattern disintegrity as a link in the relationship between stress and illness. *Advances in Nursing Science, 11*(2), 1-11.

Dubos, R. (1959). *Mirage of health.* New York: Harper and Row.

Dunn, H. L. (1961). *High level of wellness.* Thorofare, N. J: Charles B. Slack.

Elliott, G. R. & Eisdorfer, C. (1982). *Stress and human health: analysis and implications of research.* New York: Springer Publishing Co.

Epp, J. (1986). *Achieving health for all.* Ottawa: Government of Canada.

Gurklis, J. A., & Menke, E. M. (1988). Identification of stressors and use of coping methods in chronic hemodialysis patients. *Nursing Research, 37*(4), 236-239.

Hayes, V. E., & Knox, J. E. (1984). The experience of stress in parents of children hospitalized with long-term disabilities. *Journal of Advanced Nursing, 9,* 333-341.

Holmes, T. H., & Rahe, R. H. (1967). The social readjustment scale. *Journal of Psychosomatic Research, 11,* 213-218.

Hughes, C. C., & Kennedy, D. D. (1983). *Beyond the germ theory: reflections on relations between medicine and the behavioral sciences.* In J. Ruffini (Ed.), Advances in medical social science, New York: Gordon and Breach.

Hughes, H., Brown, B. W., & Lawlis, G. F. (1983). Treatment of acne vulgaris by biofeedback, relaxation, and cognitive imagery. *Journal of Psychosomatic Research, 27*(3), 185-191.

Hyman, R. B., Feldman, H. R., Harris, R. B., Levin, R. F., & Malloy, G. B. (1989). The effects of relaxation training on clinical symptoms: a meta-analysis. *Nursing Research, 38*(4), 216-220.

Jasmin, S., & Trygstad, L. N. (1979). *Behavioral concepts and the nursing process.* St. Louis: C. V. Mosby.

LaLonde, M. (1974). *A new perspective on the health of Canadians.* Ottawa: Government of Canada.

Lambert, V. A. (1985). Study of factors associated with psychological well-being in rheumatoid arthritic women. *Image, 18*(2), 50-53.

Lazarus, R. (1966). *Psychological stress and the coping process.* New York: McGraw-Hill.

Mast, D. E. (1986). Effects of imagery. Image, 18(3), 118-120.

Mercer, R. T., & Ferketich, S. L. (1988). Stress and social support as predictors of anxiety and depression during pregnancy, *Advances in Nursing Science, 10*(2), 26-39.

Neuman, B (1974). The Betty Neuman Health care systems model: A total person approach to patient problems. In J. P. Riehl, & C. Roy (Eds.), *Conceptual Models for Nursing Practice* (pp. 99-114) New York: Appleton-Century-Crofts.

Neuman, B. (1989). The Neuman Systems model (2nd ed.) Norwalk, Ct: Appleton & Lange.

Newman, M. (1986). *Health as expanding consciousness.* St. Louis: C. V. Mosby.

Oberst, M. T., & Scott, D. M. (1988). Postdischarge distress in surgically treated cancer patients and their spouses. *Research in Nursing and Health, 11*(4), 223-233.

Parse, R. R. (1981). *Man-Living-Health: a theory of nursing.* New York: Wiley.

Riegel, B. (1989). Social support and psychological adjustment to chronic coronary heart disease: operationalization of Johnson's behavioral systems model. *Advances in Nursing Science, 11*(2), 74-84.

Roberts, S.J., (1988). Social support and helpseeking: A review of the literature. *Advances in Nursing Science. 10*(2), 1-11.

Robinson, K. M. (1989). A social skills training program for adult caregivers. *Advances in Nursing Science, 10*(2), 59-72.

Selye, H. (1974). *Stress without distress.* Philadelphia: J. B. Lippincott.

Thibodeau, J. A. (1983). *Nursing models: analysis and evaluation.* Monterey, Calif.: Wadsworth.

Visintainer, M. (1986). The nature of knowledge and theory in nursing, *Image, 18*(2), 32-38.

# 19

# Sensory Perceptual Alterations

Glenda B. Kelman

## OBJECTIVES

*At the completion of this chapter, the reader will be able to:*

◆ Demonstrate knowledge and understanding of the concept of sensory perceptual alteration.

◆ Demonstrate knowledge of the sensory process.

◆ Analyze the concept of perception in relation to selected nursing frameworks.

◆ Assess clients with sensory perceptual alterations and identify effective nursing intervention strategies.

Individuals interact constantly with the environment through their ability to receive, organize, and transmit sensory stimuli. This reception and organization of stimuli is collectively known as *sensory perception*. Aging, illness, or a change in environment (i.e., hospitalization, institutionalization) can alter or impair this process and have an impact on the individual's ability to learn new patterns in order to respond appropriately. Sensory perceptual alterations are becoming more commonplace with the increase in the elderly population and increase in health technology and information that needs to be processed by individuals receiving health care.

The purpose of this chapter is to explore the concept of sensory perceptual alterations, identify common alterations, and generate nursing strategies for clients with sensory perceptual alterations.

## ❖ OVERVIEW OF THE CONCEPT OF SENSORY PERCEPTUAL ALTERATIONS

According to Carpenito, (1987, 1989) *sensory and perceptual alteration* is defined as a condition in which an individual or group experiences or is at risk for experiencing a change in the amount, pattern, or interpretation of incoming stimuli. Sensory and perceptual alteration is usually subdivided into six categories: visual, auditory, kinesthetic (perception), gustatory (taste), tactile, and olfactory. Doenges and Moorhouse (1985) describe sensory and perceptual alteration as a condition in which the usual and accustomed sensory stimuli are not experienced or recognized and interpreted accurately.

Carrieri and colleagues (1986) define *sensation* as a subjective perception or feeling associated with the stimulation of sensory receptors or sense organs. Sensations, however, may be synonymous with symptoms representing pathological states such as dyspnea, fatigue, and pain.

Flynn (1988) defines *sensation* or use of the senses as a primary means by which a person receives input from his or her environment. The senses allow an individual to experience physical sensations to which he or she can respond. The skin receives signals about temperature, humidity, touch, pressure, and pain. Eyes receive visual stimuli, ears receive sound, the nose receives odors, and the mouth distinguishes taste. A special aspect of sensation is the individual's level of consciousness and responsiveness, and the body's recognition of pain or discomfort.

*Perception* occurs when sensory input is received, decoded (synthesized), and interpreted by the cortex. When interpretation occurs, a conscious awareness of sensation begins. Perception provides the individual with an awareness of reality and a basis to determine if an adaptive or maintenance action is required (Phipps, Long, & Woods, 1987).

These definitions may represent a more traditional, mechanistic view of the concept of sensory-perceptual alterations resulting in a limited and restricted perspective. The concept of perception has also been reviewed by Bunting (1988) who suggests that perception is a process where the mind takes sensory data, interprets the data, and "makes sense" of it. This expanded view assumes a process of interaction between the environmental stimuli, and the cognitions of the individual that result in the experience of the perception. "The implication is that both the environmental stimuli and an internal process are sufficient and necessary conditions required in order for perception to occur" (pp. 168-169).

## Historical Overview

A brief review of the historical perspective of perception supports the notion that there is something "out there" (the stimulus), but its relevance and interpretation rest in the mind of the perceiver. Aristotle postulated that human minds construct images after receiving sensations, but in the process of selection, they omit contingent data (Reese, 1980). The perceiver engages in the process of selection.

During the Middle Ages, St. Thomas Aquinas proposed that the individual abstracts universal meanings from sense experience by means of *phantasms* (perceptions or illusions) (Kneale, 1971). Locke and Descartes also tried to convey the same concept using the term *ideas of sense.* Aquinas, however, further postulated that the process of perception involved two functions; the passive intellect that received the "phantasm," and the active intellect that grasped the abstracted meaning (Reese, 1980).

Descartes, a seventeenth century Greek philosopher, considered perception to be an intellectual act through which one could posit the existence of an external world. The external world included both the mind and body; thought was an attribute of the mind, and extension was the attribute of the body, and they were clearly distinct from one another. Also included in the attribute of thought were imagination, sensation, and will. Senses, therefore, could be believed only after objective scientific observations have been considered (Reese, 1980).

Philosopher John Locke was an advocate of the sense datum theory. Experience writes its message on the blank tablet or *tabula rasa* of the human mind (Locke, 1690/1975). In his quest to explain the connection between an individual's ideas and the outer world, he developed a theory of primary and secondary qualities of sensation. Primary qualities existed in the object itself, while the secondary qualities were elicited in one's mind by attending to the primary qualities. This concept was supported by Descartes and is still currently shared by psychologists and philosophers (Lian, 1981). This separate distinction between mind and body and the external and internal process of perception continues to influence nursing paradigms and theories.

Current definitions of perception reflect the various scientific and philosophical viewpoints previously discussed. Chaplin (1975) defines perception as "awareness of organic processes; a group of sensations to which meaning is added from past experience; an intervening variable inferred from the organism's ability to discriminate among stimuli; an intuitive awareness of truth or immediate belief about something" (p. 376). Perception is interrelated and dependent on stimulus factors. The meaning of the objective event results from the conditions of the stimulus and the perceiver.

However, Gestalt psychologists purport that perception of the total situation does not reflect the summation of the individual components. Perception is greater than the sum of stimuli. Perception does not take place in the sensory organs but is synthesized at some higher mental level (Cummings, 1972). This is a complex active process as the perceiver interacts with the stimuli.

This view is supported by Combs, Richards, and Richards (1976) who define perception as "any differentiation a person is capable of making in his perceptual field whether or not an objectively observable stimulus is present" (p. 17). Therefore, activities of seeing, hearing, smell, and touch are in the same category as awareness, knowing, and understanding.

This brief review of the literature reveals a lack of consensus regarding the concept of perception. Perception has been described as a passive process where the perceiver is acted upon by the environment, or as an active process in which the individual selects perceptions and assigns personal meaning. It may denote a simplistic, mechanistic process, or an integrated holistic interaction with the environment (Bunting, 1988). Locke (1975) and Reese (1980) incorporate the idea that both the active and passive function of the perceiver cause integration and interpretation of the information in a unique way.

What evolves then is a definition of perception that imposes meaning on selected experiences, which become part of the world view of

Sensation
(Awareness of external and internal stimuli)

↓

Selection of stimuli

↓

Assimilation

↓

Interpretation of the experience

❖ **Fig. 19-1**   Defining characteristics of perception.

the perceiver. Defining characteristics of perception according to Bunting (1988) include sensation or awareness of external and internal stimuli, selection of stimuli, assimilation, and interpretation of the experience (Fig. 19-1).

## ❖ FOUR NURSING MODELS VIEWS OF PERCEPTION

Several nursing frameworks incorporate the concept of sensory-perceptual alterations and will be briefly presented with specific examples.

### King: Goal Attainment

King defines perception as "each human being's representation of reality" (1981, p. 61). King postulates that sensory experiences provide individuals with raw data that assist them to shape particular and universal ideas as a way of knowing about the world. She further states that perception assists in organizing, interpreting, and transforming information from sense data and memory. Perception is an active process of human transaction with the environment and gives meaning to experiences, is representative of reality, and influences one's behavior.

King (1981) identifies five steps in the perceptive process: "(1) the import of energy from the environment organized by information, (2) transforming of energy, (3) processing of information, (4) storing of information, and (5) exporting of information in the form of overt behaviors" (p. 146). In addition, perception is discussed in one of her assumptions: "Individuals are perceiving beings" (p. 143), and in the first proposition "If perceptual accuracy is present in nurse-client interactions, transactions will occur" (p. 149).

King identifies perception as an essential, vital link necessary for reaction, interaction, and transaction to occur between the client, nurse, and environment. Transactions require perceptual accuracy in nurse-client interactions, congruence between role performance, and role expectations for the nurse and the client.

Each individual then has a personal world of reality based on his or her own perceptions. According to King's framework, the role of the nurse is to focus on the patient's perception of his or her health status and the patient's ability to adapt to stress and use resources to achieve optimum potential. The nurse and client focus on mutual goal setting.

## Orem: Self Care

Orem (1979) categorizes the concept of self-perception as one of the basic capabilities of the self-care agent (individual). Orem views perception as both active and passive. Perception is inferred when Orem refers to incoming sensory knowledge and awareness of the reality of the situation. The agent's purpose is based on this awareness and reflection. The nurse and self-care agent focus on assessing and optimizing the self-care abilities of the individual.

## Roy: Adaptation

Roy's adaptation model addresses coping with stressors by way of two subsystems: the regulator and cognator. The regulator subsystem responds automatically through neural, chemical, and endocrine coping processes, and the cognator subsystem responds through per-

ceptual and information processing, learning, judgment, and emotional channels (Roy, 1976; Andrew and Roy, 1986).

Perception is actually the process that links the two subsystems. This occurs when neural input from the environment (e.g., increase in environmental temperature) is received into the regulator, corresponding to the sensation characteristic of the definition. The body responds by perspiring, and the neural impulse is transformed into a perception (feeling warm or hot) (Tiedeman, 1983). Perception, according to Roy, is unique, and is influenced by somatic, social, cultural, and experiential factors (Meleis, 1985).

The receiver is a passive recipient of sense data, and interpretation is more of an automatic than active process (Bunting, 1988). Perception, therefore, in Roy's model is viewed from more of a reductionist, mechanistic approach. It is, however, an essential concept linking the regulator and cognator subsystems facilitating the process of adaptation.

## Rogers: Unitary Human Beings

Rogers' science of unitary human beings addresses the concept of perception from a phenomenological perspective, in contrast to previous theorists who define perception as a cause and effect relationship between the stimuli and perceiver. Causality is a contradiction of open systems. Building blocks fundamental to the science of unitary human beings are postulated to include energy fields, a universe of open systems, pattern, and four-dimensionality (Rogers, 1988).

Pattern is an abstraction that gives identity to human and environmental fields. Field pattern is always new, diverse, and changes continuously. According to Rogers, one perceives manifestations of field pattern, but one does not perceive field pattern itself. Unitary human beings are an irreducible, four-dimensional energy field identified by pattern and manifesting characteristics that are specific to the whole and

❖  **Table 19-1**
Sensory perceptual alterations case study: A comparison of four nursing models

*History:* Ms. S. is 28 years old and has given birth to her first child, a son who was born yesterday. Ms. S. is married and lives in an apartment with her husband in a large city. She has been blind since the age of 5. The nurse has initiated a teaching plan for discharge.

The following example selects only one aspect of care, but applies the process to four different nursing models.

| Theorist | Theoretical process to achieve goal | Intervention | Evaluation |
|----------|-------------------------------------|--------------|------------|
| King | Nurse validates clients' perceptions of ability to care for son at home. | Mutual goal setting | Client demonstrates ability to feed son and meets safety and comfort needs of child and self |
| | Transaction occurs to achieve congruence between role performance and role expectation. | Assisting mother and father to care for son. | |
| Orem | Nurse assists the partly compensatory role of mother and addresses wholly compensatory role of child. | Promoting self-care activities for the mother<br>Monitoring mother and father's role | Client demonstrates awareness of situation and ability as a self-care agent to provide care in partly compensatory role and ability to seek additional community resources. |
| Roy | Nurse assists client to cope with stress of new child via regulator system (physiological response) and cognator system (provides support and information) | Teaching mother and father adaptive behaviors to manipulate environment<br>Validate perception linking regulator and cognator | Mother and father adapt to role and ability to care for son. |
| Rogers | Validates parents' perception of pattern manifestation and interaction with environment | Validating parents' perception that their interaction with their child is continuously changing | Parents accept that although they may perceive similar patterns of interactions with their child, they will continue to change. |
| | Recognizes that humans are unique, diverse patterns increasing in complexity and diversity. | Assuring parents that each child is unique and different (i.e. different sleep/wake and feeding patterns) | |

cannot be predicted from knowledge of the parts (Rogers, 1988). Rogers purports that the human and environmental field are engaged in mutual, simultaneous interaction (principle of integrality).

Perception based on Rogers' model involves pattern recognition to uncover human-environment patterns of wholeness. The abstract system represents a new way to view (perceive) the universe manifested by increasing diversity and accelerating evolution of non-repeating rhythmicities. The nurse interacts with the client and environment perceiving field pattern manifestations.

The concept of perception has been reviewed from the perspective of four models and is an essential concept in nursing research and theory development. Phillips (1988) notes that there is more to be known than what is ascertained through the five senses. He postulates that in order to perceive the other side of the looking glass, nursing models that lead to pattern recognition must use relativistic, rather than mechanistic modes of inquiry. Qualitative research methods that uncover human-environment patterns of wholeness must be developed in order to move toward developing a science of wholeness. Nurses must be sensitized to the other side of the looking glass and research human-environment patterns of wholeness.

Table 19-1 provides a synopsis of the four nursing models as applied to a case study. This table provides direction to nurses in developing a theory-based practice.

### ❖ REVIEW OF THE SENSORY PROCESS

In order to understand clients with sensory-perceptual alterations, a brief review of the sensory process will be presented. The human nervous system consists of the brain, spinal cord, cranial nerves, and the peripheral nerves. The peripheral nerves act as gatherers of sensory information and transport it along nerve fibers.

Nerve fibers carry sensory information to the cortex of the brain where it is interpreted, and a response is initiated. Collateral fibers pass to the reticular activating system (RAS). Research supports that the RAS plays an important role in the efficient processing of stimuli and the resulting behavior. The RAS is comprised of a dense network of neurons, the reticular formation, which extends from the medulla to the thalamus (Fig. 19-2). The RAS controls the overall level of central nervous system activity, including the degree of wakefulness or sleep, and the ability to direct attention or focus on

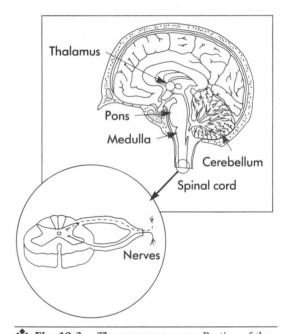

❖ **Fig. 19-2**  The sensory process. Portion of the sensory system that transmits stimuli from the receptors to higher centers (RAS). *(From Flynn, J. (1988). Sensory alterations. In J. Flynn & P. Heffron, (Eds.). Nursing: From Concept to Practice. Norwalk Ct.: Appleton & Lange, p. 462. Reprinted with permission.)*

specific parts of the environment. The activity of the RAS is influenced by stimuli from the senses and the cerebral cortex (Gioiella and Bevil, 1985).

According to Schultz (1965) the RAS monitors incoming and outgoing stimuli and becomes attuned to a certain level of activity, which is projected to the cortex. The RAS functions optimally only within this range or pace of stimulation. Schultz postulated that this specific range or level is required for normal perception, learning, and emotion. When there is a disturbance in sensory input including increases, decreases, and distortions of stimuli, the organism is no longer able to project a normal level of activation to the cortex. If compensatory adjustments fail to regain equilibrium, behavior becomes disorganized.

Schultz also theorized that the arousal state of the RAS is a general drive state he called *sensoristasis*. The organism attempts to maintain a balance in stimulus variation to the cortex as mediated by the RAS. Individuals behave in ways that maintain an optimal arousal level; some individuals seek to increase stimulation, and some seek to reduce stimulation. There also is evidence that supports a considerable variation in the amount of stimuli that different individuals consider optimal. The individual's response to stimuli is influenced by external factors in the environment as well as internal factors within the individual. Therefore, it is not only the quantity of stimulation that is important for cortical arousal, but also quality as reflected by the degree to which it is meaningful to that individual (Gioiella, 1985).

## ❖ CHARACTERISTICS OF SENSORY AND PERCEPTUAL CHANGES

Snyder (1985) notes that sensory-perceptual changes may be a result of a dysfunction of the primary sensory system, the inability to recognize and comprehend sensory stimuli (agnosia), or misinterpretation or distortion of the stimulus, such as illusions or hallucinations.

### Gnosis

*Gnosis,* the ability to comprehend and recognize sensory stimuli, involves two stages. The stimulus initially reaches the primary cortical sensory area, but then must be recognized, and its meaning comprehended in the specific association area (i.e., visual, hearing, tactile). If the stimulus is blocked or prevented from reaching the association area, recognition, interpretation, and subsequent elaboration into meaning cannot occur (Snyder, 1985).

### Agnosia

An individual unable to recognize and comprehend stimuli and its meaning has a form of *agnosia,* even though the primary receptors and sensorium remain intact. Visual and tactile agnosia is common in Alzheimers disease, and other forms of agnosia are exhibited in individual's with cerebral vascular accidents and brain neoplasms (Esberger, 1989; Fabiszewski, 1989). The individual is unable to recognize or identify objects or other individuals and may be unaware of the left side of the body and left visual space (anosognosia) and may have some form of aphasia and other deficits (Hahn, 1987).

### Hallucinations

*Hallucinations* are sensory perceptions that occur in the absence of sensory stimuli. Visual and auditory hallucinations are the most common (e.g., large monsters staring through the window or voices giving commands). Tactile hallucinations also can occur and may consist of frightening sensations of insects or other objects touching the individual (Snyder, 1983). Even if the client can say that the hallucination is not real, it may be a very disconcerting and frightening experience for the individual.

**Table 19-2**
Descriptions of agnosias and nursing assessment

| Agnosias | Description of behavior | Nursing assessment |
|---|---|---|
| Auditory | Wernicke's aphasia; unable to differentiate sounds of speech due to damage to auditory cortex; has difficulty identifying sounds. | Ask client to repeat what is said by nurse. Ask client to identify sounds with eyes closed such as a siren, ringing bell, or whistling. |
| Prosopagnosia | Unable to recognize familiar faces. | Observe if client recognizes familiar faces. |
| Tactile | Unable to recognize objects by touch with eyes closed; related to lesions of parietal lobe. | Have client close eyes, and ask to identify familiar objects placed in the hand (i.e., a pen, keys, hairbrush). |
| Unilateral asomatognosia | Unaware of left side of body and left visual space, usually related to lesions of nondominant (right) hemisphere. | Ask client to touch parts of body to assess for neglect; observe for signs of body part denial and denial of paralysis; observe for left (rarely right) unilateral neglect. Client will ignore objects, stimuli, etc. on left side. |
| Visual | Difficulty naming or recognizing familiar objects related to damage to visual cortex. | Ask client to identify objects or pictures of objects, and/or colors of objects |
| Visual-spatial | Difficulty finding way in familiar surroundings; usually related to nondominant parietal lobe involvement; difficulty with right-left orientation; unable to manipulate clothing or objects because of poor spatial relationships. | Ask client to identify right from left; observe client walk toward left side of room; observe client put on shirt. Ask client to draw a house floor plan; assess if client loses sense of direction when, for example, client walks to the shower or bathroom. |

## Pseudohallucinations

Misinterpretations or misperceptions of sensory stimuli, such as radio voices that are interpreted as people in the attic, are labeled *pseudohallucinations* or illusions (Hall, 1988). The most common types of illusions are visual and auditory (Adams & Victory, 1981). Visual illusions are visual distortions of objects that appear to be smaller (micropsia) larger (macropsia) or moving. The vertical or horizontal orientation of an object may be changed (a table is perceived to be vertical rather than hor- izontal). Auditory illusions are misinterpreta- tions of sounds; a refrigerator humming noise is interpreted as people whispering. Table 19-2 identifies several common forms of agnosia and nursing assessment of clients to differentiate the agnosias.

## ❖ SENSORY DEPRIVATION

There has been little agreement in the use and definition of sensory deprivation. Accord- ing to the literature (Brownfield, 1965; Rossi,

1969), at least 25 terms have been used interchangeably with the term sensory deprivation. The problem of definition has been further complicated by the research studies that adopt experimental conditions to "induce" the phenomenon of sensory deprivation artificially (Kim, 1983).

There are two broad categories of *sensory deprivation* generally addressed that focus either on the environment or the individual experiencing the deprivation. Suedfeld (1969) categorizes sensory deprivation based on the reduction of stimulus-input levels, the reduction of stimulus-variability, and sensory-social isolation and confinement. Kim (1983) specifies that these three characteristics, although distinct, are circular in meaning and interrelated. A reduction of stimulus-variability that is produced by monotonous stimulation will result in a reduction of stimulus-input levels, and vice versa. Additionally, sensory-social isolation and confinement commonly accompany both a reduction of stimulus-variability and a reduction of stimulus-input levels.

The concept of isolation, although somewhat similar, is broader in nature than sensory deprivation. *Isolation* encompasses social and psychological separation, while sensory deprivation is associated with the characteristics of the environment in terms of sensory stimulation. Sensory deprivation is likely to occur, however, when a person is placed in isolation.

As previously discussed, a major consequence of sensory deprivation identified in the literature is hallucinatory activity. Zuckerman (1969) theorizes that hallucinations are self-aroused images perceived by an individual because of a lack of competing sensory inputs. A person in an environment without patterned and changing stimulation may eventually become sensitized to more organized images arising from higher centers within the nervous system. These may be intensified by a high state of arousal or by reduction in competing stimuli, appearing as visual images in space in front of the person. In addition, biochemical changes, especially steroid and endorphin levels, suggest a linkage between sensory deprivation and behavioral changes mediated by internal processes of biochemical synthesis (Prescott, 1980).

If the health care environment is a potential source or contributing factor to sensory deprivation, nursing research needs to focus on sensory deprivation as a phenomenon of the client's environment.

## ❖ SENSORY OVERLOAD

Sensory overload is a condition of highly intense stimulation that is not patterned (Kenner et al, 1985). Individuals are bombarded with stimuli at a rate greater than they can integrate. Once the individual's integrative capacities have been maximized, additional sensory input is processed selectively and erratically, with the mind blocking all remaining stimuli. The result is a distortion of sensory and cognitive perceptions.

Delirium or intensive care unit (ICU) psychosis is often categorized as a sensory-perceptual alteration related to sensory overload (Easton & MacKenzie, 1988). It is estimated that 12% to 38% of conscious patients admitted to critical care settings experience this phenomenon (Belitz, 1983). The highest incidence of ICU psychosis has been reported in the surgical intensive care unit (SICU), followed by the medical intensive care unit (MICU), the coronary care unit (CCU), and general medical-surgical wards (Lipowski, 1980).

Patients with ICU psychosis may exhibit a fluctuating state of consciousness characterized by fatigue, distraction, confusion, disorientation, restlessness, incoherence, fear, anxiety, excitement, hallucinations, illusions, and delusions (Beck, 1988). Etiological and contributing factors may include individuals with a history of drug or alcohol abuse, chronic cardiovascular, metabolic, respiratory, or renal illness, or cerebral damage (Lipowski, 1980). Individuals with previous psychiatric histories (e.g., depression or paranoia) may also be more prone to development of delirium (Dubin et al., 1979).

Other contributing factors to the development of ICU psychosis include drug therapy such as anticonvulsants, digitalis preparations, morphine, antibiotics, albuterol, lidocaine, methyldopa, atropine, and corticosteroids, which may have the potential to cause delirium.

It is well documented that the hospital environment may be a major contributor to ICU psychosis. Sleep deprivation related to noise, constant lighting, immobilization, and the constant interruptions for monitoring and treatment have all been cited in the literature (Ballard, 1981).

Easton and MacKenzie (1988), in their review of the literature on ICU psychosis, suggest three themes that emerge: sensory perceptual alterations, perceptual alterations, and sensory alterations. Although some factors may be uncontrollable in the ICU setting, other factors such as client and family education, monitoring of drug therapy regimens, and reducing sensory perceptual overload may reduce the incidence and severity of delirium in ICU psychosis.

## ❖ NURSING STRATEGIES FOR SENSORY PERCEPTUAL ALTERATIONS

As previously noted, sensory perceptual alterations may arise from a broad range of etiologies. The box that follows summarizes some of the common etiological factors.

---

## ❖ SENSORY AND PERCEPTUAL ALTERATIONS: COMMON CONTRIBUTING AND ETIOLOGICAL RISK FACTORS

**PATHOPHYSIOLOGICAL**

Alterations in sensory organs (e.g., cataracts, blindness)
Neurological (e.g., accident, C. V. A., neuropathies)
Metabolic (e.g., elevated bun, hypercalcemia, acidosis, alkalosis, fluid imbalance)
Impaired $O_2$ transport (e.g., anemia, confusion, dyspnea)
Musculoskeletal changes (e.g., paraplegia, quadriplegia).

**TREATMENT-RELATED**

Amputation (e.g., mastectomy, lower limb amputation)
Drug therapy (e.g., cancer chemotherapy, sedatives)
Surgery (e.g., detached retina, glaucoma)
Radiation therapy (e.g., radiation therapy to head and neck region)
Activity or mobility restrictions (e.g., traction, radiation implants)

**SITUATIONAL**

Anxiety
Pain
Social isolation
Stress
Noise

Carpenito, L. (1989); Doenges M. & Moorhouse, M. (1988).

## Application to Practice

Major foci in a care plan for a client with sensory perceptual alterations include assessment of causative and contributing factors, identification of nursing diagnoses, planning and implementing appropriate intervention strategies, and evaluating the effectiveness of the plan of care.

## Assessment

A comprehensive data base for a client with sensory perceptual alterations includes both objective and subjective data derived from the assessment of intrapersonal, environmental, and interpersonal stressors. To gather data on intrapersonal stressors, the nurse can:

1. Assess visual, auditory, olfactory, gustatory, tactile, and kinesthetic senses. For example, consider whether the client wears glasses or uses a hearing aid or other corrective devices. Can the client perceive changes in temperature, sense painful stimuli, and discriminate odors and taste sensations? Can the client define placement or position in space?
2. Assess the client's neurological and motor status by determining level of consciousness and ability to move independently.
3. Assess the client's ability to perceive, process, and communicate in an appropriate and purposeful manner.
4. Obtain the client's age and assess the developmental level.
5. Assess psychological and behavioral status by determining coping behaviors, specific stressors, and history of alcohol or drug use.
6. Assess cultural impact in relation to health care practices, touch, expectations related to pain management, and other health care issues.

To obtain data on environmental stressors:

Assess stimulus input by determining the amount, intensity, variability, and duration of input. For example, consider the impact of hospitalization on a client who is deaf. What is the level of stimulus input for this client? Community-based stimulus input data include whether the client lives alone, the availability of support systems and contacts, and the geographic accessibility of community resources. Of particular concern with an elderly client is the extent of social isolation.

To gain an understanding of interpersonal stressors:

Relate intrapersonal stressors to interpersonal interactions. For example, consider the impact on family and significant other relationships for an elderly deaf client who fractures his hip and has a frail wife who is unable to drive or care for him at home.

## Nursing Diagnoses

Analysis of subjective and objective data derived from the assessment of intrapersonal, environmental, and interpersonal stressors results in the identification of nursing diagnoses descriptive of sensory perceptual alterations. Relevant nursing diagnoses may include:

Altered verbal communication
Impaired social interaction
Social isolation
Altered thought processes
Altered family processes
Ineffective coping
Potential for injury
Impaired physical mobility
Sleep pattern disturbance

## Planning

In the planning stage, realistic long-term and short-term goals that are measurable, observable, and definable are identified. Specific objectives that are incremental and progressive and that lead to goal achievement may also be identified. If the client is able, planning can be a mutual endeavor whereby the nurse and client agree on goals, objectives, and nursing interventions.

# ❖ NURSING CARE PLAN

**CLIENT:** Ms. J.

**MEDICAL DIAGNOSIS:** Multiple fractures; respiratory distress.

**NURSING DIAGNOSES:** Sleep pattern disturbance related to lights and noise in ICU environment.

Excessive environmental stimuli and decreased input of meaningful stimuli secondary to treatment.

Impaired verbal communication related to inability to speak secondary to intubation and decreased hearing.

Fear related to functional loss and potential inability to care for husband at home.

| GOALS | INTERVENTIONS |
|---|---|
| Ms. J. will experience____hours of uninterrupted sleep per shift. | ◆ Schedule care (procedures, treatments, and medications) to permit uninterrupted sleep.<br>◆ Reduce unnecessary environmental stimuli. |
| Ms. J. will verbalize information that is appropriate to time and surroundings.<br>Ms. J. will demonstrate ability to communicate using alternate method. | ◆ Orient client to surroundings.<br>◆ Explain sounds related to equipment and alarms.<br>◆ Place "magic slate," call bell/light within client's reach.<br>◆ Determine client's ability to seek assistance.<br>◆ When speaking, face client and speak slowly. |
| Fear, related to potential inability to care for husband, will be expressed and/or minimized. | ◆ Encourage client to communicate fears.<br>◆ Discuss available resources, initiate referrals based on client/family needs. |

**EVALUATION:**

Ms. J. sleeps for two uninterrupted hours, and this amount is expected to increase as her condition improves. Ms. J. responds to questions in a manner that indicates orientation to person, place, and time. She successfully uses the alternative forms of communication available to her. Ms. J. expresses fear about her inability to care for her husband and identifies at least one community resource available to her for caregiving assistance.

## Intervention

Nursing interventions are aimed at alleviating etiological or contributing factors as specified by nursing diagnoses. Some interventions to address sensory perceptual alterations include providing or assisting in providing for client safety, establishing structure and routine to promote pattern and meaning, enhancing and using remaining sensory perceptual function to maximize optimal rehabilitation and quality of life through mutual goal setting, and providing education and information to the client and family based on their level of cognition and readiness to learn.

## Evaluation

The goals and objectives provide the criteria for evaluation. The extent to which they are achieved determines whether the plan of care was effective, appropriate, and adequate. For example, if the goals have not been achieved, it may be that the assessment data was inadequate, the nursing diagnoses were inappropriate, the goals were not realistic, or the interventions were ineffective. Identifying specific areas that were problematic is essential to making appropriate recommendations or revising the plan of care.

## ❖ CASE STUDY

Ms. J. is a 70-year-old widow who lives alone in her own home in a rural community. She was walking across the street when she was struck by a car. She has multiple long bone fractures, a history of glaucoma in her left eye, and decreased hearing in her left ear (but she does not wear a hearing aid). She is admitted to the ICU for stabilization and monitoring. The nurse reviews the admission history and discovers that Mrs. Jones cares for her 80-year-old husband who has Alzheimer's disease and is currently residing with their daughter on an interim basis. She has a 50-year history of smoking and is temporarily intubated. The care plan on

p. 342 focuses primarily on Ms. J's sensory-perceptual disruptions.

## ❖ SUMMARY

Manifestations of sensory and perceptual alterations are universal, regardless of the diagnosis or health care setting. Understanding these alterations is an integral component of nursing practice, research, and theory development. Increased understanding of sensory and perceptual alterations is crucial to providing the nurse with the "vision" to "make sense" of the client and environment.

## ❖ APPLYING KNOWLEDGE TO PRACTICE

1. Identify the defining characteristics of perception and apply them to a client recovering at home from a left sided CVA.
2. What factors would be important to assess when orienting a blind client to the hospital environment?
3. How does the nurse assess and determine appropriate levels of stimulation for the client with senile dementia of the Alzheimer's type?

### REFERENCES

Adams, R., & Victor, M. (1981). *Principles of Neurology* (2nd ed.). New York: McGraw-Hill.

Andrews, H. A., & Roy, C. (1986). *Essentials of the Roy Adaptation Model.* Norwalk, Ct.: Appleton-Century-Crofts.

Ballard, K. (1981). Identification of environmental stressors for patients in a surgical intensive care unit. *Issues in Mental Health Nursing, 3,* 89-108.

Beck, C., Rawlins, R., & Williams, S. (Eds.). (1984). *Mental Health Psychiatric Nursing: A Holistic Life-Cycle Approach.* St. Louis: C. V. Mosby.

Belitz, J. (1983). Minimizing the psychological complications of patients who require mechanical ventilation. *Critical Care Nurse, 3* (3), 42-46.

Brownfield, C. (1965). *Isolation: Clinical and Experimental Approaches.* New York: Random House.

Bunting, S. (1988). The concept of Perception in selected Nursing Theories. *Nursing Science Quarterly, 1* (4), 168-174.

Carpenito, L. (1987). *Nursing Diagnosis: Application to Clinical Practice.* New York: J. B. Lippincott.

Carpenito, L. (1989). *Handbook of Nursing Diagnosis, 1989-90.* Philadelphia: J. B. Lippincott.

Carrieri, V., Lindsay, A., & West, C. (1986). *Pathophysiological Phenomena in Nursing: Human Responses to Illness.* Philadelphia: W. B. Saunders.

Chaplin, J. P. (1975). *Dictionary of Psychology.* New York: Dell.

Combs, A. W., Richards, A. C., & Richards, F. (1976). *Perceptual Psychology.* New York: Harper and Row.

Cummings, J. (Ed.). (1972). *Encyclopedia of Psychology.* New York: Herder and Herder.

Doenges, M., & Moorhouse, M. (1988). *Nurse's Pocket Guide: Nursing Diagnoses with Interventions.* Philadelphia: F. A. Davis.

Dubin, W., Field, H., & Gastfriend, D. (1979). Postcardiotomy delirium: A critical review. *Journal of Thoracic and Cardiovascular Surgery, 77,* 586-594.

Easton, C., & MacKenzie, F. (1988). Sensory perceptual alterations: Delirium in the intensive care unit. *Heart & Lung, 17* (3), 229-235.

Esberger, K. & Hughes, S. (1989). *Nursing Care of the Aged.* Norwalk, Ct.: Appleton & Lange.

Fabiszewski, K. (1989). Alzheimer's disease: Overview and progression. *Journal of Advanced Medical-Surgical Nursing. 1* (2), 1-17.

Flynn, J. & P. Heffron (1988). Sensory alterations. In J. Flynn & P. Heffron (Eds). *Nursing: From Concept to Practice.* (pp. 459-475). Bowie, MD: Prentice-Hall.

Gioiella, E. & C. Bevil (1985). *Nursing Care of the Aging Client: Promoting Healthy Adaptation.* Norwalk, Ct.: Appleton-Century-Crofts.

Hahn, K. (1987). Left vs Right: What a difference the side makes in stroke. *Nursing 87, 17* (9), 44-47.

Hall, G. (1988). Alterations in Thought Process. *Journal of Gerontological Nursing. 14* (3), 30-37.

Kenner, C., Gussetta, C. & Dossey, B. (1985). *Critical Care Nursing: Body-Mind-Spirit.* Boston: Little, Brown & Company.

Kim, H. (1983). *The Nature of Theoretical Thinking in Nursing.* Norwalk, Ct.: Appleton-Century-Crofts.

King, I. (1981). *A theory for Nursing: Systems, concepts and process.* New York: Wiley.

Kneale, W. (1971). An analysis of perceiving. In F. F. N. Sibleu (Ed.), *Perception: A philosophical symposium* (pp. 65-81). London: Methuen.

Lian, A. (1981). *The psychological study of object perception.* New York: Academic.

Lipowski, Z. (1980). *Delirium-acute brain failure in man.* Springfield, Ill.: Charles Thomas.

Locke, J. (1690/1975). *An essay concerning human understanding.* London: Oxford University Press.

Meleis, A. I. (1985). *Theoretical Nursing: Development and Progress.* Philadelphia: J. B. Lippincott.

Orem, D. (1979). *Concept formalization in process and product.* Boston: Little, Brown.

Phillips, J. (1988). The Looking Glass of Nursing Research. *Nursing Science Quarterly, 1* (3), 96.

Phipps, W., Long, B., & N. Woods (1983). *Medical-Surgical Nursing: Concepts and Clinical Practice.* St. Louis: C. V. Mosby.

Prescott, J. (1980). Somatosensory Affectional Deprivation (SAD) Theory of Drug and Alcohol Use. *National Institute Drug Abuse Research Monograph Series.* 30, 286-296.

Reese, W. L. (1980). *Dictionary of philosophy and religion: Eastern and Western Thought.* Atlantic Highlands, New Jersey: Humanities Press.

Rogers, M. E. (1988). Nursing Science and Art: A prospective. *Nursing Science Quarterly, 1* (3), 99-102.

Rossi, A. (1969). General Methodological Considerations. In J. P. Zubek (Ed.), *Sensory Deprivation: Fifteen Years of Research.* New York: Appleton-Century-Crofts.

Roy, C. (1976). *Introduction to Nursing: An Adaptation Model.* New Jersey: Prentice-Hall.

Schultz, D. (1965). *Sensory Restriction: Effects on Behavior.* New York: Academic.

Snyder, M. (Ed.) (1983). *A Guide to Neurological and Neurosurgical Nursing.* New York: John Wiley & Sons.

Suedfeld, P. (1969). Introduction and Historical Background: and Theoretical Formulations II. In J. P. Zubek (Ed.),: *Sensory Deprivation: Fifteen Years of Research.* New York: Appleton-Century-Crofts.

Tiedman, M. E. (1983). The Roy Adaptation Model. In, J. J. Fitzpatrick & A. L. Whall (Eds.). *Conceptual models of Nursing: Analysis and Application* (pp. 157-180). Bowie, Md: R. J. Brady Co.

Zuckerman, M. (1969). Hallucinations, Reported Sensations and Image: and Theoretical Formulations I. In J. P. Zubek (Ed.),: *Sensory Deprivation: Fifteen Years of Research.* New York: Appleton-Century-Crofts.

# 20 Pain

Betty Rolling Ferrell ◆ Connie J. Leek

## OBJECTIVES

*At the completion of this chapter, the reader will be able to:*

- ◆ **Define the concept of pain.**
- ◆ **Discuss the importance of the assessment phase in pain management.**
- ◆ **Discuss pharmacological and nonpharmacological methods of pain management.**
- ◆ **Discuss the nurse's role in pain management.**

## ❖ OVERVIEW OF CONCEPT OF PAIN

Pain is a personal experience of hurt and an event that consumes the individual experiencing it. Pain is a physiological and psychological event affecting virtually every aspect of quality of life (Ferrell, Wisdom, & Wenzl, 1989a). The advent of palliative care and the hospice movement in the United States, which are based in the art of comfort, have created a new awareness among health care professionals and the public that pain can be relieved. We are, in many ways, in the midst of a knowledge boom in the understanding of pain and its treatment. This focus on pain comes at an appropriate time when the incidence of chronic illnesses is increasing and the population is aging.

Nurses are familiar with the words of McCaffery (1979) that "Pain is what the patient says it is and exists when the patient says it does." We agree with this conceptualization of pain as the first-person experience of the patient and add that *pain management is the*

*first-person experience and responsibility of the nurse.*

This chapter focuses on the role of the professional nurse in pain management. It is not a beginning reference on principles of pain control; instead, it builds on basic knowledge to advance the nursing practice of treating individuals with pain. More comprehensive and basic references can be found in texts by McCaffery (1979), McCaffery and Beebe (1989), Wall and Melzalk (1984), Foley and Payne (1989).

Pain is in fact a component of a larger goal of comfort. Patients with pain have a number of associated symptoms such as fatigue, anxiety, sleep disturbance, and analgesia-induced nausea and constipation. To achieve pain management is not sufficient. The goal of nursing action is to provide optimal comfort. The nurse, as the primary care provider of the patient, is in the ideal position to direct pain relief efforts.

In the following pages we review key terms associated with the concept of pain, discuss pain as a multidimensional concept, and explore drug and non-drug interventions for pain to provide a basis for application to nursing practice. We also assert that pain is not simply a clinical issue delegated to the staff nurse or clinical specialist. Pain is the responsibility of nurse managers, administrators, investigators, and clinicians.

## ❖ DEFINITION OF KEY TERMS

The concept of pain by its nature is an emotionally laden term. Because pain is a subjective experience, it is difficult to measure and label. Another major influence in the confusion regarding pain concepts is the social problem of drug abuse. The massive antidrug campaign of "Just Say No to Drugs" has been of questionable benefit to recreational drug abusers but has had a dramatic impact on the fears and concerns of patients in pain (Hill, 1989). Even patients who are terminally ill frequently refuse to take pain medications to avoid the social stigma of dying as an addict. There is a great deal of confusion about physical pain versus psychological pain, drug addiction, drug tolerance, and pain behavior. These terms are confusing to nurses and other health care professionals and are therefore even more confusing to patients and their families. Establishing accurate knowledge and skills in pain management is essential for the professional nurse.

First the major concepts related to pain must be clarified (American Pain Society, 1989). It often helps to classify pain as either acute or chronic. *Acute pain* is of brief duration, usually lasting less than 3 to 6 months. It has a known cause such as surgery or injury. Acute pain often serves a purpose by alerting the person to danger (e.g., abdominal pain may signal appendicitis).

*Chronic pain* is of longer duration, usually lasting beyond 6 months. Chronic pain may occur intermittently (e.g., in a patient with osteoarthritis who has periods of pain inter-

spersed with days of no pain). Chronic pain also may occur in a constant pattern, with virtually no period of relief. It may be either malignant pain (i.e., associated with cancer and often lasting until the person's death) or of benign origin such as neuropathic or low back pain.

*Pain behaviors* are outward expressions of pain such as vocal behaviors of crying, whining, or moaning or actions such as facial grimacing and body tensing. These pain behaviors have been documented in children (McGrath et al, 1985; Ross, 1984) and in adults by research by Wilkie et al (1988). It is important that nurses be alert to these behaviors to recognize pain, particularly in cases of young children or cognitively impaired elderly who may not be able to express their pain verbally. However, the absence of pain behaviors does not mean that the person is free of pain. Review of hospital charts frequently reveals the phrase "patient sleeping—no pain," assuming that a resting or sleeping individual is not experiencing pain. Pain is a fatiguing experience, and many people have no outward expression of pain.

## ❖ EXPLORATION OF THE CONCEPT
### Physiological Basis of Pain

Wall (1984) challenged us to continue the study of pain in saying, "So long as one person remains in pain and we cannot help, our knowledge of pain remains inadequate."

Although we believe that pain exists whenever and wherever a person says it does, it is helpful to explore briefly the physiology involved in the transmission of pain stimuli. A greater understanding of specific pain theories and pain relief methods based on theory may enhance the quality of pain management by health care professionals, especially nurses.

Although the transmission of pain stimuli and the perception of pain are still not completely understood, several theories attempt to explain these phenomena. The *gate-control theory* is based on complex neurophysiological processes (Melzack & Wall, 1965). The theory hypothesizes that the modulation of pain is affected by impulses transmitted by the two neural systems ascending from the spinal cord to the brain and proposes that the neurophysiological mechanisms in the dorsal horns of the spinal cord act as a gate that can increase or decrease the flow of nerve impulses from peripheral fibers to the central nervous system. When the gate is open, pain impulses flow easily; when the gate is closed, no pain impulses can pass. When the gate is partially open, only some of the pain impulses can pass. The degree to which the gate increases or decreases sensory transmission is determined by the activity of both large- and small-diameter fibers and by descending influences from the brain. This portion of the theory helps explain why tactile stimuli sometimes relieve pain.

A central process is also imposed on this local mechanism at the cord level. These two act together as another set of pain modifiers. Thus attention, anxiety, anticipation, and past experiences are able to exert their effects directly on the pain process. The central processes are involved in identifying signals from the body, evaluating these signals in terms of actions responsible for pain perception, and initiating a response. This theory emphasizes the "tremendous role of psychological variables and how they affect the reaction to pain" (Weisenberg, 1984). Many pain relief methods involve manipulating the sensory input to the individual. Relaxation and guided imagery are both examples of this manipulation.

Further research has yielded new discoveries about the complexity of the gating system in its transmission of pain messages. Portions of the theory have been restated by Wall (1984). Even though total support has not been awarded to the gate-control theory relative to the specific anatomical positioning of the gate and to the vagueness of the theory itself, the theory is still considered conceptually sound (Weisenberg, 1984). The important fact for nurses interested in pain management is that pain messages are transmitted through the spinal cord (Wall, 1984). Since several locations are involved and the size of the nerve fibers is a factor in the perception of pain, various pain relief methods may be effective. Closing the gate decreases pain intensity and can be accomplished by several methods. Activity in large-diameter nerve fibers may relieve pain. Since the skin is heavily endowed with these fibers, many types of tactile stimulation such as touch, massage, or vibration have the potential for causing pain relief (McCaffery & Beebe, 1989).

The study of *endorphins* is another theory about the basis of pain. Endorphins, morphine-like substances secreted by the body, were identified by Snyder (1977) in the 1970s. Snyder proposed that an impulse from the brain triggers the release of endorphins, which adhere to narcotic receptors located at the nerve endings in the brain and spinal cord. This action blocks the transmission of a pain signal, preventing the impulse from reaching the conscious level.

Researchers have found that pain perception and the need for medication to control pain differ from one person to another. Varying amounts of endorphins in persons, as well as other factors that might influence the amount of endorphins present, may help explain why some individuals perceive greater intensities of pain than others (Janal et al, 1984; Tamsen et al, 1982; Cahill, 1989). Examples of other factors that may increase or decrease endorphin levels are prolonged pain, recurrent stress and the prolonged use of morphine or alcohol, brief pain or stress, physical exercise, massive trauma, and some types of acupuncture and transcutaneous electric nerve stimulation (TENS).

The relatively new *multiple opioid receptor theory* has been presented as a theory related to pain relief. Narcotics relieve pain in a variety of ways that are not fully understood at this time. This theory suggests that narcotics may bind to or occupy multiple opioid receptor sites at the ends of nerves (Houde, 1979; Jaffee & Martin, 1985). Because of the differences in receptor sites, the activities of the sites vary; thus the side effects of the narcotics may vary. One important difference is that with certain narcotics acting at specific sites, there is no physical dependence or respiratory depression. This is an important nursing consideration because many narcotics produce respiratory depression. As this theory is further explored and validated with research, significant future changes may be anticipated for pain management. This theory will be useful in designing alternate routes of administration for various opioids (Offermeier, 1984).

The above theories represent examples of the physiological work continuing in the study of pain. Nurse researchers are contributing to this knowledge base. The theories are useful in guiding clinical practice to provide a foundation for interventions.

## Pain as a Multidimensional Concept

Pain cannot in actual practice be separated into physical pain and psychological pain; rather, the concept of pain represents a human response to a stimulus that has many dimensions. Pain is associated with a number of other physical symptoms such as anxiety, depression, and fatigue. Our research (Ferrell, Wenzl, & Wisdom, 1989) has illustrated the relationship between the individual's pain, functional status, and overall quality of life. The occurrence of pain interferes with almost every other body function, including sleep, appetite, and mobility.

The meaning of the pain to the individual must also be recognized. Recent research has examined the meaning of pain to the patient and the concept of suffering. Suffering represents the emotional component of pain. Work in the area of suffering has demonstrated that pain holds significant meaning to the patient.

One of the most distressing issues regarding pain is the public perception of this symptom. Pain is generally considered untreatable and an unavoidable problem with chronic illness. Patients and their families therefore often have no expectation that pain should be aggressively treated. A very impressive and comprehensive project is in progress by the World Health Organization (WHO) to combat this expectation. WHO has designated the state of Wisconsin as the site for a demonstration project for use as a model of comprehensive pain education for health care professionals and the public. This effort has been fostered by nursing involvement (Diekmann, Engber, & Wassem, 1989). The Wisconsin Pain Initiative Project includes a major public education program to deliver the message to patients and families that pain can indeed be relieved.

Thus pain is best considered as a multidimensional concept that is a physiological event influenced by numerous psychological and social variables. Optimal nursing care is based on an understanding of these various dimensions and a plan of care that incorporates drug and non-drug intervention.

## Pharmacological Management of Pain

A number of terms related to pharmacological management of pain have taken on emotional tones as a result of the social problem of drug use. These terms warrant clarification to distinguish recreational drug use from medicinal use by persons with pain. *Drug addiction* refers to the compulsive behaviors of drug seeking and drug use for psychic effects rather than for prescribed medical use. The incidence of patients with medical illness becoming addicted is grossly overestimated. In a recent study (McCaffery et al, 1989) involving 2459 nurses across 14 states, results indicated that more than 28% of the nurses surveyed believed that drug addiction occurred in at least one in four (25%) medical patients taking narcotic analgesics. The incidence is in fact less than 1% as has been documented in studies by Porter and Jick (1980) and Marks and Sachar (1973).

*Drug tolerance* is another misunderstood term and, when used, is generally considered to indicate that a person is addicted. However, drug tolerance occurs when a larger dose of medication than formerly was needed is required to relieve pain after repeated use of that medication. It is a physiological event and does not indicate addiction (Foley, 1985). Drug tolerance can be minimized by using appropriate doses of medications and by maintaining the oral route as long as possible. An excellent article by Paice (1988) is available to guide nurses in dealing with drug tolerance.

*Physical dependence* means that withdrawal symptoms occur if the narcotic analgesic is discontinued. Dependence is a physiological event. Guidelines for appropriate withdrawal of opioids are available to avoid the sudden discontinuation of narcotic agents (McCaffery & Beebe, 1989; Jaffe & Martin, 1985).

Another major concern of nurses and patients is the respiratory depression caused by opioids. Nurses undertreat pain because of fears of respiratory depression, and patients and their caregivers are even more concerned about this issue. Research has demonstrated that tolerance to respiratory-depressant effects of drugs develops at the same rate as tolerance to analgesia (Jaffe & Martin, 1985). Thus patients requiring high doses of analgesics will develop an increased respiratory tolerance. The most important nursing consideration is to observe the individual. If mild respiratory depression occurs, it can usually be remedied by gentle stimulation of the patient.

One of the important advances in drug treatment of pain has been the recognition of routine analgesic administration rather than as-needed dosing (Foley, 1985; McGuire, 1987). In previous years pain was viewed as an unpreventable response; therefore pain medications were given only when the person was in pain. Numerous researchers and clinicians have doc-

umented the benefits of using a preventive approach to avoid severe pain. This has been applied primarily for chronic malignant pain but has also been adopted in other predictable acute pain situations such as the postoperative period. Through administration of medications around the clock (e.g., every 4 hours), pain can be prevented, and patients can achieve a steady state of comfort rather than alternating episodes of severe pain with episodes of exhaustion when pain relief is finally achieved.

It is beyond the scope of this chapter fully to address the medications available to treat pain. A number of excellent sources exist for that purpose (McCaffery & Beebe, 1989; Foley & Payne, 1989; American Pain Society, 1989). A brief overview of pharmacological management of pain is provided. Although in most settings nurses do not prescribe pain medications, nurses are centrally involved in many decisions about the use of pain medications, including monitoring the individual's response to medications, consulting with the physician to change medications, suggesting alternative forms and doses of medications, and teaching the patient about medications. It is therefore critical that nurses have a good understanding of drugs used to treat pain.

The three major classifications of medications to treat pain include (1) the nonsteroidal antiinflammatory drugs (NSAIDs) and nonnarcotic medications; (2) the narcotic or opioid analgesics; and (3) a class referred to as adjunct analgesics. Use of the NSAIDs and nonnarcotic medications is indicated for treating mild pain, and these drugs also have good antiinflammatory effects (Foley, 1985). This classification includes aspirin, acetaminophen, ibuprofen (Motrin, Advil, and Nuprin), and indomethacin (Indocin) to name just a few. These drugs vary in their antiinflammatory, antipyretic, and analgesic effects, and choice of a particular drug should be based on these considerations. These drugs act on the peripheral nervous system, interfering with the pain message at that level.

The narcotic agents or opioids work at the

**Table 20-1**
Equianalgesic chart: approximate equivalent doses of IM and PO analgesics
for moderate and severe pain*

| Analgesic | IM route (mg)[†] | PO route (mg)[‡] | Comments |
|---|---|---|---|
| Morphine | 10 | 60 (30)[§] | Both IM and PO doses of morphine have a duration of action of about 4 to 6 hr. Sustained-release tablets, rectal suppositories, and preservative-free for spinal analgesia are also available. The PO dose is 3 to 6 times the IM dose. The lower PO dose is suggested by several clinicians (Lipman, 1980, 1982: Walsh, 1984) and is based on anecdotal evidence, not experimental research (Kaiko, 1986); it may be appropriate for some patients, especially elderly patients with chronic cancer pain. *All IM and PO doses in this chart are considered equivalent to 10 mg of IM morphine in analgesic effect.* |
| Buprenorphine (Buprenex) | 0.4 (0.3) | — | A narcotic agonist-antagonist that may precipitate withdrawal in patients very physically dependent on narcotics. Dose for the sublingual form (not available in the U.S.) is 0.8 mg. Compared with morphine, this drug is longer acting and more likely to produce nausea and vomiting (Bradley, 1984). Respiratory depression is rare but serious because it is not readily reversed by naloxone (Buprenorphine, 1986). Not available in Canada. |
| Butorphanol (Stadol) | 2 | — | A narcotic agonist-antagonist that may produce withdrawal in patients physically dependent on narcotics. May also produce psychotomimetic effects such as hallucinations. Not available in Canada. |
| Codeine | 130 | 200 | Relatively more toxic in hugh doses than morphine, causing more nausea and vomiting and considerable constipation. The PO dose is about 1.5 times the IM dose. |
| Fentanyl (Sublimaze) | 0.05 | — | Most common use is for anesthesia, given IV. Onset of action when given IM is about 15 min. duration of action, about 90 min. Analgesic effect is not significantly increased by droperidol (Jaffee and Martin, 1985). Has been used as a substitute for high-dose IV morphine in terminally ill patients when morphine caused excitation. Used IV in neonates and for brief procedures. |

May be duplicated for use in clinical practice. From McCaffery, M. and Beebe, A.: Pain: clinical manual for nursing practice, St. Louis, 1989, The CV Mosby Co.

*The equianalgesic doses in this chart are based primarily on recommendations of the Analgesic Study Section, Sloan-Kettering Institute for Cancer Research, New York, based on double-blind analgesic research (Houde, 1979). This format is adapted from McCaffery, M.: A practical, portable chart of equianalgesic doses, *Nursing* 17:56-57, Aug. 1987.
†Based on clinical experience, many consider the IM and IV doses equianalgesic (Portenoy, 1987). However, some recommend using one half the IM dose for the IV dose (American Pain Society, 1987).
†Initial PO doses are usually lower than those listed here, especially for mild to moderate pain.
§Values in parentheses refer to differences of opinion among clinicians.

**Table 20-1 (cont.)**

Equianalgesic chart: approximate equivalent doses of IM and PO analgesics
for moderate and severe pain*—cont'd

| Analgesic | IM route (mg)† | PO route (mg)‡ | Comments |
|---|---|---|---|
| Hydromorphone (Dilaudid) | 1.5 | 7.5 | Somewhat shorter acting than morphine. Also available as rectal suppository and in high-potency injectable form (10 mg/ml). The PO dose is 5 times the IM dose. |
| Levorphanol (Levo-Dromoran) | 2 | 4 | Longer acting than morphine when given in repeated, regular doses. Useful alternative to PO methodone. Careful titration required because drug accumulates; both dose and interval must be adjusted. Onset of action with PO dose occurs within 1½ hr. Because drug accumulates, analgesic effect may increase with repeated doses. *Initial* PO dose is twice the injectable dose. (The SC route is recommended over the IM route.) |
| Meperidine (Demerol) | 75 | 300 | Shorter acting (2 to 4 hr) than morphine. Watch for toxic effects on the central nervous system (CNS) caused by accumulation of the active metabolite normeperidine, which produces neuroexcitability. Use with caution in patients with renal disease. *Because of the risk to the CNS, 300 mg PO is not recommended.* Since normeperidine has a long half-life (15 hr or longer), decreasing the dose in patients exhibiting a toxic reaction may increase CNS excitability, causing seizures. Effects of normeperidine are increased (not reversed) by naloxone (Kaiko et al, 1983). The PO dose is 4 times the IM dose. |
| Methadone (Dolophine) | 10 | 20 | Longer acting than morphine when given in repeated, regular doses. Careful titration required because drug accumulates; both dose and interval must be adjusted. Onset with PO dose occurs within 1 hr. Because drug accumulates, analgesic effect may increase with repeated doses. *Initial* PO dose is twice the IM dose. |
| Methotrimeprazine (Levoprome) | 20 | — | A phenothiazine (nonnarcotic) drug. Duration of action is 4 to 5 hr. Common adverse effect is hypotension; not recommended for ambulatory patients (McGee and Alexander, 1979). |

*A guide to using the equianalgesic chart*

- Equianalgesic means approximately the same pain relief. Onset, peak effect, and duration of analgesia for each drug often differ and may also vary with individual people.
- Variability among individuals may be due to differences in absorption, organ dysfunction, or tolerance to one narcotic and not to another.
- An equianalgesic chart is a *guideline*. The individual patient's response must be observed. Doses and intervals between doses are then titrated according to the individual's response.
- An equianalgesic chart is helpful when (1) switching from one drug to another or (2) switching from one route of administration to another.
- Dosages in this chart are *not* necessarily starting doses. They suggest the *ratio* for comparing the analgesia of one drug with another.
- Based on clinical experience, the IV dose is approximately the same as the IM dose. Dose adjustments are then made according to the individual's response. Some clinicians suggest approximately one half the IM dose equals the IV dose.

**Table 20-1 (cont.)**
Equianalgesic chart: approximate equivalent doses of IM and PO analgesics
for moderate and severe pain*—cont'd

| Analgesic | IM route (mg)[†] | PO route (mg)[‡] | Comments |
|---|---|---|---|
| Nalbuphine (Nubain) | 10 (20) | — | A narcotic agonist-antagonist that may produce withdrawal in patients physically dependent on narcotics. Longer acting and less likely to cause hypotension than morphine. In doses above 10 mg/70kg, it causes no additional respiratory depression (Romagnoli and Keats, 1980; Vernier and Schmidt, 1985), so patient may be started on a high dose. |
| Opium (Pantopon opium tincture) | 20 (13.3) | (6 ml) | Infrequently used. Pantopon is the injectable form; opium tincture, the oral form. Pantopon, 20 mg, equals 10 mg of IM morphine (Beaver, 1980) or 15 mg of IM morphine (Narcotic Agonists and Analgesics, 1986). Opium tincture contains 1% morphine, that is, 0.6 ml equals 6 mg of PO morphine. Therefore 6 ml equals 60 mg of PO morphine (Jaffe and Martin, 1985). |

*Table references*

American Pain Society. Principles of analgesic use in the treatment of acute pain and chronic cancer pain a concise guide to medical practice. Washington, DC, 1987. The Society.

Beaver, W.: Management of cancer pain with parenteral medication. JAMA 244:2653-2657, Dec. 12, 1980.

Beaver, W. and Feise, G.: A comparison of analgesic effect of oxymorphone by rectal suppository and intramuscular injection in patients with postoperative pain, *J Clin Pharmacol* 17:276-291, May/June 1977.

Bradley, J.: A comparison of morphine and buprenorphine for analgesia after abdominal surgery. *Annesth Intens Care* 12:303-310, Nov. 1984.

Buprenorphine. *Med Lett Drugs Ther* 28:56, May 23, 1986.

Houde, R.W.: Systemic analgesics and related drugs: narcotic analgesics. In Bonica, J.J., and Ventafridda, V. eds: Advances in pain research and therapy, vol. 2, pp. 263-273, New York, 1979, Raven Press.

Jaffe, J. and Martin, W.: Opioid analgesics and antagonists. In Gilman, A., et al, eds: The pharmacological basis of therapeutics, ed 7, pp. 491-531, New York, 1985, Macmillan Publishing Co.

Kaiko, R.: Controversy in the management of chronic cancer pain: therapeutic equivalents of I.M. and P.O. morphine, *J Pain Sympt Manag* 1:42-45, Winter 1986.

Kaiko, R., et al: Central nervous system excitatory effects of meperidine in cancer patients, *Ann Neurol* 13:180-185, Feb. 1983.

Kantor, T., et al: Adverse effects of commonly ordered oral narcotics, *J Clin Pharmacol* 21:1-8, Jan. 1981.

central nervous system level at the opioid receptor sites of the brain and spine and are indicated for treating moderate to severe pain. The critical issue is that *how* these medications are used is as important as *which* drug is used. It is estimated that more than 90% of patients with cancer pain could achieve relief with oral analgesics if they were used properly.

A critical concept to nurses is the principle of *equianalgesia*, which refers to equivalence of doses. Nurses are frequently involved in decisions regarding changing a patient from one route to another or from one drug to another, and the approximate equivalence of doses must be known. For example, a patient who is taking hydromorphine by mouth may

### Table 20-1 (cont.)

Equianalgesic chart: approximate equivalent doses of IM and PO analgesics for moderate and severe pain*—cont'd

| Analgesic | IM route (mg)[†] | PO route (mg)[‡] | Comments |
|---|---|---|---|
| Oxycodone | — | 30 (15) | Has faster onset and higher peak effect than most PO narcotics; duration of action is up to 6 hr. In one study of postoperative pain, a preparation similar to the old formulation of Percodan (containing oxycodone, aspirin, phenacetin, and caffeine) was more effective and caused fewer adverse reactions than 90 mg of PO codeine or 75 mg of PO pentazocine and was almost equivalent to 12.5 mg of IM morphine (Kantor et al, 1981). |
| Oxymorphone (Numorphan) | 1 (1.5) | — | Also available as rectal suppository: 10 mg given rectally equals 10 mg of IM morphine (Beaver and Feise, 1977). Up to 1.5 mg IM is now recommended as equal to 10 mg of IM morphine (Jaffe and Martin, 1985). |
| Pentazocine (Tahvin) | 60 | 180 | Narcotic agonist-antagonist that may produce withdrawal in patients physically dependent on narcotics. Could produce psychotomimetic effects. The PO dose is 3 times the IM dose. |
| Propoxyphene HCl (Darvon) | — | 500 | The one recognized use is for mild to moderate pain unrelieved by nonnarcotics. *Never give as much as 500 mg PO:* only low PO doses (65 to 130 mg) are recommended. The IM form is not available in the U.S. |

*Table references—cont'd*

Lipman, A.: Comment on pain cocktail article, *Drug Intell Clin Pharm* 16:332, Apr. 1982.
Lipman, A.: Drug therapy in cancer pain, *Cancer Nursing* 3:39-46, Feb. 1980.
McGee, J. and Alexander, M.: Phenothiazine analgesia—fact or fantasy? *Am J Hosp Pharm* 36:633-640, May 1979.
Narcotic agonists and analgesics. In Facts and comparisons: drug information, 242b, Philadelphia, 1986, JB Lippincott Co.
Portenoy, R.K.: Continuous intravenous infusion of opioid drugs, *Med Clin North Am* 71:233-241, Mar. 1987.
Romagnoli, A., and Keats, A.: Ceiling effect for respiratory depression by nalbuphine, *Clin Pharmacol Ther* 27:478-485, Apr. 1980.
Vernier, V., and Schmidt, W.: The preclinical pharmacology of nalbuphine. In Gomez, Q., ed: Nalbuphine as a component of surgical anesthesia, pp. 1-9 Princeton, NJ, 1985, Excerpta Medica.
Walsh, T.: Oral morphine in chronic cancer pain, *Pain* 18:1-11, Jan. 1984.

become nauseated and require a temporary change to intravenous hydromorphone. The patient must receive a dose that will provide equal pain relief.

A number of resources exist to guide the nurse and physician in decisions about *equianalgesia*. Table 20-1, reprinted from the work of McCaffery and Beebe (1989), includes the major opioid analgesics and guidelines for their use.

The adjuvant analgesics represent medications that are not classified as analgesics but actually are drugs such as antianxiety medications, antidepressants, or anticonvulsants that can contribute to pain control. Antidepressants and anticonvulsants play a role in neuropathic pain, and antipsychotic agents or benzodiazepines are useful in managing symptoms associated with pain such as anxiety and sleep disturbance (American Pain Society, 1989; Foley & Payne, 1989).

Two final comments should be noted. The first is that drug management of pain is best accomplished through a combination of agents. Recent work has cited the benefits of administering narcotic agents with NSAIDs to achieve a combined approach. The second concerns the assessment of associated symptoms. Individuals often complain of pain as a generic term to express their overall feeling of discomfort. Very often in our clinical experience it is in fact another symptom such as constipation or nausea that requires attention. Nurses need to assess carefully for associated symptoms and to intervene accordingly.

There are so many innovations in pharmacological pain management that we are entering a "high-tech" stage in pain control. Patient-controlled analgesia (PCA) use of various ambulatory infusion pumps, subcutaneous infusions of analgesics, and sublingual and rectal analgesics are currently in use. These approaches may offer benefits to many people. However, the vast majority of pain can be treated with existing oral analgesics. One innovation in this area is the advent of longer-acting oral analgesics providing 8 to 12 hours of pain relief. Two such brand-name products currently available are MS Contin and Roxanol SR (Ferrell, in press; Ferrell, Wisdom, & Wenzl, 1989).

## Non-Drug Management of Pain

Non-drug strategies for pain relief comprise an important adjunct to drug management of pain, but, unfortunately, they are very underused. The rationale for using non-drug pain relief is based on some of the pain theories described in the preceding pages. For example, using the gate-control theory, the gate can be closed by increasing activity in the large-diameter nerve fibers through skin stimulation such as by back rub or massage. The gate can be opened by increasing activity in small-diameter nerve fibers as a result of tissue trauma or facilitory impulses from the brainstem caused by insufficient input from a monotonous environment (McCaffery & Beebe, 1989). Inhibitory impulses from the brainstem caused by sufficient sensory input from distraction or guided imagery can help to reduce pain in some instances.

Although pain relief methods vary with individuals, a variety of methods is available. These methods may be behaviorally oriented or may include external stimuli of some type. They may be influenced favorably or unfavorably by classical conditioning. In classical conditioning two stimuli are paired, one conditioned and the other unconditioned. If these two stimuli occur together often enough, the presence of the unconditioned stimuli alone may result in the same response elicited by the conditioned stimuli (McCaffery, 1979). An example in clinical practice of conditioned response with the relief of pain is seen when a patient experiences pain relief almost immediately after ingestion of aspirin for a headache. In addition, certain pain relief measures may result in pain relief often enough for classical conditioning to occur. This knowledge can be used to pair pain relief measures. An example would be the use of relaxation technique in conjunction with the use of aspirin for pain relief. The use of two pain relief measures simultaneously often has an additive effect to increase pain relief. Also, with pairing one method alone may in time have the effect of both (McCaffery, 1979).

Operant conditioning methods are based on the general principle that the frequency of a behavior may be increased by positive reinforcement or decreased by nonreinforcement. When an individual has used a particular pain relief method and has consistently received pain relief, the frequency with which he or she uses that particular method will probably increase. Knowing this is helpful in understanding why the patient may resist changing from one pain relief method of proven effectiveness to one of unknown efficacy in spite of the practitioner's conviction that the new method would provide equal or better pain relief or would have fewer side effects.

The patient may learn to avoid certain activities because of pain, an adverse consequence. Physical exercise that causes pain may lead to inactivity, which may be reinforced by pain relief. Our research has documented that the primary thing patients do to relieve pain besides taking medication is to immobilize themselves (Ferrell & Schneider, 1988). Activity was cited as a major factor influencing pain.

Our research has also demonstrated that, although most nurses agree that non-drug pain management is important, few non-drug interventions are actually used. An important part of operant conditioning is giving praise and attention to the patient when he or she tries new pain relief methods. Some pain relief measures such as guided imagery require practice before they result in pain relief. Praise for these positive behaviors helps to achieve the long-term goal of reduced pain.

Many nondrug pain relief measures result from direct physical changes within the body such as production of heat, which dilates vessels and increases circulation to the affected area. Cutaneous stimulation such as massage may block transmission of pain impulses. Use of ice packs can reduce swelling through vasoconstriction. Relaxation techniques can decrease tension and prevent muscle spasm, whereas guided imagery serves as a distraction and has been documented to produce changes in physiological functioning. The use of relaxation is an intervention that helps interrupt the cycle of muscle spasm and pain by decreasing anxiety. Music provides another important and helpful

pain relief method. The patient may have some favorite selections that bring pleasant memories to mind, or specially composed musical selections may facilitate relaxation or healing. A number of excellent references provide additional information about non-drug pain management (Donovan, 1980; McCaffery, 1980; Achterberg, 1982; Snyder M, 1985).

A number of other treatments exist for pain, including TENS (Manheimer & Lampe, 1984). This method provides a low voltage electrical stimulus from a small battery-operated device using electrodes attached to the skin. TENS therapy is often initiated by a physical therapist and is a good example of the need for an interdisciplinary approach to pain control. Social workers, physical and occupational therapists, and clinical psychologists can offer a great deal in the way of non-drug pain management.

As can be seen from the preceding discussion, there are many ways in which nurses can be instrumental with prescriptive interventions for pain relief and consultation or recommendations to other members of the health care team. A summary of non-drug pain interventions is provided in the box on p. 356. It is important to remember that the patient is the center of this team. The suggested methods must be congruent with his or her beliefs and values in order for him or her to participate fully. Nurses must also examine their own values and beliefs about pain itself and about the various methods of pain relief. The American Nurses' Association (ANA) Code for Nurses reminds us that "the nurse provides services with respect for human dignity and the uniqueness of the client unrestricted by considerations of social or economic status, personal attributes, or the nature of health problems" (ANA, 1976). Comfort is certainly an important component of the services nurses provide to their patients and as such is an appropriate goal to achieve. The relief of pain is a major link in achieving a level of comfort that is acceptable to the patient, his or her family, and the caregiver.

## ❖ NON-DRUG PAIN INTERVENTIONS

**BEHAVIORAL APPROACHES**
Relaxation exercises
Rhythmic breathing
Relaxation through music
Specific posturing positions (including changing position)
Specific activities (walking, riding in car)
Guided imagery
Distraction through social interactions with others

**COGNITIVE APPROACHES**
Understanding the pain by providing accurate information about the cause and relief of pain
Exploring beliefs/values about pain relief methods with the patient to understand his or her personal
  attitudes about pain
Coping mechanisms (exploring with the patient how he or she has coped with pain in previous
  situations)

**EXTERNAL PHYSICAL CHANGES**
Tactile stimulation (hand-holding, massage, back rubs)
Temperature variances (heat applications, cold applications)
Nerve stimulation (TENS, acupuncture, acupressure)
Sensory input (increasing stimuli with guided imagery)

## ❖ PAIN MANAGEMENT IN PROFESSIONAL NURSING PRACTICE

### Pain Assessment

The first step to improved pain control is accurate pain assessment. We cannot hope to improve pain until we can measure and document it in such a way that it can be communicated between patient, family, physician, nurse, and other team members. It is typical to read in a patient's chart a comment by the physician that the patient has "no pain," a notation by the day shift nurse that the patient has "increased pain," no notation by the evening shift, and a night shift note of "complains of pain" with no hint of the intensity.

We recommend adopting a standard format that can be used consistently. Examples of pain tools are illustrated in Fig. 20-1. The 100 mm visual analog scale has been used extensively and provides a range to detect sensitive changes in pain. It is far more precise to report that the patient complains of pain of 88 than to rely on the individual nurse's estimate of "some pain." A standard of assessment is also important for evaluation. If the patient reports a pain of 86, an intervention is implemented such as administering a medication or applying a TENS unit; if the pain intensity is then reported at 38, there are good data to evaluate the effectiveness of that intervention. Whichever tool is selected, it must be consistently used.

Several pain-rating scales are available for the pediatric population. The "faces" pain scale developed by Whaley and Wong (1989) is very useful for pain assessment with children. The pictures of faces range from very happy to very sad, representing the range of no pain to the

Examples of
pain intensity scales

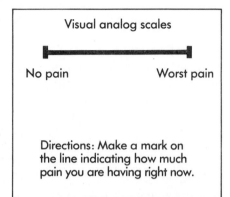

| Word descriptor scale | Visual analog scales |
|---|---|
| 0 No pain | No pain                    Worst pain |
| 1 Mild | |
| 2 Moderate | |
| 3 Severe | Directions: Make a mark on |
| 4 Excruciating | the line indicating how much pain you are having right now. |

❖ **Fig. 20-1**    Examples of pain intensity scales.

   0       1       2       3       4       5

❖ **Fig. 20-2**    Faces pain rating scale. *(From Whaley LF and Wong DL (1989). Essentials of pediatric nursing: (ed 3) St Louis: The CV Mosby Co.)*

worst pain possible. The child simply chooses the picture that best represents his or her level of comfort (Fig. 20-2).

Quality of care and patient comfort are important goals that nurses continually strive to achieve. Accurate assessment of pain is an important link in achieving a high degree of quality and patient satisfaction. The use of a valid instrument for measuring the quantity of pain an individual experiences provides a communication tool for all members of the health care team, particularly the patient. No matter which tool is selected, it must be used consistently.

## Family Involvement

Our research to date (Ferrell & Schneider, 1988) has documented the important role of the family in pain management. Although the home is considered the desired place for care and patients generally prefer being there, pain in fact is often not managed well at home. This is due to many factors such as family fears about drug addiction and tolerance and the family's inadequate knowledge about basic pain management principles. Our studies revealed several instances in which caregivers denied the patient was in pain to avoid confronting the reality that the patient's condition was worse. Family members often fear that they will administer a dose of medication that will result in death.

Caregivers can also be a tremendous asset in managing the patient's pain. Significant others can be involved in pain assessment, administering medications, and in providing non-drug pain interventions such as massage or applying heat or cold.

## The Nursing Process

The Social Policy Statement of the American Nurses' Association (ANA, 1980) provides a framework for study of the nursing care of patients with pain. The following discussion includes the assessment, nursing diagnosis, planning, implementation, and evaluation phases of this process to enable the reader to apply the information presented in a practical manner.

The assessment phase is critical in pain management. Not only is it important to do a complete physical assessment, but also an assessment of the history of pain and an evaluation of the psychosocial status of the patient add important dimensions to this multidimensional experience of the client (Ferrell, 1988; Foley, 1986). It is important during the initial assessment to explore with the individual his or her attitudes and beliefs about pain and pain management and to discuss any previous experience with pain relief he or she might have had. The cause of the pain should be determined if possible, although this information is not always immediately known. It is critical that the patient is believed whenever and wherever he or she says pain exists. Although some persons might capitalize on this underlying assumption, most persons can be trusted. Those who are manipulative are "discovered" very early in the process and represent a very small percent of patients. The pain assessment should include location, intensity, and severity.

Once the pain assessment has been made, an appropriate nursing diagnosis can be established. The North American Nursing Diagnosis Association (NANDA) has provided two categories under which nursing diagnoses related to clients with pain can be determined (Kim, 1989). "Alteration in comfort: acute pain" and "alteration in comfort: chronic pain" are the diagnoses commonly used for persons in pain.

A goal that is mutually agreed upon by the patient and the nurse is then established. This goal should be one that is objective and measurable. Many of the available pain-assessment tools are objective and provide a very precise measurement of the quantity of pain the patient perceives as existing at that moment in time.

With the determination of goals, interventions can be designed to accomplish those goals. Since some methods will work and some will not, it is helpful to have a variety of simple methods that are noninvasive such as relaxation tapes, massage, back rubs, and distraction. It is best to start with simple noninvasive and inexpensive methods that the patient can initiate independently. This promotes health restoration and self-care and adds to the individual's feelings of self-worth and independence. If these methods are ineffective, other more sophisticated approaches can be used. A sample care plan for a patient in pain follows.

## Nursing Roles

As indicated previously, pain management is the responsibility of professional nurses at all levels of practice. We believe that pain control cannot be delegated to the staff nurse or be the sole responsibility of the nurse manager. Rather, effective pain management requires a unified approach.

Nurse clinicians provide the front line of pain control. The staff nurse is the most important link to pain control because it is this position that interacts most closely with the patient and provides ongoing evaluation. Clinical spe-

# ❖ NURSING CARE PLAN

**PATIENT:** Barbara M.

**MEDICAL DIAGNOSIS:** Recurrent breast cancer with bone metastasis; hypercalcemia

**NURSING DIAGNOSIS:** Comfort, alteration in: pain (chronic)
Altered bowel elimination: constipation secondary to analgesic use
Impaired physical mobility: related to pain

| GOALS | NURSING INTERVENTIONS |
|---|---|
| Barbara will experience decreased pain intensity. | ◆ Implement a pain log and scale to better assess her pain. <br> ◆ Discuss with the physician Barbara's analgesic use with possible change in medications. <br> ◆ Evaluate current non-drug pain relief and assist Barbara with selection of alternates, such as music and exercise. |
| Barbara will resume normal elimination. | ◆ Implement use of a stool softener. <br> ◆ Encourage increased intake of fluids and higher fiber foods. <br> ◆ Suggest a mild laxative each day if there is no bowel movement. <br> ◆ Instruct patient to notify nurse if there is no bowel movement in any 48-hour period to implement additional laxatives/enemas. |
| Barbara will maintain physical mobility as long as possible. | ◆ Instruct patient to take pain medication before ambulation. <br> ◆ Instruct patient regarding active range of motion exercises. <br> ◆ Evaluate environment to determine need for walker or cane. <br> ◆ Encourage short walks and sitting in chair QID. |

## EVALUATION

Barbara reports decreased pain intensity in the pain log and uses analgesics on schedule. Her normal elimination pattern is reestablished with increased intake of fluids and high fiber foods. She maintains physical mobility by engaging in daily physical activities such as performing bed exercises and getting out of bed to sit in a chair or walk to the bathroom.

❖ **TWENTY-THREE THINGS *YOU* CAN DO TO IMPROVE PAIN MANAGEMENT IN YOUR SETTING**

1. Do a pain audit. The first step toward change is demonstrating that a problem exists.
2. Create an awareness of the status of pain management in your institution. Inform physicians, nursing staff, and administrators of the state of pain control and areas in need of improvement.
3. Designate an "expert nurse" on each shift as the consultant to colleagues on pain. Support that nurse in getting additional pain education and in becoming the unit "watchdog" for untreated pain.
4. Educate the physicians. Circulate articles, monographs, or audio tapes of interest. Work to sponsor a continuing medical education offering on pain management.
5. Adopt a uniform pain assessment tool for use during admission to the unit of any patient with pain as a significant problem.
6. Adopt an ongoing system for pain assessment (i.e., a visual analog scale).
7. Establish standards of care. You do not accept uncontrolled infection rates, extravasations, and falls, so why accept uncontrolled pain?
8. Involve others in pain management. Develop an army of supporters, i.e., workers from physical therapy, occupational therapy, social service, and the pharmacy plus the chaplain and volunteers.
9. Educate the patients. Patients must know that pain is preventable and treatable. Pain management should become a consumer issue, and patients should not settle for unrelieved pain.
10. Involve families in every aspect of pain management. Family members can be the greatest asset to pain relief or the greatest barrier.
11. Develop a "bag of tricks" for non-drug pain management, e.g., music, video tapes for relaxation, heat and cold therapy, instructions for breathing exercises, and audio tapes for imagery or relaxation.
12. Educate the nursing staff about basic principles of pain management.
13. Post equianalgesic charts on the unit. They are required nursing knowledge.
14. Develop a friend in the pharmacy. Develop a pharmacy advocate for pain management.
15. Include pain management in new employee orientation.
16. Develop a pocket card for every nurse and include a pain assessment scale and equianalgesia guides.
17. Make pain management accessible. Does you pharmacy stock appropriate medications and doses of drugs? Promote the use of longer-acting analgesics.
18. Develop an expectation in the unit that PAIN CAN BE RELIEVED. The vast majority of nurses and patients believe that cancer pain is inevitable and uncontrollable.
19. Plan for continuity in pain management. Coordinate pain efforts between inpatient units, the outpatient area, physician offices, and homes or hospices.
20. Document pain assessment. The patient's pain experience must be effectively communicated among all disciplines involved.
21. Evaluate your efforts.
22. Ask the patient. The patient remains the best authority on his or her pain and our treatment of it.
23. Provide the kind of pain management that you would seek for your own family member.

cialists can provide expertise in pain control and can serve as consultants to the nursing staff.

Nurse administrators and managers must become more involved in pain control. There is a tremendous need for establishing standards of care for pain. Nurse managers can contribute by ensuring staff education, conducting pain audits on nursing units, and fostering non-drug pain management in the setting.

Nurse researchers have made a major contribution to the current knowledge boom and to advances in pain treatment. Further research is needed to describe the prevalence of pain in understudied groups such as the elderly and to conduct trials to test nursing interventions that to date have been largely anecdotal. The box on p. 360 is intended as a very practical "to do" list for changing pain management in a setting.

## ❖ SUMMARY

Pain is a human response to illness and injury that has devastating effects on the physical and psychological well-being of the person experiencing it. Nurses have a tremendous ability to affect pain management through pharmacological and nonpharmacological interventions. Professional nursing practice at every level must be based on a solid knowledge base and on systematic assessment, planning, intervention, and evaluation.

The current focus on pain has been cited as a new health care trend reflecting societal concern for quality of life amid a health care technology that has created tremendous strides in quantity of life. Nursing care of the patient in pain is in fact founded in the most basic of nursing principles: the art of comfort. Nursing professionals can combine the historical roots of comfort nursing with the scholarly work of nursing science to achieve relief for persons in pain.

## ❖ APPLYING KNOWLEDGE TO PRACTICE

1. Identify the distinct roles of nurse clinicians, managers, and researchers in advancing pain management.
2. Identify strategies for increasing nonpharmacologic management of pain in your setting.
3. Discuss interventions to increase caregivers' involvement in pain management.
4. Explore specific strategies for evaluating the effectiveness of pain interventions.

**REFERENCES**

Achterberg, J., and Lawlis, F. (1982). Imagery and health intervention. *Topics in Clinical Nursing 3,* 55-60.

American Pain Society (1989). *Principles of analgesic use in the treatment of acute pain and chronic cancer pain: a concise guide to medical practice.* Skokie, Ill.: American Pain Society.

ANA (1976). *Code for nurses with interpretive statements.* Kansas City: ANA.

ANA (1980). *Nursing: A social policy statement.* Kansas City: ANA.

Cahill, C. (1989) Beta endorphin levels during pregnancy and labor: a role in pain modulation. *Nursing Research* 38 (4), 200-203.

Diekmann, J., Engber, D., & Wassem, R. (1989). Cancer pain control; one state's experience. *Oncology Nursing Forum 16* (2), 219-224.

Donovan, M. (1980). Relaxation with guided imagery: a useful technique. *Cancer Nursing 3,* 27-32.

Ferrell, B. (in press). Nursing implications of controlled release analgesics. *Nursing 90.*

Ferrell, B., Wisdom, C., & Wenzl, C. (1989a). Quality of life as an outcome variable in management of cancer pain. *Cancer 63* (11), 2321-2327.

Ferrell, B., Wisdom, C., & Wenzl, C., (1988). Evolution and evaluation of pain management. *Oncology Nursing Forum 15 (3), 285-289.*

Ferrell, B.R. & Schneider, C. (1988). Experience and management of cancer pain at home. *Cancer Nursing 11* (2), 84-90.

Ferrell, B., Wisdom, C., & Wenzl, C., & Brown, J. (1989). Effects of controlled release morphine on quality of life for cancer pain. *Oncology Nursing Forum 16* (4), 521-526.

Foley, K. (1985). The treatment of cancer pain. *New England Journal of Medicine. 313,* 84-95.

Foley, K., & Payne, R. (1989). *Current Therapy of Pain.* Philadelphia: B.C. Decker.

Hester, N., & Barcus, C. (1986). Assessment and management of pain in children. *Pediatric Nursing Update 1,* 2-7.

Hill, C.S., & Fields, W. (1989). *Advances in Pain Research and Therapy.* New York: Raven Press.

Houde, R.W. (1979). Analgesic effectiveness of the narcotic agonist-antagonists. *British Journal of Clinical Pharmacology* 7, 297S-308S.

Jaffe, J.H., & Martin, W.R. (1985). Opioid analgesics and antagonists. In A.G. Gillman, L.S. Goodman, T.W. Rall, & F. Murad (Eds.). *The pharmacologic basis of therapeutics.* New York: Macmillan Publishing Co.

Janal, M., Colt, E., Clark, W., & Glusman, M. (1984). Pain sensitivity, mood and plasma endocrine levels in man following long distance running: effects of naloxone. *Pain 19,* 13-25.

Kim, M., McFarland, G., & McLane, A. (1989). *Pocket Guide to Nursing Diagnosis.* St. Louis: CV Mosby.

Mannheimer, J., & Lampe G. (1984). *Clinical transcutaneous electrical nerve stimulation.* Philadelphia: FA Davis Co.

Marks, R., & Sachar E. (1973). Undertreatment of medical inpatients with narcotic analgesics. *Ann Intern Med* 78, 173-181.

McCaffery, M. (1979). *Nursing Management of the patient with pain* (2nd ed.) New York: Lippincott.

McCaffery, M. (1980). Relieving pain with noninvasive techniques. *Nursing 10,* 55-57.

McCaffery, M., & Beebe, A. (1989). *Pain: Clinical manual for nursing* St. Louis: CV Mosby.

McCaffery, M., Ferrell, B.R., O'Neil-Page, E., Lester, M., & Ferrell, BA. (1990). Nurses knowledge of opioid analgesics and addiction. *Cancer Nursing 13,* (1) 21-27.

McGrath, P.J., Johnson, G., Goodman, J.T., Schillinger, J., Dunn, J. & Chapman, J. (1985). The CHEOPS: A behavioral scale to measure postoperative pain in children. In H.I. Fields, R. Dubner, and F. Cervero (Eds.): *Advances in pain research and therapy,* (vol. 9, pp. 395-402,) New York: Raven.

McGuire, D., & Yarbro, C. (1987). *Cancer pain management.* New York: Grune & Stratton.

Melzack, R. & Wall, P. (1965). Pain mechanisms: a new theory. *Science.* 150, 971-979.

Mohinde, EA., Royle, J., Montemuro, M., Porterfield, P., Scott, J., & Tugwell, P. (1988). Assessing the quality of cancer pain management. *J Palliative Care 4* (3), 9-15.

Offermeier, J., & Van Rooyen, J.M. (1984). Opioid drugs and their receptors: A present state of knowledge. *S Afr Med Jour. 66,* 299-305.

Paice, J.A. (1988). The phenomenon of analgesic tolerance in cancer pain management. *Oncology Nursing Forum 15,* 455-460.

Porter, J. & Jick, H. (1980). Addiction rare in patients treated with narcotics. *N Engl J Med* 302, 123.

Ross, D., & Ross, S. (1984). Childhood pain: the school aged child's viewpoint, *Pain 20,* 179-191.

Snyder, M. (1985). *Independent nursing interventions* New York: John Wiley & Sons.

Snyder, S.H. (1977). Opiate receptors and internal opiates. *Scientific America. 236,* 44-56.

Tamsen, A., Sakurada, T., Wahlstrom, A., et al. (1982). Postoperative demand for analgesics in relation to individual levels of endorphins and substance P in cerebrospinal fluid. *Pain 13,* 171-183.

Wall, P., & Melzack, R. (1984). *Textbook of pain.* New York: Churchill Livingstone.

Whaley, L.F. & Wong, D.L. (1989). *Essentials of pediatric nursing* (3rd ed.). St. Louis: CV Mosby.

Wiesenberg, M. (1984). Cognitive aspects of pain. In P. Wall, & R. Melzack (Eds.), *Textbook of pain* (pp. 162-172). New York: Churchill Livingstone.

Wilkie, D., Lovejoy, N., Dodd, M., & Teslwer, M. (1988). Cancer pain control behaviors: description and correlation with pain intensity. *Oncology Nursing Forum,* 15 (6), 723-731.

# 21 Chronicity

Joyce H. Johnson

## OBJECTIVES

*At the completion of this chapter, the reader will be able to:*

◆ Understand the scope and nature of chronic health problems.

◆ Understand the impact of chronicity on the individual, family, and health care system.

◆ Apply chronicity theory and research to individuals with chronic health problems.

Chronicity is defined in *Webster's New World Dictionary* as diseases that last a long time or recur often and resist all efforts to eradicate them. Chronicity includes not only chronic illnesses such as heart disease, diabetes mellitus, and arthritis but also permanent disabilities resulting from trauma or birth defects. An array of associated social, economic, and behavioral problems that often result from chronic health problems affect the person, the family, and the community. This chapter describes the scope and characteristics of chronicity and the impact chronicity has on all aspects of society. Factors influencing the dynamics of chronicity such as developmental and adjustment patterns of the individual and family and the impact of chronicity on the health care system are included. Nursing diagnoses frequently associated with chronicity are discussed, using the nursing process as the framework.

## ❖ SCOPE OF CHRONICITY

Chronicity is currently the number one health problem in the United States. More than 110 million people in the United States are afflicted with one or more chronic conditions. Among them are more than 32 million people limited to some degree in their normal daily activities as a result of their condition. Although we are an aging population in which chronic disease and disability are endemic, chronicity is not limited to older age groups but is prevalent across the life span. Approximately 114,000 children between 6 and 17 years of age, 410,000 young adults between 18 and 45 years of age, and 3 million adults 45 years of age and over need help in one basic physical activity because of a chronic health problem (National Center, 1985).

## Defining Chronicity

Determining a definition of chronicity that encompasses all aspects of chronic illness and disability is complex and difficult. Definitions generally include the nature of the pathological condition, a time dimension, and medical intervention. Fewer definitions encompass the impact on the human element, interdisciplinary involvement including nursing, and an emphasis on self-care and health promotion.

In 1949 the Commission of Chronic Diseases described chronic diseases as "all impairments or deviations from normal which have the following characteristics: permanency, residual disability, caused by nonreversible pathological alteration, require rehabilitation, and may require a long period of supervision, observation, or care" (Roberts, 1954). Later, the National Conference on Care of the Long-Term Patient included a more definitive time dimension in relation to hospitalization and/or rehabilitation: at least 30 acute hospital days or 3 months of medical supervision and/or rehabilitation (Roberts, 1954). Other definitions address the impact of chronic illness (Feldman, 1974), the requirement for interdisciplinary involvement (Feldman, 1974; Cluff, 1981), and an emphasis on self-care and self-responsibility (Cluff, 1981; Mazzuca, 1982).

Lubkin (1986, p. 6) identified a more comprehensive and flexible definition of chronicity. She states that "chronic illness is the irreversible presence, accumulation, or latency of disease states or impairments that involve the total human environment for supportive care and self-care, maintenance, and prevention of further disability." The one aspect omitted from this definition is maximizing the person's functional ability.

## Disablement Model

Traditionally, the emphasis of health care professionals has been on the curative aspects of the disease process. Such an approach is in-adequate when caring for individuals with one or more chronic health problems. A "disablement model" that provides a functional approach to health care for the chronically ill and disabled was derived from the World Health Organization's Classification System on Impairment, Disability and Handicap (Granger, 1986).

*Impairment* is defined as "any loss or abnormality of anatomic structure or physiological or psychological function at the organ level" (Granger, 1986, p. 29). Disability results when the impairment is sufficient to lead to difficulty or inability to perform daily living activities. A person may have a chronic condition such as rheumatoid arthritis or hypertension, but as long as there is no limitation in performing skills and fulfilling social roles, the person is not considered to have a disability or handicap. *Disability* then occurs "at the person level and represents any restriction or lack of ability (resulting from an impairment) to perform an activity in the manner or within the range considered normal for a person of the same age, culture, and education" (Granger, 1986, p. 29). Individuals with a disability often require adaptive equipment to fulfill functional roles. The person with rheumatoid arthritis, for example, may require a cane or walker to ambulate. However, another person with emphysema may not require assistive devices but is considered disabled if diminished oxygen reserves interfere with daily activities and functional abilities.

The term *handicap* is used when societal norms and social policy interfere with the performance or fulfillment of social roles. Handicap "occurs at the societal level when conditions are imposed upon the person in such a way, through disadvantageous social norms and policy, that limits the individual in fulfillment of expected social roles" (Granger, 1986, p. 29). For example, limited accessibility to public transportation may prevent or hamper a disabled person from attaining vocational or educational goals, resulting in a handicap. Societal attitudes toward certain conditions such as epilepsy and cancer may limit participation in certain activities and job opportunities.

The above definitions of chronicity underscore the multidimensional nature of the concept. An analysis of the concept is necessary to understand the impact of chronicity on the individual, family, and health care system.

## ❖ CONCEPTUAL ANALYSES OF CHRONICITY

Chronicity takes on different patterns and shapes and is seen as different problems. These problems require different organizational strategies and family arrangements to manage and cope with the effects of chronicity. Considerable interactional and organizational skill and financial, medical, and family resources are needed over the course of the condition. If any of these arrangements are interrupted, client and family disruption may result.

Moos and Tsu (1977) provide a framework to help understand how chronicity affects the life of an individual (Fig. 21-1). In this model three major categories of variables influence the response to chronicity: (1) background and personal variables (age, sex, socioeconomic status, personality traits), (2) illness-related variables (phase, trajectory, symptoms), and (3) physical and social environmental factors (social support, home environment, culture). These three categories interact with each other to influence the client's cognitive appraisal or meaning of the illness, the adaptive tasks or problems associated with the chronic condition that affect the client's life, and coping skills or the ways in which the client deals with the adaptive tasks. All of these factors interact with each other to influence the eventual outcomes and adjustment to the chronic condition.

### Illness-Related Influences

The course and impact of chronicity depend on the severity of the illness or injury, the symptoms it presents, the possibility and degree of remission or comeback, the variation of symptoms, and the life-style or activity in which one wishes to engage. The phrase "illness trajectory" has been used to describe not only these variations in the physiological unfolding of a chronic condition but also the organization and work in managing the condition and the impact on those directly or indirectly affected (Strauss et al, 1985). An interdisciplinary health care model is essential to provide support and

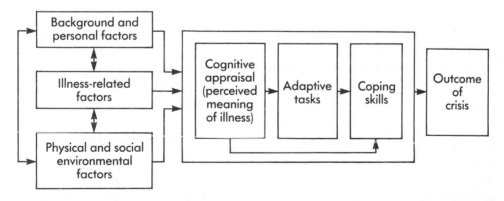

❖ **Fig. 21-1**    Conceptual model for understanding the crisis of physical illness. *(Redrawn from Moos RH and Tsu VD, editors: The crisis of physical illness: an overview. New York, 1977, Plenum Medical. Reprinted with permission.)*

resources to the individual and family throughout all phases of the illness trajectory.

Chronicity trajectories, unlike an acute illness, can have considerable variability in shape and can be broken down into phases: acute, comeback, stable, unstable, and downward (Corbin and Strauss, 1988). As an example, a person with appendicitis may have a single acute episode that is treated by surgical removal of the appendix followed by complete recovery. However, the trajectory shape for chronic conditions may show considerable variation within the same condition as well as between different conditions. Two people with multiple sclerosis can demonstrate considerable variation in the manifestations of the disease. One may have repeated episodes of exacerbations and remission, with considerable return over the course of 20 years, whereas another person may have a series of exacerbations with little evidence of remission, resulting in progressive deterioration over a period of 5 years. The illness trajectory of a person with diabetes mellitus may have a relative period of stability interrupted by brief periods of acute episodes with a more gradual decline in function. Similarly, individuals with cardiac disease, stroke, and kidney disease may show considerable variation in trajectory shapes within those conditions as well as between them.

It is this variability in the trajectory of chronic conditions that contributes to health care personnel, family members, and friends all having their own perception of what that illness trajectory is (Corbin & Strauss, 1988). These perceptions are influenced by past experiences with the chronic condition, the knowledge and understanding of the course of the condition, and the actual experiences encountered in managing the work of the client's condition. The client and family may develop effective strategies in managing the work of the chronicity over time; however, the majority of health care professionals only see the client during an acute exacerbation or remission. Involvement

with the client at different phases and to different degrees during the course of the chronic condition can influence how one projects the illness trajectory of that client. This may account for some of the differences in illness trajectories projected by the physician, the nurse, the client, and the primary caregiver.

Thus variability in the actual shape of the illness trajectory of chronicity is not dependent solely on the physiological manifestations of the condition. Other influences on the trajectory shape include the nature of the condition, the client's physical and emotional response to the condition, schemes or strategies to manage the condition, and other biographical contingencies that might affect the trajectory. Biographical contingencies include (1) contextualizing (incorporating the illness trajectory into one's life), (2) coming to terms (arriving at some degree of understanding and acceptance of the consequences), (3) reconstituting identity (reintegrating one's identity into a new conceptualization of self around the limitations imposed by the condition), and (4) recasting biography (giving new direction to one's biography or life). Thus the interplay between the influences on trajectory perceptions, trajectory perceptions of key individuals, and the influences on the trajectory shape all contribute to the actual outcome or shape of the trajectory (Table 21-1). These dynamics affect the course of the illness and the eventual unfolding of the ultimate shape of the trajectory, which cannot be known until the end of the person's life (Corbin & Strauss, 1988).

## Background and Personal Influences

**Developmental patterns and chronicity.** One of the major dimensions in which individuals with chronicity can differ is that of age group (Sutkin, 1984). Erikson (1963) identified a series of stages throughout the life span in

❖ **Table 21-1**
Chronicity trajectory

| Influences on trajectory perceptions | | Trajectory perceptions | | Influences on trajectory | | Actual trajectory |
|---|---|---|---|---|---|---|
| Past experiences with condition<br>Knowledge and understanding of condition | → | Health care professional<br>Client/patient | → | Nature of condition<br>Client's response to condition | → | |
| Actual experience in managing work of condition | | Family members<br>Friends | | Management schemes<br>Biographical processes | | |

←———————————————— Phase of chronic condition ————————————————→
(acute, comeback, stable, unstable, downward)

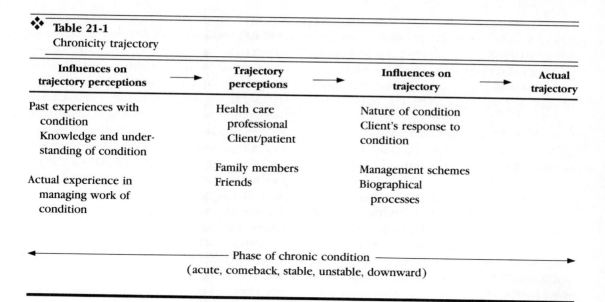

which developmental changes occur. Normal development is thought to occur when tasks of each life stage are mastered before passage to the next stage. Chronicity interacts with these normative psychosocial (Erikson, 1963) and cognitive (Piaget, 1952) developmental tasks of a child or an adult, possibly delaying or hindering the transition from one life stage to the next. Nursing interventions, therefore, that take into account not only the chronic condition but also the person's developmental stage will likely be more effective.

*Infancy.* Trust, the basic developmental task of infancy, is developed through the consistent availability of the mother to provide for the infant's basic needs and to bring comfort. A number of chronic conditions—congenital anomalies, developmental disabilities, respiratory disorders, premature birth—affecting the neonate and infant can disrupt the bonding of a trusting relationship between mother and infant. Cognitive development may also be slowed if motor or sensory impairments prevent the infant from exploring his or her environment.

Parental reaction to the infant's illness can influence subsequent behavior. Feelings of ma-

ternal failure, guilt, and anger may interfere with the usual feelings of love and nurturing associated with the birth of a child. There is also little in the environment of a neonatal intensive care unit that promotes trust. The overall noise level and repetitive diagnostic and treatment procedures interfere with providing any sustained continuity in environmental stimuli and development of a loving and trusting relationship. Subsequent behavior disturbances manifested by feeding and sleep disturbances can result. Studies, however, have shown that early supplemental stimulation and "tender loving care" by nurses and other members of the health care team have a positive effect on development and parental perceptions (Field, 1979).

*Childhood.* With the establishment of trust in infancy, preschool children proceed through the developmental stages of autonomy versus shame and guilt, initiative versus guilt, and industry versus inferiority (Erikson, 1963). The major transition of preschool to school-aged children is the entry into school, which allows them to function in an area beyond their home and parental guidance and protection. A child with a chronic condition may be prevented from proceeding normally through these developmental stages by overprotective and permissive parents and differential treatment by teachers and classmates. Inappropriate behavior, feelings of inferiority, learned helplessness, and an eventual "sick role" life-style may result. Wright (1983) emphasizes the importance during this period of a person close to the child discussing matters related to the disability or chronic condition within a coping framework. This is best done as the situation comes up naturally. Helping the child to understand the restrictions that a chronicity imposes while avoiding any value judgments can help the child identify and develop strategies to cope with the condition. It is much better for the child to realize the displeasing aspects of chronicity in a warm and supportive environment.

The child's understanding of the chronic condition and treatment procedures is postulated to parallel the stages of intellectual development (Whitt, 1984). Explanations must take into account the cognitive development stage of the child. For the very young child up to 4 years of age, emotional support and a caring approach by nurses may be more important than the explanations and/or reasons given about a condition or treatment. The operationally concrete child, however, will begin to understand the relationship between one observable occurrence, e.g., the cause of the chronic condition, and a perceptual cue or symptom resulting from the chronic condition if explanations are more visually and perceptually oriented (Whitt, 1984). It is not until the child reaches 11 or 12 years of age with the onset of more formal operational thinking that he or she understands the nature of the condition and the interrelationship between the cause of chronicity and the effect on the body in more abstract terms. Until this time the nurse must be especially alert for misconceptions and distortions about the meaning of the illness to the child.

*Adolescence.* Erikson (1963) identifies the developmental task of adolescence as the search for identity. Chronicity may delay the adolescent's passage into full adulthood status marked by economic independence and marriage or a separate household (Wright, 1983). Such circumstances then prolong the tenuous position of the adolescent between childhood and adulthood, resulting in parental conflicts and inconsistent emotional behavior. The adolescent with a chronic condition has to cope with two overlapping situations: the situation caused by chronicity and the situation related to the passage from childhood to adulthood (Wright, 1983).

Despite the additional stress of chronicity, studies indicate that adolescents with chronic illnesses are essentially healthy psychologically and generally have positive outlooks (Blumberg, Lewis, & Susman, 1984). This in part may be due to the adolescent's feelings of indestructibility and encouragement by the caregivers to continue with as many activities as possible.

*Young adulthood.* During young adulthood the primary development goal is related to the formation of mature interpersonal relationships (Erikson, 1963). Chronicity only increases the complexity of developing close friends, choosing a career, and developing a close, meaningful sexual relationship.

Glueckauf and Quittner (1984) identified four areas of interpersonal functioning altered by chronicity. First, public attitudes about physical disability may exclude the young adults from employment and educational opportunities and from recreational and social activities even though they have the requisite ability. Interpersonal functioning is also affected by the differential behavior patterns of the able-bodied toward the disabled. The disabled are often subject to two different and often conflicting expectations at the same time (Wright, 1983). On one hand they are considered disabled and are expected to act accordingly; but at the same time they are expected to behave just like an able-bodied person. A third area of concern is embarrassing social situations related to specific conditions. Social situations can be complicated by individuals who act as if the disabled person is not present or cannot hear. For example, it is not unusual for someone who is blind to be ignored while an able-bodied friend is asked what the blind person wants. The fear of an unexpected bowel movement, urinary incontinence, and falling as a result of gait disturbances has been shown to increase levels of discomfort and anxiety during social encounters (Dunn, 1977). The last area concerns the reinforcement of dependent behaviors by health care personnel. Chronicity often requires frequent hospitalization during crises and exacerbations. All too often nurses and other health care personnel encourage dependent behavior. The problem-solving and social skills necessary for the young adult to cope with chronicity are never acquired. Greater emphasis must be placed on developing self-care and problem-solving behaviors necessary for community reintegration.

*Adulthood and middle age.* The developmental tasks of middle age are closely associated with the family. Erikson (1963) called this period generativity, i.e., a concern for others and care, nurturance, and guidance of the younger generation. Studies have indicated that the years of childrearing through the time children leave the home are the most stressful (Rustad, 1984).

Crisis in adaptation during this period generally occurs as a result of an unexpected event. As an example, a husband develops chronic renal failure necessitating extensive treatment and early retirement. Such an event not only places additional financial strain on the family but also may necessitate additional role responsibilities on the part of the wife. Decreased marital satisfaction has been reported by clients and spouses.

*Old age.* Erikson (1963) identified ego integrity as the major developmental task of old age. It is the primary time when one must face a series of losses: loss of health, loss of physical ability, loss of spouse, loss of friends, and loss of living independently at home. The stresses the older adult faces are not any less than those of any other life-stage, only different.

Chronicity is prevalent as one grows older. Eighty percent or more of persons over the age of 65 have at least one chronic disease (Williams, 1986). Elderly persons seem more vulnerable to the stresses associated with chronicity. The difficulties seem to result from the intense, personal feelings that accompany increased disability; the attempt to preserve self-esteem; and trying to incorporate the additional changes and losses into an established life-style (Kemp, 1986). The normal physiological changes resulting from aging may further diminish the older adult's ability to respond to these additional stressors. Maladaptive responses to chronicity may be manifested by various affective disorders, including depression, lack of motivation or interest, stress-related disorders, including alcoholism, and social isolation.

## Social Environmental Influences

**Requirement for mourning.** Society often expects individuals to respond to chronicity in a predetermined manner. Wright (1983) talks of three aspects of the requirement of mourning that others may impose on the person with a chronic illness or disability. The empathetic requirement of mourning arises from the expectation of suffering resulting from a chronic illness or disability. One may feel sorry for the person or if expected suffering does not become evident, may wonder "why not?" The self-aggrandizing requirement of mourning occurs when the motive is the need to preserve one's own status. By placing the disabled person in a position of the unfortunate, one maintains superiority. An able-bodied person may then feel threatened if the disabled person does not show evidence of suffering. The third type, the "ought" requirement of mourning, stems from the need to preserve how one ought to feel and act. In each of the above instances the observer exaggerates suffering on the part of a person considered unfortunate. Health care providers often expect a client to react or behave in a certain way. When a client fails to do so, they may label the person as being in denial and dismiss evidence concerning the adequacy of the adjustment. Coping with chronicity is influenced, therefore, not only by prior patterns of coping and personality traits but also by the particular circumstances of the situation.

**Illness Roles.** During illness societal role expectations must accommodate a changing health status. Parsons (1951) developed a model to explain society's response to persons who are ill. In this model the sick person is exempted from normal role responsibilities, providing the illness has been legitimized by others and by a physician, and has the right to receive care. The obligations of the sick person include a desire to get well, to obtain competent medical help, and to cooperate with health professionals. Parsons' model is limited in explaining behavior related to chronicity in which the individual is expected to assume normative social roles. For example, persons with chronic low back pain may be viewed as malingerers because the pathological aspects of the condition cannot be legitimized by usual diagnostic techniques. Other conditions for which legitimization for release of role responsibilities can be difficult include alcoholism and mental illness.

### Cognitive Appraisal

The perception or subjective meaning of chronicity is influenced by the personal, illness-related, and social environmental variables pre-

viously discussed. The extent that chronicity threatens an important life goal or value can influence the individual's perception, coping behaviors, and adjustment. As an example, a seemingly inconsequential loss of an index finger may significantly disrupt a person's life. Although not crucial to most people, it would significantly affect the ability of a concert violinist to continue his or her professional career.

Attractiveness and physique, although judged by different standards, are important attributes in all cultures. Body experience and awareness, however, generally recede in consciousness except when some disruption occurs. Shontz (1975) describes seven psychological functions of body experience that can be disrupted by chronic conditions. They are the body as a sensory register, an instrument for action, source of drives, stimulus to self, stimulus to others, private world of experience, and expressive instrument. Murray (1972) notes that the connection with body image is decreased more when an attribute is viewed as a tool than when it is looked on as a personal characteristic. However, it is often difficult to separate the personal aspect of an attribute from its use as a tool. Body experience need not be prominent to be important, even crucial, to a given person or in a given situation. It is the meaning that the individual and society attach to alterations that determines the affect on the person (Norris, 1978).

### ❖ ADAPTIVE TASKS OR PROBLEMS
### Impact of Chronicity on the Individual

Chronicity potentially causes multiple problems, often requiring a restructuring of a person's entire life-style. Strauss (1975) detailed the interaction between the physical, social, and psychological problems that persons with a chronic condition must face in their daily lives. These problems include (1) prevention and management of medical crises; (2)

control of symptoms; (3) managing prescribed medical regimens; (4) prevention of, or living with, social isolation; (5) adjustment to changes in the course of the disease; (6) attempts to normalize the interactions with others and lifestyle; and (7) obtaining funding for treatments or survival. These problems and resulting lifestyle changes can affect role behavior, body image perceptions, sense of control or powerlessness, and adherence to the health care regimen.

**Role behavior.** Role conflict can emerge when chronically ill or disabled persons enter the acute hospital setting because of an exacerbation of symptoms or superimposed acute illness. The traditional sick role model assumes that the client is in a state of illness that renders him or her helpless and dependent on physicians and nurses for care. Chronically ill clients, therefore, may be viewed as uncooperative and problem clients if they attempt to control their hospital care by requesting special treatments or routines. Nurses, as well as physicians, must acknowledge the practical experience a person has attained through day-to-day management of symptoms and health regimens. The nurse should encourage the active involvement and participation in care to the extent that the client's physical and psychological reserves allow. At the same time nurses must not expect that the clients are knowledgeable about other aspects of their care unrelated to their chronic condition.

**Body image.** Feelings of being different and inferior can result when the impairment is visible. Joint swelling resulting from rheumatic diseases, loss of function associated with paralysis, or loss of a body part such as a breast can significantly threaten one's body image. Even less obvious or visible changes may threaten a person's body image. The peril to life imposed by a myocardial infarction can threaten a person's body image. The more meaning or importance a person attaches to a body part or func-

tion, the greater will be the impact on body image as a result of loss or disfigurement associated with chronic illness or disability.

**Stigma.** Whereas body image relates primarily to one's perception of self, *stigma* relates to the devaluation by society of persons who deviate from social norms or fail to live up to socially accepted standards. Goffman (1963, p. 3) defines a stigma as "undesirable attributes incongruous with our stereotype of what a given individual should be." That is, stigma is the discrepancy between what is desired and what is actual. Society often ascribes an underprivileged status to persons with chronic conditions. Wright (1983) cautions that we should not concentrate solely on the negative attitudes ascribed by society to the disabled but should consider the positive attitudes of the public as well. Wright suggests that social encounters that take into account the individual as a unique complement of interests, abilities, personality traits, and life circumstances beyond the labeled disability result in more positive attitudes.

Wright (1983) discusses the concept of *spread* in which the power of single characteristics evokes inferences about a person. As an example, a deaf and mute child is often thought of as mentally retarded even though intelligence tests and performance levels indicate otherwise. Because of spread, the extent of the impairment or disability is often perceived as more severe than it actually is.

Stigmatized individuals respond in a variety of ways (Lubkin, 1986). Individuals may elect to ignore or disregard the incident, identify and associate with similarly afflicted people, look for secondary gains, speak out or challenge the rules, conceal any signs of the stigmatizing feature, or de-emphasize or attempt to make the defect seem insignificant. As an example, Tom and Ken, two spinal cord injured persons with similar functional levels, responded differently. Tom elected to de-emphasize his disability by identifying and associating primarily with non-disabled persons, whereas Ken identified with individuals with similar disabilities, becoming actively involved in a number of groups of disabled persons. Each learned to respond to the stigmatizing aspects of his disability in different ways. Both the length and nature of the condition as well as individual personality characteristics can influence how an individual deals with stigma.

**Powerlessness.** *Powerlessness* is defined by Miller (1983, p. 38) as "the perception that one's own actions will not significantly affect an outcome." Powerlessness can result from chronicity when the client perceives the lack of control over his or her immediate situation. Stapleton (1983a) categorized four groups of stressors in clients with chronic renal failure that contribute to powerlessness: (1) physiological stressors such as lack of control over symptoms and uncertainty of disease course; (2) psychological stressors related to changes in body image, fear of death, frustration of basic drives, and dependence-independence conflict; (3) role disturbances in social, occupational, or family group; and (4) life-style changes associated with financial insecurity, limitation of activity, and time required for dialysis. Many of these same stressors can be found in other chronic conditions. Prolonged powerlessness can lead to anxiety, depression, hopelessness, and eventually physiological deterioration.

Pfister-Minogue (1983) and Stapleton (1983b) identified enabling strategies that can be used by nurses to increase a client's sense of control and power. These strategies include client education, individualized approach to client care, behavior modification, modification of the environment, involvement of significant others, and facilitating the verbalization of feelings.

**Compliance.** An expectation of health professions is that medical regimens will be meticulously followed. Clients who do not adhere to the prescribed regimen are frequently desig-

nated as uncooperative. *Compliance* has been defined as "the extent to which a person's behavior (in terms of taking medications, following diets, or executing life-style changes) coincides with medical or health advice" (Haynes, 1979, p. 1). Concerns have been voiced about the appropriateness of the use of these terms (Quigley & Giovinco, 1988). Unfavorable connotations have been associated with the concept of compliance: (1) exertion of power or control by the health professional over the client; and (2) passivity and lack of autonomy by the client. Given and Given (1984) extended the definition of compliance to include behaviors that the client demonstrates at the suggestion of, with the encouragement of, or in joint agreement with a health care provider to maintain his or her health status. This definition implies client involvement in determination of the health care regimen. Adherence and nonadherence have received some acceptability as alternative terms. Whichever term is used, it is important in treating clients with chronicity that we do not label or stereotype clients as noncompliant without first determining the cause of the behavior.

Notwithstanding methodological and conceptual problems that characterize compliance research, the prevalence of high noncompliance in chronicity has been consistently reported. Noncompliance not only can contribute to a client's deteriorating health status but also to health care costs through more frequent hospitalizations and extensive and expensive treatments.

Noncompliant clients frequently are regarded as foolish, stupid, and uncooperative by health care personnel. However, the issue is that clients with chronic conditions must manage their health regimen in the context of a specific set of social and financial conditions that may vary from day to day. Strauss (1975) listed 10 regimen characteristics that influence compliance: (1) the ease or difficulty to learn and carry out; (2) amount of time needed; (3) amount of discomfort or pain it causes; (4)

presence or absence of side effects, especially if they entail high risk; (5) amount of energy or effort needed to carry out; (6) visibility of regimen to others; (7) possibility of stigmatizing the person if known; (8) perceived efficiency of regimen; (9) amount of expense; and (10) extent the regimen leads to increased social isolation. Generally, the more difficult the regimen and the more the person's life-style is affected, the less likely it is he or she will comply completely with the regimen. In many instances the treatment regimen may be seen as more of a problem than the chronic condition itself.

Lubkin (1986) identified three additional aspects that can influence compliant behavior. First, the manner of the client-provider interactions can influence compliance. The acute care model ascribes the client to the sick role with the provider of care being dominant as the professional expert and manager of the condition. Because the client assumes extensive responsibility in the management of a chronic condition, a more complementary role that takes into account the client's perspective is appropriate. Second, lack of motivation has been often ascribed as a reason for noncompliance. However, compliance with a treatment regimen competes with other tasks, roles, or relationships. Without taking the client's perspective into account, health care providers may simply label the client as having low motivation. Negotiation and compromise by both the client and provider of care may increase compliance. Third, education has frequently been identified as the key to compliance. Simply imparting knowledge about the condition or treatment regimen, however, does not ensure compliance. The actual participation of the client and significant other, if warranted, in the treatment regimen must be included as part of the teaching protocol. Consideration of the client's cultural values, educational level, learning, and memory abilities are other variables that need consideration.

More important than labeling a client simply as noncompliant is determining the cause or contributing factors that lead to the noncompliant behavior. These factors may vary from complexity of or lack of confidence in the regimen to inability to perform tasks or lack of understanding of the regimen. To foster compliance nurses must tailor the regimen to the daily routine of the client. Medication regimens can often be associated with specific daily activities, e.g., mealtimes. Simplifying the regimen as much as possible has been associated with improved compliance. Memory aids such as cue cards, visual reminders, or alarm clocks can be useful, particularly for the elderly.

## Impact of Chronicity on Significant Others

Chronicity not only directly affects the afflicted member but also the entire family constellation. Demands such as job responsibilities, child rearing, or spousal expectations often compete with caregiving responsibilities. Even when family members do not assume any caregiving responsibilities, the chronic condition and demands of the treatment regimen may seriously affect family dynamics. Kemp (1986) identified seven problems associated with family adaptive patterns: (1) families who are uninformed about the condition or sources of help; (2) another unidentified family member also ill from a medical or mental health problem; (3) families who "demote" the disabled person from usual roles or responsibilities; (4) the overburdened or stressed families often associated with dementia or severely disabling conditions; (5) families in which there is considerable disagreement over the course of action to be taken; (6) families with a long-standing history of conflict that prevents effective cooperation; and (7) families lacking in affection who provide care in a cold, business-like manner.

Assessment of the impact of chronicity on the family relationship has most often been viewed as a dyadic relationship (client/family and physician/client) or a therapeutic triangle (client, family members, and the health care team). Rolland (1988) has extended this to a therapeutic quadrangle with the inclusion of psychosocial illness types as the fourth member of four interlocking triangles. With this conceptualization, the original therapeutic triangle (client, family, health team) can be analyzed from the perspective of the "personality" associated with different illness types (onset, course, outcome, degree of incapacitation, and predictability) and the developmental life course of a disease (phases of chronicity, e.g., crisis, chronic, and terminal). For example, the demands on the family of a client with a rapidly progressive disease such as cancer of the lung are much different from the demands of a slowly progressive illness such as chronic obstructive pulmonary disease. The former requires continual adaptive changes and ever-new demands, whereas the latter places a higher premium on stamina over a long period of time. The therapeutic quadrangle provides a framework for assessment and clinical intervention in a family facing chronicity. The strengths and weaknesses of various components of family functioning can be analyzed in relation to the life cycle of the chronic condition.

**Impact on the spouse.** Most chronic conditions create the necessity for role changes and adjustments in the marital relationship (Sutkin, 1984). A young spouse may not have the capacity to accept the additional responsibilities that a partner's chronic condition requires. Because of the limitations of a disabled partner, the opportunity to share experiences is significantly affected, resulting in a less balanced relationship.

Spousal relations during the middle years are particularly affected because the chronic condition strikes during the most productive period in a person's life. Wives may find themselves assuming increased responsibilities as the breadwinner in addition to their usual child-rearing responsibilities. This is at a time when demands related to parent-caring may also be substantially increased. Such a woman has been described as in the "sandwich generation" because of family responsibilities for her own children as well as for parents. The conflict between assuming the dual role of marital partner and caregiver can place substantial stress on marital relationships, particularly on the intimacy related to sexual relations. Loneliness and isolation have been reported as sequelae in both the disabled and the able-bodied spouse.

Chronic conditions in the older adult can potentially disrupt their shared life if the able-bodied spouse is unable to meet the additional demands brought about by chronic illness or disability. Frequently it is the onset of a physical disability or cognitive impairment that causes the greatest disruption. Placement into a nursing home may be the only alternative.

**Impact on siblings.** Siblings of children with chronic conditions are affected by chronicity. Initially, siblings experience high levels of anxiety and feelings of vulnerability to chronic illness. Siemon (1984) identified two aspects that influence sibling responses: (1) the consequence of the chronic condition and (2) the nature of a sibling's relationship. Limited emotional and financial resources may be taxed by the demands of one chronically ill child. Families must continually struggle with balancing the needs of one with the good for all. Siblings must learn to adjust and adapt to the consequences and compromises these decisions entail.

Having a sibling with special needs results in ambivalence and emotional struggles. Within the family structure each child strives to be special, while outside the family children strive to be just like other children. Having a sibling with a chronic condition can result in fears of rejection and stigmatization. Sibling responses can also be affected by the inequality of the relationship. The dependency disabled children have on their parents prevents the normal play and secrets that siblings share. Role relationships are altered when a chronically ill older child assumes the role of the youngest. Older siblings may have to assume additional responsibilities, including caregiving, and younger siblings must subordinate their needs to those of the chronically ill child. Feelings of jealousy, anger, guilt, and resentment, which can contribute to long-term personality defects, may surface.

**Impact on children.** Children of chronically ill and disabled parents can be vulnerable to stress, especially during the period immediately after the onset of a condition. Hospitalization of the ill parent and concerns of the healthy parent about his or her spouse may deprive younger children of the closeness and support that they need. Parents may contribute to the stress by withholding information from younger children to "protect them." Although older children have a better understanding of the situation, they also experience anxiety about the short- and long-term effects of the illness. Older children who are about to leave home may experience conflict between their desire for freedom and autonomy and additional responsibilities they must assume in the home. Parents should be encouraged to explain to children what is happening and should include them in decision making at a level appropriate for their age. Parental disability, however, was found not to affect children adversely in a sample of children whose fathers became paralyzed as a result of spinal cord trauma (Buck & Hohmann, 1981).

**Impact on caregivers.** Caregiving encompasses two roles: the provision of actual physical care and the management of care. It is essential that primary caregivers develop management and communication skills to organize daily activities and obtain services through the health care system. Nurses and other health professionals can assist the caregiver in negotiating the maze of health care services and organizing the daily caregiving tasks. Even relatively modest suggestions to decrease the dependency needs of the care recipient can substantially reduce the caregiver's work.

Although research has shown that the caregiver role can be both burdensome and satisfying, all too often the effects of chronic health problems are overwhelming. Emotional, physical, and financial strain have been documented as long-term effects of caregiving. Emotional strain can be manifested as feelings of isolation, anxiety, guilt, resentment, and frustration. Guilt results from the anger and resentment that may occur when the caregiving role interferes with usual activities. Long-standing physical and emotional strain can result in physical illness in the caregiver. Four variables appear especially important in determining the impact of caregiving: the client's level of disability and dependence; the caregiver's health and functional mobility; the presence or absence of other informal supports; and the caregiver's other roles and responsibilities.

### ❖ COPING SKILLS

Responses of individuals to the demands may vary within and between various chronic conditions, resulting in different patterns of coping. Cognitive appraisal of the event determines to a great extent the nature and degree of coping behaviors used by the individual to maintain a state of equilibrium. Coping behaviors are also influenced by antecedent variables: background and personality, illness-related events, and social environmental factors.

Cohen and Lazarus (1979) have identified five main coping strategies that may be used to change the stressful situation for the better or to manage the physiological and psychological outcomes of stress-related emotions so that they do not overwhelm the person. These strategies are information seeking, direct action, inhibition of action, intrapsychic processes, and turning to others.

**Information seeking.** Nurses must be aware of information-seeking behaviors by clients and families and the type of information sought. Generally, when teaching is directed toward areas clients view as problematic, client education is more effective (Burckhardt, 1987).

**Direct action.** Direct action is any behavior that the client does to handle a stressful situation. Such action may be viewed as positive by health professionals (adherence to treatment regimen) or detrimental (noncompliance to treatment regimen). The client, however, views both types of action as beneficial. The nurse can help the client evaluate the impact of direct action behaviors on outcomes.

**Inhibition of action.** Inhibition of action relates to avoiding those behaviors that have potential harm. A housewife with multiple sclerosis may have to relinquish certain household tasks because of physical limitations and potential injury. The inhibition of an action, however, is not always beneficial to the client, for relinquishing certain household tasks may reduce the risk for injury or excess fatigue but may be detrimental to the client's self-esteem. The nurse should assess the meaning of relinquishing an action on client outcomes. Perhaps an alternative approach would allow the client to continue doing a particular task.

**Intrapsychic processes.** Intrapsychic processes are those cognitive processes people use to regulate their emotions. They include the various defense mechanisms such as denial, cognitive strategies such as relaxation techniques, and the meaning given to the situation. Intrapsychic processes become maladaptive when they adversely affect the treatment regimen or outcomes. The nurse must evaluate the overall short- and long-term benefits of the intrapsychic

process used by the client. Use of other modes to increase the client's sense of control (relaxation techniques, biofeedback, self-management of pain medication) can be suggested to reduce emotional stress.

**Turning to others.** The support of others is necessary to cope with the long-term effects of chronicity. Support can be formal (health care professionals and agencies) or informal (family and friends). Generally, both formal and informal supports are available during the acute and rehabilitative phases of a chronic condition; however, changes in available supports may occur with the passage of time. Where informal support networks are inadequate or nonexistent, accessing the formal health care network may be necessary. Nurses must continually evaluate the amount, type, and adequacy of supports desired and needed by the client.

## ❖ OUTCOMES AND ADJUSTMENT TO CHRONICITY

Whenever stressful events such as the diagnosis or exacerbation of a chronic condition occur, some degree of disequilibrium results, with the potential for a crisis. The additional demands of chronicity also place the client in an ongoing state of potential threat or stress. Aguilera (Aguilera & Messick, 1989) sees three balancing factors that influence the state of equilibrium between the onset of a perceived stressful situation and the resolution of the problem. These three factors, similar to those of Moos and Tsu (1977), are the perception of the event, available situational supports, and coping mechanisms. Strengths or weaknesses in any one of these factors can determine the presence or absence of crisis.

Studies of individual responses to chronic illness or disability have identified anticipated behavior patterns. Shontz (1975) identified a series of stages through which people proceed as they deal with physical illness or disability:

shock, encounter, retreat, and reality testing. These stages imply that adaptation occurs sequentially in a series of steps. Adjustment in chronicity, however, is not a single event but a series of repeated encounters. For example, the remissions and exacerbations of multiple sclerosis and the complications secondary to the chronic condition require repeated adjustments. In reality, then, the adjustment process involves continual shifting back and forth between encounter or struggle and retreat or denial.

Total disruption of life can often be endured if the illness is short and the aftereffects negligible. Pervasiveness, the extent an illness or disability disrupts the total life of the individual, and permanence of the condition are critical variables. Success or failure in dealing effectively with situational crises related to chronicity determines whether the person has successfully adjusted to the presence of a chronic condition.

## ❖ APPLICATION OF NURSING PROCESS IN CHRONICITY

Chronicity imposes a lifelong process of adjustment on the person. It requires nurses who are sensitive and have the expertise to deal with the physical-psychosocial-cultural values of the individual conducive to attaining or maintaining his or her optimal functional level. Emphasis must be placed on illness prevention, health promotion, and health maintenance rather than the disease orientation of the acute care model.

### Self-Care and Chronicity

Strauss (1975) and Wright (1983) view the client as manager or co-manager of his or her chronic condition and associated regimens. In either case the emphasis is placed on self-care. The vast majority of the time the client resides in the home and is the primary person responsible for directing or managing care. A self-care approach includes not only activities to cope

❖ **Table 21-2**
Model of self-care in chronic illness

| Predisposing factors | Enabling factors |
|---|---|
| Self-concept | Client characteristics |
| Health motivations | Psychological status |
| Perceptions | Regimen characteristics |
| Seriousness | Cues to action |
| Vulnerability | Social support |
| Efficacy | System characteristics |

Self-care behaviors

From "Self-care and the Chronically Ill Patient" by C. E. Connelly, 1987, *Nurs Clin North Am, 22,* p. 21. Reprinted with permission.

with the chronic condition but also encompasses a broad range of health-related behaviors.

The client's active participation in care and decision making is a key essential to effective self-care (Connelly, 1987). In this approach the nurse assumes the role of facilitator of care by the client rather than the actual provider of care. The goals of nursing are to stimulate and enhance effective self-care; to reduce barriers to self-care; and to reinforce and support self-care behaviors. Connelly identified a model of self-care in chronic illness (Table 21-2), which includes predisposing factors and enabling factors. Predisposing factors to engaging in self-care behaviors include self-concept, health motivation, and the client's perception of the seriousness of the condition, his or her vulnerability to complications, and the efficacy of the treatment regimen. Enabling factors include client characteristics, psychological status, regimen characteristics, cues to action, social support, and system characteristics. This model has been suggested as a guide to nurses in assessing the client's potential for self-care behaviors.

**Health care resources.** Access to formal and informal health care resources is necessary to enable the client to participate in self-care behaviors. Advances in health care technology have resulted in persons with chronic conditions living longer and requiring more support services to maintain their independence. However, the health care delivery system is still primarily organized to meet the demands of acute illness rather than chronicity. Government-sponsored insurance and private insurance often fail to provide follow-up services, including home care support. Health care for long-term care remains meagerly funded and fragmented. Available resources are often limited and difficult to access through the maze of agencies. The nurse must be knowledgeable about the availability of and means to access the needed resources.

*Chronic care providers.* The complexity of the problems associated with chronicity require the efforts of health care personnel from a wide range of disciplines. They include nurses, physicians, physical therapists, psychologists, speech pathologists, social workers, and vocational rehabilitation counselors. However, health care providers are often task oriented and sometimes have difficulty in working together. Even in well-defined teams such as are seen in rehabilitation settings, the individual members tend to focus on their own areas of practice. Such a myopic view is the difference between a multidisciplinary approach and that of an interdisciplinary team. A true interdisciplinary team approach involves not only discipline-oriented activities but also reflects a team commitment to resolving the health care problems.

Probably the key member of the team is the client as an active participant or co-manager. Despite the general acceptance of the active participation on the part of the client, Wright (1983) identifies several impediments to implementation in practice. The helping relationship tends to reinforce the attitude that the health care expert has the answers and hinders the active participation of the client. Other impediments include the preference of the health professional for an authoritarian relationship and the time and energy frequently required to involve the client in a co-manager role.

*Chronic care settings.* The continuum of care is reflected in the settings providing care to the chronically ill and disabled. Although home care is the most prominent setting, families must frequently seek formal health support services.

The *acute care hospital* is most likely the setting for the diagnostic workup, diagnosis, and treatment of the initial phase of the chronic condition and during periods of exacerbation of symptoms. However, conditions such as arthritis are frequently diagnosed and treated in physicians' offices and clinics without acute hospitalization.

The *rehabilitation setting* provides comprehensive services, primarily to the physically disabled for the purpose of restoring them to their fullest physical, mental, social, and vocational potential possible. The chronically ill have been less a focus for rehabilitation services; however, in recent years pulmonary, cardiac, and alcohol rehabilitation programs have become more prevalent. Certainly many individuals, both young and old, with impairments resulting from chronic disease, could benefit from these services.

A variety of facilities provide long-term institutional care. The *skilled nursing facility* provides 24-hour service to individuals requiring the specialized training of a registered nurse, physical therapist, occupational therapist, or speech therapist. The *intermediate care facility* provides 24-hour service to individuals requiring considerable nursing care. The health needs of the residents tend to be chronic, often requiring both assistance and supervision. A *care home* is a licensed facility that provides 24-hour care to individuals requiring assistance or supervision of activities in daily living. Residents are usually ambulatory or semi-ambulatory. Generally these facilities primarily serve the elderly population.

Several types of providers of care support the family in providing home care. *Home health care* provides multidisciplinary services to the client in the home. Supportive services may include the skills of registered nurses and home health aides under the supervision of a community health nurse, personal care and homemaking, chore services, and transportation.

*Adult day care, respite care,* and *hospice care* are additional services available to the chronically ill and disabled. Adult day-care centers provide a variety of health, social, and related support services in a noninstitutionalized ambulatory care program. The majority of adult day-care centers offer unstructured programs aimed primarily at recreation and socialization. Some day-care centers offer a program of intensive rehabilitation. Respite care is any service that provides intervals of rest and relief for the family and caregiver. These services can range from several hours to several weeks and can occur either in the home or an institution. Hospice care, although not uniformly available, provides nursing care and support services to the client and his or her family during the terminal phase of a chronic illness.

### Public policy, legislation, and funding.

Program development and funding allocation decisions that affect the chronically ill and disabled reflect the values of society through the political process. Brody (1986) identifies the attitudes toward the disabled and elderly on which public policy is based: (1) the physically sick role has been assigned to the disabled and elderly; (2) health needs of the disabled and elderly require a high-tech medical response; (3) disability relates to medical diagnostic categories; (4) independence is good and dependency bad; (5) disability is a personal limitation; and (6) the disabled and elderly are a disadvantaged minority. The result of these attitudes has been substantial federal support that provides access to rehabilitation and skilled nursing care through medical insurance for acute care but provides much less support for home health care.

Financial assistance and services for long-term care are often fragmented, inadequate, and difficult to access. Three main categories of services are provided: income maintenance, medical insurance, and social programs, including housing, education, and transportation.

Income maintenance is provided through *Social Security Disability Insurance* (SSDI) and *Supplemental Security Income* (SSI) (Social Security Administration, 1988). SSDI eligibility requirements are narrowly defined as tied to the individual's capacity to work and his or her expected duration of employment. Inclusion criteria are a history of gainful employment and a physical or mental impairment expected to last 12 months or end in death. Benefits are available to disabled workers before age 65, to widows and widowers who are disabled and caring for dependent children, to dependent children under the age of 22, or to disabled individuals under age 22. SSI provides monthly income support to the needy aged (age 65 and over), the blind, and the disabled with income and assets below federal standards. SSI also often qualifies recipients for Medicaid, food stamps, rehabilitation, and home care programs.

Medical insurance programs include Medicare and Medicaid, which were enacted in 1965 as amendments to the Social Security Act (Social Security Administration, 1988). *Medicare Part A* provides reimbursement for acute care hospitalization for persons age 65 and over. Skilled nursing facilities are also covered for a limited number of days, but only after acute hospitalization. Long-term supportive care for the elderly is not included under the coverage. *Medicare Part B* is a voluntary medical insurance supplement for those individuals who pay a specified monthly premium. Part B covers "reasonable" charges for outpatient services, including home health services, physical and speech therapy, physician services, medical supplies, diagnostic tests, and use of an ambulance. *Medicaid,* legislated under Title XIX of the Social Security Act, provides medical care to the eligible poor and indigent. Medicaid is both state and federally funded, so the amount and kind of coverage varies by state.

Social service needs of the chronically ill and disabled are addressed through a variety of federal, state, and community programs. *Title XX,* as part of the 1974 Social Security Act, is operated by both state and federal levels. Eligibility is determined by financial need. Services provided include use of a homemaker, health aide, day care, home-delivered or congregate meals, use of senior activity centers, legal aid, and transportation. The *Older Americans Act* of 1965 is specifically targeted to individuals over age 60. Covered services include social services, nutrition services, senior center facilities, training, research, and demonstration activities.

Information about agencies may be obtained through local health care agencies and institutions. The local telephone directory can be useful in identifying specific agencies such as the local chapter of the Multiple Sclerosis Society, the Muscular Dystrophy Association, American Heart Association, and Department of Vocational Rehabilitation and support groups such as Reach for Recovery and ones for clients who have had a stroke or for families of clients who have Alzheimer's disease. Access Living, a national organization with local offices throughout the country, acts as an advocacy group for the disabled. The local library often serves as a repository of information on agencies and resources. The *Encyclopedia of Associations,* available in most libraries, provides information on various agencies for the chronically ill and disabled. At the national level the *National Health Information Clearing House* in Washington, D.C., assists consumers and health pro-

fessionals to locate resources. The various local Area Agencies on Aging act as information centers about services and programs for the elderly.

## Chronicity and Nursing Research

Considerable research has been generated by nurses investigating chronic health conditions and associated problems. The majority of the research has been related to specific chronic illnesses, client education strategies, and phenomena associated with the adaptation to chronicity. Fewer studies have focused on health promotion directed toward the prevention of chronic health problems.

Pollock (1987) analyzed the contribution of nursing research to understanding responses to chronic illness. A total of 54 articles were published in *Nursing Research, Research in Nursing and Health, Western Journal of Nursing Research,* and *Advances in Nursing Science* between 1980 to 1986. She concluded that intervention studies that involved the client in his or her program of care positively affected the client's compliance and health status. More than 25 of the studies related to a variety of phenomena concerned with adaptation to chronicity, including control, hope, life satisfaction, compliance, anxiety and depression, and family adjustment. These studies can provide direction for planning nursing care by directing assessment toward physiological, psychological, and sociological factors that enhance development of the phenomena. Nursing interventions can then be designed to alleviate or take into account the cause of the problem.

Client education is accepted by nurses as an established component of self-care management in chronicity. However, several reviews of the research literature have shown that client education alone is not sufficient to improve compliance and the trajectory of chronicity. Mazzuca (1982) reviewed 30 articles about controlled experiments of client education in chronic disease. Although he found that client education was the most successful in altering compliance, behaviorally oriented programs that paid special attention to changing the environment in which clients cared for themselves were more successful in improving the course of the disease. Pollock (1987), Hogue (1979), and Haynes (1976) all concluded that behaviorally oriented approaches that took into account the client's particular regimen and circumstances were superior to providing information alone. Characteristics of chronicity include long duration, complexity, and high degree of behavioral change; all of these factors have been associated with noncompliance as well. In chronicity, education programs designed to help the client adapt to his or her unique self-care plan are much more likely to improve compliance and the course of the disease.

The above studies indicate the importance of incorporating research findings into clinical practice. Information about research can be found in the previously cited nursing research journals and in many clinically oriented nursing journals. Findings from other disciplines such as medicine, physical therapy, and psychology can often be applied in nursing practice.

## Chronicity and Selected Nursing Diagnoses

Previous sections of this chapter have indicated the complex nature of chronicity, which results in varied and multiple health care problems. One study identified 50 valid nursing diagnoses in a chronically ill population (Hoskins et al, 1986). The nursing diagnoses selected for discussion address patterns of health management, self-perception, and role relationships, diagnoses frequently identified in chronicity.

**Altered health maintenance.** "Altered health maintenance is the inability to identify, manage, and/or seek out help to maintain health" (McFarland & McFarlane, 1989, p. 29). This diagnosis is identified most often in the community setting and can be related to predisposing risk factors of chronicity and to the consequence of chronicity. Factors contributing to the diagnosis include ineffective coping, inadequate resources, changing support system, lack of access to health care services, and inappropriate health practice behaviors such as smoking and alcohol or drug abuse. The nurse must first identify the factor contributing to the diagnosis before appropriate interventions can be identified and implemented.

CASE STUDY: Mary and Frank Martin are an elderly couple living independently in their own home. Their only family members reside in a city several hundred miles away and visit infrequently. They live on a fixed income primarily derived from Social Security Income benefits. Mary recently was discharged from a skilled care nursing home following recovery from a fractured hip. Frank visited daily and often ate lunch with Mary.

On discharge a referral was made to the local home health care agency to evaluate the home situation and provide follow-up care. The nurse's priority during the first visit was to determine whether Mary and Frank were managing their health care in the home. Initial assessment determined poor nutritional intake related to difficulty in obtaining food and in the preparation of food. Both voiced concerns that they will not be able to manage in their home much longer. Mary still required some assistance in dressing and moving about. Frank, who is approaching 90 years of age, was barely able to manage his own care. A nursing diagnosis of "Altered Health Maintenance related to lack of adequate resources and support system" was made by the home health care nurse.

Nursing intervention must be directed toward maintaining Mary and Frank in their home through mobilizing formal and informal support networks. Formal support services might include mobile meal delivery to the home, use of a home health aide to assist with daily hygiene, and provision of lifeline services for emergency help. The nurse should explore with Mary and Frank possible informal support networks (friends and neighbors, churches, local organizations) that might provide shopping services, take out the garbage, or provide free loaner equipment such as canes, walkers, and wheelchairs. A sample nursing care plan follows that provides for Mary's immediate health care needs in the home.

**Noncompliance.** "Noncompliance (specify) is the state in which an individual who has expressed the desire and intent to adhere to a therapeutic recommendation does not adhere to the recommendation" (McFarland & McFarlane, 1989, p. 37). Noncompliance has been frequently reported in chronicity when adherence to lifetime regimens is necessary. Determination of the factors contributing to noncompliant behavior is essential. Assessment should include personal factors (e.g., values and beliefs about health, motivation, cultural beliefs, developmental level), interpersonal factors (adequacy and nature of supportive relationships), and environmental factors (nontherapeutic environment to carry out regimen).

CASE STUDY: Tom is 15 years old and beginning his first year of high school. He was diagnosed with juvenile diabetes mellitus at the age of 11. During the past 4 years he has managed his diet, insulin injections, and activity levels without difficulty. Blood sugar levels have remained at acceptable levels. However, recently he has become noncompliant with his diabetic regimen. Two days ago he was admitted to the hospital in a diabetic coma. On questioning, Tom admits that he has not followed his diet and insulin regimen.

Further assessment reveals that Tom has recently moved. He voices fears that his peers at the new school will not accept him if they know of his diabetic condition. He admits he has been eating the wrong foods to be just "one of the guys." He also indicates that he eats lunch at the school cafeteria, which often serves foods that are not on his diet. Tom also voices fears that he might not be able to participate fully in sports. He had been actively involved in football and baseball at his previous school. A nursing diagnosis of "Noncompliance related to fear of being rejected by peers and nontherapeutic environment at school" is made.

Interventions must be directed toward helping Tom allay his fears and adjust to the new environment. The nurse must explore with Tom, his parents, and the school nurse solutions that are acceptable to Tom. The nurse might also discuss strategies with Tom on how to manage questions from his "friends" about his condition. Tom and his parents should be encouraged to talk with the coach about his participation in sports. By directing the solutions to the causes of noncompliant behavior, the nursing diagnosis is often resolved.

**Powerlessness.** "Powerlessness is the perceived lack of control over a current situation, immediate happening, or future outcome" (McFarland & McFarlane, 1989, p. 621). Powerlessness is often seen in chronicity when a person does not perceive he or she has control or can affect an outcome or decision. Assessment must identify the source of actual or perceived powerlessness. Possible indicators include expressions or behaviors indicating diminished or lack of control or influence over situations, outcomes, self-care, physical condition, or passivity (Miller, 1983).

CASE STUDY: Mike, 20 years old and married within the past year, suffered a $C_6$ spinal cord injury in a car accident. He had not been wearing a seatbelt. After 3 months of intensive rehabilitation therapy, Tom's discharge date has been set for 2 weeks. Throughout his hospitalization Mike has insisted he would "walk out." He is knowledgeable about his care but recently has been "forgetting" to follow the position change or self-catheterization schedule. He recently said to his nurse, "I guess Jane and I will be living with my parents now. They are going to remodel the

# NURSING CARE PLAN

**CLIENT:** Mary M

**MEDICAL DIAGNOSIS:** Fractured hip

**NURSING DIAGNOSIS:** Altered health maintenance: related to lack of adequate resources

Impaired physical mobility: related to fractured hip, age, and decreased strength and endurance

Self-care deficit: dressing and bathing related to musculoskeletal impairment

| GOALS | NURSING INTERVENTIONS |
|---|---|
| Mary will obtain the necessary resources to meet health needs in the home. | ◆ Discuss and facilitate obtaining formal health care services (e.g., meals-on-wheels and a home health aide). <br> ◆ Assist Mary to identify and arrange for informal supports (e.g., friends, neighbors, relatives to run errands, go to the doctor, etc.). |
| Mary will walk independently with a walker in the home. | ◆ Teach Mary exercises to increase strength of her arms and legs. <br> ◆ Teach Mary proper positioning and range-of-motion exercises to prevent contractures. <br> ◆ Instruct Mary to ambulate with her walker at least three times a day with informal caregiver's or health aide's assistance. <br> ◆ Make referral to physical therapist. |
| Mary will require minimal assistance in dressing and bathing. | ◆ Obtain necessary equipment to facilitate independence in dressing and bathing—grab bars and tub seat, elevated toilet seat and arm supports, and arm extender for dressing. <br> ◆ Teach Mary and Frank techniques to increase Mary's independence in dressing and bathing. <br> ◆ Obtain home health aide and/or friends and family to help with dressing and bathing until Mary is independent or requires minimal assistance. |

## EVALUATION

Mary identifies and mobilizes family and community resources to meet current home health needs. She reports increasing levels of independence in ambulating with a walker as a result of a regular exercise program and in-home physical therapy. On a long-term basis, Mary reports a decreased level of assistance needed in bathing and dressing as her physical mobility improves.

basement so we can have our own place. I guess that's best. I don't know what I'm going to do about school. My parents don't think I should go back to college. I suppose this is best. It will take some pressure off of Jane."

Chronicity results in major life-style changes. The client may feel decisions are being made that are outside of his or her control. As a result of his injury, Mike's future plans and goals may seem impossible. Assessment reveals that Mike feels he has no control over decisions that are being made by his family regarding discharge. He is afraid he will not be able to continue his college education and career goal in design and drawing. A nursing diagnosis of "Powerlessness related to changes in health status" is made. The nurse arranges for a family conference to include Mike, his wife, and his parents. A referral is also made to the Vocational Rehabilitation Department to address Mike's concerns about college and career. If Mike is agreeable, arranging for a peer counselor with a similar disability and life-style might be of help. These measures will allow Mike more control over decisions affecting his postdischarge plans.

**Altered role performance.** "Altered role performance is an actual or perceived disparity seen by self or others in meeting role obligations or expectations" (McFarland & McFarlane, 1989, p. 693). Changes in health status associated with chronicity are likely to affect roles. Assessment of altered role performance should focus on identifying alterations resulting from the assumption of new roles, conflict or incompatibility between roles, ineffectiveness in performing role functions, or not experiencing satisfaction with one's role.

CASE STUDY: Ron was in his mid-forties when he developed end-stage renal disease and has been on biweekly hemodialysis for the past 3 months. Up to the time of his illness he had successfully managed a small appliance store. He and his wife, Barbara, have three children 10 to 17 years of age. She teaches in the local high school. For the past several months Barbara has found it necessary to be absent from school several days to take Ron for his treatments or to oversee activities at the store. The principal of the school has been understanding but recently voiced concern about her increasing number of absences. Although both Ron and Barbara indicate they have a close relationship, arguments have been more frequent since Ron's illness.

Chronicity often makes additional demands on family members that can place a strain on family relationships. Ron is likely experiencing feelings of role failure. Increasing demands of his illness prevent his maintaining previously successful roles as husband, father, and provider. Barbara's frustration is a result of not being able to meet the additional demands resulting from Ron's illness. A nursing diagnosis of "Altered Role Performance related to changed expectations" is made. The nurse arranges for a time to meet with Ron and Barbara to discuss and clarify their feelings and expectations. Verbalization of feelings can lead to a sharing and mutual understanding of the conflict between perceived role expectations and role performance. Open communication between Ron and Barbara will help them to set realistic goals and expectations. Identifying and exploring each task associated with various roles can lead to solutions and resolution of role conflict and strain.

### ❖ SUMMARY

Chronicity has become the number one health problem. With the advances in health technology, individuals are surviving longer with chronic conditions than ever before. However, chronicity has generated less interest and involvement by nurses than has the acute phase of illness. Yet this is an area in which nurses, by the nature of their emphasis on caring and advocacy, can have a significant impact. The complexity of chronicity requires the knowledge, experience, and care of a professional nurse. Opportunities in areas of prevention of chronicity and its management are going to increase over the next decades.

Chronicity offers a challenge, not only to all health care workers but also to society in general. Finding alternative and creative means of meeting the health care needs of the chronically ill, including funding, will allow them to assume a more productive and satisfying role in society. Providing opportunities for the disabled to pursue employment, recreation, and education goals within the limitations of his or her condition benefits not only the individual but also society in general. Nurses can work toward increasing the public's awareness of the needs of the chronically ill and disabled.

### ❖ APPLYING KNOWLEDGE TO PRACTICE

Select two clients you have taken care of recently, one with an acute illness and one with a chronic illness or disability. Discuss the following questions in relation to the two clients you have identified:

1. Compare the trajectory of the conditions of the two clients. What factors influence the trajectory of the illness? How does the trajectory of the illness influence the nurse's involvement and approach to client care?

2. How does the type of illness (acute or chronic) affect the individual's adaptation? What coping strategies are used by each client? Are the coping strategies similar or different? Would your approach to facilitate coping for the client with a chronic condition be different? If so, how?

3. Consider the developmental stage of the client. Does the developmental stage affect the client's reaction to chronic illness differently from that to acute illness? How does it affect client/ family relationships? Nurse/client relationships? Nurse/family relationships?

4. What do you need to consider in preparing the two clients for discharge? How does discharge planning differ for the client with a chronic condition? Consider the concepts of powerlessness, compliance, and client education. What resources are available in the client's community to provide support after discharge (e.g., funding, health care, emotional assistance)?

## REFERENCES

Aguilera, D. C., & Messick, J. M. (1989). *Crisis intervention theory and methodology* (4th. ed.). St. Louis: C.V. Mosby.

Blumberg, B. D., Lewis, J., & Susman, E. J. (1984). Adolescence: A time of transition. In M. G. Eisenberg, L. C. Sutkin, & M. S. Jansen (Eds.), *Chronic illness and disability through the life span* (pp. 133–149). New York: Springer.

Brody, S. J. (1986). Impact of the formal support system on rehabilitation of the elderly. In S. J. Brody & G. E. Ruff (Eds.), *Aging and rehabilitation* (pp. 62–88). New York: Springer.

Buck, F. M., & Hohmann, G. W. (1981). Personality, behavior, values and family relations of children of fathers with spinal cord injury. *Archives of Physical Medicine and Rehabilitation, 62,* 432–438.

Burckhardt, C. S. (1987). Coping strategies of the chronically ill. *Nursing Clinics of North America, 22,* 543–550.

Cluff, L. (1981). Chronic disease, function and the quality of care, editorial. *Journal of Chronic Diseases, 34,* 299–304.

Cohen, F., & Lazarus, R. S. (1979). Coping with the stresses of illness. In G. C. Stone, F. Cohen, & N. E. Adler (Eds). *Health psychology: A handbook.* San Francisco: Jossey-Bass.

Connelly, C. E. (1987). Self-care and the chronically ill patient. *Nursing Clinics of North America, 22,* 621–629.

Corbin, J. M., & Strauss, A. (1988). Unending work and care. San Francisco: Jossey-Bass.

Dunn, M. (1977). Social discomfort in the patient with spinal cord injury. *Archives of Physical Medicine and Rehabilitation, 58,* 257–260.

Erikson, E. H. (1963). *Childhood and society* (2nd ed.). New York: Norton.

Feldman, D. (1974). Chronic disabling illness: A holistic view. *Journal of Chronic Diseases, 27,* 287–291.

Field, T. (1979). Interaction patterns of preterm and term infants. In T. Field, A. Sostek, S. Goldberg, & H. Shuman (Eds.), *Infants born at risk,* Jamaica, N.Y.: Spectrum.

Given, B. A., & Given, C. W. (1984). Creating a climate for compliance. *Cancer Nursing, 7,* 139–147.

Glueckauf, R. L., & Quittner, A. L. (1984). Facing physical disability as a young adult: Psychological issues and approaches. In S. J. Brody & G. E. Ruff (Eds.), *Aging and rehabilitation* (pp. 167–183). New York: Springer.

Goffman, E. (1963). *Stigma: Notes on management of spoiled identity.* Englewood Cliffs, N.J.: Prentice-Hall.

Granger, C. V. (1986). Goals of rehabilitation of the disabled elderly. In S. J. Brody & G. E. Ruff (Eds.), *Aging and rehabilitation* (pp. 27–35). New York: Springer.

Haynes, R. B. (1976). Strategies for improving compliance. In D. L. Sackett & R. B. Haynes (Eds.) *Compliance with therapeutic regimens* (pp. 69–82). Baltimore: John Hopkins University Press.

Hogue, C. C. (1979). Nursing and compliance. In R. B. Haynes, D. W. Taylor, & D. L. Sackett (Eds.). *Compliance in health care* (pp. 247–259). Baltimore: John Hopkins University Press.

Hoskins, L. M., McFarlane, E. A., Rubenfeld, M. G., Walsh, M. B., & Schreier, A. M. (1986). Nursing diagnosis in the chronically ill: Methodology for clinical validation. *Advances in Nursing Science, 8,* 80–89.

Kemp, B. (1986). Psychosocial and mental health issues in rehabilitation of older persons. In S. J. Brody & G. E. Ruff (Eds.), *Aging and rehabilitation* (pp. 122–158). New York: Springer.

Lubkin, I. M. (1986). *Chronic illness: Impact and interventions.* Boston: Jones & Bartlett.

Mazzuca, S. (1982). Does patient education in chronic disease have therapeutic value? *Journal of Chronic Diseases, 35,* 521–529.

Miller, J. F. (1983). *Coping with chronic illness: Overcoming powerlessness.* Philadelphia: F. A. Davis.

McFarland, G. K., & McFarlane, E. A. (1989). *Nursing diagnosis & intervention.* St. Louis: C.V. Mosby.

Moos, R. H., & Tsu, V. D. (1977). The crisis of physical illness: An overview. In R. H. Moos (Ed.), *Coping with physical illness* (pp. 3–21). New York: Plenum Medical.

Murray, R. L. E. (1972). Body image development in adulthood. *Nursing Clinics of North America, 7,* 617–630.

National Center for Health Statistics estimates from the National Health Interview Survey U.S., 1982. (1985). *Vital and health statistics* (Series 10, DHHS Publication No. PHS 85-1578). Washington, DC: U.S. Government Printing Office.

Norris, C. M. (1978). Body image: Its relevance to professional nursing. In C. Carison & B. Blackwell (Eds.), *Behavioral concepts and nursing intervention* (pp. 5–36). New York: Lippincott.

Parsons, T. (1951). *Social system.* Glencoe, Ill.: Free Press.

Pfister-Minogue, K. (1983). Enabling strategies. In J. M. Miller, (ed.). *Coping with chronic illness* (235–256). Philadelphia: F. A. Davis.

Piaget, J. (1973). *The child and reality* (R. Rosin, Trans.). New York: Grossman.

Pollock, S. E. (1987). Adaptation to chronic illness. Analysis of nursing research. *Nursing Clinics of North America, 22,* 631–644.

Quigley, P., & Giovinco, G. (1988). Nurses' use of the terms compliance and non-compliance in rehabilitation nursing practice. *Rehabilitation Nursing, 13,* 90–91.

Roberts, D. (1954). The over-all picture of long-term illness. *Journal of Chronic Diseases, 8,* 149–159.

Rolland, J. S. (1988). A conceptual model of chronic and life-threatening illness and its impact on families. In C. S. Chilman, R. W. Nunnally, & F. M. Cox (Eds.), *Chronic illness and disability: Vol. 2. Families in trouble series.* Newbury Park: Sage.

Rustad, L. C. (1984). Family adjustment to chronic illness and disability in mid-life. In M. G. Eisenberg, L. C. Sutkin, & M. S. Jansen (Eds.), *Chronic illness and disability through the life span* (pp. 222–242). New York: Springer.

Shontz, F. C. (1975). *The psychological aspects of physical illness and disability.* New York: Macmillan.

Siemon, M. (1984). Siblings of the chronically ill or disabled child. *Nursing Clinics of North America, 19,* 295–307.

Social Security Administration (1988). *Social security handbook 1988* (10th ed.). (SSA Publication No. 05-10135). Washington, DC: U.S. Government Printing Office.

Stapleton, S. (1983a). Recognizing powerlessness: Causes and indicators in patients with chronic renal failure. In J. M. Miller (Ed.), *Coping with chronic illness* (pp. 135–148). Philadelphia: F. A. Davis.

Stapleton, S. (1983b). Decreasing powerlessness in the chronically ill: A prototype. In J. M. Miller (Ed.), *Coping with chronic illness* (pp. 257–274). Philadelphia: F. A. Davis.

Strauss, A. L. (1975). *Chronic illness and the quality of life.* St. Louis: C.V. Mosby.

Strauss, A., Fagerhaugh, S., Suczek, B., & Wiener, C. (1982). The work of hospitalized patients. *Social Science and Medicine, 16,* 977–986.

Sutkin, L. C. (1984). Introduction. In M. G. Eisenberg, L. C. Sutkin, & M. S. Jansen (Eds.), *Chronic illness and disability through the life span* (pp. 1–19). New York: Springer.

Whitt, J. K. (1984). Children's adaptation to chronic illness and handicapping conditions. In M. G. Eisenberg, L. C. Sutkin, & M. S. Jansen (Eds.), *Chronic illness and disability through the life span* (pp. 69–102). New York: Springer.

Williams, T. F. (1986). The aging process: Biological and psychosocial considerations. In S. J. Brody & G. E. Ruff (Eds.) *Aging and rehabilitation* (pp. 13–18). New York: Springer.

Wright, B. A. (1983). *Physical disability—A psychosocial approach* (2nd ed.). New York: Harper & Row.

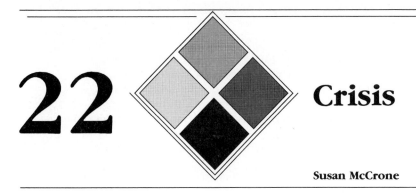

# 22  Crisis

Susan McCrone

## OBJECTIVES

*At the completion of this chapter the reader will be able to:*

◆ Describe the evolution of crisis theory.

◆ Define crisis and discuss the effect of balancing factors in a stressful event.

◆ Discuss the etiology of three types of crises.

◆ Explain crisis intervention and its application to nursing practice.

*A small trouble is like a pebble. Hold it too close to your eyes, and it fills the whole world and puts everything out of focus. Hold it at proper viewing distance, and it can be examined and properly classified. Throw it at your feet, and it can be seen in its true setting just one more tiny bump on the pathway to eternity.*

CELIA LUCE

The study of the concept of crisis involves two parts, crisis theory and crisis intervention. In the first part of this chapter the theoretical ideas surrounding the concept of crisis are reviewed. In the second part crisis intervention and its application are discussed.

Crisis is an inevitable part of human existence. Individuals are continually faced with potentially crisis-producing situations that threaten their level of functioning. The rapidity and diversity of change and the stress of today's society combine to test a person's ability to use problem-solving behaviors effectively to maintain equilibrium. Any stressful event can precipitate a crisis for an individual, depending on his or her perception of the event, coping skills, and available sup-

ports. Regardless of the area in which they are working, nurses are in a unique position to identify clients who are in a potential state of crisis and to intervene with clients who are experiencing a crisis.

The word crisis is derived from the Greek word *krinen,* "to decide." In Chinese two characters are used to write the word crisis; one is the character for danger, and the other is the character for opportunity. As a danger, crisis threatens to overwhelm the individual; as an opportunity, it prompts development of new coping skills. An important aspect of the crisis period is that it is a time of increased vulnerability that can produce increased growth in the individual. If, however, the crisis is not resolved

## ❖ DEFINITION OF KEY TERMS

*Crisis:* An event experienced when a person faces an obstacle to important life goals, i.e., insurmountable for a time through the use of customary methods of problem solving (Caplan, 1964); an internal disturbance that results from a stressful event or perceived threat

*Stress:* The body's arousal response to any demand, change, or perceived threat

*Maturational crisis:* Transitional or developmental periods within a person's life when his or her psychological equilibrium is upset

*Situational crisis:* A crisis that occurs when a specific external event upsets an individual's psychological equilibrium

*Adventitious crisis:* An accidental, uncommon, and unexpected crisis that may result in multiple losses and gross environmental changes

*Primary prevention:* Biological, social, or psychological intervention that promotes health and well-being or reduces the incidence of illness in a community by altering the causative factors before they have the opportunity to do harm

*Secondary prevention:* A type of prevention that seeks to reduce the prevalence of illness through interventions that provide for early detection and treatment of problems

*Tertiary prevention:* Measures designed to reduce the severity, disability, or residual impairment resulting from illness through rehabilitation

*Crisis intervention:* A short-term active mode of therapy that focuses on solving the client's immediate problem and reestablishing psychological equilibrium

Modified from Stuart and Sundeen, 1987.

successfully, the result may be poor functioning.

A crisis is a life-turning point or juncture in which customary problem-solving or decision-making methods are not adequate. Caplan (1964) believes that the essential factor influencing the occurrence of a crisis is an imbalance between the difficulty and the importance of the problem and the resources immediately available to deal with it. Definitions of the key terms associated with the concept of crisis are presented in the above box.

## ❖ THE CONCEPT OF CRISIS

In the discussion of crisis, certain areas are critical to a comprehensive overview of the concept. The concept of crisis must be placed in historical perspective. From this perspective a clearer delineation of the terminology such as phases of the crisis, the crisis sequence, and types of crisis emerge.

## Historical Perspective

Crisis theory developed as an outgrowth of psychoanalytical theory. Freud believed in the principle of causality as it related to psychic determinism. In simple terms every act of human behavior has its cause or source in the history and experience of the individual, with the crucial foundation laid in infancy and early childhood. Those theorists who developed preventive psychiatry used psychoanalytical concepts to develop crisis theory. They supported the idea that by intervening briefly during stressful periods, the therapist could help the client to resolve problems in an adaptive or positive way.

Building on the work of the psychoanalytical theory, Erik Erikson (1963) integrated biological, cultural, and deterministic theories into a developmental theory. He believed that the ego develops through a series of eight phases in an orderly and sequential manner. In this progression each stage with its concomitant physiological and social changes represents a crisis for the individual. Successful completion of one stage is dependent on the successful completion of the previous stage. Erikson believed that during a time of upheaval, or "crisis," the individual is the most vulnerable and the most open to change. Erikson's work became the basis for the development of ideas about maturational crises, situational crises, and individual adaptation to current environmental dilemmas.

Two contributions in the 1940s added to the body of knowledge about crisis theory. Military psychiatrists in World War II noted that many battle weary and emotionally upset soldiers who received help at the front lines were able to return to duty but those soldiers who did not receive immediate treatment needed admission to inpatient psychiatric facilities. This observation was further substantiated in the Korean War.

The second contribution came from the work of Eric Lindemann (1944) who studied bereavement. He studied 101 clients in crisis. Included in his sample were psychoneurotic clients who lost a relative during the course of treatment, relatives of clients who died in hospitals, bereaved disaster victims from the Coconut Grove nightclub fire, and relatives of members of the armed forces. Through his work he was able to differentiate normal grief from the symptomatology of a morbid grief reaction. Bereaved individuals experiencing normal grief showed signs of somatic distress and sensorium alterations, preoccupation with the image of the deceased, hostile reactions, guilt, and changes in patterns of activity, and they sometimes took on the characteristics of the dead person. The normal grief response was acute, with an identifiable onset. It was also time-limited and occurred through a predictable sequence of stages. Unlike the individual with normal grief reactions, the individual experiencing morbid grief reactions demonstrated either delayed or distorted reactions, including overactivity without a sense of loss, acquisition of symptoms of the last illness

of the deceased, development of a medical disease, alteration in relationships to friends and relatives, development of furious hostility, and, frequently, clinically agitated depression.

Lindemann described the role of the mental health worker as assisting the client to extricate himself or herself from the ties to the deceased and to develop new patterns of fulfilling interaction. He generalized the concepts applicable to bereavement to interventions during other stressful periods such as marriage and birth. His ideas became the precursors to the generic approach to crisis intervention. He believed strongly in the prevention of psychiatric disorders in the community through the use of a model similar to the public health model. In collaboration with Gerald Caplan, Lindemann established a community mental health clinic in Massachusetts that used crisis intervention.

In 1958 Tyhurst studied reactions of individuals and groups to natural disasters and to upsets produced by migration and industrial retirement. He identified three overlapping phases in response to disaster—impact, recoil, and posttrauma. According to Tyhurst, in the first phase 75% of the victims experience shock, confusion, and fear. During recoil the initial stress of the disaster is over, and victims usually express dependency needs. The full impact of the losses come in the third stage, posttrauma. Grief is a predominant response as the survivors begin the process of mourning.

The theorist most widely known in the development of crisis theory and crisis intervention is Gerald Caplan. Caplan stresses the growth potential for the client inherent in a crisis state. He views the individual as living in a state of emotional equilibrium, with the goal of maintaining or returning to this state. A crisis ensues when the obstacle to be faced is insurmountable through the use of customary methods of problem solving. The outcome of the crisis depends on the kind of interaction that takes place between the individual and the key figures in his or her emotional milieu. In 1964 Caplan formally introduced concepts of community mental health practice. He clearly defined crisis theory and described crisis intervention as a formal therapy.

Caplan defined the concepts of primary, secondary, and tertiary prevention. *Primary prevention* involves social and interpersonal actions that help a community deal with potential crises. Examples of primary prevention include education programs and nutrition incentives. Crisis therapy is a primary prevention concept and has developed into an effective method of preventing mental disorders. The aim of *secondary prevention* is to decrease the number of existing cases through early detection and effective treatment. Early referrals and screening programs are examples of secondary prevention. *Tertiary prevention* involves reduction in the rate of disability after the mental disorder has been treated. Rehabilitation programs come under the category of tertiary prevention.

In 1961 the report of the Joint Commission of Mental Illness and Health added impetus to and eventually, funding for crisis therapy. Conclusions related to crisis theory included the following:

> People in crisis were not receiving immediate help but were instead put on lengthy waiting lists.
>
> When they did receive help, it was often through lengthy and expensive psychotherapy.
>
> Extended or late psychotherapy was often not helpful to people in crisis.
>
> When people in crisis needed help, almost 50% sought out clergy, family physicians, or nonmental health professionals.
>
> Interested people with minimal training could be helpful to people in crisis.
>
> A large number of interested people in the community had been neglected as a resource for helping people in crisis (Wilson & Kneisl, 1983, p. 274).

Soon after the publication of the report, large amounts of federal funds were made available for community-based mental health programs, giving an enormous impetus to the establishment of crisis intervention services throughout the country.

Building on the work of Lindemann, Caplan, and theorists such as Parad and Resnik (1975) and Rapoport (1962), Jacobson (1965) and Aguilera (1986) have refined crisis theory and developed assessment and treatment models for crises in marital and family conflict and in suicide prevention. In establishing treatment parameters Caplan's (1964) phases of a crisis have been used.

## ❖ PHASES OF A CRISIS

A crisis is an internal disturbance that results from a stressful event or a perceived threat to self. In response to the threat or precipitating event, the individual's anxiety rises and Caplan's (1964) four phases of a crisis occur. In the first phase the individual's coping mechanisms are called into action by the stimulus of anxiety. If relief is not obtained by using these coping mechanisms and there is inadequate situational support, the individual progresses to the second phase. This phase is identified by an increase in anxiety incurred by the failure of coping mechanisms. In the third phase the individual tries out new coping mechanisms or redefines the threat to use the old mechanisms. As a result of these behaviors, resolution may occur in this phase. If resolution is unsuccessful, the individual enters the fourth phase in which continuation of very high anxiety may lead to psychological disorganization.

Aguilera and Messick (1989) identify certain balancing factors that determine the outcome of the phases described by Caplan. These factors include the perception of the event, the individual's coping mechanisms, and the availability of situational supports. Successful resolution of the crisis is more likely to occur if the individual's perception of the threat is realistic, if he or she has adequate coping mechanisms, and if there are situational supports available. These balancing factors are represented in a paradigm developed by Aguilera and Messick (Fig. 22-1).

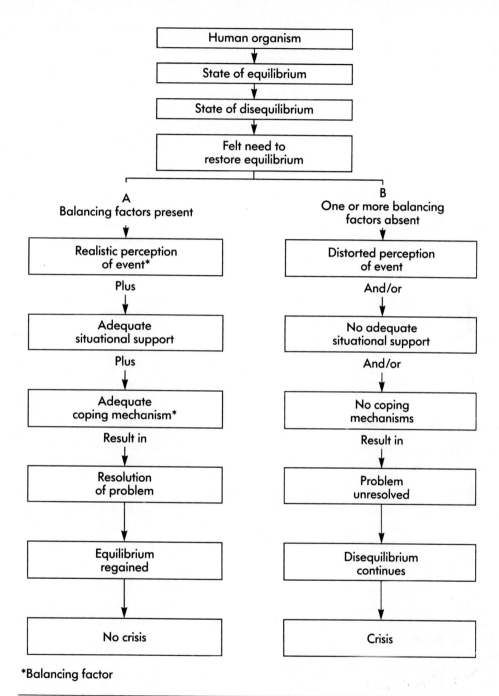

*Balancing factor

❖ **Fig. 22-1**    Effect of balancing factors in a stressful event. *(From Aguilera, D. C. & Messick, J. M. (1989). Crisis intervention: theory and methodology, (ed. 6,) St. Louis: C. V. Mosby.)*

Many symptoms are experienced by people in a crisis. They can include anxiety, depression, confusion, anger, helplessness, withdrawal, somatic symptoms, inefficiency, and hopelessness. People involved in a crisis situation may have suicidal or homicidal thoughts. Feelings of alienation also occur frequently.

Crises are generally self-limiting and find resolution with or without intervention. Support generally aids in creating a positive resolution. An important aspect of crisis theory is that the period of intense conflict is also a time of increased vulnerability that may lead to growth. People in crisis experience turmoil and are ready to accept help from others to help them in their return to psychological equilibrium. It is important for nurses to identify the growth-producing part of crisis in working with clients in these situations. For example, a person experiencing a crisis with the death of a parent may be able to resolve feelings of guilt and hence may be better prepared to deal with death of other family members in the future.

## ❖ THE CRISIS SEQUENCE

Parad and Resnik (1975) developed the crisis sequence based on time periods experienced around a crisis. These include the precrisis, the crisis or upset, and the postcrisis periods. During the *precrisis* period the individual maintains equilibrium through the use of his or her usual coping skills. The individual may perceive minor stresses, but they are not perceived as threatening to life goals, which relate to basic security needs such as body integrity, love, or sense of security. When a person perceives an event as threatening to life goals and unmanageable based on current coping mechanisms, he or she enters the *crisis* period. This period begins at the time of the impact of the crisis. During the crisis period the individual experiences disorganization, tension, and anxiety. In an attempt to regain equilibrium, he or she uses various trial and error responses to

resolve the crisis. With the development of effective and adaptive coping mechanisms, *crisis resolution* occurs. The individual then enters the *postcrisis* period. This period is characterized by a return to equilibrium. Depending on the effectiveness of the crisis resolution, the individual may resume his or her precrisis level of functioning, attain a higher level of functioning, or function at a lower level (Fig. 22-2).

## ❖ TYPES OF CRISES

Crises can be divided into three types—maturational (developmental), situational, and adventitious.

### Maturational Crisis (Developmental)

*Maturational crises* are precipitated by the normal stress created by the social, psychological, and behavioral changes associated with development. Erikson (1963) described eight critical periods in his theory of psychosocial development in which there is a predictable increase in anxiety or stress that could precipitate a maturational or developmental crisis. These periods include birth, toilet training, starting school, puberty, leaving home, marriage, parenthood, and retirement. Development at any stage is dependent on successful completion of the previous stages. What differentiates a person who develops a maturational crisis from one who does not is his or her ability to make role changes necessary for a new maturational level. Patterson (1986) identifies three main reasons why an individual may not be able to prevent a maturational crisis:

1. The person may not be able to visualize himself or herself in a new role because of inadequate role models. *Example: A female child reared without a mother may have difficulty assuming a maternal role with her child.*
2. The individual may lack the interpersonal resources to make necessary and appropriate

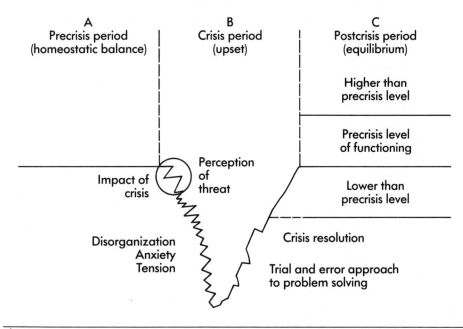

A
Precrisis period
(homeostatic balance)

B
Crisis period
(upset)

C
Postcrisis period
(equilibrium)

Higher than
precrisis level

Precrisis level
of functioning

Impact of
crisis

Perception
of
threat

Lower than
precrisis level

Disorganization
Anxiety
Tension

Crisis resolution

Trial and error approach
to problem solving

❖ **Fig. 22-2**    Crisis sequence diagram. *(From Beck, C. M., Rawlings, R. P. & Williams, S. R. (1984). Mental health-psychiatric nursing. St. Louis: C. V. Mosby, p. 494.)*

changes. *Example: A retired person may have no social network if his or her previous network revolved around work.*

3. Other people may refuse to acknowledge the individual's maturational role. *Example: Parents may fail to recognize their toddler's need for independence.*

Because maturational events are predictable and occur gradually, the individual has time to prepare. Anticipatory guidance can be effective in circumventing a crisis. This is considered primary prevention and may take the form of premarital counseling, parenting groups, or retirement planning.

CASE EXAMPLE: Mr. K. is a 27-year-old black employed male who came to the clinic for a routine physical examination. He complained of a feeling of lethargy, early morning awakening, poor appetite, and a loss of interest in his usual activities. He explained that his wife had delivered a baby 6 weeks ago and that since that time he believed that she had lost interest in their relationship. Mr. K. believes that all of his wife's time is taken caring for the baby. He feels guilty when he asks her to spend time with him. He went on to explain that the baby was the result of a planned pregnancy, but now he has doubts about his ability to be a good father. He begins to cry when he explains that he really resents the child. Mr. K. described his childhood as difficult because of the loss of his father at age 2 in an automobile accident. Because of this, he feels strongly that he wants to be a good father to his child, but he believes that he is incapable of doing so.

### Situational Crisis

A *situational crisis* occurs as a response to a traumatic event that is usually sudden and unavoidable. The external event threatens the physical, psychological, or social integrity of the individual and disrupts equilibrium. Because the definition of self comes from the various roles that one assumes, the threat of loss or loss of a role viewed as necessary to maintain one's self-image will usually lead to a situational crisis. Examples of situational crises include loss of job, loss of a loved one, unwanted pregnancy, onset or exacerbation of a medical illness, or divorce.

CASE EXAMPLE: Mrs. P., a 34-year-old married white female, was admitted to a surgical unit for a biopsy of a suspicious lump in her left breast. She became very tearful the night before surgery when the nurse entered to give her a sleeping pill. Mrs. P. explained to the nurse that she feared that her husband would leave her if she had cancer and needed a mastectomy. She was not sure that she wanted to live if he left. Mrs. P. stated that she believed that she would only be half a woman without her breast. She always prided herself on her appearance and believed that without her breast she would be ugly and undesirable to everyone. She explained that she had not slept for a week since the diagnosis of the lump and had lost all interest in food. She had not shared her concern with her husband because she did not want to worry him. She was also unable to discuss her fears with the doctor because she believed that he was too busy.

## Adventitious Crisis

An *adventitious crisis* results from an accidental, uncommon, or unexpected event involving multiple losses or gross environmental changes. Adventitious crises may result from fires, earthquakes, floods, mass tragedies (e.g., airline crashes), group kidnappings, and nuclear accidents. Fortunately, these crises do not occur in the lives of everyone as they challenge every coping mechanisms because of the severity and number of stressors encountered. Disaster-precipitated problems often surface weeks or months after the occurrence. Frederick and Garrison (1981) expanded the work of Tyhurst and identified five phases of human disaster response (Table 22-1).

Garmezy (1986) described three approaches to disaster research: clinical-descriptive, epidemi-

ological, and quasi-experimental. The clinical-descriptive research is based on observations of professionals personally involved in relief efforts and has set the stage for studies of victim reactions described at Buffalo Creek, West Virginia (1972), Three Mile Island, Pennsylvania (1980), Mount St. Helens in Washington (1982), and Armero, Columbia (1985).

CASE EXAMPLE: On November 13, 1985, the Nevado del Ruiz volcano in north central Columbia erupted. The explosion dumped tons of ice, snow, and volcanic material into several river beds that originated at the base of the volcano. One river curved around to the town of Armero approximately 30 miles away. Armero received the brunt of the mile-wide avalanche of gray ash, mud, rocks, tree trunks, and everything in the path of the river.

Within hours the catastrophe had left 22,000 people of the town and the surrounding area dead or missing under 50,000 million cubic feet of boiling mud. Thousands more were injured, orphaned, or homeless. Some victims were able to reach high locations. Others were able to keep their heads just inches above the surface of the mud. Many were buried up to their necks or were entwined in trees. All were covered with hardened mud and volcanic material. Only after the victims were washed was the damage to skin, bone, and muscles discovered.

To identify postdisaster behavior of hospitalized victims, the personnel had to differentiate the manifestations of medical shock and reactions to rescue procedures from psychological trauma. All clients showed signs of psychological distress. Children had large pupils and constant, intense stares, signs of autonomic arousal. Clients reported different signs of anxiety such as fluctuating sensations of warmth, perspiration, and fear. A large number reported sleep disturbances and a lack of dreams. Others reported an inability to relax and make decisions. Victims stated that familiar patterns of social interaction had lost value. Early signs of psychic trauma included ambivalence about learning the details about the avalanche and the losses and periods of aggressive and explosive behavior. Early symptomatology of grief reactions was identified by the continuation of apathy, feelings of unreality, preoccupation with details, emotional distancing from people, and persistent irritability (Cohen, 1987).

❖ **Table 22-1**
Five phases of human disaster responses

| Phase | Responses |
|---|---|
| Impact | Includes the event itself and is characterized by shock, panic, or extreme fear; the person's judgment and assessment of reality factors are very poor, and self-destructive behavior may be seen. |
| Heroic | A cooperative spirit exists between friends, neighbors, and emergency teams; constructive activity at this time can help to overcome feelings of anxiety and depression, but over-activity can lead to "burnout." |
| Honeymoon | Begins to appear 1 week to several months after the disaster; the need to help others is sustained, and the money, resources, and support received from various agencies cause life to begin again in the community; psychological and behavioral problems may be overlooked. |
| Disillusionment | Lasts from approximately 2 months to 1 year; a time of disappointment, resentment, frustration, and anger; victims often begin to compare their neighbors' plights with their own and may start to resent, envy, or show hostility toward others. |
| Reconstruction and reorganization | Individuals recognize that they must come to grips with their own problems; they begin to rebuild their homes, businesses, and lives in a constructive fashion; this period may last for years after the disaster. |

From Stuart, G., and Sundeen, S. (1987). Principles and Practice of Psychiatric Nursing, (ed. 3.) St. Louis: C.V. Mosby Co, p. 294.

## ❖ CRISIS INTERVENTION

Crisis theory has been placed in operation through the development of crisis intervention, for crisis intervention involves the use of crisis theory to guide practice. Crisis intervention has been clearly defined and identified as useful in a variety of settings. It can be useful with individuals, families, and groups and has also been used on telephone hotlines.

Aguilera and Messick (1989) describe crisis intervention as a treatment strategy that can offer immediate help to a person in crisis to re-establish equilibrium. It is an inexpensive, short-term treatment that focuses on solving the immediate problem.

Clients requiring crisis intervention are generally dealing with a sudden life-situation that requires attention and is beyond the coping mechanisms of the person. Some authors limit the selection of people for crisis intervention to well-integrated individuals with normal health and social adjustment and no previous psychiatric history. In so doing, these authors define an emotional crisis as a normal event in the life of a well-adjusted individual rather than as a signal drawing attention to an underlying illness. Other authors describe successful interventions with chronically mentally ill patients who are experiencing a temporary crisis.

The criteria that most authors identify for

successful use of crisis intervention strategies are clients with problems amenable to short-term problem-solving techniques and motivation of the client to solve the problem.

## Settings for Crisis Intervention

Nurses, because of the variety of settings in which they practice, are in a unique position to identify people in crisis and to intervene. For example, clinics provide nurses an arena in which to assess people in maturational crises such as during obstetrical visits, pediatric visits, and annual physical examinations.

Hospitalization may create a situational crisis for many clients and their families. Psychological stressors in hospitalized clients include fears of the following:

Loss of life
Loss of body part
Limitation of activity
Loss of control
Loss of independence
Strangers
Separation from loved ones
Loss of love and approval
Reactivation of guilt or shame
Retaliation

Another area in which nurses assess clients in crisis is in the emergency room. These clients may include rape victims, individuals who have attempted suicide, psychosomatic clients, or families of accident victims. Careful assessment and triage in these situations may prevent a potential crisis from becoming an actual crisis. Referral sources include inpatient psychiatric units, outpatient services, and psychiatric nurse clinicians. Recently, mobile treatment teams have been used in emergency rooms. Bengelsdorf and Alden (1987) describe the function of one multidisciplinary team based in the emergency room of a county hospital. Seventy percent of the clients seen by this team were treated without hospitalization. The team identifies and resolves problems not only with clients and their families but also with referring therapists and agencies as well.

Nurses in the community are in an excellent position to identify people in crisis. Clearly, the role of crisis intervention has been well established as part of the services offered in the community mental health system. In a less definitive way nurses in public health and home health care identify, evaluate, and intervene with clients in crisis. These situations may include refusal by children to go to school, an illness in the family, or the presence of a dying family member. The nurse must often be flexible and assume a variety of roles such as resource person, teacher, or family liaison in re-establishing the client's equilibrium.

Some communities have established residential crisis services to provide people in a crisis with a protective and supportive setting in which to stay temporarily while they regain equilibrium. Residential services are appealing because they provide less restrictive and more normative environments than inpatient units in which to treat persons experiencing acute psychiatric crises. These settings potentially can provide less stigmatized and less disruptive care that also meets the need for cost containment. The programs in this area can be divided into two types: those that provide treatment to one or two individuals at a time, usually within a family-based crisis home, and those that treat clients in groups in group residences. Primarily two groups of patients are treated with these residential services—individuals with long-term mental illnesses who are experiencing an episodic recurrence of acute illness and people experiencing acute crises without prior mental illness.

Another area of community involvement for the nurse is in consultation with school systems. With the increasing incidence of childhood and adolescent mental disorders, the nurse's role in schools becomes essential. Schonfeld (1989) describes a model of intervention in schools for bereavement support both for specific death and for death education aimed at providing information in a preventive mental health capacity.

A study in the community on bereavement intervention was completed by Constantino (1988), comparing levels of depression and socialization among three groups. The three groups used for intervention included a bereavement crisis intervention group, a social activities group, and a control group. The mean score on depression and socialization scales decreased for the bereavement crisis intervention group, increased for the social adjustment group, and remained fairly constant for the control group.

## Modalities

Crisis intervention has been successfully used as a framework for a variety of treatment modalities. Individual interventions include both the generic and individual approach. Family theorists support the use of crisis intervention with families as the focus. Group crisis intervention is also a viable treatment modality. Finally, crisis intervention has become the treatment of choice on telephone hotlines.

**Individual intervention.** Crisis counseling with an individual is usually short in duration (five or six sessions) and issue oriented. Intervention with an individual is divided into two types—the generic approach and the individual approach.

The *generic approach* is a type of crisis intervention based on a public health model and is derived from the idea that certain common psychological tasks and problem-solving behaviors must be achieved to resolve a crisis. It is designed to reach high-risk individuals and large numbers of people facing a crisis quickly by providing a specific intervention effective for all clients experiencing a particular type of crisis. An example of a generic approach to crisis intervention would be bereavement counseling based on Lindemann's work. There are several benefits to this approach:

1. It is easily practiced across disciplines and by nonprofessionals because the interventions are based on anticipated patterns of behavior.
2. It is easily taught.
3. It provides a theoretical base for the development of preventive programs.

The second type of individual intervention is the *individual approach.* This approach follows the medical model of diagnosis and treatment of a specific problem in a specific client. The nurse using this method must understand the psychodynamics of the present crisis and must have the ability to assess, plan, implement, and evaluate treatment. Situations most amenable to the individual approach include the following:

1. A combination of maturational and situational crises
2. A client with suicidal or homicidal ideation
3. A client not responding to the generic approach
4. A crisis in which a theoretical formulation of the crisis has not been established

Every nurse brings individual strengths and style to an interaction with a client in crisis. Hoff (1978, p. 237) describes some techniques that nurses may use to help the client achieve healthy coping skills:

1. Listen actively and with concern.
2. Encourage open expression of feelings.
3. Help the client gain an understanding of the crisis.
4. Help the client gradually accept reality.
5. Help the client explore new ways of coping with the problem.
6. Link the client to a social network.
7. Engage in decision counseling or problem solving.
8. Reinforce newly learned coping skills.
9. Follow-up after the crisis resolution.

**Family intervention.** Family theorists identify a crisis as a family problem regardless of the identified client and favor using a family-based approach to intervention. This orientation cites role problems as causing disequilibrium in the family. A growing body of research identifies the critical role played by the psychosocial kinship system in determining the ability of the family to adapt to potential maturational or situational crises. Gutstein et al (1988) describe a study to test the effectiveness of one family treatment model. The treatment involved three components in dealing with adolescent situational crises seen in the emergency room: (1) the provision of an immediate emergency response to stabilize family anxiety; (2) the mobilization of extended family members; and (3) the restructuring of the kinship system to provide long-term solutions to the current crisis. The study determined that care could be provided safely on an outpatient basis without institutionalization and that the program could alleviate the sense of crisis within the family. It further noted that the program was successful in training the family to deal better with future stresses and transitions.

**Group intervention.** Aguilera and Messick (1989) describe a crisis group as a collection of individuals, unknown and unrelated, who meet with a therapist to work toward the resolution of the individuals' crises. Referral to a group rather than individual crisis counseling is often based on the client's need for increased interaction with peers. People whose problems may be treatable with group intervention include the following:

1. People with problems of social isolation
2. People with low self-esteem
3. People with poor self-images
4. People with difficulty accepting advice from professionals

The role of the therapist in group crisis intervention is active, direct, and present oriented; often the manner in which people function in a group clearly depicts the areas of faulty coping skills and can be identified by the therapist and group members. One of the disadvantages of group crisis intervention is that it is an individually focused group with each person working on his or her own crisis and time becomes a factor.

**Telephone hotlines.** With the dramatic increase in crisis intervention services throughout the United States came the demand for methods to reach people unwilling to come to centers for help. By 1977 there were more than 600 suicide and crisis hotlines in operation in the United States with as many as 12 million people using these services annually (Rosenbaum & Calhoun, 1977). Without visual cues, listening skills became an essential quality for triaging calls. In response to the need for more accurate assessment of callers, courses were developed to train hotline personnel, and training manuals were created with suicide rating scales, community resource referrals, and drug information. In an effort to evaluate the effectiveness of hotline intervention, Bonneson and Hartsough (1987) developed a crisis call outcome rating scale (CCORS) for caller behavior. This 26-item scale has the potential for application in the evaluation of hotline effectiveness.

In an attempt to reach other potentially suicidal individuals, the Dutchess County Department of Mental Hygiene and the New York State Bridge Authority jointly established a suicide prevention phone connected to a 24-hour psychiatric emergency service on a bridge known as a place of frequent suicide attempts. After 2 years of operation, the phone has been used 30 times, with 23 of those people brought in for psychiatric services.

## Application of Crisis Intervention

There are four steps in the process of crisis intervention that are similar to the nursing process—assessment, planning, implementation, and evaluation.

**Assessment.** Assessment is the first phase of crisis intervention. It is during this step that the nurse begins to establish a positive working relationship with the client. The nurse collects data on the nature of the crisis and its effect on the client. Balancing factors, important to the development and resolution of the crisis, are identified:

1. The precipitating event
2. The client's perception of the event
3. The nature and strength of the client's support systems
4. The client's previous strengths and coping mechanisms

*Precipitating event.* There are three areas of assessment under the category of precipitating event: the client's perception of threat to needs, the onset of symptoms, and past associations connected with the event (Benter, 1987). Benter also identifies four types of needs: biological functioning, sexual role mastery, self-esteem, and dependency.

Biological functioning involves the client's perception of life as safe and without threat. Sexual mastery is achieved when the individual attains vocational, sexual, and parental role successes. Self-esteem needs involve successful role experiences, and dependency needs are satisfied when interdependent relationships are achieved.

In assessing these areas the nurse questions the client about the fulfillment of his or her needs. For example, does the client feel safe, are relationships satisfying, and are there areas in the client's life in which he or she feels successful? The nurse then helps the client identify obstacles to the fulfillment of needs.

*Perception of the event.* The point at which previous coping skills become ineffective and symptoms appear is often after the occurrence of the stressful event. Individual perception of the event plays a major role in determining if the client enters a crisis. As the client connects life events with the breakdown in coping mechanisms, an understanding of the precipitating event can materialize. Clues to the

nature of the precipitating event are provided by recurrent themes and surfacing memories. Some crisis theorists believe that current issues are symbolically connected to past issues. Since most crises involve losses or threats of loss, the theme of loss is common.

*Support systems.* The nurse must assess the support systems of the client. Information is sought about present and potential sources of support. Areas needing assessment include the following:

1. Living arrangements
2. Close relationships
3. Family composition and proximity
4. Religious support
5. Networks and/or affiliations

Assessment of support systems provides vital information for disposition, (e.g., a referral to family therapy to strengthen family ties or to group therapy for a person who needs to enhance peer support). Finally, hospitalization may be needed to protect the client or others from suicidal or homicidal risks.

*Coping mechanisms.* The last area for assessment of balancing factors is coping mechanisms. The client must identify how he or she has handled previous crises in life, what strategies were used (e.g., talking problems out, leaving the situation, or crying), and what strategies the client has tried in the present situation.

**Nursing diagnosis.** After the assessment has been completed, the data are compiled in the form of nursing diagnoses (see box, p. 402).

**Planning.** The second step in the process of crisis intervention is planning the intervention. This involves the development of short- and long-term goals and outcome criteria.

**Intervention.** Interventions are targeted at the reestablishment of equilibrium for the client. They include environmental manipulations, general support, or referral for a crisis intervention, either as an individual, family, or group.

## ❖ NURSING DIAGNOSES RELATED TO CRISIS INTERVENTION

**PRIMARY NANDA NURSING DIAGNOSES**
Coping ineffective, individual
Coping ineffective, family; compromised
Family process, alteration in

**EXAMPLES OF COMPLETE NURSING DIAGNOSIS**
Ineffective individual coping related to child's illness evidenced by limited ability to concentrate and psychomotor agitation
Ineffective individual coping related to daughter's death evidenced by inability to recall events pertaining to the car accident
Ineffective family coping, compromised, related to separation from husband evidenced by excessive dependency on friends and preoccupation with having husband return home
Ineffective family coping, compromised, related to wife's cancer diagnosis evidenced by feelings of grief, fear, and guilt
Alteration in family process related to move to a new town evidenced by social withdrawal and rejection of help from others
Alteration in family process related to marriage of daughter evidenced by unclear family boundaries and distorted communication patterns

From Stuart, G., & Sundeen, S (1986). Principles and Practice of Psychiatric Nursing, (ed. 3.) St. Louis: The C.V. Mosby Co. (p. 297).

Environmental manipulation includes those interventions that directly change the client's physical or interpersonal situation to provide situational support or to remove stress. An example might be the use of respite care for an older relative when the caregiver needs a break from care responsibilities.

General support includes interventions identifying the advocacy position of the nurse for the client with family and health resources. The nurse's use of warmth, acceptance, empathy, and caring provides a therapeutic relationship in which the advocacy can be developed.

Types of crisis intervention for referral are described in detail in the section, "Modalities."

**Evaluation.** The last step in crisis intervention is evaluation. It is in this phase that the nurse and client collaborate to determine the effectiveness of the intervention. Evaluation is made in the following areas:

1. Level of the individual in the postcrisis period—the same, higher, or lower than in the precrisis state
2. Satisfaction of unmet needs threatened by the crisis
3. Alleviation of symptoms of ineffective coping
4. Revitalization or establishment of effective coping mechanisms
5. Activation or reactivation of support systems

The nurse reinforces the client's own effectiveness in bringing about the changes that have occurred and helps the client generalize the learned strategies to future situations. If the goals have not been met, the process returns to the assessment phase.

CASE EXAMPLE: Ms. R. is a 45-year-old, married, white female with three children. She came to the clinic in November with vague complaints of sleeplessness, early morning awakening, lack of interest in usual activities, and weight loss. The nurse collecting the intake information obtained the following history.

Ms. R. had worked as a teacher until the past June. During the summer Ms. R.'s 80-year-old mother, Mrs. T. had suffered a stroke and was unable to live alone. After a brief hospitalization, Mrs. T. moved into Ms. R.'s home in what was thought to be a temporary arrangement, but Mrs. T. has not regained enough mobility to return to her home. Ms. R. has taken a leave of absence from her job to care for her mother. Ms. R.'s symptoms started in September and have not improved in the last month, so she is seeking medical help.

Ms. R. was the oldest of three children. Her two younger brothers live within close proximity. Growing up, the children were fairly close, but her father seemed to favor the boys as evidenced by his paying for their college education and believing Ms. R. did not need college training. Ms. R. was close to her mother and believed that her mother had been an excellent role model for her. Her father died several years ago. Until this summer her mother had been in excellent health and very active. She stated that her brothers had never felt any responsibility for the care of their parents. Family history revealed no history of chronic illness or mental illness.

Ms. R.'s nuclear family includes her husband, Mr. R., and her three children, Lisa (14), Toby (12), and Tommy (9). She described her relationship with her husband as excellent, although in the last few months there has been more conflict than usual. Ms. R. identified her husband as a strong source of support. Her relationships with her children are warm and loving. She admitted that adolescence was not her favorite stage of the children's lives. Ms. R. described a small network of friends, most of whom were teachers in the school in which she had taught.

Ms. R. recently had her yearly physical examination and was found to be in excellent health. A gynecological examination at that time indicated no problems.

Ms. R. complained of feeling sad but not really depressed. She felt tense and nervous all of the time. She stated that she was not sleeping well and was irritable with her husband and children. She did not believe that the care of her mother was a burden and stated that it was the least that she could do. She stated that finances so far are not a major concern because her mother is contributing her social security check to the household. She said that she could not understand why she had these feelings now.

Ms. R. demonstrated good comprehension, above-average intelligence, a good capacity for introspection, and an adequate memory. Her thought processes were organized, and there was no evidence of a perceptual disorder. Although Ms. R. had many symptoms of depression, her score on the Beck Depression inventory was within normal range.

Ms. R.'s usual means for coping was talking problems out with her husband and friends. She believed that she and her husband had not had much time alone together recently. She had enjoyed aerobics class in the past but seemed too busy to go to class now. The family had enjoyed outings, but the children recently had become more interested in spending time with their friends than with the family.

Ms. R. showed strong motivation for working on her problems, although she was not sure what they were. She was clearly reaching out for help.

*Assessment.* Using the crisis model (see Fig. 22-1) as the framework for assessment, data are presented in Table 22-2, with relevant nursing diagnoses listed in the box that follows.

*Planning.* Ms. R. was in a situational crisis, an internal disturbance that resulted from a perceived threat. The precipitating event in this case was the stroke of her mother and her subsequent inability to live alone. Another factor was Ms. R's decision not to resume teaching in the fall. These events affected Ms. R.'s self-esteem because they significantly decreased her ability to fulfill her social roles. They affected the area of sexual role mastery in affecting both her vocational role and her parental role and also posed a threat to her dependency needs by creating conflict in her most significant interdependent relationship with her husband. Ms. R.'s previous coping mechanisms, talking and exercise, had been interrupted because of her perception of time restraints. As her coping became ineffective, her symptoms of anxiety and depression appeared. Memories of her father's preferential treatment of her brothers resurfaced, as did her strong feelings of obligation to her mother. Support systems had been diminished because of conflictual problems with her

❖ **Table 22-2**
Assessment of Ms. R using balancing factors

| Balancing factors | Threat | Assessment data |
|---|---|---|
| Precipitating event | Threat to dependency | Mother's stroke |
| | | Mother's inability to return to independent living |
| | Threat to self-mastery (vocational success) | Decision to take a leave of absence from teaching |
| | Threat to self-esteem | Conflict with husband |
| Perception of event | | Unclear as to linkage of symptoms with current stressors |
| Coping mechanism | | Talking with husband |
| | | Physical exercise |
| Support systems | | Living with husband, children, and mother |
| | | Close relationship with husband |
| | | Religious affiliation not mentioned |
| | | Network or affiliation—friends at school |

❖ **NURSING DIAGNOSES**

Ineffective individual coping related to sleeplessness, anorexia, anxiety, and depression secondary to mother's stroke and entrance into family system

Ineffective family coping related to increased marital conflict secondary to limited time to work on relationships

Alteration in family processes related to conflict and tension secondary to change in composition of family with addition of mother

Alteration in nutrition related to anorexia secondary to stress (no physiological basis documented by physical examination)

Alteration in sleep-pattern disturbance related to sleeplessness and early morning awakening secondary to stress (no physiological basis documented by physical examination)

husband and her lack of contact with her school friends.

The overall goal of treatment was to have Ms. R. return to at least her precrisis level of functioning and ideally to a higher level. A crisis intervention model was decided on jointly by the client and the nurse. The client demonstrated potential for problem solving and strong motivation to improve as rapidly as possible.

Short-term plans included the following:

1. Respite care for Mrs. T. so that Mr. and Ms. R. might resume a less conflictual relationship
2. A family meeting to determine if Ms. R. might be able to delegate some care to her children and husband
3. A meeting with Ms. R.'s brothers to determine if they could provide any resources

Long-term plans were as follows:

1. Increasing Ms. R.'s intellectual understanding of the crisis (by understanding the source of her anxiety, the client could be helped to problem solve potential solutions)
2. Reinforcing old coping mechanisms and modifying her schedule to allow for the use of these mechanisms
3. Learning new strategies to allow time for self without feelings of guilt
4. Increasing support systems by participating in a caregivers' group.

*Intervention.* The intervention used by the nurse was the individual approach, which included environmental manipulation, general support, and the generic approach. The individual approach was chosen because there is no developed theory delineating a crisis resulting from caregiving stress. Environmental manipulation was achieved by Ms. R.'s discussion of delegation of caregiving responsibilities in a family meeting shortly after her first visit to the nurse. The family was surprised that Ms. R. had not asked sooner and were pleased to have a role in caring for Mrs. T. Arrangements were made so that Mr. and Ms. R. could resume time alone together and so that Ms. R. could attend aerobics class.

General support was given by the nurse who provided warmth, empathy, caring, reassurance, and optimism. The client and the nurse explored Ms. R.'s feelings about caregiving and giving up her job. The nurse provided literature on caregiving options. They discussed Ms. R.'s feelings, and the nurse let her know that she understood them.

The generic approach was used through the nurse's supplying Ms. R. with information on respite care and support groups for caregivers. The nurse helped her understand the concept of anxiety and interventions such as using relaxation to combat anxiety.

The individual approach was used in assessing Ms. R.'s specific problems. She responded well to the nurse's suggestions and was given a list of individual and family therapists to use if she believed she needed further counseling.

*Evaluation.* The nurse and Ms. R. evaluated the interventions when she returned for her biweekly appointments. Ms. R. was pleased with the response that she had received from her husband and children. Mrs. T. was thoroughly enjoying the time that she was spending with her grandchildren and had commented to Ms. R. how much more rested she looked. The tension in the family had significantly subsided, and Ms. R. was sleeping and eating better. She had decided not to meet with her brothers at this time but hoped that she would have the courage to do so in the future. She was investigating the prospect of substitute teaching the next semester at her old school and had resumed contact with her teacher friends. Finally, Ms. R. had joined a caregivers' group and was realizing that she was not alone in the problems that she was facing.

Ms. R. and the nurse discussed how Ms. R. could use the methods of problem solving that she had used during this crisis in future situations. A sample care plan for Ms. R. follows.

### ❖ SUMMARY

Crisis is an inevitable part of human existence. Any stressful event can precipitate a crisis in an individual, depending on the person's perception of the event, his or her coping skills, and the support systems available. Crisis theory and intervention developed as an outgrowth of psychoanalytical theory and preventive psychiatry. Lindemann and Caplan pioneered the definition of crisis theory and the practice of crisis therapy.

A crisis can be classified as maturational

---

## ❖ NURSING CARE PLAN

---

**CLIENT:** Ms. R.

**NURSING DIAGNOSIS:** Ineffective individual coping related to sleeplessness, anorexia, anxiety, and depression secondary to mother's stroke and entrance into the family system

| GOALS | INTERVENTIONS |
|---|---|
| Ms. R will return to her precrisis level of functioning. | ◆ Identify other members within the family system who will be able to assist Ms. R. in the care of her mother. |
| | ◆ Assist Ms. R. in identifying previous coping strategies such as aerobics to deal with her current situation. |
| | ◆ Discuss available caregivers' support groups and determine if Ms. R. is interested in attending. |
| Ms. R will demonstrate understanding of the concept of crisis and be able to identify future times when intervention is needed. | ◆ Discuss crisis concepts such as precipitating events, balancing factors, support systems, and coping mechanisms. |
| | ◆ Assist Ms. R. in applying these ideas to her personal situation. |
| | ◆ Reassure Ms. R. of the normalcy of her responses and encourage her to seek assistance early in any future crisis. |

### EVALUATION

Ms. R. returns to her precrisis level of functioning as she uses previous coping strategies such as regular attendance at aerobics classes and the identification of at least one other family member to assist in the care of her mother. Ms. R. demonstrates understanding of the concept of crisis by describing how the concepts apply to her current personal situation. She is able to apply the ideas to future crisis situations and acknowledges the need to seek assistance early in the process.

(developmental), situational, or adventitious. A maturational crisis is precipitated by the normal stress of developmental transitions. A situational crisis occurs as a response to a traumatic event that is usually sudden and unavoidable. An adventitious crisis results from an accidental, uncommon, or unexpected event involving multiple losses or gross environmental change.

Crisis intervention is an inexpensive, short-term treatment that focuses on solving the immediate problem. Clients with problems amenable to short-term problem-solving techniques and with good motivation are excellent candidates for crisis intervention. Modalities for crisis intervention include the generic approach, the individual approach, family intervention, group intervention, and telephone hotlines. Nurses, because of the variety of settings in which they practice, are in a unique position to identify people in crisis and to intervene.

## ❖ APPLYING KNOWLEDGE TO PRACTICE

1. How have the contributions of various crisis theorists influenced the practice of crisis intervention?
2. In developing protocol for clients facing a death in the family, what assessment questions should be included?
3. Using the case examples for maturational, situational, and adventitious crises given in this chapter, develop a plan of crisis intervention.

## REFERENCES

Aguilera, D. C. & Messick, J. M. (1989). *Crisis intervention. Theory and methodology,* (2nd ed.) St. Louis: CV Mosby.

Beck, C. M., Rawlins, R. P., & Williams, S. R. (1984). *Mental health-psychiatric nursing,* St. Louis: C. V. Mosby.

Bengelsdorf, H., & Alden, D. C. (1987). A mobile crisis unit in the psychiatric emergency room. *Hospital and Community Psychiatry, 38*(6), 662-665.

Benter, S. E. (1987). Crisis Intervention. In G. W. Stuart & S. J. Sundeen (Eds.). *Principles and practice of psychiatric nursing,* (pp. 287-312), St. Louis: C. V. Mosby.

Bonneson, M. E., & Harsough, D. M. (1987). Development of the crisis call outcome rating scale. *Journal of Counsulting and Clinical Psychology, 55*(4) 612-614.

Caplan, G. (1964). *Principles of preventive psychiatry,* Boni Books, USA.

Cohen, R. E. (1987). The Armero tragedy: Lessons for mental health professionals. *Hospital and Community Psychiatry, 38*(12), 1316-1321.

Constantino, R. E. (1988). Comparison of two group interventions for the bereaved. *Image: Journal of Nursing Scholarship, 20*(2), 83-87.

Erikson, E. (1963). *Childhood and Society.* New York: W. W. Norton & Co.

Frederick, C., & Garrison, J. (1981). Behav Today 12:32, Aug.

Garmezy, N. (1986). Children under severe stress: Critique and commentary. *Journal of the American Academy of Child Psychiatry, 25,* 384-392.

Glott, K. M. (1987). Helpline: suicide prevention at a suicide site. *Suicide and Life-Threatening Behavior, 17*(4), 299-309.

Gutstein, S. E., Rudd, M. D., Graham, J. C., & Rayha, L. L. (1988). Systemic crisis intervention as a response to adolescent crisis: An outcome study. *Family Process,* 27, 201-211.

Hoff, L. A. (1978). *People in crisis: Understanding and helping.* California: Addison-Wesley.

Hradek, E. A. (1988). Crisis intervention & suicide. *Journal of Psychosocial Nursing, 26*(5), 24-27.

Jacobson, G. F. (1965). Crisis theory and treatment strategy: Some sociocultural and psychodynamic considerations. *Journal of Nervous Mental Disorders, 141,* 209-218.

Joint Commission on Mental Illness & Health (1961). *Action for mental health,* New York: Basic Books.

Lindemann, E. (1944). Symptomatology and management of acute grief. *American Journal of Psychiatry, 101,* 101.

Parad, H. J., & Resnik, H.L.P. (1975). The practice of crisis intervention in emergency care. In H.L.P Resnik, H. L. Ruben, & D. D. Ruben (Eds.). *Emergency psychiatric care: the management of mental health crisis,* Charles Press, MD.

Patterson, S. L. (1986). Crisis theory and intervention. In B. S. Johnson (Ed.), *Psychiatric-mental health nursing,* (pp. 489-502). Philadelphia: J. B. Lippincott.

Rapoport, L. (1962). The state of crisis: some theoretical considerations *Social Science Review, 36,* 211-217.

Rosenbaum, A. & Calhoun, J. F. (1977). The use of telephone hotline in crisis intervention: A review, *Journal of Community Psychology, 5,* 325-339.

Schonfeld, D. J. (1989). Crisis intervention for bereavement support. *Clinical Pediatrics, 28*(1), 27-33.

Stroul, B. A. (1988). Residential crisis services: A review. *Hospital & Community Psychiatry, 39*(10), 1095-1099.

Stuart, G., & Sundeen, S. (1986). Principles and practice of psychiatric nursing, ed. 3, St. Louis: C. V. Mosby.

Williams, S. R., & Aguilera, D. C. (1988). Crisis Intervention. In C. K. Beck, R. P. Rawlins, & S. R. Williams (Eds.). *Mental health-psychiatric nursing,* (pp. 490-508), St. Louis: C. V. Mosby.

Wilson, H. S., & Kneisl, C. R. (1983). Life turning points: Crisis theory, assessment and intervention. In H. S. Wilson & C. R. Kneisl (Eds.), *Psychiatric nursing,* (pp. 270-294), Reading: Addison Wesley.

# 23

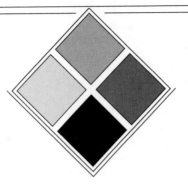

# Substance Abuse and Dependence

Cecelia M. Taylor ◆ Mary Ellen Wewers
Barbara Parker

## OBJECTIVES

*At the completion of this chapter, the reader will be able to:*

◆ Discuss the underlying factors that contribute to an individual's use of specific substances.

◆ Describe specific symptoms that result from the use of various substances.

◆ Identify alterations in motor activity, sleep and arousal patterns, cognition, and feeling states from the use of specific substances.

◆ Develop a plan of care for an individual with a substance abuse problem.

The use of chemical substances to alter moods and feeling states is a practice as old as humanity itself. Undoubtedly, the first human beings discovered the mood-altering properties of certain substances and the healing properties of other substances by accident. The widespread production of illicit drugs and the pharmaceutical industry grew from these primitive trial-and-error beginnings. Although the purposeful ingestion of chemicals for their therapeutic effects has increased the length and quality of life, when the therapeutic use of chemicals extends to nontherapeutic purposes or a person becomes physically or emotionally dependent on the substance, the length and quality of life become threatened.

Very few human behaviors have consequences as far-reaching as do those of individuals who abuse or are dependent on chemical substances. In addition to affecting their own physical, emotional, and social well-being, the behavior of these persons affects the well-being of their families and society. For example, alcoholism is one of the primary reasons for lost time and productivity, both on the assembly line and in the executive suite, and is a significant factor in the economic health of the nation.

To the extent that the substance on which the individual is dependent is illegal, the individual inevitably becomes involved in criminal activity and secondarily contributes to the maintenance of organized crime. At the very least, the cost of such abuse and dependence diverts money from more fruitful ventures such as providing adequate food, clothing, and shelter for the family.

## ❖ DEFINITION OF ABUSE AND DEPENDENCY

Although the terms *abuse* and *dependency* are often used interchangeably by the lay public and even some health professionals, it is important to differentiate between the two forms of substance usage. Although both definitions include components of the use of substances in a deleterious manner, dependence includes specific symptoms of withdrawal from the substance.

The *Diagnostic and Statistical Manual of Mental Disorders* (third edition, 1987) of the American Psychiatric Association assists in clarifying the differentiation between abuse of psychoactive substances and dependence on these substances. The diagnostic criteria for substance dependence are that at least three of the following apply and some symptoms of the disturbance have persisted for at least 1 month or have occurred repeatedly over a longer period of time:

1. Substance often taken in larger amounts or over a longer period than the person intended
2. Persistent desire or one or more unsuccessful efforts to reduce or control substance use
3. A great deal of time spent in activities necessary to get the substance (e.g., theft), taking the substance (e.g., chain smoking), or recovering from its effects
4. Frequent intoxication or withdrawal symptoms when expected to fulfill major role obligations at work, school, or home (e.g., does not go to work because hung over, goes to school or work "high," intoxicated while caring for his or her children) or when substance use is physically hazardous (e.g., drives when intoxicated)
5. Important social, occupational, or recreational activities given up or reduced because of substance use
6. Continued substance use despite knowledge of having a persistent or recurrent social, psychological, or physical problem that is caused or exacerbated by the use of the substance (e.g., continues using heroin despite family arguments about it, cocaine-induced depres-

sion, or having an ulcer made worse by drinking)
7. Marked tolerance: need for markedly increased amounts of the substance (i.e., at least a 50% increase) to achieve intoxication or desired effect or markedly diminished effect with continued use of the same amount
NOTE: The following items may not apply to use of cannabis, hallucinogens, or phencyclidine (PCP)
8. Characteristic withdrawal symptoms
9. Substance often taken to relieve or avoid withdrawal symptoms

The diagnostic criteria for substance abuse are some symptoms of the disturbance have persisted for at least 1 month or have occurred repeatedly over a longer period of time; the individual has never met the criteria for substance dependence for this substance; and at least one of the following applies:

1. Continued use despite knowledge of having a persistent or recurrent social, occupational, psychological, or physical problem that is caused or exacerbated by use of the psychoactive substance
2. Recurrent use in situations in which use is physically hazardous (e.g., driving while intoxicated)

## ❖ BEHAVIORS ASSOCIATED WITH SUBSTANCE ABUSE AND DEPENDENCY

Behaviors associated with substance abuse and dependence can be categorized into four phases: acquisition, maintenance, cessation, and relapse. However, these categories are artificial delineations in that the behavior of the substance-abusing or substance-dependent person is dynamic and moves back and forth from one phase to another (Lichtenstein, 1979).

The *acquisition phase,* or initiation of substance abuse, is often characterized by exploratory behaviors and typically takes place when people are young. Peer influences apparently are the most important single factor in initial experimental acquisition of psychoactive substances. Often a secondary motivation is curiosity about the drug's effects combined with a desire for new, pleasurable, thrilling, and even dangerous experiences (Ghodse, 1989). Substance abuse in adults often begins as attempts at self-medication with alcohol or over-the-counter or prescribed drugs.

The *maintenance phase* is characterized by the regular day-to-day routine use of the substance and often leads to or reflects substance dependence. Experts offer various explanations of substance dependence. However, all agree multiple factors are involved. They include individual physiological predispositions to dependence such as that demonstrated in alcoholism; differing psychological responses to the substance; environmental and familial expectations; and cultural expectations. Fig. 23-1 illustrates the interrelationships between the individual, the substance, and the setting.

When the user is in a physical and social environment that supports substance use and when he or she believes that the substance produces feelings of ease and relaxation or provides escape from immediate problems, the behavior persists, and the maintenance phase

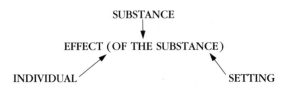

*Substance variables:* The dosage, route, and frequency of administration, purity, drug, food, and chemical interactions
*Individual variables:* The individual's age, weight, state of health, genetic background, state of mind, and mood at time of use
*Setting variables:* The social and environmental expectations of behaviors while using the substance

---

❖ **Fig. 23-1** Interrelationship between the substance, the individual, and the setting.

continues. Some experts (Compton, 1989; Milkman & Frosch, 1973; Khantzian, 1985) believe that the probability of substance abuse and dependence increases when there is a "fit" between the specific effects of the drug and the psychological needs of the individual. For example, opiates help control feelings of rage, and cocaine lifts feelings of fatigue and depression. Compton (1989) describes this phenomenon using Orem's ideas of self-care deficit. In this perspective substances are used by the client to handle painful feelings or as "ego-soothing" behaviors.

The *cessation phase* is characterized by the user's increased awareness of the deleterious effects of substance use and his or her attempts to control, diminish, or cease use of the substance. Unfortunately, these attempts are frequently unsuccessful unless accompanied by the assistance of others who are knowledgeable about the particular type of substance dependence. Even in these instances, *relapse,* the fourth phase, is common. For example, relapse rates for persons treated for heroin, nicotine, and alcohol dependence show similarities over time. At 3 months after treatment, the relapse rate for all three forms of substance dependence is approximately 60%. At 1 year, 67% to 75% of these persons have relapsed (Hunt, Barnett, & Branch, 1971).

❖ **TYPES OF SUBSTANCE DEPENDENCY**

Although there are commonalities among the various forms of substance dependence, substances vary in the physical consequences of their use, presenting symptoms, and treatment protocols. Following is a discussion of the major categories of substances on which persons are dependent.

### Nicotine

Nicotine dependence most commonly occurs as a result of inhaling cigarette smoke. Although legal, cigarette smoking is considered a serious form of substance dependence since the nicotine in tobacco causes pharmacological and behavioral processes that are similar to drugs such as heroin and cocaine (USDHHS, 1988). For example, the nicotine-dependent individual will run to the store at midnight to purchase cigarettes or will experience feelings of panic when no cigarettes are available. The heavy cigarette smoker will experience symptoms of withdrawal within 2 hours after the last cigarette. These symptoms include a craving for nicotine; irritability, frustration, or anger; anxiety; difficulty concentrating; restlessness; decreased heart rate; and increased appetite. These symptoms increase in severity for the first 24 hours and then decrease over a period of 2 to 14 days. However, some former cigarette smokers report continued craving for nicotine for many months or even years after cessation.

### Narcotics

Narcotics are general depressants of the central nervous system and are medically used to relieve moderate and severe pain. Most narcotics are in the chemical class termed *opiates.* Morphine, heroin, and codeine are derivatives of opium; demerol and methadone are synthetic substitutes. Although some opiate-dependent persons use morphine or demerol, most do not have access to these drugs and therefore use heroin, which is readily available on the streets of many cities. However, health care providers often have access to morphine and demerol, and an increasing number have become dependent on these drugs.

Opiates are parenterally administered and produce a temporary state of well-being. The individual feels temporarily free from anxiety and pain. Ever-increasing amounts of the drug are needed to produce this exhilaration, and eventually the heroin user may require as much as 15 to 20 grains daily. Withdrawal symptoms

include tearing, sneezing, coryza, yawning, irritability, and restlessness. Within 24 hours these symptoms are followed by abdominal cramps, vomiting, diarrhea, headaches, sweating, and pains in the muscles and joints. On the third day of abstinence the individual becomes hysterical and noisy and may destroy objects within his or her reach. Within a week most of the withdrawal symptoms disappear.

Withdrawal from opiates has been made more humane through the use of methadone, a synthetic substitute. The use of methadone is somewhat controversial because it substitutes one dependence for another, albeit a medically prescribed substance. However, methadone eliminates the criminal activity involved in obtaining illegal drugs. In addition, methadone is relatively inexpensive, and the person on methadone maintenance can usually hold a job and function as a responsible citizen. Methadone clinics, from which the individual receives his or her daily dose of methadone, are available in most large cities. Most clinics require proof that the person is not continuing to use heroin by making urine testing mandatory.

### Alcohol

Alcohol is a central nervous system depressant. The amount required to produce a demonstrable effect varies according to the interrelationship of such variables as the percentage of alcohol in the beverage, the tolerance the individual has developed, the individual's physical and emotional state of health, and the environment in which the person is drinking. In addition, the amount and type of food in the stomach are major factors that affect the rate of absorption. Alcohol consumed by a person unaccustomed to drinking and who is emotionally upset, has not eaten all day, and is in the company of people who are accepting of intoxication is certain to produce a rapid effect.

Once alcohol is absorbed into the bloodstream, it affects all body tissues, but its immediate effects are caused by its action on the brain. At a level of 0.05% of alcohol in the blood, inhibitions are diminished, and the individual may act in a manner different from when he or she is sober. As noted in Chapter 24, an individual's behavior while intoxicated is socially and culturally derived. Intoxicated persons generally act in the manner they believe is expected by others.

At a level of 0.10% of alcohol in the blood, motor and speech activity is impaired. It is for this reason that driving a motor vehicle or operating equipment is very dangerous when a person has been consuming alcohol.

Alcohol dependence takes many forms. A "chronic alcoholic" drinks excessively and is incapacitated most of the time. A "periodic alcoholic" drinks excessively at certain times of his or her life but during other periods may not drink at all. A third type of alcoholism is exhibited by an individual who drinks large quantities of alcohol daily over a period of years. Slowly and insidiously, physical, mental, and emotional deterioration occurs. Eventually this person may be described as suffering from alcoholic deterioration.

Short-term, immediate treatment of the alcohol-dependent person is focused on withdrawing him or her from this substance and assisting him or her to regain physical health. This is accomplished by symptomatic treatment of the anxiety, tremors, nausea, and diaphoresis that accompany withdrawal. Seizures and delirium tremens are serious, life-threatening conditions that may occur during detoxification.

## Central Nervous System Stimulants

The most frequently abused drugs in this category are cocaine, crack, and amphetamines, with cocaine and crack use increasing in the past few years. Cocaine was used for medical purposes in the late 1800s. It acts directly on the cerebral cortex and initially increases the sensation of mental and physical well-being.

Physically, it speeds heart rate, raises the blood pressure, and causes the pupils to dilate (Mittleman, Mittleman, & Elser, 1984).

Crack, a derivative of cocaine, was first seen in urban areas of the United States in the early 1980s. Unlike cocaine, crack is generally smoked rather than snorted or injected. Its use has become widespread throughout the nation, very likely because its effects are more intense than those of cocaine and its price is lower.

Cocaine is absorbed very rapidly: 2 to 3 minutes when snorted, 30 to 60 seconds when injected, and 3 to 5 seconds when smoked (House, 1990). It metabolizes so quickly that users may take the drug every 20 to 30 minutes to maintain their high (Vandegaer, 1989). Crack has an even shorter period of effect than cocaine, lasting only 5 to 7 minutes. The intensity of the euphoria created by crack, combined with the shortness of its duration, is largely responsible for the fast and intense dependency on this drug that users frequently report.

Cocaine and crack are commonly believed to be "safe" drugs because they do not always produce definitive withdrawal symptoms. However, depression is common after withdrawal and may be severe enough to precipitate a suicidal attempt. This phenomenon is called "crashing" by users. Cocaine has been described as more toxic than heroin and is linked to cardiac arrests, seizures, bacteremia, renal and intestinal infarction, and respiratory ailments (Gold & Giannini, 1989). Between 1976 and 1981 there was a 300% increase in emergency room visits and a 400% increase in deaths from cocaine (Gold & Giannini, 1989). Cocaine-related deaths often result from the user's inadvertently overdosing by unknowingly purchasing cocaine that is more pure than that previously used. An additional potential problem is that many cocaine and crack users also take other drugs in an attempt to control the fluctuating feelings and effects of the drug and its withdrawal. Drugs commonly used to mediate the negative effects of cocaine include chlordiazepoxide (Librium), diazepam (Valium), and alcohol (Vandegaer, 1989).

The most commonly abused amphetamines are amphetamine sulfate (Benzedrine) and methamphetamine (Desoxyn). In the past these drugs have been used legitimately in small doses to treat depression and as appetite suppressants. Individuals who take these drugs to become "high" take 6 to 200 times the daily dose usually prescribed by a physician. Intravenous amphetamines are known as "speed" in street language.

The physiological effect of these drugs is to raise blood pressure, sometimes to dangerous levels. Large amounts have been known to cause immediate death, accounting for the saying among drug users that "speed kills."

Individuals who use amphetamines think these drugs increase their physical energy, sharpen their physical and sexual reactions, and increase their confidence. Thus a period of frantic activity results from the ingestion of large amounts of amphetamines. This is followed by a great letdown in which the fatigue and depression are so great that the user is apt to seek release by taking the drug again. Chronic use of amphetamines can lead to a schizophrenic-like psychosis with paranoid features. This reaction is a result of the drug and is not related to a premorbid personality trait. In addition, prolonged use at high dosages can lead to massive, irreversible brain damage that may result in death (Arif & Westermeyer, 1988).

## Hallucinogens

Lysergic acid diethylamide (LSD or acid) is the most commonly abused hallucinogen. It was first used in research studies in an attempt to discover the cause of schizophrenia. Ingestion of reasonably small doses produces temporary hallucinations and other schizophrenic-like symptoms. The user experiences waves of color, and vibrations seem to pass through the head. Individuals believe that they have had an almost mystical experience in which the nature

of emotional conflicts becomes clear.

Although there is little evidence that the use of LSD causes physical dependence, it is dangerous for several reasons. First, the substance causes some people to believe that they have supernatural powers, and they may be injured by attempting to undertake such activities as flying off a building. Second, although there is no withdrawal reaction even after prolonged, high-dosage use, a panic reaction may occur, particularly in the first-time user. This reaction is known as a "bad trip" and may last as long as a week. In such instances the user can be helped by being "talked down" by a trusted friend who remains with him or her and points out reality. Third, "flashbacks" in which the user experiences hallucinations days or weeks after using a hallucinogen can also occur (Moreines, 1989).

## Phencyclidine

Phencyclidine (PCP) has historically been classified as a hallucinogen; however, it does not have hallucinogenic effects at low to moderate doses. Rather, low doses produce mild depression and then stimulation (McCoy, Rice, & McFadden, 1981). High doses, however, can produce a schizophrenic-like psychosis with paranoid delusions and hallucinations. The route of administration of PCP plays a significant role in the severity of intoxication. The onset of symptoms from oral ingestion occurs in approximately 1 hour. If taken intravenously, sniffed, or smoked, the onset of symptoms may develop within 5 minutes. The cardinal signals of PCP ingestion include a "blank stare" appearance, ataxia, muscular rigidity, vertical and horizontal nystagmus, tendencies toward violence, and generalized anesthesia (McCoy, Rice, & McFadden, 1981).

## Marijuana

Until recently marijuana was an easily obtained and relatively inexpensive drug. It is a crude preparation from the whole *Cannabis sativa* plant, which grows wild in Mexico and is easily cultivated in the United States. It is usually absorbed into the body through smoking cigarettes called "reefers." Hashish is prepared by scraping resin from the tops of the hemp plant. The active ingredient in both marijuana and hashish is tetrahydrocannabinol, with hashish being more potent.

Inhalation of marijuana causes a state of exhilaration or euphoria. Under its influence the user feels light in body as if he or she were floating through space, and his or her behavior is not unlike that with a mild mania. Marijuana is not an aphrodisiac, but it can lower inhibitions and intensify sexual pleasure. It seems to make many users temporarily passive in contrast to alcohol, which releases aggression in certain situations. Marijuana affects the individual's sense of time and results in diminished concentration and attention span, impaired balance, and decreased coordination. These effects impair the individual's operation of motorized vehicles for 12 to 24 hours after usage (Klahr, Roerich, & Miller, 1989). Users become psychologically dependent on marijuana but do not become physically addicted as with morphine.

Currently a great deal of attention is being given to marijuana by the government because its use has risen dramatically. Official arguments have been carried in the press about the relative dangers of marijuana and the appropriate penalties that should or should not be levied against people who use it. Unfortunately, there is a limited amount of research on which to base a scientific, unbiased judgment about the immediate and long-term effects of using this drug.

## ❖ IMPLICATIONS FOR NURSING PRACTICE
### Nursing Assessment

Although abuse of or dependence on each substance has unique features, it is possible to cite some commonalities about all people suffering from substance abuse or dependence. Although behaviors in each category are presented as separate entities, they are highly interrelated and are adaptations to similar stressors. Further, in many instances behavior designed as an adaptation to one stressor becomes a stressor itself in another dimension.

Nursing assessment in all settings must include questions and observations related to substance dependence and abuse. The nurse practicing in the acute-care, general hospital must be particularly alert to the possibility of the client's being substance dependent even though he or she is being treated for a seemingly unrelated illness. One assessment approach suggests raising questions in a nonthreatening, logical manner by stating that the history contains questions regarding prescription and nonprescription drug use. The nurse begins these questions by asking what physician-prescribed drugs the client has taken in the past 2 months. The next question ascertains what nonprescription drugs such as those ingested in response to a cold or minor ailment have been taken in the past 2 months. The next questions center on drugs or substances such as caffeine, nicotine, alcohol, marijuana, or cocaine used consistently by the client as self-medication. This progression of questions may enhance the cooperation of the client (Smith, 1983).

If the client acknowledges substance abuse or dependence, the nurse must attempt to determine the amount of the substance normally taken on a daily basis and the time and amount of the dose last taken. Experienced nurses report that individuals who are alcohol dependent tend to minimize their consumption by 50% whereas drug-dependent persons exaggerate the extent of their habit by 50% in an effort to ensure receiving an amount of the drug sufficient to prevent withdrawal symptoms.

Regardless of whether or not the client acknowledges substance abuse or dependence, the nurse must raise the question of substance dependence if the client exhibits signs and symptoms characteristic of substance withdrawal but uncharacteristic of the illness for which the client is being treated. Therefore, in addition to asking direct questions, the nursing assessment should include observations of the client's motor activity, sleep and arousal patterns, cognition, and feeling states.

The motor activity of a substance-dependent individual is always affected when the substance (e.g., opiates, alcohol, barbiturates, and amphetamines) affects the central nervous system. In the case of intoxication with opiates, alcohol, and barbiturates psychomotor retardation will be observed. Even small amounts of alcohol and low doses of barbiturates will produce incoordination and an unsteady gait in most users. In contrast, intoxication with amphetamines results in psychomotor hyperactivity.

Sleep and arousal patterns are often impaired when a person abuses or is dependent on substances affecting the central nervous system. Central nervous system depressants allow the person to fall into a stuporous sleep but cause a "rebound" effect approximately 4 hours later when the person awakes with a start, often with tachycardia. Central nervous system stimulants cause insomnia and are often taken initially to achieve this affect.

Cognition is almost always altered by substance abuse. Acute intoxication produces alterations in decision making, judgment, memory, and thought processes. The permanency of these changes depends on whether the drug has destroyed brain tissue. For example, long-term alcohol abusers show evidence of diminution of cognitive processes even after years of abstinence.

Feeling states are often altered during intoxication, and this alteration is the conscious goal of initial substance use. As previously noted, individuals use narcotics to create a feeling of "normalcy," sedative hypnotics to create a feeling of calm, and central nervous system stimulants to create a feeling of euphoria. Furthermore, during periods when they are not using the drug, many people experience guilt, sadness, and shame about their behavior when they were intoxicated.

### Nursing Diagnosis

The next stage in the nursing process identifies appropriate nursing diagnoses. The box

❖ **POTENTIAL NURSING DIAGNOSES FOR CLIENTS WITH A KNOWN OR SUSPECTED PROBLEM WITH SUBSTANCE ABUSE OR DEPENDENCY**

1. Altered Nutrition: less than body requirements.
2. Impaired Social Interaction.
3. Ineffective Denial related to acknowledgment of substance abuse/dependency.
4. Chronic Low Self-Esteem related to history of substance abuse.
5. Compromised Family Coping.
6. Family Process, Altered, related to member who has a problem with substance abuse.
7. Grieving related to loss of substance as a coping mechanism.
8. Health Maintenance, Altered related to tobacco use.
9. Hopelessness related to relapse in program of sobriety.
10. Sensory/Perceptual Alterations.
11. Situational Low Self-Esteem related to acknowledgment of problem with substance abuse.
12. Sleep Pattern Disturbance related to use of psychoactive substances.
13. Spiritual Distress.
14. Violence, Potential for related to recent use of central nervous system stimulants.

lists potential nursing diagnoses for a client with a known or suspected problem with substance abuse.

## Nursing Intervention

The plan for intervention is derived from the nursing diagnosis and must be highly individualized to be effective. In general, the objectives of care relate to assisting the client to regain physiological homeostasis, increase self-esteem, and develop functional methods of coping with stress.

Past beliefs about intervention with substance-abusing people included the long-standing conviction that the person had to "hit bottom" before treatment would be effective. This belief came from the view that abstaining from the use of a chemical that provided a desirable sensation would not occur as long as the pleasure or relief derived from its use exceeded the unpleasant consequences (Twerski, 1983). A newly developed strategy, however, is to design an "intervention" that essentially confronts the substance abuser with his or her behavior and its consequences before irreversible physical and social problems occur. In this approach the substance abuser is confronted by significant people in his or her life, i.e., family members, friends, employers, and a health care professional. The people involved in the intervention state clearly and without anger those behaviors they have observed and what actions they plan to take if the abuser does not immediately seek help. This type of intervention has been used successfully to assist substance-dependent individuals, but it must be carefully planned before its use. Decisions to make include who should be present, who should talk, what should be said, and planned replies to potential responses from the substance abuser. A few cardinal rules include confronting the individual with specific behaviors rather than generalities or vague statements, not threatening an action unless the person is willing to take it, and having a treatment facility prepared to admit the substance abuser

that day if desired. For example, a spouse should not threaten to leave or evict the substance abuser unless he or she is prepared to take that action. Honesty of all participants is crucial for success (Haack & Hughes, 1989). Responses to an intervention may range from outright denial and rationalization to relief that someone cares enough to help with a problem that the person feels incapable of being able to handle.

The substance-dependent client who no longer has access to drugs often will express a great deal of anxiety. These feelings must be taken seriously because the client is accustomed to coping with stressful events by blunting or altering emotional responses with chemicals. It may be helpful to explore these fears with the client and to assist him or her in developing potential responses to fearful situations. These would include responses when offered a drink (for an alcoholic), when returning to work (for a cocaine user), or when in a stressful situation (for a former smoker). Throughout the process of planning for the future, additional concerns may involve finding a place to live and employment and developing a social network that is drug free.

The client must be helped to plan realistically for a future life without drugs. The first step in this process is to help the client explore what drugs mean to him or her and to identify and grieve for the losses he or she will experience without them. These losses may be concrete such as friends and activities, or they may be abstract such as a way of life. Carruth and Pugh (1982) discuss the grieving process in recovering from alcohol abuse. They note that friends, relatives, and even health professionals often assume that the recovering person will feel relieved to be free of alcohol and its associated problems. In contrast, however, the recovering alcoholic frequently grieves the loss of alcohol as a substance that had become an important coping mechanism.

Families are also in dire need of intervention. It is well known that substance dependence affects not only the individual but also his or her family and the family system as a whole. In fact, family members of substance-dependent individuals are sometimes referred to as "co-dependents" since their behavior inadvertently supports the substance dependence by protecting the dependent member in a struggle to maintain the stability of the family system. Thus it is not unusual for the wife of an alcohol-dependent man who is hung over to call his office voluntarily with the excuse that he cannot come to work because he is ill. This behavior serves to deny the seriousness of the situation and lengthens the time before the person experiences the consequences of his substance dependence.

Perhaps the most unfortunate victims of a family in which there is substance abuse are the children. Children in a substance-abusing family spend their formative years in an environment in which reality dictates the concealment of genuine feelings to maintain family stability. In addition, physical and emotional abuse is common and is often interpreted by the child as his or her fault. These and many other factors contribute to the long-lasting effects of growing up in a family in which there is substance abuse.

Group counseling and lay self-help groups have proven inestimably helpful in the treatment of not only the substance abuser but also his or her spouse and children. Among the most helpful are Alcoholics Anonymous, Narcotics Anonymous, and Women for Sobriety (for users); Al-Anon (for spouses); Alateen (for children of users); and Adult Children of Alcoholics (A.C.O.A.). Information on these organizations is listed in the box below.

These groups assist individuals not only to deal with past events but also to cope effectively with family changes in the present. In referring clients and families to self-help groups, the nurse must recognize that many of these groups have a unique focus or may vary within different meetings of the same organization. Clients or families who do not feel comfortable with one group should consider finding an alternative meeting or group rather than abandoning the self-help approach.

The nursing process with substance-abusing clients will vary, depending on the setting and the client's acknowledgment of the problem. The nursing care plan that follows describes a sample plan for a client with an unacknowledged problem of substance dependency.

❖ **NATIONAL RESOURCES FOR INDIVIDUALS AND FAMILIES WITH A CURRENT OR PAST PROBLEM WITH SUBSTANCE ABUSE**

Alcoholics Anonymous (A.A.)
  468 Park Avenue South
  New York, NY 10016
  (212) 686-1100

Al-Anon/Alateen
P.O. Box 862
Midtown Station
New York, NY 10018
(800) 344-2666

Adult Children of Alcoholics (A.C.O.A.)
  555 Madison Avenue
  New York, NY 10022
  (212) 351-2680

Cocaine Hotline
(800) COCAINE

Women for Sobriety
P.O. Box 618
Quakertown, PA 18951
(215) 536-8026

## ❖ NURSING CARE PLAN

**CLIENT:** Virginia Jones

**CLINICAL DESCRIPTION:** Virginia Jones is a 45-year-old attorney who was admitted to the medical unit with the diagnosis of acute pancreatitis. This is her second admission in 3 months with this diagnosis. She describes herself as a "social drinker" and denies any problems with alcohol.

**MEDICAL DIAGNOSIS:** Acute pancreatitis

**NURSING DIAGNOSIS:** Ineffective denial related to acknowledgment of substance abuse/dependency

| GOALS | INTERVENTIONS |
| --- | --- |
| Virginia will maintain physical safety throughout hospitalization. | ◆ Observe for early signs of withdrawal (agitation, tremors, diaphoresis).<br>◆ Prevent access to substances; monitor visitors and belongings.<br>◆ Assess for suicide potential. |
| Virginia will acknowledge dependence on alcohol as a coping mechanism. | ◆ Maintain a nonjudgmental, positive approach in interactions.<br>◆ Provide information about the disease process of alcoholism, emphasizing that alcoholism is a disease and not a moral problem or a lack of self-control.<br>◆ Assess Virginia's current use of alcohol, including amount, setting, and frequency (recognize that underestimation may occur). |
| Virginia will attend an appropriate counseling group. | ◆ Assist Virginia in identifying an appropriate group for counseling. Discuss pros and cons of self-help groups and professionally led groups. Identify if a group limited to women is appropriate.<br>◆ Determine if Virginia is willing to be visited by a recovering alcoholic while in the acute hospital. Identify reasons for resistance. |

*Continued.*

## ❖   NURSING CARE PLAN—cont'd

### EVALUATION

On a short-term basis Virginia expresses recognition that she depends on alcohol as a way to "relax" after a busy day and usually drinks from the time she gets home until she falls into bed. She states that her past attempts at controlling her drinking have failed and that she needs the support of other people with the same problem. She is visited by a woman from Women for Sobriety and agrees to attend a meeting. On a long-term basis, Virginia abstains from alcohol and other psychoactive substances.

Although only some nurses are in a position to assess, diagnose, and intervene with individuals and families who are dependent on illicit drugs, all nurses have frequent contact with people who are dependent on legal substances such as nicotine and caffeine. Despite the fact that nurses are seen by the public as highly credible health professionals, there is little in the literature in regard to nursing interventions with individuals who are dependent on nicotine and caffeine. Exceptions to this lack of information are the studies by Wewars (1988, 1989) that discuss postcessation stressors and cigarette craving among former smokers. Nursing should seize the opportunity to incorporate smoking and caffeine assessment tools into data bases since nurses can easily obtain pertinent information about client history, reasons for such dependence, level of dependence, withdrawal symptoms, social support, and perceived stress levels. Based on this assessment data, effective cessation interventions could be designed and implemented congruent with nursing's mission of fostering health-promoting behaviors.

### Evaluation

Evaluating successful outcomes with substance-abusing clients involves both a short- and a long-term perspective. On a short-term basis, the client's acknowledgment of a problem and attendance at appropriate meetings would indicate beginning goal attainment. However, as previously noted, most clients experience difficulty in abstaining from psychoactive substances, and relapse rates after 1 year are as high as 85% (Hunt, Barnett, & Branch, 1971). It may also be difficult to measure successful outcomes if the person is motivated to falsify his or her use of substances if criminal activity is involved or if his or her job is in jeopardy. Long-term success therefore is best measured by lifestyle changes and the development of new coping skills. The person must develop a supportive network of friends and family and learn to spend his or her time in healthy, constructive activities.

### ❖ SUMMARY

Substance abuse and dependence are preventable contributors to premature death and disability. Commonly abused substances include nicotine, narcotics, alcohol, cocaine and crack, amphetamines, hallucinogens, PCP, and marijuana. Substance abuse and dependence are disorders that are complex, multidimensional, and motivated by a variety of factors. Understanding the motivations, behaviors, and treatments of individuals and families who are affected by substance abuse and dependence is a significant challenge facing all professional nurses, regardless of their clinical setting.

## ❖ APPLYING KNOWLEDGE TO PRACTICE

1. Describe a client for whom you have cared who had a substance-abuse problem. What interventions were particularly effective? What specific problems did you encounter? How did the substance abuse affect the family?

2. Many nurses use the substances of tobacco and caffeine. Do you think this is a problem? How might it interfere with health teaching?

3. Some experts in the field have suggested that all illicit substances should be legalized and dispensed in clinics as a way to eliminate the criminal activity involved in the profits from the sales of illicit drugs. Do you agree with this approach? Debate the issue, with people taking both sides of the argument.

## REFERENCES

American Psychiatric Association (1987). *Diagnostic & Statistical Manual of Mental Disorders III R.* (3rd ed.). Washington D.C. APA.

Arif, A., & Westermeyer, J. (1988). *Manual of Drug and Alcohol Abuse.* New York: Plenum.

Carruth, G., & Pugh, J. B. (1982). Grieving the loss of alcohol. A crisis in recovery. *Journal of Psychosocial Mental Health Nursing, 20*(18), 18-21.

Compton, P. (1989). Drug abuse: A self-care deficit. *Journal of Psychosocial Nursing. 27*(3), 22-26.

Ghodse, H. (1989). *Drugs and addictive behavior.* Boston: Blackwell Scientific Publications.

Gold, M., & Giannini, A. (1989). Cocaine and Cocaine Addiction. In A. Giannini & A. Slaby, (Eds). *Drugs of abuse.* Oradell, N.J.: Medical Economics Books.

Haack, M., & Hughes, T., (1989). *Addiction in the nursing profession.* New York: Springer.

House, M. (1990). Cocaine. *American Journal of Nursing. 90*(4), 41-45.

Hunt, W. A., Barnett, L. W., & Branch, L. G. (1971). Relapse rates in addiction programs. *Journal of Clinical Psychology. 27,* 455-456.

Jacobs, M. R., & Fehr, K. O. (1987). *Drugs and drug abuse: A reference text.* Alcohol and Drug Addiction Research Foundation. Toronto.

Khantzian, E. (1985). The self-medication hypothesis of addictive disorders: Focus on heroin and cocaine dependence. *The American Journal of Psychiatry. 142*(11), 1259-1264.

Klahr, A., Roehrich, H., Miller, N. (1989). Marijuana. In A Giannini & A. Slaby, (Eds.). *Drugs of Abuse.* Oradell, N.J.: Medical Economics Books.

Lichtenstein, E. (1979). Social learning, smoking, and substance abuse. *NIDA Research Monograph Series. 23:*114-127.

Marlatt, G. A., & Gordon, J. R. (1980). Determinants of relapse: Implications for the maintenance of behavior change. In P. O. Davidson & S. M. Davidson (Eds.). *Behavioral medicine: changing health lifestyles.* New York: Brunner/Mazel.

McCoy, S., Rice, M., & McFadden, K. (1981). PCP intoxication. Psychiatric issues of nursing care. *Journal of Psychosocial Mental Health Nursing. 19*(17), 17-23.

Milkman, H., & Frosch, W. (1973). On the preferential abuse of heroin and amphetamine. *Journal of Nervous and Mental Disorders. 156,* 242-248.

Mittleman, H. & Mittleman, R., Elser, B. (1984). Cocaine. *American Journal of Nursing. 84,* 1092-1094.

Moreines, R. (1989). The Psychedelics. In A. Giannini & A. Slaby, (Eds.). *Drugs of Abuse.* Oradell, N.J.: Medical Economics Books.

Smith, J. (1983). Diagnosing alcoholism. *Hospital and Community Psychiatry. 34*(11), 1017-1021.

Twerski, A. (1983). Early intervention in alcoholism: Confrontational techniques. *Hospital and Community Psychiatry. 34*(11), 1027-1030.

U.S. Department Health and Human Services (1988). *The health consequences of smoking: nicotine addiction.* Rockville, Md., U. S. Government Printing Office.

Vandegaer, F. (1989). Cocaine: The deadliest addiction. *Nursing 89 19*(2), 72-73.

Wewars, M. E. (1988). The role of post-cessation factors in tobacco abstinence: stressful events and coping responses. *Addictive Behaviors. 13,* 297-302.

Wewars, M. E., & Gonyon, D. (1989). Cigarette craving during the immediate postcessation period. *Applied Nursing Research. 2,* 46-48.

# 24 Violence

Barbara Parker

## OBJECTIVES

*At the completion of this chapter, the reader will be able to:*

♦ Describe selected theories on the cause of violent behavior.

♦ Describe common responses of people who have survived a violent incident.

♦ Identify appropriate nursing interventions in working with survivors of several types of violence.

Violence and potential violence are major stressors for individuals, families, and communities. Although most registered nurses have some awareness of the impact of family violence, in reality nurses confront violence or potential violence in almost every area of practice. Violence and abuse are not new concerns but are now recognized as a public health problem (Surgeon General's Workshop on Violence and Public Health Report, 1986).

Historically, the two leading causes of early or premature death have been infectious diseases and violence. Through the use of antibiotics, improved nutrition, sanitation, and education, premature deaths from infectious diseases have greatly decreased. Violence, however, "has defied the best minds in health, politics, religion and law enforcement and has often appeared to be inevitable" (Foege, 1986).

Violence is a major influence in America and is reflected in the health care system when victims are cared for in emergency rooms, intensive care units, and psychiatric units. The management of violence between individuals and within families is one of the most difficult challenges facing nursing today.

The concept of violence must also be addressed from the perspective of the nurse. The fear of violence can be a major factor in a nurse's choice of work settings, specialty area, and hours of employment. This chapter focuses on violence and aggressive behavior as it affects clients and families, staff, and the nurse.

Violence as a concept is sometimes difficult for health professionals to study for several reasons. First, thinking about violence sometimes reminds people of painful personal experiences or of their own potential vulnerability. With 16% to 20% of married women being physically abused by their husbands (Straus, Gelles, & Steinmetz, 1980) and 1.5 million children per year experiencing maltreatment (U.S. Department of Health and Human Services, 1988), many nurses have personal experiences that may or may not be resolved. In addition, thinking about rape or sexual assault may evoke powerful feelings of fear and vulnerability within the nurse, especially if the nurse is a woman.

Second, thoughts of violence and aggression evoke fear and repugnance that may promote the use of denial. Lion (1987, p. 882) suggests that violence is the dark side of mental illness and that "rather than call attention to patients who would be better off in jail, clinicians prefer to focus their energy on treating the nobler entities of depression or schizophrenia." Nurses who have worked to establish group homes or halfway houses in communities find that the potential for violence is a major fear and hindrance in community acceptance, even though violent clients are generally ineligible for community placement.

Because violence is relatively unusual, there is some tendency to ignore or minimize it. Unfortunately, however, recent epidemics of drug abuse, especially of crack cocaine, which seems to intensify violent behavior, makes the issue of violence one that can no longer be ignored in nursing.

Interpersonal violence is generally conceptualized as an interaction between individual factors and factors within the society. Societal factors promoting violence include societal norms legitimizing the use of violence, economic conditions (especially poverty and unemployment), and the prevalence of violence in the media. Individual factors that may lead to ongoing violent behaviors include the person's past experiences, especially victimization or having inappropriate role models as a child, substance abuse, and psychiatric or organic diseases.

Several questions about violence and aggressive behavior are unanswered. Are children born aggressive or do they learn aggressiveness? Is the potential for violence innate? Is violent behavior simply a lack of impulse control? Can violent reactions be controlled? Violence and violent behavior have been studied by individuals in widely divergent disciplines, generating a number of theories on the causes, con-

sequences, and prevention of violence and aggressive behavior.

## ❖ FACTORS CAUSING VIOLENCE
### Temperature-Aggression Theory

One mode of inquiry into violent behavior has examined the effects of temperature on aggressive behavior and violence. This question has been studied for more than 80 years because police officials noticed an increase in violent crimes during hot weather. Anderson (1989) recently published a review article examining and summarizing a vast number of studies. He concluded that "Clearly, hot temperatures produce increases in aggressive motives and tendencies. Hotter regions of the world have more aggression, . . . hotter years, quarters of years, seasons, months and days all yield relatively more aggressive behaviors such as murders, rapes, assaults, riots and wife beating." An interesting component of the temperature-aggression research is that, although field studies show a direct relationship, laboratory studies have inconsistent findings. Anderson speculates that the differences are related to issues of internal validity in experimental studies. Specifically, individuals in an uncomfortably hot laboratory setting may recognize that aggression is being tested and behave differently from individuals in a normal temperature room.

The temperature-aggression theory has implications for nursing in the prevention of aggressive behaviors in an inpatient setting. Since temperature is a factor of milieu, these studies indicate the importance of keeping the unit temperature at a cool setting. Nurses in the community might also increase their vigilance for themselves during hot weather and in screening for victims.

### The Cycle of Violence

A pervasive finding in research on violence and violent behaviors is the concept of a cycle of violence. Specifically, children who are abused or who witness abuse become violent and abusive adults. Although several theories have been postulated about this phenomenon, the most enduring is the social learning theory, in which violence is viewed as a learned behavior.

Social learning postulates that a child learns to be violent in the family setting in which a violent parent has been taken as a role model. In this perspective violence and victimization are learned behaviors as a result of exposure to violence in childhood. This exposure teaches both the means and the approval of violence, for children who witness violence not only learn specific aggressive behaviors but also acquire the belief that violence is a legitimate way to solve problems. When frustrated or angry as an adult, the individual relies on this learned behavior and responds with violence.

Social learning theory was first applied to child abuse when it was noted that many child abusers were themselves abused as children (Kempe & Helfer, 1980). A number of authors have also examined this process with wife abuse, noting the incidence of violence in the family of both the survivors and the abusers (Parker & Schumacher, 1977). An extensive literature review conducted by Hotaling and Sugerman (1986) noted that witnessing parental violence during childhood or adolescence was one of the strongest risk factors for the abuse of wives in adulthood. To date there is limited empirical evidence of intergenerational transmission of violence in elder abuse. Pillemer and Suitor (1988), however, postulate that elder abuse could be the result of formerly abused children displaying both retaliatory and imitative behavior or of their modeling the behavior observed between their parents and grandparents. Many treatment modalities, especially cognitive approaches, are based on the social learning model that states that violent reactions can be unlearned and replaced with constructive responses to conflict.

Recently Widom (1989) studied the cycle of violence and all criminal behavior. This study, with a prospective design, examined criminal arrest records of adults who had been identified as abused or neglected as a child by the court system 20 years before the time of data collection. When compared to nonabused controls matched on sex, age, race, family socioeconomic conditions, neighborhood, and school, the adult who had been abused as a child had significantly more arrests as a juvenile and as an adult and a greater number of total offenses. Widom concluded that "early childhood victimization has demonstrable, long-term consequences for delinquency, adult criminality, and violent criminal behavior" (p. 164). Thus the cycle of violence is an issue in both family and stranger assaults. These findings validate the importance of aggressively intervening with clients in ongoing violence as a method of primary prevention for the future.

## Alcohol and Drug Use

The relationship between substance use and abuse and violence has been the subject of much speculation. Victims of family violence frequently report concurrent substance abuse by the abuser. However, most researchers deny that substance abuse is a direct causative factor in violence because it does not meet the criteria of stability, consensus, and consistency. That is, people who abuse alcohol are not consistently violent, and people who are violent are not always intoxicated. Instead, it has been suggested that rather than acting violent because one is drunk, the person uses alcohol as a means of deviance disavowal (Berk et al, 1983). In this perspective drinking provides a socially acceptable reason for engaging in otherwise inappropriate behaviors, which the aggressor can later excuse by claiming that he or she was intoxicated. Family and friends may also attribute the conduct to the effects of alcohol, which to some extent mitigates the degree of blame. An additional relationship is that for some people

the use of alcohol or drugs reduces fear or inhibitions and creates a lessened perception of
the impact of their behavior.

Cross-cultural studies suggest that behavior
while drinking varies from culture to culture. In
societies in which it is believed that alcohol is a
disinhibitor, people become disinhibited. If
they believe it is a depressant, they become depressed when drinking. If people in the United
States believe that normal rules of behavior are
suspended when one is drinking, people will
act in an antisocial manner (Gelles & Cornell,
1985).

Recently Lenord and Jacob (1988) conducted an extensive literature review of the relationship between alcohol abuse and family violence. They concluded that there was some
evidence implicating alcohol use and alcoholism in marital violence, although the evidence
related to child abuse was much weaker. In addition, with marital violence, confounding variables such as the stress of alcoholism on the
family system or familial expectations that
drinking will increase aggressive behavior have
not been adequately controlled in research
studies.

## ❖ WORKING WITH VIOLENT CLIENTS

Perhaps the most difficult challenge a nurse
experiences is working with a violent or aggressive client. In general, psychiatric and drug-
abusing clients are the most aggressive as a
group; however, violence is also a risk with alcoholic, confused, or elderly clients.

Winger et al (1987) in a study of 101 clients in a Veterans Administration long-term
care unit found that 84% of nursing home clients and 66% of intermediate care clients had
aggressive behaviors that endangered themselves or others. Carmel and Hunter (1989)
studied staff injuries from inpatient violence at
a state forensic hospital and found a rate of injury to nursing staff of 16 injuries per 100 nursing staff. Most injuries occurred when nursing

staff were containing or attempting to control a
violent client. The remaining injuries were the
result of direct client attacks. Carmel and
Hunter found that those most likely to be injured were recently hired, male nursing staff.

Morrison (1989) tested theoretical causal
factors contributing to psychiatric client violence. The nursing framework examined variables identified from a prior qualitative study
and psychiatric nurses' prior experiences with
violent clients. Morrison reported that demographic variables predicting client violence
were the length of stay (possibly a measure of
chronicity), a history of violence toward others,
and the client's diagnosis. Clients with psychotic symptomatology such as hallucinations
or delusions were not violent, but substance-
abusing clients were. A nursing management
variable that was significant in predicting violence was inconsistency in enforcing social
rules such as those related to smoking or visitors. Because this was not an experimental
study, however, this finding could be attributed
to the nurse's decision not to enforce a social
rule if the client was agitated or upset and the
nurse's belief that rigid adherence would further provoke the client. As noted by Morrison,
nursing must continue to develop a body of
knowledge on this important aspect of care.

Recently research on the incidence of assaultive client behaviors, including antecedent
conditions, has been facilitated by the use of
videotape recordings of the dayroom in psychiatric settings (Brizer et al, 1988). The use of
videotaping has advantages in increasing detection rates when compared to official incident
reports and in increasing the ability to analyze
behaviors occurring in an emotionally charged,
rapidly changing situation. In addition, inter-
rater reliability can be established in terms of
environmental and social antecedents by re-
playing the event in a neutral environment. This
methodology has potential for nursing research
directed toward increasing understanding of violent client behavior and differentiating be-

tween interventions that are effective and those that escalate the situation.

Managing aggressive clients is primarily a nursing responsibility. When aggression is controlled, there is increased quality of life for the client, safety for the staff and other clients, and a reduction in employee injuries. Most registered nurses will have studied the management of violent and aggressive clients in their basic psychiatric nursing education, so this chapter only briefly reviews critical aspects of this issue.

Registered nurses working with violent clients often work in a supervisory capacity, directing the care of others. This makes an understanding of violence even more critical because the supervisor's attitudes and beliefs about violent clients will be reflected by the entire nursing staff. In addition, when client altercations occur, the supervisor is usually summoned and must manage the situation in a professional manner.

Several violence management programs are available to train staff members in the management of aggressive clients. These programs include instructions on verbal "talk down" techniques, escape procedures such as escaping from a choke hold, and physical restraint techniques. Nurses working with violent and aggressive clients should consider knowing these techniques as important as the ability to do cardiopulmonary resuscitation.

The best nursing interventions for managing assaultive behaviors are anticipation and prevention. Some violent attacks occur impulsively and without warning. Often, however, the client will give cues that violence is about to erupt. Agitation, verbal threats, and gestures should be taken seriously and should be viewed as pleas for help when the client fears losing control.

In addition, with newly admitted clients, performing a thorough nursing assessment will give indicators of clients who may be prone to violent attacks. Assessment should ascertain any past history of assaultive behaviors, arrests, or criminal activities. Clients with past or current alcohol or drug abuse should also be carefully observed for signs of potential violence. Additional questions to probe for potential violence would include inquiries on how clients relieve stress or what they do when they are angry or upset. A sample care plan for a potentially violent client follows.

## ❖ MANAGEMENT OF AN AGGRESSIVE CLIENT

Aggressive clients frequently evoke fear in the nursing and ancillary staff and must be managed in a direct and immediate manner. There are several guidelines to remember in intervening with a violent or agitated client. One of the most important considerations is that adequate help must be available before interventions are attempted. This does not necessarily mean that the client is surrounded by a group of attendants, but adequate numbers of personnel must be visible and available for immediate assistance if necessary.

Maintaining a distance of at least an arm's length will avoid territorial intrusion into the client's space and may protect the nurse from unexpected blows. Touching the client in any way, including a touch intended to be calming, should be avoided because the client may misinterpret any moves as threatening. The tone of voice should be calm but firm, assuring the client that the nurse is in control.

If particular people or objects appear to be threatening to the client, they should be removed. The most important consideration in the entire process is to strengthen the client's ability to control himself or herself by whatever method is necessary. At the same time, the principle of least restrictiveness is important. This means that efforts at control must first include verbal persuasion, and these attempts must be documented. When verbal techniques are insufficient to control the situation, the use of restraints, medications, or seclusion may be required.

## ❖  NURSING CARE PLAN

**CLIENT:**  William Jones

**MEDICAL DIAGNOSIS:**  History of cocaine use

**NURSING DIAGNOSIS:**  Potential for violence related to history of drug abuse

| GOALS | INTERVENTIONS |
|---|---|
| William will control his aggressive outbursts with assistance from others. | ◆ Closely observe for early signs of agitation or withdrawal.<br>◆ Acknowledge William's feelings (e.g., "you are having a rough time").<br>◆ Set clear limits on William's behavior, using concise, clear terminology.<br>◆ Establish a unit environment that is quiet and nonthreatening to William. |
| William will increase his ability to verbally express his needs. | ◆ When he is not agitated, encourage William to identify and discuss his response to various activities.<br>◆ Assist William in identifying his feelings and describing both positive and negative feelings.<br>◆ Provide positive feedback for all of William's attempts to discuss his feelings verbally. |

### EVALUATION

With close monitoring by others, William controls aggressive outbursts as evidenced by a decrease in the number and intensity of verbal and physical attacks. William becomes increasingly more able to state verbally when he is feeling upset and to undertake alternative activities (e.g., physical exercise) when he recognizes that he is upset.

## ❖ FAMILY VIOLENCE

In addition to working with violent and aggressive clients in the hospital and community, registered nurses must have thorough understanding of family violence. It is now recognized that, regardless of the setting, registered nurses work with victims (survivors) of family violence. Although the health care system has recognized family violence since the 1960s when child abuse was identified as a health care problem, the problem is far from being solved, and indeed, often less than totally comprehensive, sensitive care is provided to families experiencing violence.

One issue to confront is the terminology used to describe people who have experienced violence. Traditionally, the term *victim* has been used, along with discussions of *syndromes*. These labels serve to distance the nurse from the person who has experienced abuse as we search for differences between ourselves and the survivors to decrease our feelings of vulnerability. Therefore in this chapter the term *survivor* is used as an attempt to emphasize that the person who has experienced abuse has many strengths and coping strategies that can be incorporated into the plan of care.

### Child Abuse

The form of family violence that was recognized earliest within the health professional literature was physical abuse to children. Although violence to children was considered a social problem in the previous century, it was not until the 1940s that it was first identified as a medical problem, indeed a unique "syndrome." In 1962 the classical article by C. Henry Kempe and his associates, "The Battered Child Syndrome," first brought sustained interest to the problem of physical abuse to children. By the end of the 1960s every state had enacted legislation mandating the reporting of suspected child abuse and neglect (JAMA,

1985). Under current regulations nurses and any other professionals providing services to children are required to report suspected incidents of child abuse and neglect.

There are many forms of abuse to children, including physical abuse or battering, emotional abuse, sexual abuse, and neglect. Although research on the many forms of child abuse has been extensive, much is still unknown about the causes, treatment, and prevention of child abuse.

The most enduring theoretical framework on the causes of child abuse is the Helfer and Kempe (1976) model of child abuse and neglect. The model incorporates both psychological and social factors and provides a more comprehensive approach than traditional medical models. The model hypothesizes that three factors are present in child abusing families: (1) a special parent, (2) a special child, and (3) stress.

*Special parent* refers to characteristics in the caregiver that generate a proneness to use violence as a way to alleviate stress or communicate displeasure. The adult may be immature (indeed may be an adolescent), may have unrealistic expectations of the child (Egeland, 1980; Fesbach, 1980), or may have been abused himself or herself as a child (Burgess, 1984). Numerous studies have suggested the intergenerational transmission of violence (Perry, Wells, & Doran, 1983; Straus, 1980), and indeed a history of victimization appears to place a parent at risk for being an abuser. However, other controlled studies (Starr, 1982) examining parental punishment history and current child abuse found no differences between abusive and nonabusive parents. Simply experiencing abuse as a child does not totally determine an adult's later behaviors. Many people who were abused as children are able to avoid violence with their own children. Straus (1980) suggests that the key factor may be the age at which the child was abused or which parent was abusive. Experiencing abuse from a father at age 4 may be a totally different experience from experiencing abuse from one's mother as an adolescent.

*Special child* refers to characteristics of the child that place it at increased risk for abuse, and in most child-abusing families abuse is directed to one "special child" (Millor, 1981). These characteristics include children with handicaps (Nesbit & Karagianis, 1982), learning disabilities, aggressive behaviors or hyperactivity, and chronic health problems (Lynch, 1975; Sherod et al, 1984). Additional features include children who are unwanted or unplanned or who may remind the parent of a disliked relative or an unhappy time of his or her life. This is not to imply that some children "deserve to be abused" but that each child brings certain self-characteristics to the parent-child interaction that interrelate with the parent's self-characteristics (Millor, 1981).

*Stress* is a subjective phenomena that is defined by the family and may or may not be apparent to the nurse. Some known stressors include unemployment (Steinberg, Catalino, & Dooley, 1981), poverty (Straus et al, 1980; Zuravin, 1989), health problems of other family members, and marital discord. Other authors have questioned the direct relationship between stress and increasing rates of child abuse (Pagelow, 1984; Straus, 1980) and have noted that the presence of resources and other mediating factors must also be considered when indicating stress as a causal factor in child abuse. Egeland (1980) found that high stress alone did not differentiate between abusing and nonabusing mothers but mothers who were both highly stressed and abusive were often unaware of the difficulties and demands of being a parent. Seagull (1987) also found that parents of abused children tended to perceive their children more negatively and derived little emotional satisfaction from the child.

The three factors seem to work together to set the stage for potential physical abuse or neglect. However, to date research has not indicated any factors that are present in all abusing and absent in all nonabusing parents (Starr, 1988).

Although physical abuse and sexual abuse of children and adolescents are dramatic and frequently recognizable behaviors, psychological abuse and neglect are important considerations to include in nursing assessment and interventions. Psychological abuse includes behaviors such as unrealistic expectations beyond the child's growth and development (e.g., unrealistic expectations about toilet training), belittling, teasing, calling the child demeaning names, and blaming the child for family problems caused by other family members. Child neglect includes withholding necessary food, shelter, clothing, and health care. An important consideration, however, in determining child neglect is to not confuse the profound effects of poverty and homelessness with child neglect. As in all forms of child abuse, the nurse who has questions about potential abuse or neglect should seek the advice of other nurses and health care professionals.

**Sexual abuse of children and adolescents.** Sexual abuse is defined as the involvement of children and adolescents in sexual activities they do not fully comprehend and to which they do not freely consent (Feinauer, 1989). Sexual abuse results in both long- and short-term problems. Short-term physical symptoms include venereal disease or infection; vaginal or rectal bleeding, itching, or soreness; recurrent urinary tract infections; or pregnancy. The presence of any of these symptoms in a child or adolescent should cue the nurse to assess further for sexual abuse, even if it is not readily disclosed by the child. Short-term emotional indicators include behavioral changes, difficulty sleeping, school problems, or chronic fears or unhappiness.

The long-term effects of sexual abuse as a child include sexual problems, difficulty trusting others, anxiety and panic attacks, depression, and substance abuse. A recent study by Feinauer (1989) of adult women who had been sexually abused as a child found that women experienced more emotional distress and long-term effects when the perpetrator was a person who was known and trusted by them. Feinauer found that the kinship relationship between the victim and the abuser was less important in creating distress than the emotional bond the victim felt toward the perpetrator. Thus a critical factor apparently is the violation of the child's trust, as well as the physical trauma.

**Nursing assessment of child abuse.** Nursing assessment of actual or potential child abuse begins with a thorough history and physical examination. Gathering a history of child abuse can be a stressful experience for both the nurse and the family. It is therefore essential that the nurse first examine his or her own values and past experiences to maintain a therapeutic and nonjudgmental clinical approach.

In obtaining a history an honest, trusting environment that is not intended to punish or shame either the child or parent must be established (Campbell & Humphreys, 1984). If the nurse recognizes that most abusive parents are genuinely embarrassed about their behavior and would like assistance in developing alternative approaches to discipline, an environment can be established that will facilitate honesty and sharing. The setting for the interview must be quiet, private, and uninterrupted.

In general, the child and the adult(s) should be separated during the initial interview. This decision is dependent on the child's age and other extenuating circumstances. The nurse should honestly describe the purpose of the interview, the type of questions being asked, and the subsequent physical examination. The approach must be calm and supportive because both the child and the family will be affected by uneasiness.

The interview with the parent(s) can begin with a discussion of the problem that first brought the child to a health care facility. During this discussion particular attention should be paid to the parent's understanding of the problem, discrepancies in the stories, and the parent's emotional responses. The interview can then be expanded to discussions of how the parent "disciplines" the child or how often he or she spanks the child. The initial interview is not the time to confront the abuser directly because measures must be taken to document thoroughly and report the abuse to ensure the child's safety.

When child abuse is suspected, the nurse must report his or her suspicions to protective services. An investigation by the state protective service agency is legally mandated and also serves to reinforce to the family the seriousness of the problem. When protective services are involved, the nurse should explain to families precisely what will happen in an investigation and the amount of time involved.

All nurses must be aware of how protective services work in the community in which they practice. It is extremely valuable to know personally the professionals at the agency to remain informed about the policies and reporting protocols and to ensure successful coordination and continuity.

## Wife Abuse

Domestic violence between adults is generally referred to as spouse abuse, regardless of the marital status of the couple. A distinction that must be clear, however, is that the problem is primarily abuse of women. Although some authors have contended that husband abuse is as prevalent as wife abuse (Steinmetz & Lucca, 1988), numerous other authors (Campbell & Humphreys, 1984; Dobash & Dobash, 1988; Stark & Flitcraft, 1988) have argued that husband abuse and wife abuse are not comparable. Studies of husband abuse do not examine the important issues of self-defense, resulting injuries, provocation, and differences in physical strength. Therefore the focus of this section is wife abuse.

The experience of being abused by a partner in an intimate relationship has profound effects on a woman's health, her children, her career, and perceptions of herself. Women can be abused by their partner at any point in the relationship; however, certain times are particularly dangerous. For example, most survivors of abuse report that their partner was not violent while they were dating. The violence generally begins after the couple is living together or is legally married or the woman becomes pregnant. Although no controlled studies currently document that pregnancy places women at increased risk for abuse, nursing research documents the incidence of wife abuse during pregnancy and the effect on maternal and infant health.

Bullock et al (1989) interviewed 593 women in the postpartum setting and reported that the women experienced blows to the abdomen, breasts, and genitals and sexual assault during their pregnancy. In addition, Bullock found that the battered women were four times more likely to deliver a low–birth-weight baby than women who did not experience abuse during their pregnancy.

**The experience of abuse for the survivor.** In working with survivors of abuse, the registered nurse must understand the process of abuse and victimization and how it subtly influences the woman's feelings and perceptions. Landenburger (1988) conducted a series of interviews with abused women and described four stages of the violent relationship and the differing themes involved in each stage of entrapment.

In the *binding,* or initial, stage of the relationship the focus is on establishing the relationship and possibly a family. In this phase the woman attempts to ignore or minimize warning signals of potential or actual violent incidents.

As problems occur, the woman tries to change her behavior to "make things right." As these attempts prove futile, she begins to question her own abilities as a wife or mother and wonders why she is unable to stop the violence. She may think about leaving the abuser but still believes that she can somehow stop the violence.

The second stage of the process, *enduring,* continues the process of self-blame and acceptance of responsibility for the abuse. She may begin to hide the signs of abuse, lose hope, and begin to feel worthless as a person. This stage can last anywhere from months to years.

The third stage, *disengaging,* often begins as the woman begins to realize that she is not alone in her problem, and she begins to identify with other women. She may seek help as she begins to gain enough confidence in herself to think about leaving the relationship. Gondoff and Fisher (1988) note that help-seeking behaviors increase when there is an escalation in the amount of wife abuse, child abuse, and other antisocial behaviors (substance abuse, arrests) by the batterer.

In the *recovering* phase, the fourth stage, the woman gradually becomes more independent. She may have residual feelings of guilt or may grieve for the loss of her partner or the relationship. Campbell (1989) found that women leaving an abusive relationship experienced stress and grief over their decision to leave their partner. She also noted that a marriage without abuse takes as long as 4 years to dissolve and usually includes attempted reconciliations. However, when survivors of abuse grieve over the termination of the relationship or attempt a reconciliation, they may be labeled as pathological or masochistic.

Although not all women experience these phases sequentially or even remain in a violent relationship beyond the binding stage (Parker & Schumacher, 1977), this conceptualization of the process is useful in understanding the phenomena and developing interventions. Counseling the abused woman should take into account the stage in which she is and her perception and hopes for the relationship.

**Assessment of the abused woman.** Nursing assessment of women who have experienced abuse must be conducted privately and with assurances of confidentiality. Many women feel ashamed or responsible for the violence, and assessment must be approached in a nonjudgmental, gentle manner. At the same time the nurse should be direct in her questions because it is unfair to expect the woman to respond to indirect or oblique communication.

Often the registered nurse first encounters the survivor of abuse in the emergency department, outpatient department, or obstetrical clinic. Frequently the only way that abuse will

be discussed is if it is a routine part of the nursing assessment form. The question must be asked directly (see the questions listed in the box that follows, which were developed by the Nursing Research Consortium on Violence and Abuse). These assessment questions were developed primarily for use with pregnant women but could be adapted for any specialty area.

Assessing for abuse carries the responsibility for intervening following a positive response. At a minimum, all agencies should have referral sources available and information on the available legal and criminal options. In working with abused women the nurse must be aware of state reporting procedures and must be available to assist the woman in filing a report if she so requests. Since shelters and intervention programs are available in most areas,

❖ **ABUSE ASSESSMENT SCREEN**

1. Have you ever been emotionally or physically abused by your partner or someone important to you?  YES  NO
2. Within the last year, have you been hit, slapped, kicked, or otherwise physically hurt by someone?  YES  NO
   If YES, by whom _____
   Number of times _____
3. Since you have been pregnant, have you been hit, slapped, kicked, or otherwise physically hurt by someone?  YES  NO
   If YES, by whom _____
   Number of times _____
   Mark the area of injury on body map.

4. Within the last year, has anyone forced you to have sexual activities?  YES  NO
   If YES, by whom _____
   Number of times _____
5. Are you afraid of your partner or anyone you listed above?  YES  NO

information on local laws and ordinances can be determined by contacting these agencies. Most programs welcome the opportunity to provide continuing education programs for nurses because they recognize that many referrals are initiated through contact between abused women and registered nurses.

A common response is for the woman to report violence but attempt to minimize the frequency or severity of its occurrence. This may take the form of blaming herself, blaming alcohol use by herself or her partner, or asserting that the violence was a temporary aberration caused by family difficulties or unemployment. Kelly (1988) notes that "forgetting" or minimizing are effective coping strategies, especially if sexual abuse is involved. She points out that if the woman believes that others will not define her problem as seriously as she does, minimizing the event in her own mind will make her feel less alienated from others.

Recently several authors have studied racial and ethnic minority women and observed some characteristics that differ from the assessment of the abuse of white women. One characteristic of both black and Hispanic women is an increased reluctance to report abuse, especially if the nurse or therapist is from a different cultural group.

Torres (1987) reported that Hispanic women were more tolerant toward abuse than white women in her study and that acts such as hitting or verbal abuse had to occur more frequently with Hispanic women before they would seek services for the violence. In addition, Torres found that a Hispanic American woman is more sensitive to perceived criticisms of herself, her family, culture, and male relatives (including her husband). White (1985) notes that for African American women a sense of racial loyalty may make it more difficult to report violence, especially if she believes the information will be used to perpetuate racist views about African American men.

**Interventions with survivors of wife abuse.** The most important consideration in the initial assessment of the survivor of wife abuse is to determine the woman's safety. Violence usually escalates over time in both frequency and severity, and assessment must carefully determine the woman's current safety.

A related concern is the need to advise the woman that the interview itself is not necessarily providing documentation of the abuse. This knowledge may be especially important for women with language difficulties or others who do not understand the official system of reporting abuse.

Intervening with survivors of wife abuse can be a difficult experience for the nurse. As noted in the Campbell study (1989), women who are abused have as much difficulty terminating a relationship as women who have not experienced abuse. Often the woman will remain in the relationship, especially if her partner is remorseful or promises to change his behavior. The practitioner must remember that the woman wants only the violence to end, not necessarily to end the relationship. Women who remain in violent relationships require as much, if not more, support and counseling than those who leave.

Intervention with survivors of abuse may entail assistance to objectively evaluate the relationship and its inherent strengths and limitations. Because the woman may be in a state of intense confusion or feel conflicting loyalties, it is important for the nurse to use problem-solving and decision-making skills.

One approach is for the nurse and the survivor to brainstorm various options jointly. The options include remaining in the home and seeking help for herself and/or her spouse; remaining in the home and attempting to anticipate the violent attacks and to protect herself and her children; or leaving the relationship either temporarily or permanently. When a complete list has been generated, the nurse and client can jointly determine the positive and negative consequences of each option and select the best alternative. If the woman decides to remain in the relationship, intervention can focus on methods of recognizing imminent violence and ways of protecting herself and her children.

If (and when) the woman decides the situation is not going to change, she may be ready to make long-term decisions. At this point the practitioner can assist the woman with practical help such as providing a list of shelters for abused women and information on local police protection and available legal resources. For example, in many states an abused woman can obtain a restraining order from the police or have police protection while she is removing her belongings from the home. Once again, it is critical for the nurse to be aware of the local laws and services.

At this point the practitioner and woman will be making decisions such as when she should leave, where she will go, and which possessions she should take. In making these decisions the nurse must be cognizant of the beginning evidence that the most dangerous time for a woman in a violent relationship is after she has left the abuser. Women apparently are at higher risk for homicide after leaving a relationship than while enduring the violence. Therefore plans to leave must be carefully made to avoid last minute crisis decisions. Obtaining information on the potential for homicide using the Danger Assessment (Campbell, 1986) might also be considered. This instrument lists 16 risk factors for homicide and/or suicide such as the presence of a gun in the house, violence outside of the home, and an increase in the incidence and severity of the violent episodes.

Often the plan for leaving a violent relationship involves the use of a shelter for battered women. Shelters are available in every state and are an important source of temporary housing and counseling. However, in planning to use a shelter the nurse must also be aware of shelter limitations. Most shelters for abused women are overcrowded and have waiting lists. This means the woman cannot wait until the next crisis and expect to find space in a shelter. She must contact the shelter before leaving and place her name on the waiting list. If her home is too dangerous, she might need to make temporary arrangements with a friend or relative or a homeless shelter while calling the shelter daily to determine space availability.

## Elder Abuse

Elder abuse includes direct physical assaults, neglect, financial abuse, psychological abuse, or acts that violate the elder's right to self-determination. Although the phenomenon of elder abuse has been known for decades, it is the area of family violence that has received the least amount of research. Authors of review articles on elder abuse (Hudson & Johnson, 1987; Pillemer & Suitor, 1988) report that there are no reliable estimates of the prevalence of elder abuse and the causes of maltreatment are generally unidentified. Thus developing assessment techniques and effective interventions is extremely difficult. This chapter focuses on caretaker abuse of the elder, although it must be recognized that elder abuse is frequently spouse abuse.

Physical abuse of elders includes both acts of commission and omission. Elder abuse frequently involves a type of benign neglect as family members withhold needed personal or medical care. A cross-sectional survey of health care professionals indicated that passive neglect (inattention or isolation) was by far the most common form of elder abuse (Hickey & Douglass, 1981). Examples include leaving nonambulatory elders unattended for long periods of time or without needed services. Frequently this form of abuse occurs in families in which the needs of the elders exceed the capacity of the families' resources (e.g., in families in which all the adults are working or there are small children).

Active physical abuse includes direct blows or shoving the elder, tying the elder to a chair when the caretaker must leave the home or is otherwise occupied, or the misuse of medications. Frequently elders are oversedated in an attempt to make them more passive and manageable (Pollick, 1987).

Financial abuse includes both direct theft and the misuse of the elder's financial assets or property. Children may visit the elder to steal the monthly Social Security check and then physically or psychologically abuse the elder when he or she objects. Families with an elder in the home may rely on the elder's Social Security to provide for all the family members and keep the elder home even when institutionalization is indicated.

Psychological abuse includes verbal assaults and threats, provocation of fear, and isolation of the elder either physically or emotionally (Beck & Furguson, 1981). This abuse includes treating elders in a manner that diminishes their personal identity or dignity. Psychological abuse may be the result of the stress of caregiving expressed in the form of emotional outbursts toward the elder. Psychological abuse is particularly complex because it generally involves the interaction of parties who have established patterns of interactions over many years.

**Documenting elder abuse.** Documenting elder abuse is complicated by several factors. Since many frail elders are also subject to falls, the cause of bruises and injuries may be difficult to differentiate. In addition, since elders may be subject to forgetfulness because of decreased cerebral circulation, obtaining a history may be difficult. Complicating these conditions is the fear of many elders that reporting abuse may lead to retaliatory violence or an unwanted placement in a nursing home. Agencies may also be reluctant to report suspected abuse because of a lack of knowledge in identifying or dealing with the problem (Pollick, 1987).

Recent research on elder abuse has focused on the influence of stress on the caregivers, especially on those caring for frail or impaired elders. Bunting (1989) noted that caregivers experience stress from restrictions on time and freedom, from economic burdens, including curtailment of employment, and from adjusting to the changing roles and capabilities of the elder. These stressors are often perpetuated by inadequate support systems for the caregivers. Frequently the elder's needs compete with the available family resources of attention, time, energy, and money, and caretakers feel torn between the needs of their children and those of their parents. If this stressful situation is compounded by a family history of violence as a means of problem solving, elder abuse can occur.

Steinmetz (1988) conducted extensive interviews with 104 caregivers of elderly kin. She found that 23% reported using physically abusive methods at some time to control the elder. Statistical analysis identified seven significant variables in predicting physical abuse: (1) stress resulting from caring for a mobile but senile elder, (2) stress from emotional dependency, (3) total mobility dependency, (4) elders who used verbal abuse, (5) elders who refused to eat or take medications, (6) elders who called the police, and (7) elders who invaded the caretaker's privacy. Steinmetz notes that a confounding aspect of abuse of elders by adult children is that it is not always possible to separate the victim from the perpetuator. Her sample, described as "caring, thoughtful, loving children who felt duty bound to care for their elderly parent," felt overburdened and overstressed by elders who hit or slapped them, threw food or refused to eat, were verbally abusive, or manipulated the caretaker through the use of guilt.

The current lack of community support facilities such as adult day-care and respite services compounds the family stress.

Registered nurses will most likely encounter victims of elder abuse in emergency departments, outpatient clinics, or the community. Because many elders are reluctant to report abuse, assessment involves careful, sensitive questioning and thorough documentation. Because requirements for reporting suspected elder abuse vary from state to state, it is important for the registered nurse to know the local reporting procedures and referral agencies.

## ❖ RAPE AND SEXUAL ASSAULT

Rape and sexual assault are concerns for individuals, families, and the community. Sexual assaults against women and children, the most prevalent victims, result in physical trauma, psychic and spiritual disruptions, and deterioration of social relationships. In addition, the fear of rape and sexual assault has major consequences in the lives of women because they restrict their activities in attempts to ensure their safety. Victims of sexual assaults include women and men of all ages, social class, race, and occupations. Sexual assault causes a disruption in every aspect of the victim's life, including social activities, interpersonal relationships, employment, and career. Although it is recognized that males can be sexually assaulted and women can be sexual offenders, in this chapter the victim is referred to as *she* and the offender as *he.* However, men and young boys are also victimized, and assessment must not be limited to women.

*Sexual assault* is generally defined as forced perpetration of an act of sexual contact with another person without his or her consent. This definition includes the lack of consent resulting from the victim's cognitive or personality development, feelings of fear or coercion, or physical or verbal threats. Most authors agree that sexual assault is not a sexual act but is instead motivated by a desire to humiliate, defile, and dominate the victim. Sexual assault has occurred for centuries but is now recognized as a social and public health problem.

The concept of consent can be conceptualized as a continuum as seen in Fig. 24-1. This continuum demonstrates gradations in coercion, including bribery, taking advantage of one's position of power or trust in a relationship, or the victim's inability to consent freely.

Most cases of sexual assault do not occur between strangers. Marital rape has recently been recognized in most states, and child sexual abuse by family members, family friends, and caretakers is being reported in record numbers.

Marital rape is frequently reported concurrently with physical abuse. Campbell (1989) found that the majority of abused women in her study reported that their husbands believed it was their right to have sex whenever they wanted, including when the women were ill, had recently given birth, or were discharged from a hospital. The women in Campbell's study reported forced vaginal intercourse, anal intercourse, being hit, burned, or kicked during sex, having objects inserted into their vagina and anus, or being forced to perform sexual acts with animals or while their children were observing. Many women were threatened with weapons or were beaten when they refused to take part in these activities. Marital rape may be especially devastating for the victim because she often must continue to interact with the rapist because of her dependence on him. In addition, many victims do not seek health care or the support of family members or friends because of embarrassment or humiliation.

Rape and sexual assault are important to nursing because nurses treat victims in the hospital and the community and because they fear for their personal safety. Several aspects of the practice of nursing places nurses at an in-

## Sexual Behavior: The Force Continuum

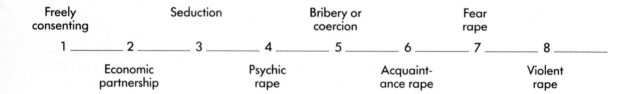

1. Freely Consenting: Partners with equal power mutually choosing sexual activity. Equal power means each partner has equal status, knowledge, and ability to consent. This includes one partner agreeing to engage in sexual activity, even if not interested, as expression of love and caring for the other person.

2. Economic Partnership. One person agrees to sexual activity as part of an economic agreement. The type of sexual behaviors permitted are mutually determined as part of the economic agreement.

3. Seduction. One party attempts to persuade the other to engage in sexual activities.

4. Psychic Rape. Assault to another person's dignity and self-respect such as verbal abuse, street harassment, or the portrayal of violence or pornography in the media.

5. Bribery or coercion. The use of emotional or psychological force to persuade the other to take part in sexual activities. This includes situations of unequal power between the individuals, especially when one person is in a position of authority.

6. Acquaintance rape. Sexual assault occurring when one party abuses the trust of a relationship and forces the other into sexual activities.

7. Fear rape. When one party engages in sexual activities out of fear of potential violence if she resists.

8. Violent rape. When violence is threatened or occurs. This includes forced sexual activity between spouses, acquaintances, or strangers.

Adapted from Stuart & Sundeen (1987).

❖❖ **Fig. 24-1**   Sexual behavior: the force continuum. *Principles and Practice of psychiatric nursing. St. Louis: C. V. Mosby.)*

creased risk for sexual assault by strangers: hours of employment, home-visiting in the community, and for some nurses, a reluctance to create a scene or defend themselves aggressively. In recent years nurses who were sexually assaulted in hospital parking lots or on hospital property have successfully sued the hospital for negligence in not providing adequate security (Regan, 1983).

People respond to sexual assault differently, depending on their past experiences, personal characteristics, amount and type of support received from significant others, health care providers, and the criminal justice system. Burgess (1985) describes a two-phased reac-

tion to sexual assault. The acute stage, immediately following the attack, is characterized by extreme confusion, fear, disorganization, and restlessness. Some victims, however, may mask these feelings and appear outwardly calm or subdued.

The second phase involves the long-term process of reorganization and generally begins several weeks after the attack. This phase may include intrusive thoughts recalling the traumatic event during the day and while asleep, and fears or phobias such as extreme fears of being alone, in a crowd, or traveling. After a sexual assault the victim frequently has a sense of living in a dangerous, unpredictable world and may become preoccupied with feelings of victimization and vulnerability. She may encounter difficulties in sexual relationships or in her ability to relate comfortably to men. Some victims develop secondary phobic reactions to people or situations that remind them of the attack. Coping strategies may include changing one's phone number or residence, talking with friends or family, or taking classes in self-defense.

### Nursing Care of the Victim of Sexual Assault

An important consideration in the treatment of victims of rape and sexual assault is the initial assessment. Although most nurses would quickly recognize the woman brought to the emergency department by the police following an attack by a stranger, many victims of sexual assault are not readily identifiable. Therefore, nursing assessments should include questions to determine current or prior sexual abuse. Since people have different definitions of rape, the assessment question must be broadly stated such as that suggested by Campbell (1989), "Has anyone ever forced you into sex that you did not wish to participate in?" This question may uncover other types of sexual trauma such as incest, date rape, or sexual abuse as a child. When the answer is affirmative, it can be gently followed with broad questions such as "Can you tell me more about it" or "How often has it happened." Often the response may be an embarrassed laugh or a hesitant or querying response. When this response occurs, the nurse can increase the client's comfort by explaining that the question is routinely included because it is not an uncommon occurrence and the nurse is available to assist the woman in obtaining legal or social services.

When assessment indicates that abuse has occurred, it cannot be ignored. As noted by Campbell (1989), disclosing sexual abuse is an indication of trust. If the nurse responds by immediately referring the client elsewhere, the message given is that the problem is too distasteful or delicate for the nurse to handle or that there are serious psychological implications. Thus assessment carries a responsibility for immediate intervention with nonjudgmental listening and psychological support. Later interventions may include referrals to survivors' groups, shelters for battered women (in instances of marital rape), or legal services.

### ❖ SUMMARY

Regardless of the setting, the practice of nursing is greatly influenced by violence and the threat of violence. Registered nurses must be prepared to intervene with violent clients, family members, and the survivors of past or current abuse.

---

### ❖ APPLYING KNOWLEDGE TO PRACTICE

1. What do you think about this chapter's terminology regarding the use of *survivor* versus *victim?* Do you agree with the author? Do you think this differentiation is true for all forms of violence?
2. Discuss experiences you have had working with survivors of abuse in the clinical setting. What nursing problems were the most difficult for you?
3. Have you ever been afraid of a client? How did you handle your fear?

**REFERENCES**

Anderson, C. (1989). Temperature and aggression: Ubiquitous effects of heat on occurrence of human violence. *Psychological Bulletin, 106*(1), 74-96. *Wife Abuse.* Newbury Park, Ca.: Sage.

Beck, C. & Ferguson, D. (1981). Aged abuse. *Journal of Gerontological Nursing, 7*(6), 333-336.

Berk, R., Berk, S., Loseke, D., & Rauma, D. (1983). Mutual combat and other family violence myths. In D. Finkelhor, R. Gelles, G. Hotaling, & M. Straus (Eds.). *The Dark Side of Families: Current Family Violence Research.* Beverly Hills, Ca.: Sage.

Bottom, W., & Lancaster, J. (1981). An ecological orientation toward human abuse. *Family and Community Health, 4,* 1-10.

Brizer, D., Crowner, M., Convit, A., & Volavka, J. (1988). Videotape recording of inpatient assaults: A pilot study. *American Journal of Psychiatry, 145,* 751-752.

Bullock, L., McFarlane, J., Bateman, L., & Miller, V. (1989). The prevalence and characteristics of battered women in a primary care setting. *The Nurse Practitioner, 14*(6), 47-52.

Bunting, S. (1989). Stress on caregivers of the elderly. *Advances in Nursing Science, 11*(2), 63-72.

Burgess, A. (1984). Intrafamilial sexual abuse. In J. Campbell & J. Humphries (Eds.). *Nursing Care of Victims of Family Violence,* Reston, Va: Reston.

Burgess, A. (1985). Rape trauma syndrome: A nursing diagnosis. *Occupational Health Nursing, 33*(8), 405-406, 419-422.

Campbell, J. & Humphreys, J. (1984). *Nursing Care of Victims of Family Violence,* Reston, Va.: Prentice-Hall.

Campbell, J. (1986). Nursing assessment for risk of homicide with battered women. *Advances in Nursing Science, 8*(4), 36-51.

Campbell, J., & Alford, P. (1989). The dark consequences of marital rape. *American Journal of Nursing, 89*(7), 946-949.

Carmel, H., & Hunter, M. (1989). Staff injuries from inpatient violence. *Hospital and Community Psychiatry, 40*(1), 41-46.

Dobash, R. E. & Dobash, R. P. (1988). Research as social action: the struggle for battered women. In K. Yllo & M. Bogard (Eds.). *Feminist Perspectives on Wife Abuse,* Newbury Park, Ca.: Sage.

Egeland, B., Breitenbucher, M., & Rosenberg, D. (1980). Prospective study of the significance of life stress in the etiology of child abuse. *Journal of Consulting and Clinical Psychology, 48,* 195-205.

Feinauer, L. (1989). Comparison of long-term effects of child abuse by type of abuse and by relationship of the offender to the victim. *American Journal of Family Therapy, 17*(1), 48-56.

Fesbach, S. (1980). Child abuse and the dynamics of human aggression and violence. In G. Gerber, C. Ross, & E. Zeigler (Eds.), *Child abuse: An agenda for action,* New York: Oxford University Press.

Foege, W. (1986). Violence and public health. In *Surgeon General's Workshop on Violence and Public Health Report.* (DHHS Publication No. HRS-D-MC 86-1, Washington D.C: U.S. Government Printing Office.

Gelles, R., & Cornell, C. (1985). *Intimate Violence in Families,* Beverly Hills, Ca.: Sage.

Gondolf, E. & Fisher, E. (1988). *Battered women as survivors: an alternative to treating learned helplessness,* Lexington, Ky.: D. C. Heath.

Helfer, R., & Kempe, C. H. (1976). *Child abuse and neglect,* Cambridge, Mass.: Harper & Row.

Hickey, T. & Douglass, R. L. (1981). Mistreatment of the elderly in the domestic setting: An exploratory study. *American Journal of Public Health, 71,* 500-507.

Hotaling, G. T. & Sugerman, D. (1986). An analysis of risk markers in husband to wife violence: The current state of knowledge. *Violence and Victims, 1,* 101-124.

*Journal of the American Medical Association* (1985). AMA diagnostic and treatment guidelines concerning child abuse and neglect. *254*(6), 796-800.

Kelly, L. (1988). How women define their experiences of violence. In K. Yllo & M. Bograd (Eds.). *Feminist Perspectives on Wife Abuse.* Newbury Park, Ca.: Sage.

Kempe, C. H. & Helfer, R. (1980). *The battered child,* Chicago: University of Chicago Press.

Kempe, C., Silverman, F., & Stelle, B. (1962). The battered child syndrome. *JAMA, 181,* 17-24.

Landenburger, K. (1988). Conflicting realities of women in abusive relationships. *Communicating Nursing Research, 21,* 15-20.

Lanza, M. L., Milner, J., & Riley, E. (1988). Predictors of patient assault on acute inpatient psychiatric units: A pilot study. *Issues in Mental Health Nursing, 9*(3), 259-270.

Leonard, K. & Jacob, T. (1988). Alcohol, alcoholism, and family violence. In V. Van Hasselt, R. Morrison, A. Bellack, & M. Hersen (Eds.). *Handbook of Family Violence,* New York: Plenum.

Lion, J. (1987). Training for battle: Thoughts on managing aggressive patients. *Hospital and Community Psychiatry, 38*(8), 882-884.

Lynch, M. (1975). Ill-health and child abuse. *Lancet, 2,* 317-319.

Maiuro, R. & Eberle, J. (1989). New developments in research on aggression: An international report. *Violence and Victims, 4*(1), 3-15.

Millor, G. (1981). A theoretical framework for nursing research in child abuse and neglect. *Nursing Research, 30,* 78-84.

Morrison, E. (1989). Theoretical modeling to predict violence in hospitalized psychiatric patients. *Research in Nursing and Health, 12*(1), 31-40.

Nesbit, W., & Karagianis, L. (1982). Child abuse: Exceptionality as a risk factor. *Alberta Journal of Educational Research, 28,* 69-76.

Newbern, V. (1989). Sexual victimization of child and adolescent patients. *Image. 21*(1), 10-13.

Pagelow, M. (1984). *Family violence.* New York: Praeger.

Parker, B., & Schumacher, D. (1977). The battered wife syndrome and violence in the nuclear family of origin: A controlled pilot study. *American Journal of Public Health, 67*(8), 760-761.

Perry, M., Wells, E., & Doran, L. (1983). Parent characteristics in abusing and non-abusing families. *Journal of Clinical Child Psychology, 12,* 329-336.

Pillemer, K., & Suitor, J. (1988). Elder abuse. In V. Van Hasselt, R. Morrison, A. Bellack, & M. Hersen (Eds.). *Handbook of Family Violence,* New York: Plenum.

Pollick, M. (1987). Abuse of the elderly: A review. *Holistic Nursing Practice. 1*(2), 43-53.

Regan, W. (1983). Rape on hospital property: Now you can sue. *RN(46),* 69-70.

Seagull, E. (1987). Child psychologist's role in assessment. In R. Helfer & R. Kempe (Eds.). *The battered child, 4th ed.* Chicago: University of Chicago Press.

Sherrod, K., O'Connor, S., Vietze, P., & Altemeier, W. (1984). Child health and maltreatment. *Child Development, 55,* 1174-1183.

Stark, E., & Flitcraft, A. (1988). Violence among intimates: An epidemiological review. In V. Van Hasselt, R. Morrison, A. Bellack, M. Hersen (Eds.). *Handbook of Family Violence.* New York: Plenum.

Starr, R. (1982). A research based approach to the prediction of child abuse prediction. In R. Starr Jr. (Ed.). *Child abuse prediction: Policy implications,* Cambridge, Mass.: Ballinger.

Starr, R. (1988). Physical abuse of children. In V. Van Hasselt, R. Morrison, A. Bellack, M. Hersen (Eds.). *Handbook of Family Violence,* New York: Plenum.

Steinberg, L. Catalano, R., & Dooley, D. (1981). Economic antecedents of child abuse and neglect. *Child Development, 52,* 975-985.

Steinmetz, S. (1988). *Duty bound: Elder abuse and family care,* Newbury Park, Ca.: Sage.

Steinmetz, S. & Lucca, J. (1988). Husband battering. In V. Van Hasselt, R. Morrison, A. Bellack, & M. Hersen (Eds.). *Handbook of Family Violence,* New York: Plenum.

Straus, M., Gelles, R., & Steinmetz, S. (1980). *Behind closed doors: Violence in the American family,* New York: Praeger.

Straus, M. (1980). Stress and child abuse. In C. Kempe & R. Helfer (Eds.), *The battered child* (3rd ed.). Chicago: University of Chicago.

Torres, S. (1987). Hispanic-American battered women: Why consider cultural differences? *Response, 10*(3), 20-21.

Surgeon General's Workshop on Violence and Public Health Report. (1986). (DHHS Publication No. HRS-D-MC 86-1, Washington, D.C.: U.S. Government Printing Office.

Tobias, C., Turns, D., Lippman, S., & Pary, R. (1988). The violent patient: What to do? *Southern Medical Journal, 81*(5), 640-643.

U.S. Department of Health and Human Services (1988). Study Findings. Study of national incidence and prevalence of child abuse and neglect. (DHHS Publication No. (OHDS) 20-01099.) Washington, D.C.: U.S. Government Printing Office.

White, E. (1985). *Chain, chain, change: For black women dealing with physical and emotional abuse,* Seattle: Seal Press.

Widom, C. (1989). The cycle of violence. *Science, 244*(4901), 160-166.

Winger, J., Schirm, V., & Stewart, D. (1987). Aggressive behavior in long term care. *Journal of Psychosocial Nursing, 25*(4), 28-33.

Zuravin, S. (1989). The ecology of child abuse and neglect: Review of the literature and presentation of data. *Violence and Victims, 4*(2), 101-120.

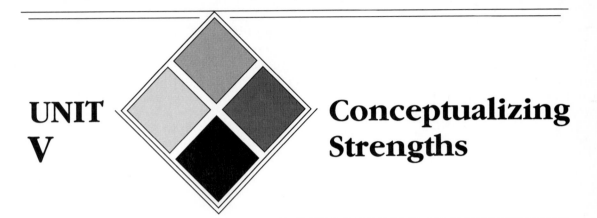

# UNIT V

# Conceptualizing Strengths

**A**SSESSING client and family strengths and assisting in the development and growth of identified strengths is an integral component of all nursing practice. All clients have strengths or potential strengths such as hope, coping, empowerment, hardiness, or humor. With some clients and families these will be readily identifiable as the nurse assesses the client's past abilities to deal with problems and accomplish life goals. With other clients, however, such as severely depressed individuals or multiproblem families, the identification of strengths may be more difficult and challenging. It is with this type of client or family that the identification of strengths is even more critical. In addition, all clients have potential social support systems that the nurse can assist in identifying and mobilizing.

The chapters in this unit describe the concept, incorporate nursing research relevant to the topic, and provide a sample nursing care plan specific to the topic. The care plans incorporate a sample medical diagnosis or clinical description, nursing diagnoses, goals, intervention, and evaluation as a model for nursing intervention. The care plans provide a beginning model for the use of the concepts in practice.

# 25 Social Support

Constance R. Uphold

## OBJECTIVES

*At the completion of this chapter, the reader will be able to:*

◆ Analyze the various mechanisms through which social support has been theorized to affect health.

◆ Compare and contrast conceptual definitions of social support.

◆ Develop nursing care plans, using Norbeck's model, for individuals when there is a mismatch between support need and support availability.

◆ Differentiate between interventions that enhance support systems and interventions that provide direct support.

◆ Describe approaches for measuring social support in the clinical area.

In the last decade there has been increasing interest in the concept of social support. Books (Cohen & Syme, 1985; Gottlieb, 1988; Sarason & Sarason, 1985), review articles (Broadhead et al, 1983; Leavy, 1983; Norbeck, 1987; Wortman, 1984), and hundreds of empirical investigations devoted to the study of social support have appeared in the literature (Ganster & Victor, 1988). Since the early 1970s when the first studies using the term *social support* were published (Norbeck, 1987), voluminous data have linked social support with various health outcomes. Consistently, social support has been found to exert a positive impact on mental health and mortality. Although empirical data are not as conclusive, there also appears to be a relationship between social support and physi-

cal illness (Ganster & Victor, 1988). It is posited that social support can be linked to health through its influence on neuroendocrine responses, immune function, health behaviors, adherence, affect, self-esteem, and personal control (Cohen, 1988).

Despite this growing volume of empirical evidence on the significance of social support, certain conceptual and methodological issues must be addressed before the mechanism through which social support affects health can be interpreted with confidence. Recent advances in social support research such as the development of reliable and valid instruments and the increase in the number of prospective and experimental studies have added to understanding of the concept. However, there is still little agreement on what social support is, how it functions, and how it should be measured and analyzed.

## ❖ DISCUSSION OF THE CONCEPT
### Conceptual Definitions

Numerous conceptual definitions of social support have been developed. One approach is to view social support as a *psychosocial resource* (Cohen & Syme, 1985). From this perspective, social support includes all environmental factors that contribute to a person's well-being. This view of social support is expansive and may include any personal asset such as self-esteem, competence, or control.

Others define social support as a *coping mechanism* or activity (Schaeffer, Coyne, & Lazarus, 1981). From this perspective, social support is a phenomenon that is always associated with stress or crisis. Social support is part of the coping process rather than an attribute of the person's social environment. More specifically, seeking help or activating one's social support system is viewed as one type of problem-solving coping (Lazarus & Folkman, 1984).

Others consider social support as serving important functions regardless of whether one is under stress. Social support is thought to exert a direct effect on an individual's well-being by gratifying needs and enabling the individual to fulfill personal goals (Thoits, 1982). Consistent with this theoretical perspective is Kaplan's opinion (1977) that social support is an interaction with others in which the person's basic needs including affection, esteem, approval, belonging, identity and security are met.

Some view social support as an action or behavior that is provided by one person (i.e., a donor) and received by another person (i.e., a recipient). For example, Caplan (1979) defines social support as an input directly provided by another person (or group) which moves the receiving person towards desired goals. This view emphasizes the actual nature or frequency of the support behaviors that are provided.

Others focus more on the reciprocity of support behaviors between individuals. Social support is defined as an interaction or transaction between two people who react and influence each other. For example, Kahn and Antonucci (1980) state that there are certain necessary interpersonal variables that affect the social support exchange. Mutual confidence, trust, and the ability to exert influence are essential to view a relationship as socially supportive.

From a different perspective, some theorists emphasize the need to determine individual's perceptions of how they view the help or actions offered by others. *Perceived social support* can refer to either the individual's belief that he or she can obtain help (i.e., availability of support) or the degree to which the person is satisfied with the support that is provided or available (i.e., adequacy of support). Researchers and theorists maintaining this position tend to view the cognitive appraisal process as the major means by which social support influences well-being. As House (1981, p. 27) states, "Social support is likely to be effective only to the extent perceived." Consistent with this theoretical perspective is Schaefer (1981) and associates' definition that social support is "evaluation or appraisal of whether and to what extent an interaction, pattern of interactions or relationships is helpful" (p. 384).

Social support can also be viewed as a *process.* For example, Leavy (1983) states that individuals develop, nurture, and then use supportive ties. Similarly, Dunkel-Sheeter (1984) contends that the amount of support provided and received depends on past experiences, perceived needs at the time, support offered, and the degree to which support resources are subject to other demands.

Heller and Swindle (1983) present a theoretical model that describes the social support process as an interaction between the environmental and personal variables occurring across time. In this model the individual is viewed as having an active role in selecting and maintaining socially supportive relationships. Social support is a function of the availability of environmental support structures and the individual's previous experience with support availability, the degree to which the individual has interpersonal skills, and the actual support-seeking behaviors undertaken by the individual during times of stress.

Previous literature suggests that social support can be broadly defined as personal assets or more specifically as a type of coping strategy. Vaux and Harrison (1985) succinctly describe social support as a meta-construct that includes psychosocial resources, behaviors, and actions provided by a donor and the perception that one is supported. Recent theoretical work that describes social support as a process seems to be a promising avenue for future explorations. Choice of a conceptual definition is dependent on the clinician's or researcher's theoretical background and purpose for exploring the concept empirically or in the practice setting.

## Types of Social Support

Most researchers and theorists agree that social support is a multidimensional concept (Thoits, 1982). Taxonomies or lists of the components of social support have been developed. Generally the types of support are related to the individual needs they fulfill. Reviewing the taxonomies, it is possible to identify psychological support and tangible support as the two main types of social support.

**Psychological support.**    Psychological support has several components. One component is *positive affect,* which includes intimacy and attachment, being able to confide in another, and expressions of empathy, trust, and concern. Affective interactions "lead the recipient to believe that she is cared for and loved" (Cobb, 1976b, p. 189). *Affirmation* is another component of psychological support and includes expressions of approval, respect, admiration, and appreciation. Interactions of affirmation or esteem support "lead the recipient to believe that

she is esteemed and valued" (Cobb, 1976b, p. 189). *Reliable alliance,* another component of psychological support, leads one to believe that he or she is secure and can rely and depend on another for help, assistance, and guidance (Weiss, 1974). In addition, social integration and opportunity for nurturance, terms coined by Weiss (1974), are two less frequently identified components of psychological support. Social integration or perceptions of belonging to a social group provide individuals with a source of enjoyable companionship and social activity. Opportunities for nurturance or the experiences of taking care of children can provide an adult with a sense of being needed.

**Tangible support.** The second main type of support is *tangible support,* which is often called instrumental or material support. Tangible support includes aid and assistance as well as the provision of material items or financial help. In most previous studies tangible support has been found less effective in promoting positive individual outcomes than psychological support. However, in certain circumstances such as after the birth of baby help with household duties (i.e., tangible support) may be needed more than psychological support (Norbeck, 1981).

The above example illustrates the importance of assessing distinct types of support. Not all types of support are equally effective in reducing distress in certain situations (Thoits, 1982). On the other hand, researchers have found that the various types of support are highly related to one another (Wortman, 1984). For example, lending money to a friend who has lost his or her job may often be perceived as a form of love or emotional support rather than a form of tangible support. Findings from factor analytical studies have failed to uncover distinct dimensions in a variety of social support instruments (Brandt & Weinert, 1981; Brown, 1986; Norbeck, Lindsey, & Carrieri, 1981), further suggesting that social support may be a unidimensional concept.

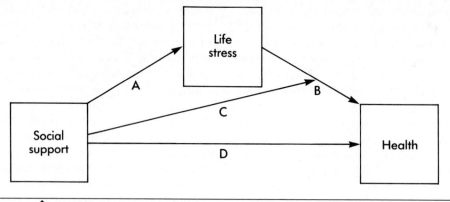

❖ **Fig. 25-1**   Relationship between social support, life stress, and health.

## Mechanisms of Social Support

**Direct and buffering effects.** In addition to the conceptual controversies, there is debate on how social support works to promote and maintain healthy functioning. Generally, there are three perspectives regarding the influence of social support on health (House, 1983). Fig. 25-1 illustrates the ways social support can affect health.

One view is that social support is an *antecedent factor* that reduces the likelihood of life changes occurring (Lin et al, 1979). Thus support may determine whether or not an individual is exposed to stressful events. Having social support may give persons a sense of self-esteem and personal efficacy, making them more resilient to change and preventing their interpreting certain events as stressful (Caplan, 1982). Support may enhance one's cognitive processing, which may facilitate effective decision making and problem solving, thereby reducing the number of stressful situations that the person must encounter (McFarlane et al, 1983). Having adequate social support may increase one's access to information about ways to avoid high-risk situations or dangerous environments (Cohen, 1988). Social support might also reduce an individual's chances of experiencing stressful life events by altering his or her mood. Positive moods can facilitate constructive coping strat-

egies, encourage relaxation, and even alter neuroendocrine response (Wortman, 1984). Graphically, this perspective views social support as having a direct, main effect on life stressors (*arrow A*, Fig. 25-1) and thereby indirectly affecting health (*arrow B*).

Another theory is that social support *buffers* the effects of stressful life events (*arrow C*, Fig. 25-1). Viewed as a buffering factor, the impact of social support follows the occurrence of a life stressor and acts to enhance adaptation by providing resources to facilitate coping or helps to make the threatening event seem less consequential (Lin et al, 1979). This buffering hypothesis implies that social support does not exert a direct effect on stress or health; instead, there is an interactional relationship between stress and social support so that positive health is most likely to occur in a situation of high support and low life stress (Lenz et al, 1986).

Finally, social support can have a *direct,* main effect on health (*arrow D*, Fig. 25-1). Most people need intimacy, social belonging, security, approval, and social contact. Social support can fulfill these important human needs, thereby exerting a direct effect on health.

**Other views.** The observed relationship between social support and health may be a result of an underlying third variable that simultaneously affects both support and health (Thoits, 1982). For example, the link between support and health may be due to sociodemographic factors. Individuals with reduced incomes may be exposed to numerous life changes that impair health and concurrently reduce support (Holahan & Moos, 1981). Similarly, social ties may enhance health for reasons other than the support they provide. Individuals caring for young children or dependent frail elderly may not obtain support from these relationships, but these caregivers may be motivated to remain well by practicing preventive health measures to meet their responsibilities (Lazarus & Folkman, 1984). Being needed by another may be a crucial asset by itself (Weiss, 1974).

Poor health and stress may lead to a reduction in social support rather than vice versa. People with chronic illness may be isolated and at risk for negative outcomes of all types. Thus it may not be social support that results in positive outcomes but illness that results in stress and reduced social support. This reversed cause-and-effect relationship was partially supported by Coyne (1976) who found that depressed persons tended to offend their potential sources of social support, thus intensifying their maladaptation.

Until more longitudinal studies are completed, the causal relationship between social support and health will remain uncertain. Clearly the relationship is complex, and different processes probably affect the link between social support and health at different stages of the health-illness cycle. Therefore it is important for nurses not only to assess clients' current levels of support and health but also to ask clients to describe their previous support patterns and physical and mental functioning.

## Structural Aspects

Structural characteristics of a person's social relationships may influence how social support is provided and received. Typically, structural analysis involves an assessment of a person's social network or the set of linkages among a particular group of people (Wortman, 1984). Frequently researchers assess the size, density, intensity, and directedness of the social network. *Size* refers to the number of individuals with whom a person has direct contact. *Network density* is the extent to which members are in contact with one another. *Loosely knit* and *close-knit* are terms that graphically describe the degree of density in a person's network. *Content* focuses on what transpires between two network members. The relationship is described as multiplex rather than uniplex when members are involved in more than one content area such as being fellow employees as well as frequent social companions. *Intensity* refers to the degree of closeness in the relationship linkage. *Directedness*, or the degree of reciprocity between network members, is an additional structural property that influences social interaction (Ellison, 1983).

Numerous instruments are available to assess social networks (see Wellman, 1981). These instruments are usually too complex and cumbersome for use by nurses in clinical settings but are described later (see "Use in Practice With the Individual"). Ellison (1983) suggests certain questions nurses can ask to obtain social network information. Measures of social networks are objective and do not ask individuals to evaluate the quality or quantity of their support. Because individuals describe rather than evaluate their networks, network analysis is less likely to be influenced by a person's mood or mental well-being than are measures of social support. However, these structural properties provide only a one-dimensional viewpoint of the social support process.

Nevertheless, significant results have been obtained by researchers focusing on social network properties. For instance, Mueller (1980) found that psychiatric clients had smaller, more asymmetrical, and more kinship–reliant networks than control subjects. In times of crisis small, close social networks have been found more supportive (Wortman, 1984). Schizophrenics who had low-density networks had the highest rate of institutional readmission (Sokolovsky & Cohen, 1981).

The differences between social support and social networks must be clarified. Provision of social support is only one of the many functions of social networks. Actions of network members provide support, and this support is communicated through the network's structure. The important point is that the network is distinct from the support the members exchange with one another (O'Reilly, 1988).

## Positive and Negative Aspects

Even though social support is provided by network members, not all people in the social network are supportive (Norbeck, 1981). This statement highlights the fact that social interactions have both costs and benefits. Relationships between network members can be valuable personal resources, but they also may be sources of stress (Lazarus & Folkman, 1984). For example, being a member of a large family may increase the number of persons available to provide support, but it also may increase one's risks of having to deal with the sick and dependent.

A network member may visit frequently and provide extensive behaviors that are intended to help the recipient. However, the behaviors may be of poor quality, ineptly provided, badly timed, interfering, and inappropriate to the context or the current needs of the person (Fisher, Nadler, & Whitcher-Alagna, 1982). Therefore many theorists suggest that the perception of the support between the recipient and the donor is the crucial element in the social support process.

One's perception of the quality of support may depend on whether the recipient believes that he or she can reciprocate the help given by the donor. *Equity theory* suggests that assistance given to one member of a relationship must equal the services offered by the other member or the relationship tends to deteriorate. Lending support to this theory is the finding that lack of reciprocity in help undermines the effective quality of adult child–parent relations (Ingersoll-Dayton & Antonucci, 1989). Beckman (1981) found that older women perceived their relationships with their offspring as distressing and dissatisfying when their children were providing them with aid they could not reciprocate.

*Reactance theory* is also helpful in explaining the process of how one evaluates the quality of social support. This theory states that individuals will experience negative feelings when their freedom of choice and their autonomy are threatened. Help that is too intense may result in negative outcomes. For example, clients in nursing homes who are provided with too much help may develop dependency on the caregivers that may lead to decreases in their self-esteem and consequential physical declines. Partially supporting the reactance theory is research that has found that recovery from an illness was impeded in the presence of well-meaning but overprotective support (Hyman, 1972; Garrity, 1973).

Another factor that can influence how one interprets help is the recipient's perception of the donor's motives or intentions for providing support. According to *attribution theory* (Kelley, 1967), when the intent of support behaviors is perceived to derive from concern rather than obligation, the recipient is likely to react favorably toward the donor (Fisher et al, 1982).

The importance of measuring perceptions of support rather than more concrete variables such as degree of association of behavioral inputs is emphasized by empirical data. Studies that have measured perceived support, social network variables, and behavioral inputs demonstrate that perceived support accounts for a greater portion of variance in psychological outcomes than the other approaches (Fiore, Becker, & Coppel, 1983; Rook, 1984; Schaeffer et al, 1982). Individual's social needs and preferences are so highly individualized that they cannot be measured solely with objective instruments. Whether or not support is effective in enhancing well-being and health ultimately depends on how the individual perceives the situation.

Social interactions that are perceived negatively are usually not defined as a form of social support. However, Shumaker and Brownell (1984, p. 13) define social support as an "exchange of resources between at least two individuals perceived by the provider or recipient to be intended to enhance the well-being of the recipient." Shumaker and Brownell explicitly state that their definition was formulated to encompass both positive and negative aspects of social support.

Regardless of how one conceptually defines social support, nurses must assess both the negative and positive aspects of relationships with instruments such as Tilden and Gaylen's Cost and Reciprocity Index (1987). Most relationships have irritating as well as gratifying qualities. Studies have shown that people rate their most satisfying relationships as also the most conflictual (Argyle & Furnham, 1983; Troll, 1980).

## Source of Support

The source of support or the relationship of the donor to the focal person may determine whether the help is interpreted positively or negatively. For instance, when a friend provides advice, it is often interpreted as a sign of caring, whereas a similar behavior from one's parents may be interpreted as meddling (Wood, 1984). As Weiss (1974) notes, relationships may be relatively specialized. Different sources of support may not be readily substituted for one another.

Five major sources of support have been identified in the literature: natural support systems, religious organizations, helping professions, organized support groups, and groups not directed by health professionals (Pender, 1987). On the other hand, some theorists argue that help offered by strangers, professionals, or casual acquaintances does not qualify as a form of social support. From this perspective, the exchange of help is only considered social support when the involved individuals belong to the same social network (Cobb, 1976; Norbeck & Tilden, 1988).

Regardless of this conceptual debate, previous research has shown that different types of relationships help to fulfill different needs. For example, Fischer (1983) found that mothers and mothers-in-law provide different types of support to their daughters or daughters-in-law. Adult women experiencing the birth of a baby sought child-rearing advice from their mothers, whereas they sought advice on their husband's habits from their mothers-in-law. Research has shown that support from one's spouse has a greater impact on well-being than support from other sources (Verbugge, 1979). Dunkel-Shetter (1984) found that cancer patients viewed advice from physicians but not family and friends as helpful.

Several investigators have explored the differences in support provided by family as opposed to friends. Generally, the studies indicate that individuals seek and accept financial and instrumental support from kin. Friends are more likely to provide social belonging and emotional support in times that do not involve intense stress (Fisher, 1982).

These studies suggest that researchers and clinicians need to explore the various types of support provided by different members of the social network. The majority of previously developed instruments for measuring social support have focused on the adequacy of support provided by the total network. There is a growing recognition that more measures are needed that ask questions specific to the type, amount, and intensity of support provided by various people (Wortman, 1984).

## Timing of Support

The source of support and the benefits derived from it may change as time progresses. Bankoff (1983) found that aged parents were the single most important source of support for recently widowed women. However, as the widowed women moved into the transition stage of grieving, the major source of support changed to single friends. It was speculated that initially widows need nurturant support from parents, but as they resolve their grief, the support of friends enables them to become integrated into single life.

There can also be changes in the effects of social support over time. For example, some friends of women about to undergo a breast biopsy recommended that herbal remedies would be more beneficial than the diagnostic procedure (Hobfoll & Wolfish, 1982). The initial effect could have been relief, whereas the long-term effect could be extremely harmful (Shumaker & Brownell, 1984).

Dimond and Jones (1983) suggest that an individual's needs for social support change with three different phases of illness. During the diagnostic period the needed help might be information and emotional support to reduce anxiety and uncertainty. During the acute stage of the illness direct aid such as help with household tasks may be needed to enable the client to rest and receive the treatments. In the recovery phase the client may need financial help to manage the costs of the illness and affirmative support to bolster his or her self-esteem in returning to previous life activities.

## Provider of Support

Another dimension of social support, which has been overlooked, is the positive and negative outcomes that evolve from providing support. Previous research and literature have focused on the beneficiaries of social support. However, social support is both given and received. In fact, research has demonstrated that those who reciprocate social support are likely to be more healthy than those who do not (Broadhead et al, 1983).

Shumaker and Brownell (1984) suggest that providing support to others is a gratifying experience because it leads to feelings that one's actions can make a difference in another person's life. Offering help to another may assure individuals their needs will be met in the future if a problem arises. One's sense of efficacy may be enhanced by the knowledge that he or she was instrumental in alleviating another's stress or pain. Studies have found that volunteers in ostomy and widow self-help groups have higher levels of acceptance of the changes or losses in their lives (Silverman, 1970; Trainor, 1981).

On the other hand, provision of support may be costly. Being available for a person in a crisis may be emotionally draining and may increase the helper's sense of vulnerability by alerting him or her to similar risks in his or her life. Numerous studies on families with chronically ill members highlight the financial, physical, and psychological problems associated with caregiving (Bunting, 1989; Haley et al, 1987; Moritz, Kasl, & Berkman, 1989).

Providing support can result in both positive and negative outcomes over time. For example, family caregivers acknowledge that providing physical care to members causes fatigue but also gives them a feeling of accomplishment that they are helping a loved one (Given et al, 1988). To understand social support fully, researchers and clinicians must assess the perceptions of both the recipient and the provider in the supportive exchange.

## Family Social Support

Family members are often the primary providers of social support. According to Caplan (1982), the family has several social support functions. First, the family acts as a collector and disseminator of information. Within the family children are socialized and develop a sense of what is socially acceptable behavior. The family often functions as a feedback guidance system in which members can discuss their behaviors and feelings while simultaneously receiving validation of the appropriateness of their actions. The family system is an important reference group in which individuals develop their own values and a strong sense of identity. The family acts as a guide and mediator in problem solving by providing help, advice, and encouragement with everyday and stressful life events. When a person is in need of service or aid, the family is a frequent source of practical assistance. During times of distress, illness, and alarm, the family often becomes a haven for rest and recuperation and a resource for emotional comfort and help with mastering the crisis.

Relationships with family members play a predominant role in most people's lives. Approximately two fifths of people's social networks consist of family members, and this proportion increases with age (Fehr & Perlman, 1985). Generally, people rate the quality of family relations positively. In particular, one's spouse is viewed as an important source of support. Married individuals enjoy better physical and mental health and have greater life satisfaction than single people (Fehr & Perlman, 1985).

The salience of family support may depend on the other sources of support available to the person. Family support was a more effective predictor of nonemployed women's well-being than employed women's well-being. Men's well-being was largely a function of the support they derived from work, whereas women's well-being was more influenced by family support (Holahan & Moos, 1981).

Nevertheless, during life transitions family members are important sources of support for most people. When individuals begin parenthood, their family members provide support in the form of visits, gifts, encouragement, aid, advice, and financial loans (Carveth & Gottlieb, 1979; Fischer, 1983). During a divorce the size of one's social network decreases because of the loss of central help from in-laws, but one's relationships with consanguinal kin often become more involved (Spicer & Hampe, 1975). As mentioned previously, recently widowed women frequently turn first to their own parents for support (Bankoff, 1983). Until parents become extremely frail and debilitated, there is a mutual exchange of support between adult children and their aging parents (Troll & Smith, 1976).

Similarly, during stress and illness families apparently are a major source of help. Family support was the most effective predictor of psychological adjustment in a sample of juvenile rheumatoid arthritis clients (Varni, Wilcox, & Hanson, 1988). Myocardial infarction victims listed family members as providing the most frequent and intense help after their crisis (Croog, Lipson, & Levine, 1972), and supportive family relationships improved stroke clients' rate of recovery (Evans et al, 1987).

The preceding studies focus on the effects of family support on individual members. Less often, researchers and theorists focus on the family as a total unit embedded in a social environment. Kane (1988) proposes that family characteristics such as esteem and stability influence the family's social support or the family's ability to maintain reciprocal helping relationships and to provide advice and intimacy. Through the process of social support the family develops versatility and resourcefulness and ultimately achieves health and resources.

Empirical studies that investigate the impact or lack of social support on the total family unit are limited. Research has shown that in times of disasters, families who have resources in the form of friends and relatives seem to adjust better than isolated families (Unger & Powell, 1980). Families who abuse their children have been found socially isolated without adequate support systems (Garbarino & Sherman,

1980). Family functioning is impaired when family caregivers of Alzheimer's disease clients have insufficient support (Scott, Robertson, & Hutton, 1986).

## Community and Public Policy

The role of the community or broader society in influencing the social support patterns of individuals and families has been largely ignored. Historically, clinicians have attempted to improve health by altering individuals' social networks and supports. However, as Brownell and Shumaker (1985) discuss, it may be more advantageous to institute broad policies that alter the environment and resources within the community and society.

At the federal level, policymakers need to consider the impact of certain bills on support systems. For example, urban-renewal projects and interstate-highway expansion projects may disrupt the normal supportive functions of networks when members are forced to relocate. Incentives for families caring for ill members and financial help for single mothers needing day care for children are examples of legislation that acknowledges the benefits of enhancing natural support systems.

State and local policymakers can also play a role in promoting social interaction. Policymakers should encourage designers to develop neighborhoods, institutions, and community buildings that facilitate the exchange of social support. Other community plans that may enhance group support include the promotion of community crime-prevention programs, development of public recreational parks, or funding for teen centers for adolescent gatherings (Brownell & Shumaker, 1985).

Research on the organizational and environmental characteristics of social support is limited. Zimring's extensive literature review of physical environment (1981) surprisingly found that individuals tended to be more sociable in institutions, dormitories, and community settings when they had well-defined private space with controlled, easy access. In another study Kaplan (1983) found that settings that limited sensory distractions enhanced the exchange of information and facilitated problem solving (Kaplan, 1983). Businesses that encourage cooperativeness as opposed to competiveness have been found to enhance the support process (Shumaker and Brownell, 1984).

## ❖ USE IN PRACTICE WITH THE INDIVIDUAL

In 1981 Norbeck proposed a model (Fig. 25-2) to guide clinical research and practice in nursing. Although only parts of this model have been empirically tested, it can serve as guide for practicing nurses who are familiar with using the nursing process in their clinical practice.

### Nursing Assessment and Analysis

In the assessment the nurse should determine whether the level of social support is adequate or inadequate. This determination involves weighing an individual's need for support versus the actual social support that is available. The support is assessed as inadequate when the available support does not match an individual's need for it. Properties of the person and the situation can influence this match between support need and availability.

Previous discussions in the literature suggest important properties of the person that influence need for support. For example, an infant who is dependent on others for feeding, warmth, and protection has greater needs for support than an adult who functions fairly independently as a worker, parent, and spouse. Poor socioeconomic status predisposes an individual to more life stressors and fewer personal resources to cope with the added pressures, thereby increasing the individual's need for support. Persons differ in the amount of social contacts most conducive for mental well-being. Introverts have a

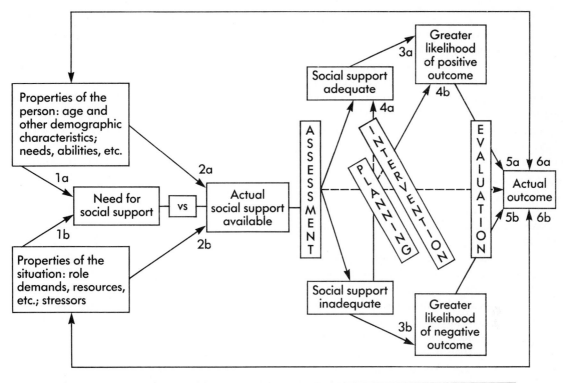

❖  **Fig. 25-2**    Norbeck's model. (From Norbeck J.S.: [1981]. Social support: a model for
clinical research and application, *Advances in Nursing Science,* 3, p. 46.)

substantially lower desire for social interaction
than extroverts (Norbeck, 1982). Cultural values that emphasize the importance of family
over individualism or cooperativeness over personal gain also influence an individual's need for
support.

Properties of the situation also influence
need for support. Individuals experiencing an
event that involves numerous role changes and
involves a diversity of stressors usually need
more support than people undergoing a minor
life event. For example, after the death of a
spouse, a person may need to assume the new
roles of bread winner, financial planner, and
household caretaker as well as deal with the
stressors of decreasing finances, relocation of

living, and lack of sleep. Thus a recent widow
would need types and amounts of support different from those of a woman who has had cataract surgery.

Assessing a client's needs for support is difficult and not well described in Norbeck's
model. A logical strategy for determining need
would be simply to ask a client how much and
what type of support he or she believes is
needed. Although this approach may yield valuable information, most clients, because of their
stress, disability, or lack of knowledge, are not
able to relay the pertinent information. Another
logical approach would be to assess clients'
level of stress, assuming that clients with signs
of depression, nervousness, withdrawal, and fa-

tigue are in need of more support. This strategy may be effective, but the nurse must remember that these signs may be related to the medication's side effects and the physiological ramifications of disease rather than social influences. Frequently nurses must rely on their diverse educational preparation in the biopsychosocial sciences to alert them to which individuals are most vulnerable to developing problems. A comprehensive data base that includes the usual demographic attributes and information on culture, role obligations, social competencies, recent life events, coping styles, and personality characteristics would be important to obtain.

The amount and type of support available is also dependent on characteristics of the person. Tamir and Antonocci (1981) found that adults in earlier stages of the life cycle had more available social support than older individuals. Other studies show that females receive more social support than males during adolescence (Burke & Weir, 1976), young adulthood (Hirsch, 1979), and old age (Lowenthal & Haven, 1968). Some people have greater ability in establishing social relationships and thus can use different numbers and types of support. Other individual differences such as physical attractiveness, coping ability, shyness, and range of recreational interests are likely to affect the pool of social support resources.

Situational demands affect the support that individuals receive from their social networks. Parents who had experienced the recent death of a child related difficulty finding people willing to provide emotional help (Chesler & Barbarin, 1984). Breast cancer clients reported that their illness led others to avoid them or to offer inappropriate forms of supports (Peters-Golden, 1982). Various life transitions such as marriage, parenthood, and retirement alter the availability of support. Upon marriage, in-laws and friends of one's spouse are often perceived as new sources of support. Cronenwett (1985) found that after the birth of a child, new parents

changed the composition of their networks by replacing some network members with individuals who were parents themselves. Retirement often results in the loss of support from work-related friends and associates.

Availability of support can be assessed more easily than need for support. Several research instruments can be modified for clinical purposes. Sometimes support availability is assessed by presenting research respondents with hypothetical crisis or stress situations and asking them about their perceptions of how much or what quality of support they can count on in each situation. The Personal Resource Questionnaire, Part One (Brandt & Weinert, 1981), which was developed by two nurses, the Social Support Questionnaire (Sarason et al, 1983), and Schaefer and associates' (1981) Social Support Questionnaire are examples of instruments that present hypothetical situations and ask respondents to whom they would turn for help.

Other instruments focus on describing the amount, type, and/or quality of support that is received rather than what support they believe would be forthcoming in given situations. For example, in the Norbeck Social Support Questionnaire (Norbeck, Lindsey, & Carrieri, 1981) respondents are asked to list up to 24 significant persons and then to rate the amount of each type of support provided by the specific network members. Similarly, in the Arizona Social Support Interview Schedule (Barrera, 1981) and the Social Support Resources (Vaux, 1982) respondents list network members who provide various support functions and then rate the adequacy of the support.

In addition, behaviorally oriented indexes of support provide information on how much and how often individuals actually receive support. In the Inventory of Socially Supportive Behaviors respondents rate the frequency with which certain specific types of support were received during 1 month (Barrera, Sandler, & Ramsay, 1981). For example, respondents are asked how often someone showed them physical affection or gave them feedback on how they were doing. Questioning clients about enacted support in addition to its availability is important in understanding the process individuals use in accessing their social networks.

Network analysis is another method for gaining insight into an individual's availability of support. Although most of the existing methods of network analysis are too complex for the clinical area, Ellison (1983) provides examples of simplified ways to assess networks. For example, the size and extent of the social networks can be obtained by asking clients to name those persons who are most important to them. Information on reciprocity can be obtained by asking clients to name those persons with whom there is an equal give and take of support. Nurses can ask clients the number of people in their networks who are in contact with one another to gather information about interconnectedness.

Various unique approaches for measuring social support may be adapted for the clinical area. A sociogram may be developed to illustrate through a series of concentric circles the immediate family, extended family, distant relatives, friends, and community sources of support (Rich, 1978). Hirsch (1979) developed a self-monitoring log on which the respondents name the network members with whom they interacted during the day and estimate the amount of time spent with each person and the degree of satisfaction with the interaction. The Kaplan Scale (Kaplan, 1977) consists of vignettes that describe people with varying degrees of social support. Individuals compare themselves to the people described in the vignette and then check the person most like themselves.

In summary, the nurse must use a variety of assessment strategies to determine whether an individual's need for support can be met by the available pool of support resources. Various personal and situational characteristics must be taken into account when assessing the match between need and availability. Research instruments can be modified for use in the clinical area.

### Planning

After data analysis establishes that the client's social support is inadequate or adequate, the nurse must determine priorities of care and goals for intervention. For the person with adequate support, nursing goals may include the following: maintaining the current available support, preventing future deterioration of the available support, and promoting a higher level of functioning of the social network than that experienced before the stressor. After an illness or hospitalization, network members may learn new coping skills, become socially closer to each other, and draw on previously unrecognized strengths. However, this high level of network functioning may be available only during the acute phase of the stressor. Thus the nurse must develop long-range care plans to address social needs with all persons, regardless of their current level of adaptation.

More intense planning is needed for the person with inadequate support. A variety of goals may be developed based on the comprehensive assessment and analysis. The goals may be to improve relationships between the client and available members in the social network, to improve the client's social skills in accessing new support systems or mobilizing support that was previously unavailable, or to increase the size of the client's social network by referring him or her to self-help groups or individual counseling.

Norbeck (1981) suggests that the nurse should consider personal and situational factors when formulating goals. In addition, other literature suggests that nurses should recognize that the type of support needed depends on when the support is offered (i.e., timing) and who would be best to provide this support (i.e., source). Encouraging reciprocity between network members is another aspect that needs consideration.

The ultimate goal of the plan is to maintain or improve the support available with only minimal disruption of the client's natural support system unless the system is pathological. In this stage the nurse must also consider whether there is a match between the family unit's and the community's availability and need for support. The nurse must be cautious in planning interventions that supplant the role of the family or key network members. For example, the nurse planning a client's discharge may enlist the aid of a home health attendant without considering the detrimental consequences this action may have on the client's large, close-knit family that resents outside help.

## Intervention

**When social support is adequate.** In Norbeck's model no intervention is needed for the person judged to have adequate support. However, it is suggested that even persons currently obtaining adequate support are in need of nursing intervention. By positively reinforcing network members for their helping behaviors and focusing on the strengths of network members, the nurse can assist people in maintaining their present level of functioning. In addition, the nurse should prevent the development of future problems in the network. Researchers have found that the amount of help available changes over time. Brocklehurst et al (1981) found that family members of stroke clients had much less support after a year of caring for their ill relative than when the stroke first occurred. Immediately after the death of a spouse, widows receive an abundance of support from family and friends but are often forced to face stressors alone after the first few weeks of grieving (Lopata, 1978). Network members must be encouraged to provide support on a long-term basis. Clients need to be given information about community programs and resources that can be accessed if

there are reductions in the help given by available network members. The nurse may also be able to help network members in developing relationships that are even more positive than ones before the stressor. For example, the nurse may be able to focus on and encourage network members to use new coping skills that were not identified before the crisis event.

**When social support is inadequate.** Norbeck's model (1981) describes two types of intervention possible for the person with inadequate support. One intervention focuses on enhancing the support system, and the other concentrates on offering direct support.

The nurse can enhance the client's support system by influencing the structure, functioning, or use of the person's natural support system. Early in the intervention the nurse should explore which persons in the social network can be enlisted to provide support. At times the nurse may need to help the client initiate a reunion with family members or close friends from whom he or she has had an extended separation. For example, during pregnancy or birth of a child a woman may experience a reawakening of positive sentiments toward her mother. If this mother-daughter relationship has been conflictual, the nurse may help resolve the dyadic problems (Norbeck, 1981).

Other types of assistance with available network members can help potentiate positive client outcomes. Ervin (1973) teaches husbands of mastectomy clients how to provide support to their wives by explaining the typical emotional reactions and needs of women after surgery. Another educational program significantly improved the knowledge level, coping skills, and competence of spouses caring for clients with Alzheimer's disease (Chiverton & Caine, 1989).

Educating network members about developmental or maturational changes may improve relationships. Parents of children about to enter adolescence may be supported by teaching about teens' needs for independence. Family members of an elderly woman who refuses to care for herself may be more supportive if they are taught about normal aging changes such as sensory losses, memory changes, and motor weaknesses.

Similarly, in times of crisis the nurse may be instrumental in assisting network members to provide appropriate support. For example, network members may have inadequate knowledge about the grieving process and may prematurely push a widow into developing new social relationships (Norbeck, 1981). Network members may inappropriately offer false hope and cheerful reassurances to a terminally ill client who wants comfort and someone in whom to confide. In addition to performing client teaching, nurses can act as role models for network members and can demonstrate therapeutic forms of interaction with distressed clients.

Changing the environment may also be helpful in improving the support offered by the network. In a nursing home residents with similar levels of orientation and social skills may be put in the same room to increase interpersonal communication. In acute care settings a staff conference room may be converted to a room in which network members may meet with clients in privacy for extended periods of time. Changes in standard hospital policies such as extending visitor hours in particular situations may also be needed.

Network members and clients may need supplementary sources of support when their needs exceed the resources that are available. Volunteer linking or establishing relationships with others who have experienced a similar crisis may enhance client and network functioning. For example, the nurse may suggest that a quadriplegic client and his or her network members visit and talk with a person who is permanently paralyzed and who has successfully coped.

Using mutual aid or self-help groups is another intervention for supplementing the support of available network members. Groups are available for individuals and families with multiple problems such as addiction, maturational stressors, life events, and medical conditions. Parents Without Partners, Alcoholics Anonymous, Reach to Recovery, and Compassionate Friends are examples of nationally organized groups.

One common characteristic of most self-help groups is that members are living through the same stressor or are in the same life situation. This commonality of experiences demonstrates that individuals are not alone in managing a problem and that others have been in similar situations and have learned to cope effectively. These groups serve an educational function that helps individuals to understand better the stressors they are experiencing. The group members offer mutual support and act as role models for adjustment (Lieberman & Borman, 1979). Contacts made at self-help groups may be integrated into one's network, thereby increasing an individual's available support resources (Fehr & Perlman, 1985). As mentioned previously, providing support to others sometimes increases one's self-esteem and gives a person a purpose for living. The added benefits of providing help to others in support groups should not be minimized.

Although self-help groups provide support in numerous ways, they may not be beneficial to some individuals. Some people prefer to handle their problems by themselves or with close family members. Others feel uncomfortable in discussing their concerns with strangers and fear that disclosure of problems will lessen their individualism and make them dependent on others. Before encouraging individuals to attend self-help groups, the nurse must assess whether the individual is a person who in the past has joined groups and is receptive to meeting new people to discuss issues (Roth, 1989).

Network therapy is another alternative to use to supplement available social support systems. Group sessions with the individual's extended network are undertaken. Together the network members discuss family secrets and attempt to help the individual reopen involvement with extended family members (Norbeck, 1982).

Provision of direct help may be required when a continuous, intense need of support has depleted all resources in the available social network such as occurs in a family that has recently relocated to a new town and is managing the care of a child with a long-term physical disability. The nurse's role may be to refer the family to a health professional such as mental health nurse, psychologist, family therapist, or religious counselor to help the family in forming and maintaining a new social network. Acting as a case manager, the nurse can also directly link the family with community resources such as organizations to help defray financial costs, health equipment stores, and facilities that provide physical therapy.

Persons with pathological relationships in their social networks also need direct intervention. For example, the main deficit in psychotic clients' social networks was the predominance of enmeshed kin relationships (Pattison et al, 1975). Helping these individuals develop more peer-level relationships and gradually loosen ties with kin would be appropriate strategies to undertake (Norbeck, 1982).

The nurse also must consider the social capabilities of the client. Individuals who lack social skills can become even more frustrated and dejected when they are encouraged to increase their network of friends or repair their relationships with emotionally separated relatives. Social skill training programs that provide guidance in gradually developing a social support network may be constructive. Problems with shyness, poor communication techniques, and fears of meeting people may be lessened with programs such as assertiveness training (Norbeck, 1981). Strategies to improve a person's physical attractiveness such as demonstrating good grooming techniques and ways to move

and stand may be helpful. Increasing the client's awareness of the need for reciprocity in developing and maintaining relationships is an important goal of intervention. Experiences that involve reciprocity in everyday life should be included in the plan (Ellison, 1983).

## Evaluation

The final step in the nursing process is evaluation. Evaluation should be a continuous procedure that addresses each phase of the nursing process. The nurse must consider whether the initial assessment of personal and situational variables related to social support was complete and must determine whether the analysis of inadequate or adequate support was accurate. Consideration should be given to whether the goals were met or are in need of revision. The interventions also must be evaluated to determine whether they were successful and acceptable to the clients. A thorough evaluation will enable the nurse to gain more information on the client's needs for support and its availability. The new information will lead to a refinement of the original goals and interventions, which will be more realistic and individualized. The nursing care plan on pp. 462 and 463 illustrates interventions related to the need for social support for a family caregiver in the community.

## ❖ THE NURSING PROCESS AND THE FAMILY

Nurses can play important roles in maintaining and promoting family and community social support with the use of the nursing process. A genogram (Fig. 25-3) is a helpful tool for assessing family relationships within and across generations. Information on age, names, divorces, marriage, births, health status, and death can be pictorially represented for three or more generations of family members. The genogram can provide insight into family patterns of dis-

Name:                                            Date:

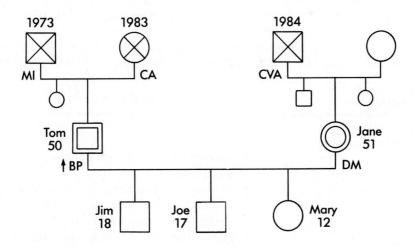

Symbols:

| | | | |
|---|---|---|---|
| Male | □ | Identified Client | ▣ or ◎ |
| Female | ○ | | |
| Marriage | □—○ | | |
| Death | ⊠ or ⊗ | | |
| Miscarriage | △ | | |
| Divorce | □—//—○ | | |
| Unmarried | ☐  ♀ | | |

❖ **Fig. 25-3**   Family genogram.

# ❖ NURSING CARE PLAN

**CLIENT:** Frederick O.

**CLINICAL DESCRIPTION:** Mr. O., 72 years old, is sole caregiver of his wife who is bedridden and confused.

**NURSING DIAGNOSES:** Social isolation related to time-consuming nature of caregiving role

Impaired home maintenance management related to stress and fatigue associated with caring for ill family member

| GOALS | INTERVENTIONS |
|---|---|
| Mr. O. will increase his number of meaningful relationships. | ◆ Encourage Mr. O. to discuss his feelings of loneliness.<br>◆ Explore his reasons for continuing to provide sole care for his wife.<br>◆ Discuss the importance of his social life in promoting his own emotional and physical strengths in caring for his wife.<br>◆ Spend time allowing Mr. O. to reminisce about his old friends and social outings with his wife. This will encourage pleasurable thoughts and help the nurse identify potential social groups and individuals with whom Mr. O. will be comfortable.<br>◆ Encourage Mr. O. to make contact with individuals or groups to expand his social interactions (e.g., previous friends, neighbors, church groups, senior citizen groups). |
| Mr. O. will express satisfaction with his caregiving role. | ◆ Validate the normalcy of his feeling sorrow and grief when his spouse has changed physically and mentally.<br>◆ Identify others from his natural support system (i.e., family and neighbors) who can help with care so he can leave home.<br>◆ Encourage Mr. O. to discuss his caregiver fatigue and problems with his only daughter who may be able to act as supportive listener, an active problem solver, and an extra hand around the house. |

## ❖    NURSING CARE PLAN—cont'd

| GOALS | INTERVENTIONS |
|-------|---------------|
| | ◆ Suggest community resources (i.e., home care, respite care, elderly day care, friendly visitors) that can provide care for his wife and allow him free time.<br><br>◆ If Mr. O. is comfortable in group situations, bring him telephone numbers and names of support groups for family caregivers.<br><br>◆ Suggest time-saving tips that can increase his leisure or rest time. For example, teach him to cook large quantities of food at one time that can be frozen into smaller portions and then easily thawed for quick meals.<br><br>◆ Positively reinforce Mr. O. for the excellent care he is providing, but at the same time discuss caregiver "burnout" and the need to lessen stress through rest, relaxation techniques, social outings, or becoming involved in a hobby or club.<br><br>◆ Allow time to talk about his fears of the future. Encourage him, along with his daughter, to formulate a plan for when his wife's condition worsens or his health declines. When he is ready, suggest that he visit adult congregate living facilities, elderly housing units, and nursing homes to explore the costs and services of the various options. |

### EVALUATION

Mr. O. reports an increased number of social interactions with friends and neighbors. He expresses greater satisfaction with his caregiving role as measured by less somatic complaints and an increase in time spent in pleasurable activities. In addition, he attends a support group for family caregivers, which provides the opportunity to make new friends and share concerns with one another.

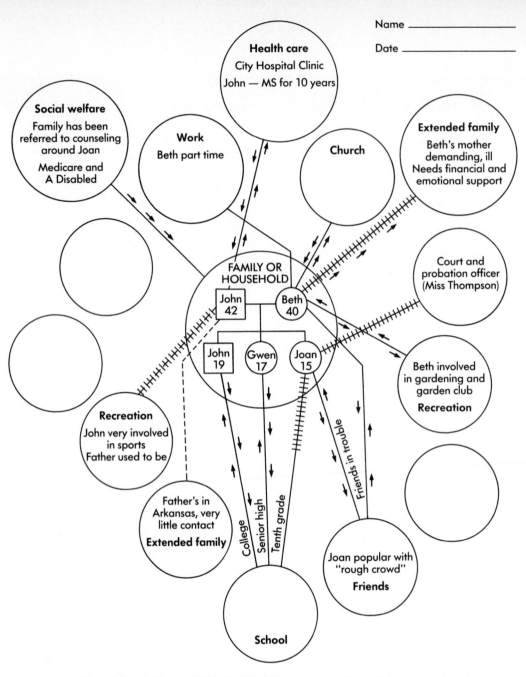

**❖ Fig. 25-4**  Ecomap. Fill in connections where they exist. Indicate nature of
connections with a descriptive word or by drawing different kinds of
lines: _____ for strong; . . . for tenuous; __//// __ for stressful. Draw
arrows along lines to signify flow of energy and resources (→ → →). Identify
significant people and fill in empty circles as needed. (From Hartman A.
(1978). Diagrammatic assessment of family relationships. *Social Casework,*
59, p. 470.)

ease, support, and coping. In addition, the genogram is an easy and fun way to involve all members in the data collection process (Wright & Leahey, 1984) and can provide an opportunity for family members to reminisce about departed members.

Nurses must assess not only the family's influence on individual members, as discussed earlier, but must also assess the family as a total unit receiving support from the wider social system. Nurses must remember when assessing families that a crisis such as the diagnosis of terminal cancer affects the client and all the family members. Trying to mobilize support from distressed members may be inappropriate and even harmful. Besides assessing the internal functioning of families, the nurse must observe how the total family interacts with its outside social network members and the community at large.

The ecomap (Fig. 25-4) is another assessment tool that provides a graphic model of family relationships to friends, neighbors, and community organizations. The family members are placed within the inner circle, and other significant relationships are placed in outer circles. Straight, dotted, and slashed lines between the inner and outer circles represent strong, tenuous, and stressful relationships, respectively. Arrows may also be drawn to show the direction in which resources and energy tend to flow. The ecomap provides a concise picture of how the family members tend to interact with their social environment (Roth, 1989).

In the planning and intervention stages the nurse must consider whether there is a match between a family's need and the availability of support. Families with adequate support can benefit from positive reinforcement of current behaviors and from teaching or counseling on how to prevent development of future problems. Programs such as marital enrichment and parenting classes are examples of health-promoting interventions for families with adequate support. Nurses can play important roles

in preventing maturational crises within families by offering information and prospective support for families who are about to experience parenthood, retirement, or an addition of an elderly relative into the household.

Network members can also be included in strategies to change health behaviors and values. For example, researchers have found that supportive family members are important in promoting compliance with health-promoting interventions (Hubbard, Muhlenkamp, & Brown, 1984). Traditionally, health professionals have attempted to change high-risk health behaviors by trying to alter the individual client's life-style. A more effective intervention may be to encourage desired health behaviors in the entire family system.

Families with inadequate support may need direct help from health professionals. Nursing interventions geared to families may include interventions that facilitate acknowledgment of loss, provision of advice on ways to promote family communication, discussion of the grieving process, and encouragement to join a self-help group. For multiproblem families such as those involved in family violence and addiction, help from mental health professionals in the form of marital therapy, family therapy, group therapy, or network therapy may be needed. Although direct help may be needed initially in unhealthy families, the long-term goal is to assist families to assess their own needs for support, to access their own natural helping systems, and to seek support independently from qualified professionals when appropriate.

## ❖ THE NURSING PROCESS AND THE COMMUNITY

Nurses can play an instrumental role in enhancing social support at the level of the community. For example, nurses can influence legislators to adopt policies that prevent the disruption of social networks and promote the functioning of natural support systems. To enact this role, the nurse must thoroughly assess the community (see Stanhope & Lancaster, 1988, for community assessment tools) to determine whether there is inadequate support in the community as a result of a mismatch between support need and support availability. For example, the nurse may determine that the community has an inadequate support system when he or she gathers data showing the high percentage of elders living in a geographic area with no long-term care facilities. By presenting this information to lay advisers, community leaders, the mass media, and local legislators, the nurse can play a critical role in influencing health policy.

## ❖ SUMMARY

There is much theoretical and empirical literature on social support, but the debate on what social support is, how it functions, and how it should be measured and analyzed still continues. Social support has been viewed as a psychosocial resource, a coping mechanism, an interaction or transaction that satisfies needs, a behavior or input provided by an individual, or a process that evolves over time. Although studies using factor analysis have failed to uncover distinct dimensions in measures, most theorists believe that social support is a multidimensional concept with both psychological and tangible components.

There are two perspectives on how social support functions to promote and maintain health. One theory is that social support buffers the effects of stressful life events, whereas another theory proposes that social support has a direct, positive effect on health. More longitudinal, well-designed studies are needed to determine the causal relationship between social support and health.

People in an individual's network provide social support, and this support is communicated through the network's structure. Thus structural analysis such as determination of the size, density, intensity, and directedness of the social network is an important assessment strategy. Relationships among the social network members may have both costs and benefits. A network member may provide frequent support, but the support may be of poor quality, ineptly provided, badly timed, interfering, and inappropriate. Equity, reactance, and attribution theories suggest explanations for why help or aid is sometimes perceived negatively.

In addition, who is providing the help (i.e., source) and when the help is offered (i.e., timing) may influence whether the help has positive or detrimental consequences. Different types of relationships (i.e., family, friend, coworker) fulfill different needs. Various types of help may be viewed positively or negatively, depending on what stage of recovery the person is experiencing.

Providing social support to another can be a gratifying experience. On the other hand, providing support may be emotionally and physically draining. The perceptions of both the recipient and provider of social support are important.

Norbeck's model (1981), which uses the framework of the nursing process, can serve as a guide for nurses in their clinical practice. According to Norbeck, properties of the person and the situation can influence whether there is a match between support need and availability. After determining whether the level of social support is adequate or inadequate, the nurse can plan an intervention that enhances the support system or provides direct support.

Social support to individuals is provided and received within the context of the family and community. Nurses must be cognizant of the dangers in disrupting natural support systems that are already in place. Changes in national policy may affect the exchange of social support at the community, family, and individual levels.

## ❖ APPLYING KNOWLEDGE TO PRACTICE

1. What are the major differences between the concepts of social support and support network?
2. Provide examples from your nursing practice that illustrate the importance of type, source, and timing of support in promoting the clients' recovery from disease or disability.
3. Which interventions would you suggest for an individual who has a continuous, intense need for support and lacks skills in developing and maintaining social relationships?

## REFERENCES

Argyle, M. & Furnham, A. (1983). Sources of satisfaction and conflict in long-term relationships. *Journal of Marriage and the Family, 45,* 481–483.

Bankoff, E. A. (1983). Social support and adaptation to widowhood. *Journal of Marriage and the Family, 45,* 827–839.

Barrera, M., Jr. (1981). Social support in the adjustment of pregnant adolescents: Assessment issues. In B. H. Gottlieb (Ed.), *Social networks and social support.* Beverly Hills, CA: Sage.

Barrera, M., Sandler, I. N., & Ramsay, T. B. (1981). Preliminary development of a scale of social support: Studies on college students. *American Journal of Community Psychology, 9,* 435–447.

Beckman, L. J. (1981). Effects of social interaction and children's relative inputs on older women's psychological well-being. *Journal of Personality and Social Psychology, 41,* 1075–1086.

Brandt, P. A. & Weinert, C. (1981). The PRQ—a social support measure. *Nursing Research, 30,* 277–280.

Broadhead, W. E., et al. (1983). The epidemiologic evidence for a relationship between social support and health. *American Journal of Epidemiology, 117*(5), 521–537.

Brocklehurst, J. C., Morris, P., Andrews, K., Richards, B., & Laycock, P. (1981). Social effects of stroke. *Social Science Medicine, 15A,* 35–39.

Brown, M. A. (1986). Social support during pregnancy: A unidimensional or multidimensional construct? *Nursing Research, 35,* 4–9.

Brownell, A. & Shumaker, S. A. (1985). Where do we go from here? The policy implications of social support. *Journal of Social Issues, 41,* 111–121.

Bunting, S. M. (1989). Stress on caregivers of the elderly. *Advances in Nursing Science, 11,* 63–73.

Burke, R. J. & Weir, T. (1976). Personality characteristics associated with giving and receiving help. *Psychological Reports, 38,* 343–353.

Caplan, G. (1982). The family as a support system. In H. I. McCubbin, A. E. Cauble, & J. M. Patterson (Eds.). *Family stress, coping and social support.* Springfield, Ill.: Charles C Thomas.

Caplan, R. D. (1979). Social support, person-environment fit and loving. In L. A. Ferman, J. P. Gordus, (Eds.). *Mental health and the economy.* Kalamazoo: Upton Institute.

Carveth, W. B. & Gottlieb, B. H. (1979). The measurement of social support and its relationship to stress. *Canadian Journal of Behavioral Science, 11,* 179–188.

Chesler, M. A. & Barbarin, O. A. (1984). Difficulties of providing help in a crisis: relationships between parents of children with cancer and their friends. *Journal of Social Issues, 40*(4), 113–134.

Chiverton, P. & Crane, E. D. (1989). Education to assist spouses in coping with Alzheimer's disease: A controlled trial. *Journal of American Geriatrics Society, 37,* 593–598.

Cobb, S. (1976). Social support as a moderator of life stress. *Psychosomatic Medicine, 38,* 300–314.

Cobb, S. (1976). Social Support and health through the life course. In H. I. McCubbin, A. E. Cauble, & J. M. Patterson (Eds.). *Family stress, coping and social support.* Springfield, Ill.: Charles C Thomas.

Cohen S. (1988). Psychosocial models of the role of social support in the etiology of physical disease. *Health Psychology, 7,* 269–297.

Cohen, S. & Syme, S. L. (Eds.). (1985). *Social support and health.* Orlando: Academic Press.

Coyne, J. C. (1976). Toward an interactional description of depression. *Psychiatry, 39,* 28–40.

Crawford, G. (1985). A theoretical model of support network conflict experienced by new mothers. *Nursing Research, 34,* 100–102.

Cronenwett, L. R. (1985). Parental network structure and perceived support after birth of first child. *Nursing Research, 34,* 347–352.

Croog, S. H. (1970). The family as a source of stress. In S. Levine & N. A. Scotch (Eds). *Social stress* pp. (19–53). Hawthorne, NY: Aldine Publishing.

Croog, S. H., Lipson, A., & Levine, S. (1972). Help patterns in severe illness: The roles of kin network, non-family resources and institutions. *Journal of Marriage and the Family, 32,* 32–41.

Dean, A. & Lin, N. (1977). The stress-buffering role of social support: Problems and prospects for systematic investigation. *Journal of Nervous and Mental Disorders, 165,* 403–417.

Dimond M., & Jones, S. L. (1983). Social support: a review and theoretical integration. In. P. Chinn (Ed.). *Advances in Nursing Theory Development.* Rockville, MD: Aspen.

Dunkel-Schetter, C. (1984). Social support and cancer: Findings based on patient interviews and their implications. *Journal of Social Issues, 40*(4), 77–98.

Ellison, E. S. (1983). Social networks and the mental health caregiving system: Implications for psychiatric nursing practice. *Journal of Psychosocial Nursing and Mental Health Services, 21,* 18–24.

Ervin, C. V. (1973). Psychological adjustment to mastectomy. *Medical Aspects of Human Sexuality, 7,* 42–65.

Evans, R. L., Bishop, D. S., & Matlock, A. (1987). Family interaction and treatment adherence after stroke. *Archives of Physiological and Medical Rehabilitation, 68,* 513–517.

Fehr, B. & Perlman, D. (1985). The family as a social network and social support. In L. L'Abate (Ed.), *The handbook of family psychology and therapy* (Vol. 1). Homewood, ILL: Dorsey Press.

Fiore, J., Becker, J. & Coppel, D. B. (1983). Social network interactions: A buffer or a stress. *American Journal of Community Psychology, 11,* 423–439.

Fisher, C. S. (1982). *To dwell among friends: Personal networks in town and city.* Chicago: University of Chicago Press.

Fischer, L. R. (1983). Mothers and mothers-in-law. *Journal of Marriage and the Family, 45,* 187–192.

Fisher, J. D., Nadler, A., & Whitcher-Alagna, S. (1982). Recipient reactions to aid. *Psychological Bulletin, 91,* 52–78.

Ganster, D. C. & Victor, B. (1988). The impact of social support on mental and physical health. *British Journal of Medical Psychology, 61,* 17–36.

Garbarino, J. (1983). Social support networks: Rx for the helping professions. In J. Whittaker & J. Garbarino (Eds.), *Social support networks: Informal helping in the human services* (pp. 3–28). New York: Aldine.

Garrity, T. (1973). Vocational adjustment after first myocardial infarction. *Social Science and Medicine, 7,* 705–717.

Given, B. A., King, S. K., Collins, C., & Given, C., W. (1988). Family caregivers of the elderly: Involvement and reactions to care. *Archives of Psychiatric Nursing, 11,* 281–288.

Gottlieb, B. H. (Ed.). (1988). *Marshaling social support: Formats, Processes, and Effects.* Newbury Park: Sage.

Haley, W. E., Levine, E. G., Brown, S. L., Berry, J. W., & Hughes, G. L. (1987). Psychological, social, and health consequences of caring for a relative with senile dementia. *Journal of American Geriatrics Society, 35,* 405–411.

Hartman, A. (1978). Diagrammatic assessment of family relationships. *Social Casework, 59,* 465–476.

Heller, K. & Swindle (1979). The effects of social support: Prevention and treatment implication. In A. P. Goldstein, F. H. Kanfer (Eds.). *Maximizing treatment gains: Transfer enhancement in psychotherapy.* New York: Academic Press.

Hirsch, B. J. (1979). Psychological dimensions of social networks: A multimethod analysis. *American Journal of Community Psychology, 7,* 263–277.

Hobfoll, S. E., & Walfisch, S. (1984). Coping with a threat to life: A longitudinal study of self concept, social support and psychological distress. *American Journal of Community Psychology, 12,* 87–100.

Holahan, C. J. & Moos, R. H. (1981). Social support and psychological distress: A longitudinal analysis. *Journal of Abnormal Psychology, 90,* 365–370.

House, J. S. (1981). *Work stress and social support.* Reading, Mass: Addison-Wesley.

Hubbard, P., Muhlenkamp, A. F., & Brown, N. (1984). The relationship between social support and self-care practices. *Nursing Research, 33,* 266–270.

Hyman, M. (1972). Social isolation and performance in rehabilitation. *Journal of Chronic Diseases, 25,* 85–97.

Ingersoll-Dayton, B. & Antonucci, T. C. (1988). Reciprocal and nonreciprocal social support: Contrasting sides of intimate relationships. *Journal of Gerontology, 43,* S65–73.

Kahn, R. & Antonucci, T. C. (1980). Convoys over the life course: Attachment, roles, and social support. In P. B. Baltes and O. C. Brim, Jr. *Life-Span Development and Behavior.* New York: Academic Press.

Kane, C. F. (1988). Family social support: Toward a conceptual model. *Advances in Nursing Science, 10,* 18–25.

Kaplan, A. (1977). *Social support: The construct and its measurement.* Unpublished bachelor's thesis. Brown University, Providence, RI.

Kaplan, S. (1983). A model of person-environment capability. *Environment and Behavior, 15,* 311–332.

Kelley, H. H. (1967). Attribution theory in social psychology. In D. Levine (Ed.), *Nebraska symposium on motivation.* (Vol. 15). Lincoln: University of Nebraska Press.

Lazarus, R. S. & Folkman, S. (1984). *Stress, appraisal and coping.* New York: Springer.

Leavy, R. L. (1983). Social support and psychological disorder: A review. *Journal of Community Psychology, 11,* 3–21.

Lenz, E., Parks, P., Jenkins, L., & Jarrett, G. (1986). Life change and instrumental support as predictors of illness in mothers of six-month-olds. *Research in Nursing and Health, 9* (1) 17–24.

Lieberman, M. A. & Borman, L. D. et al. (1979). *Self-help groups for coping with crisis.* San Francisco: Jossey-Bass.

Lin, N., Simeone, R. S., Ensel, W. M., & Kuo, W. (1979). Social support, stressful life events, and illness: A model and an empirical test. *Journal of Health and Social Behavior, 20,* 108–119.

Lopata, H. (1978). Contributions of extended families to support of metropolitan area widows: Limitations of modified kin network. *Journal of Marriage and the Family, 40,* 355–366.

Lowenthal, M. & Haven, C. (1968). Interaction and adaptation: Intimacy as a critical variable. *American Sociological Review, 33,* 20–30.

McFarlane, A. H., Norman, G. R., Streiner, D. L., & Roy, G. (1983). The process of social stress: Stable, reciprocol and mediating relationships. *Journal of Health and Social Behavior, 24,* 160–173.

Mishler, E. & Waxler, N. (1965). Family interaction patterns and schizophrenia: A review of current theories. *Merrill Palmer Quarterly, 11,* 269–315.

Moritz, D. J., Kasl, S. V., & Berkman, L. F. (1989). The health impact of living with a cognitively impaired elderly spouse: Depressive symptoms and social functioning. *Journal of Gerontology, 44,* 517–527.

Mueller, D. (1980). Social networks: A promising direction for research on the social environment of psychiatric disorder. *Social Science and Medicine, 14A,* 147–161.

Norbeck, J. S. (1981). Social support: A model for clinical research and application. *Advances in Nursing Science, 3,* 43–59.

Norbeck, J. S. (1982). The use of social support in clinical practice. *Journal of Psychosocial Nursing and Mental Health Services, 20,* 22–29.

Norbeck, J. S. (1987). Social Support. In J. J. Fitzpatrick, R. L. Taunton, & J. Q. Benoliel. *Annual Review of Nursing Research.* Vol. 6 (pp. 85–110), New York: Springer.

Norbeck, J. S., Lindsey, A. M. & Carrieri, V. L. (1981). The development of an instrument to measure social support. *Nursing Research, 30,* 264–269.

Norbeck, J. S. & Tilden, V. P. (1988). International nursing research in social support: Theoretical and methodological issues. *Journal of Advanced Nursing, 13,* 173–178.

O'Reilly, P. (1988). Methodological issues in social support and social network research. *Social Science Medicine, 26,* 863–873.

Pattison, E. J., Defrancisco, D., Wood, P., Frazier, H., & Crowder, J. A. (1975). A psychosocial kinship model for family therapy. *American Journal of Psychiatry, 132,* 1246–1251.

Pender, N. J. (1987). *Health promotion in nursing practice.* Norwalk, Conn.: Appleton & Lange.

Peters-Golden, H. (1982). Breast cancer: Varied perceptions of social support in the illness experience. *Social Science and Medicine, 16,* 483–491.

Rich, O. J. (1978). The sociogram: A tool for depicting support in pregnancy. *Maternal Child Nursing Journal, 7,* 1–9.

Rook, K. S. (1984). The negative side of social interaction: Impact on psychological well-being. *Journal of Personality and Social Psychology, 46,* 1097–1108.

Roth, P. (1989). Family social support. In P. J. Bomar (Ed.), *Nurses and family health promotion: Concepts, assessment, and interventions.* Baltimore: Williams & Wilkins.

Sanford, J. R. A. Tolerance of debility in elderly dependents by supporters at home: Its significance for hospital practice. *British Medical Journal, 3,* 471.

Sarason, I. G., Levine, H. M., Basham, R. B., & Sarason, B. R. (1983). Assessing social support: The social support questionnaire. *Journal of Personality and Social Psychology, 44,* 127–139.

Sarason, I. G., & Sarason, B. R. (Eds.). (1983). *Social support: Theory, research and applications.* Dordrecht: Martinus Nijhoff Publishers.

Schaefer, C., Coyne, J. C., & Lazarus, R. S. (1981). The health-related functions of social support. *Journal of Behavioral Medicine, 4,* 381–406.

Scott, J. P., Roberto, K. A. & Hutton, T. (1986). Families of Alzheimer's victims: Family support to the caregivers. *Journal of the American Geriatrics Society, 34,* 348–354.

Shumaker, S. A. & Brownell, A. (1984). Toward a theory of social support: Closing conceptual gaps. *Journal of Social Issues, 40*(4), 11–36.

Silverman, P. R. (1970). The widow as a caregiver in a program of preventive intervention with other widows. *Mental Hygiene, 54,* 540–547.

Sokolovsky, J. & Cohen, C. (1981). Toward a resolution of methodological dilemmas in network mapping. *Schizophrenia Bulletin, 7,* 109–116.

Spicer, J. W. & Hampe, G. D. (1975). Kinship interaction after divorce. *Journal of Marriage and the Family, 37,* 113–119.

Stanhope, M., & Lancaster, J. (1988). *Community health nursing: Process and practice for promoting health.* St. Louis: C. V. Mosby.

Tamir, L. M. & Antonucci, T. C. (1981). Self-perception, motivation, and social support through the family life course. *Journal of Marriage and the Family, 43,* 151–160.

Thoits, P. A. (1982). Conceptual, methodological and theoretical problems in studying social support as a buffer against life stress. *Journal of Health and Social Behavior, 23,* 145–159.

Tilden, V. P. & Gaylen, R. D. (1987). Cost and conflict: The darker side of social support. *Western Journal of Nursing Research, 9,* 8–18.

Trainor, M. A. (1982). Acceptance of ostomy and the visitor role in a self-help group for ostomy patients. *Nursing Research, 31,* 102–106.

Troll, L. E. (1980). Intergenerational relations in later life: a family system approach. In N. Datan & N. Lohmann (Eds.), *Transtions of aging.* New York: Academic Press.

Troll, L. E. & Smith, J. (1976). Attachment through the life span: Some questions about dyadic bonds among adults. *Human Development, 19,* 156–170.

Unger, D. G. & Powell, D. R. (1980). Supporting families under stress: The role of social networks. *Family Relations, 29,* 566–574.

Varni, J. W., Wilcos, K. T. & Hanson, V. (1988). Mediating effects of family social support on child psychological adjustment in juvenile rheumatoid arthritis. *Health Psychology, 7,* 421–431.

Vaux, A. (1982). Measures of three levels of social support: resources, behaviors and feelings. Unpublished manuscript.

Vaux, A. & Harrison, D. (1985). Support network characteristics associated with support satisfaction and perceived support. *American Journal of Community Psychology, 13,* 245–268.

Verbrugge, L. M. (1979). Marital status and health. *Journal of Marriage and the Family, 41,* 267–285.

Weiss, R. S. (1974). The provision of social relationships. In Z. Rubin (Ed.). *Doing onto others.* Englewood Cliffs, NJ: Prentice-Hall.

Wood, Y. R. (1984). Social support and networks: Nature and measurement. In P. McReynolds & G. J. Chelune (Eds.), *Advances in psychological assessment* (Vol. 6), San Francisco: Jossey-Bass.

Wortman, C. B. (May 15, 1984). Social support and the cancer patient: Conceptual and methodologic issues. *Cancer,* May 15 Supplement, *53,* 2339–2360.

Wright, L. & Leahey, L. (1984). *Nurses and families.* Philadelphia: F. A. Davis.

Zimmings, C. (1982). Stress and the designed environment. In G. W. Evans (Ed.), *Environmental stress.* (pp. 151–178). New York: Cambridge University Press.

# 26

# Coping

Jane Ehlinger Sherman

## OBJECTIVES

*At the completion of this chapter, the reader will be able to:*

♦ Discuss the multiple dimensions of the concept of coping.

♦ Describe the factors affecting coping and the relationship between coping and adaptation.

♦ Appreciate the situation-specific, unique, and highly personal nature of coping in the planning and delivery of nursing care.

The concept of coping is one with which most people are somewhat familiar. It is used by many individuals, both lay and professional, in a generic sense, similar to the use of terms such as *stress* and *burnout*. There is a certain casualness to the notion of coping as women, men, and children go about the business of dealing with issues that confront them day to day. Coping can be viewed as something that is done on a continuing basis; one copes with the weather, family, job, health, and holidays.

Although it can be argued that there is familiarity with the concept and most people would admit to having experienced it, the essence of the concept is more elusive. What comprises the concept of coping? What are the distinguishing features of the concept? What are the hallmarks or characteristics of coping? What are its dimensions?

Beyond these questions, why focus on the concept within the context of nursing? What is the importance or utility of the concept to pro-

fessional practice? By addressing these and additional questions, this chapter explores the concept of coping, examines the many dimensions of coping, and discusses the relevance of the concept of coping to the practice of nursing.

Two concepts closely related to coping are stress and crisis. They are discussed briefly in this chapter; however, for an in-depth presentation of stress and crisis, the reader is referred to Chapters 17 and 22 in this book.

## ❖ CONCEPT OF COPING
### What Is Coping?

One approach toward developing an understanding and appreciation of the concept of coping is to examine its various definitions. Richard Lazarus and his associate, Susan Folkman, are well known for their research into the psychological aspects of coping. Historically, Lazarus (Lazarus, 1979; Lazarus, Averill, & Opton,

1974) studied coping within the confines of the laboratory setting in which his experimentation was carefully controlled and consequently was very *unlike* the real world in which coping takes place. More recently, Lazarus and Folkman (1980, 1984) directed their attention to the study of coping as it unfolds within the context of specific everyday life situations. They define coping as the "constantly changing cognitive and behavioral efforts to manage specific external and/or internal demands that are appraised as taxing or exceeding the resources of the person" (Lazarus & Folkman, 1984, p. 141). Coping is described in terms of what people think and what they do to make things better and as a process that changes over time.

McCubbin (1980) studied coping as it relates to the family. His work focused on the identification of coping behaviors in women whose husbands were missing in action in Vietnam, parents whose children were chronically ill, and couples undergoing separation and divorce. McCubbin (1979) defined coping as a "strategy for managing stress" (p. 238) and as the overt and covert behaviors used to deal with stress (1981). In McCubbin's scheme coping included using any resources that were available. These resources included assets or characteristics of the individual, the family, or the community that would be helpful in managing the stressful situation (e.g., financial resources, social support, community organizations).

In nursing literature Benner and Wrubel (1989) discussed stress as "the experience of the disruption of meanings, understanding and smooth functioning. Coping is what one does about that disruption" (p. 62). They view coping as being influenced by what the particular situation means to, and holds for, the individual. Consequently, every coping encounter is unique, highly personal, and dependent on the person's interpretation as to how stressful it is.

Scott, Oberst, and Dropkin (1980), who also are nurses, described coping as "a process characterized by continuous use of goal-directed strategies that are initiated and maintained over time and across encounters by means of cognitive appraisal and regulation of emotion and physiologic response" (p. 16). This definition highlights the goal-oriented nature of coping (that coping efforts are activated in relation to a specific situation) and reiterates the importance of appraisal (what is at stake for the individual) as part of the process. Additionally, this definition includes a physiological response, which is probably reflective of the authors' nursing perspective. It would seem appropriate that a coping model developed by nurses would place importance on physiological variables equal to that of the affective and behavioral variables emphasized in the psychological and sociological models.

Along with discussion and definition of coping, theorists also give attention to the concept of adaptation and how it relates to coping. Coping and adaptation are very different, yet related, concepts. Most authors (Goosen & Bush, 1979; Lazarus & Folkman, 1984; McCubbin & Patterson, 1981; Scott, Oberst, & Dropkin, 1980) agree that coping is the process that leads to adaptation as the outcome. Coping is viewed as the link between stress and adaptation. Coping is what one does, the efforts one initiates to deal with stressful encounters with the expectation of adaptation as the end result.

By examining these few selected definitions of coping, some of the key features begin to emerge. As suggested by the preceding discussion, coping:

1. Is goal-oriented
2. Is a process
3. Includes cognitive and behavioral components
4. Activates resources
5. Is situation specific
6. Has emotional and physiological components
7. Forms the linkage with adaptation

❖ **Table 26-1**
Definitions of key terms

| Term | Definition |
| --- | --- |
| Stressor | The event, combination of events, or circumstances that have the potential to produce stress |
| Cognitive appraisal | The process by which the individual evaluates a stressor as threatening or nonthreatening and considers what his or her coping options might be |
| Stress | The relationship between the person and the environment that is appraised by the individual as threatening (Lazarus & Folkman, 1984) |
| Coping | Behaviors that alter the impact of the stressor; behaviors aimed at changing the situation or changing the emotional response to the situation |
| Coping resources | Psychological, social, interpersonal, and material attributes of the individual, family, and community that are perceived by the individual as having the actual or potential ability to alter the impact of a stressor (McCubbin & Patterson, 1981) |
| Reappraisal | Reevaluation of the stressful person-environment relationship and the effectiveness of initial coping efforts; may include implementation of new or additional coping strategies |

Coping is a complex concept with many dimensions. Each of these several dimensions are addressed more fully as the chapter progresses. Because of the multidimensional nature of the concept and the limited scope of this particular chapter, the focus is primarily on the psychosocial aspects of coping and much less on the biophysiological aspects.

## Relevance of Coping to Nursing

The Commission on Nursing Research (1980) advocated giving priority to the study of coping behaviors of individuals and families with emphasis on "decreasing the negative impact of health problems on coping abilities, productivity, and life satisfaction" (p. 219). Carpenito (1987), Doenges and Moorhouse (1988), and McFarland and McFarlane (1989) include nursing diagnoses related to coping in their nursing texts. Assessment of coping skills and abilities and the subsequent enabling of coping strategies should form essential parts of the practice of nursing. To explore more fully the utility of the concept of coping in the practice of nursing, certain key terms are defined, key features and dimensions of the concept are elaborated, and an example of using the concept in practice is provided.

## Definitions of Key Terms

A beginning understanding of key terms is helpful in appreciating the material that follows (Table 26-1). Some of the terms have already been used and briefly discussed in this chapter.

## ❖ ANALYSIS OF THE CONCEPT OF COPING

Several definitions of coping have been presented, and from them several key features and dimensions of coping have been identified. A discussion of some of the previously mentioned dimensions of coping follows.

## Coping Is Goal-Oriented

Coping is purposeful behavior focused toward improving the troubled person-environment relationship. The person finds himself or herself in a situation that calls for action and to which he or she needs to respond. Typically the goal or purpose of the coping efforts serves to change or handle the circumstances surrounding the situation, to change or handle the emotional response generated from the situation, or both.

Lazarus (1979) called these two types of efforts direct action and palliation. *Direct action* refers to those efforts that have the potential to change the situation. *Palliation* refers to those efforts that have the potential to reduce the stress or discomfort associated with the situation. The latter, rather than changing the situation, changes the impact of the situation and makes it more bearable. Folkman and Lazarus (1980) viewed such coping efforts as serving two main functions: (1) changing or managing the person-environment relationship that generated the stress and (2) changing or managing the stressful emotions. Similarly, Pearlin and Schooler (1978) characterized coping as altering or allaying the emotional impact of stressors.

For example, Ms. Miles, age 68 years, was experiencing some unusual skin changes on her vulva. The changes varied from red to purple to blue color with some denuded and excoriated areas. The changes had been present over several months, but Ms. Miles did not mention them. She was convinced that she had cancer, was terribly upset with the prognosis as she saw it (i.e., she was dying, with no hope for any treatment), and wished that she were someone else because then she would not have to deal with the problem.

Ms. Miles' "wishing she were someone else" could be considered a goal-oriented action directed toward changing and relieving—at least temporarily—the stressful emotions associated with her situation. After exploring the feelings surrounding her illness with the nurse, Ms. Miles agreed to a consultation with a gynecologist. This latter behavior could be considered a goal-oriented action directed toward changing and relieving the stressful situation, itself.

Coping efforts should not be equated with coping outcomes. *Coping efforts* are strategies for managing the stressful situations and stressful emotions. In the example above, Ms. Miles' wishful thinking might be construed by some as inappropriate and unhealthy. However, for her it provided some temporary relief from the very stressful emotions she was experiencing, and in that sense it was helpful.

Identification of coping behaviors that were helpful to women whose husbands were acutely, critically ill was the focus of a study by Sherman (1985/1986). The study focused on development of The Sherman Coping Tool, an instrument that contains 50 coping behaviors that are ranked by the wives in terms of helpfulness. Respondents were women whose husbands had a suspected or documented myocardial infarction. Of the 50 items on the tool, 49 were identified as helpful in coping with the husband's illness. Not all women ranked the items similarly, giving credence to the notion that what is helpful to one person may differ from what is helpful to another.

## Coping as a Process

Conceptualizing coping as a process highlights its active, dynamic nature. Coping as a process demands that the individual be intimately involved in the encounter. As such, the person considers the situation, whether or not it is threatening, and the coping options available and activates coping choices based on the foregoing assessment.

Coping as a process involves *appraisal,* which is a key feature in many conceptualizations of coping (Folkman & Lazarus, 1980; Goosen & Bush, 1979; Lazarus & Folkman, 1984; Scott, Oberst, & Dropkin, 1980; Sherman, 1985/1986). It is during the process of appraisal that the individual determines whether or not the stressor is harmful. If the stressor is deemed harmful or threatening, coping options are reviewed, and coping choices are initiated to deal with the stressor.

The appraisal process consists of three discrete, yet interacting, aspects: primary appraisal, secondary appraisal, and reappraisal (Fig. 26-1). *Primary appraisal* refers to the individual's initial assessment that the stressor is irrelevant, benign/positive, or stressful. If the primary appraisal process indicates that the stressor is irrelevant or benign/positive, no further action is necessary. If the stressor is assessed as stressful, *secondary appraisal* ensues. During the process of secondary appraisal the individual considers what, if anything, can and might be done, what is at stake, and what coping options are available. In the process of *reappraisal* the original situation is reviewed in

light of the results of initial coping efforts and any new or additional information, and a decision is made to continue or discontinue the current coping efforts or initiate new coping behaviors.

For example, Mr. Ruff, age 43 years, started having symptoms of sneezing, coughing, and rhinorrhea while at work. These symptoms constituted the stressor that prompted him to engage in primary appraisal of the stressor. During this process he assessed whether the stressor (i.e., the symptoms of sneezing, coughing, and rhinorrhea) was irrelevant, benign/positive, or stressful. He decided it was stressful. This decision enabled him to move into the secondary appraisal process. In secondary appraisal he considered what coping options were available to him, i.e., leaving work and going home to bed, asking his secretary to go to the corner drugstore for some cough medicine, increasing

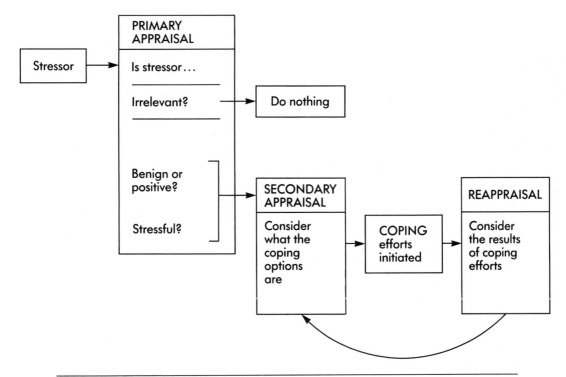

❖ **Fig. 26-1**    Relationships among stressor and three aspects of appraisal and coping.

his fluid intake, or removing the new wool sweater he was wearing because he might be allergic to it.

Considering his history of allergy to wool, he removed the sweater and did nothing else. Thirty minutes later his symptoms subsided. At this point he activated the reappraisal process. During reappraisal he reviewed what prompted the coping encounter, the results of his coping action, and whether or not he needed to continue with the current coping action, terminate the current coping action, or initiate different coping actions. Given the original situation (i.e., the symptoms of coughing, sneezing and rhinorrhea), the subsequent coping action of removing the sweater, the results of the coping action (i.e., the symptoms subsided), he decided that he would not wear the sweater and no further coping actions would be required.

Although three aspects of appraisal are identified and are initiated in sequential order, there is considerable interaction between and among them. No one aspect takes precedence over or is more important than either of the others.

## Coping Includes Cognitive and Behavioral Components

One of the definitions presented earlier described coping as the "cognitive and behavioral efforts made to master, tolerate or reduce external and internal demands and conflicts among them" (Folkman & Lazarus, 1980, p. 223). *Cognitive efforts* refer to coping that focuses on solving the problem by changing the situation. *Behavioral efforts* refer to coping that focuses on regulating or managing the stressful emotions that surround a particular situation.

It is simplistic to categorize coping efforts as exclusively cognitive or behavioral. However, for purposes of examining and understanding the many dimensions of coping, it is useful to consider coping in terms of what people think and what they do. Folkman and Lazarus (1980) conducted

a study among 100 middle-aged men and women engaged in stressful encounters of daily living and attempted to categorize the coping behaviors as problem focused (cognitive) or emotion focused (behavioral). The stressful encounters were identified as those day-to-day situations involving health, work, and family matters. In 98% of the 1332 coping episodes analyzed, both types of coping were used to deal with the stressful encounter. Consequently, the authors suggest there is probably more overlap and less distinction between the two types of coping than originally believed. Thoughts and actions used for coping tend to serve more than one purpose and as such cannot be categorized exclusively as cognitive or behavioral efforts. However, in stressful encounters related to work situations more problem-focused coping was used, whereas in stressful encounters related to health situations, more emotion-focused coping efforts were used.

Several nursing studies conceptualized coping as having cognitive and behavioral components. Although some of the researchers used terms other than cognitive and behavioral to describe coping, the essence of coping is identified as what people think and what they do to manage stressful encounters.

Jalowiec and Powers (1981) compared the life stresses and coping behaviors of emergency room clients with nonserious acute illness with those of newly diagnosed hypertensive clients. Coping was measured by a tool developed by Jalowiec, consisting of 40 coping strategies rated on a five-point scale. Each coping behavior was categorized as either problem-oriented or affective-oriented. Problem-oriented behaviors were directed toward dealing with the problem or stressful situation; affective-oriented behaviors focused on dealing with the emotions generated by the situation. An example of a problem-oriented choice is "Set specific goals to help solve the problem," whereas an affective-oriented choice is "Don't worry about it, everything will probably work out fine" (Jalowiec & Powers, 1981, p. 13). The authors found that the hypertensive clients used significantly more problem-oriented coping behaviors than did the emergency room clients. The former group used religion and physical activity to cope, and the latter group was more apt to use daydreaming or past experiences to deal with the situation. These findings support the notion that affective-oriented coping is often used in situations in which nothing can be done to change the circumstances, so reducing the emotional impact becomes the focus of the coping efforts. It is conceivable that the emergency room clients construed their situation as one that could not be changed and therefore used more emotion-focused coping to alter the impact of the stressor. Conversely, the hypertensive clients viewed their situation as one that was alterable—it is possible to reduce blood pressure to normal levels—so they elected to use more problem-focused coping.

Walker (1988) conducted a study to identify and describe cognitive and behavioral coping strategies used by siblings of children with cancer. She interviewed the well children and asked them to indicate what things they "did or thought" or how they "handled" their sibling's illness. Parents were interviewed and asked to identify the kinds of coping strategies they thought the well children were using. Walker identified three domains or aspects of cognitive and behavioral coping: "intrapsychic (being within the individual's mind), interpersonal (relating to others or involving relationships with others), and intellectual (guided or developed by the intellect rather than emotions)" (pp. 210-211). As an example of cognitive coping, Walker cites how a 10-year-old girl dealt with her brother's illness: "When I think about his being so sick, I tell myself to stop it and think about Christmas or my birthday" (p. 210). The three domains of behavioral strategies were "self-focusing (behaviors directed toward or involving self), distraction (behaviors to divert oneself), and exclusion (behaviors that bar oneself from contact with the stressor)" (p. 211).

Examples of behavioral coping include playing alone, eating, or getting involved in strenuous activity.

In the Sherman Coping Tool described earlier, coping was conceptualized as having cognitive and motor behaviors. Women whose husbands were diagnosed with a documented or suspected myocardial infarction were interviewed while the husband was hospitalized and were asked to reveal what kinds of things they "thought" or "did" that made it easier for them to deal with the husband's illness. More than 100 coping behaviors were identified and categorized as either cognitive or motor behaviors. Thoughts and beliefs that helped the wife deal with her husband's illness were categorized as cognitive behaviors, and physical actions or activities that helped her were classified as motor behaviors. An example of a cognitive behavior is "believing that I am strong"; an example of a motor behavior is "walking or exercising" (pp. 105-106). Although it is acknowledged there might be some overlap between the two categories, the distinction was a useful one to measure helpful coping in women whose husbands were acutely critically ill.

## Coping Activates Resources

*Resources* refer to the coping options that are available to the individual and as such are different from coping responses. Resources for coping are the many alternatives from which a person makes a selection or choice. The process of making a selection from among the possible choices and using that selection constitutes a *coping response.*

Sherman (1985/1986) conceptualized coping as consisting of cognitive and motor behaviors. Additionally, she characterized coping as the process of activating resources—of selecting one or more coping options related to one of three resources: (1) personal, (2) family, and (3) community. The relationship of coping options to cognitive and motor behaviors and to

**Table 26-2**
Coping resources and associated coping behaviors

| Resources | Behaviors | |
| --- | --- | --- |
| | Cognitive | Motor |
| Personal | Thoughts and beliefs the individual has about himself or herself (e.g., "Believing that I will get through all of this") | Actions the individual performs alone (e.g., "Exercising by myself") |
| Family | Thoughts and beliefs related to the family (e.g., "Knowing the family will have the strength to survive") | Actions the individual performs with the family (e.g., "Eating meals with the family") |
| Community | Thoughts and beliefs related to the community (e.g., "Knowing there is a hospital nearby") | Actions the individual performs with the community (e.g., "Attending the Bible study group") |

the three kinds of coping resources is presented in Table 26-2.

*Personal resources* include the psychological, social, interpersonal, and material attributes of the individual involved in the coping encounter. A personal resource, for example, is the availability of financial assets or a belief that one has the strength to survive the situation.

*Family resources* refer to the psychological, social, interpersonal, and material attributes of the family members who are available to the individual involved in the coping encounter. Included are the characteristics of the family such as the degree of closeness, the amount of kinship support, and the ability to solve problems. An example of a family resource is the ability to discuss a problem with a family member or relative or knowing that no matter what happens, there will always be a family member or relative there for support.

*Community resources* refer to the psychological, social, interpersonal, and material attributes of individuals or groups outside of the family that are available to the individual involved in the coping encounter. Such resources include friendships, professional services, agencies, and support groups. An example of a com-

munity resource is a religious organization or a health care provider such as a nurse.

These resources are perceived as having the potential to alter the course of the stressful encounter. It is the process of activating one or more of these resources that constitutes a coping response.

Recall that the process of cognitive appraisal, described earlier, included primary appraisal, secondary appraisal, and reappraisal. It is during the secondary appraisal phase that the individual is confronted with deciding what, if anything, can be done to deal with the situation. In other words, the person reviews his or her available options to deal with the situation and makes a selection. This selection constitutes activation of coping resources and initiates what is then known as a coping effort or response.

## Coping Is Situation Specific

Coping efforts are instituted when a stressor is appraised as actually or potentially harmful or threatening. It is the particular situation that generates the need for coping. Each and every situation is different; hence coping efforts are specific to that particular situation. Similarly, each situation is different for each individual, and it is the individual that determines whether or not a situation is actually or potentially stressful.

Benner and Wrubel (1989) portrayed the person in the situation as being very involved. They indicate that "there is no situationless involvement" (Benner & Wrubel, 1989, p. 82). How a person is "engaged" and "involved" in a situation is critical to how that person will cope with the situation.

Folkman and Lazarus (1980, 1984) discouraged the notion that coping behaviors are simply personality traits that are consistent over time and over situations. Instead, they advocate a conceptualization of coping that is linked with and strongly influenced by the situation. The idea that coping efforts are related to the situation does not discount the usefulness of previous coping behaviors since those behaviors may be appropriate and beneficial in subsequent coping encounters. What is emphasized is the dynamic nature of coping as each situation unfolds, and coping efforts are called into play based on the specific requirements of the particular situation.

Given the same situation, what generates stress and in turn the need for coping efforts for one person might indeed be different from that which generates stress and the need for coping in another. For example, two clients are scheduled for breast biopsy. The first client wants to have the procedure as soon as possible, get the results as soon as they are available, and proceed with any treatment immediately. Additionally, she seeks as much as information as she can about the details of the procedure and about her options if the biopsy reveals a malignancy. The second client consents to the biopsy only after thinking about it for a month. Initially she said that she did not want to know if the biopsy revealed a malignancy and indicated that if she learned she had cancer, she would refuse any treatment. It is inappropriate to judge one coping effort as better or superior to the other.

However, it is possible to ascertain that, given the same situation of needing a breast biopsy, coping efforts for each of these women were specific to her personal appraisal of the situation.

Coping efforts are influenced not only by the situation but also by the dynamics within the situation as it unfolds. As the situation changes, so do the coping requirements. In any given situation, once coping choices are initiated, the implementation of those very coping efforts changes the situation. Subsequently, the now-changed situation generates the need for reappraisal and the need to decide whether to continue or discontinue the same coping efforts or add new ones.

An example of changes within a situation often occurs during the course of an illness. Benner and Wrubel (1989) indicated that "different phases in an illness are literally different situations" (p. 83). As these different phases are revealed, different coping efforts are required. For example, an illness such as an acute myocardial infarction begins with a critical and life-threatening onset. At this phase coping efforts might include going to the emergency room, getting immediate medical attention, and telling oneself that "it must be indigestion ... I can't be having a heart attack." After 3 days in the coronary care unit and transfer to a step-down unit, the situation changes; it is less ominous and begins to take on some aspects of a long-term and less harmful health problem. During this phase coping efforts might include reviewing one's diet and exercise habits and resolving to initiate new or revised ones, planning to incorporate more leisure and stress-reduction activities into one's life, and vowing to attend church services on a regular basis. Without judging the value or utility of any of the aforementioned coping efforts, it becomes clear that coping choices change as the situation changes.

Because each coping encounter is dynamic and fluid and in that sense unpredictable, coping efforts must be flexible and unique. There is no set of predetermined coping efforts that automatically enables the individual to manage the stress related to a myocardial in-farction, a breast biopsy, or the birth of a child. Rather, coping choices are initially linked to and influenced by the situation and subsequently to the dynamics of that situation as it unfolds.

### ❖ FACTORS AFFECTING COPING

Throughout this discussion of coping an effort has been made to avoid portraying coping as a stress-response phenomenon but rather to consider coping as influenced by many factors. Characterizing coping as a stress-response sequence relegates it to a simplistic, unidimensional, static entity and denies its dynamic process and situation-specific nature. Part of the challenge related to understanding coping has to do with this complexity. Coping can be envisioned as multidimensional, multifaceted, and multiinfluenced.

One way to examine the many factors affecting coping is to consider variables related to the stressor, the person, and the environment (Lazarus & Folkman, 1984; Moos & Schaefer, 1984; Panzarine, 1985). Factors related to the *stressor* refer to special features of the stressor. For instance, if the stressor is an illness, the appraisal of how life-threatening or serious the illness is will influence or affect the choice of coping effort. *Personal factors* include the individual's values, beliefs, assets, and sense of control. For example, a person may believe that no matter what happens, she or he will be able to handle it because of a strong faith in God. *Environmental factors* include the circumstances surrounding the situation and features of the environment that enhance or impede coping efforts. For instance, if a person sustains a severe injury in an automobile accident, the coping choices and outcome might be different if the accident occurred on a well-traveled, ma-

jor highway as opposed to a rarely used, geographically remote country road.

This set of three factors exerts its influence on coping choice through the previously described cognitive appraisal process (see Fig. 26-1). Coping efforts can be affected at any or all phases of the appraisal process.

Benner and Wrubel (1989) discuss the concept of *concern* and how it influences what is meaningful for the individual. When a person is concerned about an issue, another person, or anything, the object of that concern has meaning for the person; concerns express what is important to the individual. This notion of concern can be viewed as affecting coping in that concern "is a meaning term that defines an involvement" (Benner & Wrubel, 1989, p. 87), and how a person is involved in a situation is critical to how that person copes in the situation.

### ❖ RELATIONSHIP BETWEEN COPING AND ADAPTATION

Most authors who write about coping also consider the concept of adaptation. *Adaptation* is portrayed as a balance, an outcome, the end result of the coping efforts. Panzarine (1985) discussed coping as "an important factor mediating the relationship between a stressor and the individual's eventual adaptation" (p. 49). Others (Goosen & Bush, 1979; McCubbin & Patterson, 1981; Scott, Oberst, & Dropkin, 1979) agree that adaptation is an outcome and coping is the process directed toward that outcome. Coping is like a bridge or connection that links stressor and adaptation.

A nursing study that investigated the relationship of coping to adaptation was done by Gass and Chang (1989). They studied appraisals of bereavement, coping, coping resources, and psychosocial health dysfunction (PHD) in widows and widowers. The level of psychosocial health was conceptualized as the outcome—as adaptation. They hypothesized that PHD was related to how the loss of the spouse was appraised, the coping behaviors used, and the coping resources available. This study is interesting and useful because it highlights and in some ways summarizes much of what has been presented in this chapter. Widows and widowers were asked to appraise their bereavement in one of three ways: (1) as a harmful loss without other losses, (2) as a loss with other anticipated losses, or (3) as a challenge. Those who appraised their bereavement as a harmful loss without other losses acknowledged experiencing a great loss with the death of their spouse but did not anticipate any other losses related to the death and believed that they would be able to manage the situation. Those who appraised their bereavement, as a loss with other anticipated losses experienced not only the great loss of their spouse but also anticipated being confronted with other losses, concerns, and problems that they would not be able to handle. Those who appraised their bereavement as a challenge believed that they had the strength to overcome the situation and considered it an opportunity for growth.

These researchers used the Folkman and Lazarus Ways of Coping Checklist, which includes 68 coping behaviors that are categorized as either problem-focused or emotion-focused. They hypothesized that both kinds of coping behaviors would directly affect PHD. They also examined what coping resources were available to widows and widowers to help them deal with the stress of bereavement. Resources included material (income), social (helpfulness of social supports), and psychological factors (belief and control over the situation).

Finally, they focused on PHD as measured by the Sickness Impact Profile. The researchers described PHD as a "type of adaptation to conjugal bereavement" (Gass & Chang, 1989, p. 32). It was hypothesized that all of the variables—appraisal of bereavement, coping choices, and coping resources—would affect PHD.

The study revealed that PHD was reduced when the bereavement appraisal was lower (i.e., appraised as harmful loss without other losses), more problem-focused and less emotion-focused coping was used, resources were greater, and clients were younger. Additionally, when bereavement appraisal was higher (i.e., appraised as loss with other anticipated losses), more problem-focused and more emotion-focused coping were used. Bereavement appraisal was lower when coping resources were greatest. The results of this study emphasize the relationship of appraisal to outcome (adaptation), the relationship of appraisal to coping choice, and the relationship of appraisal to coping resources and underscore the interrelatedness of appraisal, coping choice, coping resources, and coping outcome.

## ❖ UNIQUE AND HOLISTIC NATURE OF COPING

If it can be argued that coping is situation specific and that coping choices are affected by features of the stressor, the person, and the environment, it would follow that coping is unique for any individual in any given set of circumstances. Each coping encounter requires the person to respond in a unique fashion to the demands inherent in and peculiar to that particular situation. Mengel (1982) cautioned that "consideration of the client as less than a whole unique person in constant interaction with a changing environment is incomplete and artificial" (p. 3). Consider some of the many influences that help shape a coping encounter—personal beliefs, assets, values, concerns, available coping resources—and how these influences involve the totality of the individual's past, present, and future experiences. The person formulates a coping effort unique to his or her respective situation—unique to that encounter. It is the collective, comprehensive nature of the individual's experience that makes each coping encounter unique and holistic.

This is not to suggest that previously used coping choices are discounted and excluded from use, but it emphasizes the need to consider each coping encounter as open to many possible influences, appraisals, and coping choices.

### ❖ APPLICATION TO PRACTICE: THE NURSING PROCESS

The first step in the nursing process is assessment, a logical place to begin to develop a nursing care plan related to coping. However, herein lies the challenge: How does the nurse assess coping? Is there an assessment tool that the nurse can use to measure a client's coping?

Although there are instruments available that assess coping, their utility in the clinical setting is questionable. For instance, the Ways of Coping Checklist developed by Folkman and Lazarus (1984) was not designed for, nor is it appropriate for use in health-related situations. Instruments that have a health-related focus such as the ones developed by Jalowiec (1981) and Sherman (1985/1986) were designed for use with specific health problems. Jalowiec's instrument focused on hypertensive and emergency room clients, and Sherman's tool focused on women whose husbands had had an acute, critical illness. Consequently, these latter two instruments have limited utility in health-

---

### ❖ CHARACTERISTICS OF COPING AS GUIDE FOR ASSESSMENT

**GOAL ORIENTED**
Is client doing something to change the situation? If so, what?
Is client doing something to change the emotional response generated from the situation? If so, what?

**PROCESS**
What does the client identify as the stressor?
How does client appraise the stressor?
 Primary appraisal: Does the client appraise the stressor as irrelevant, benign/positive, stressful?
 Secondary appraisal: What has the client done to cope with the stressor?
 Reappraisal: What are the results thus far of coping efforts?
  Has the situation changed as a result of coping?
  Have coping efforts changed as the situation changed?
  What coping efforts has the client continued?
  What coping efforts has the client discontinued?

**COGNITIVE AND BEHAVIORAL COMPONENTS**
What kinds of things is the client "thinking" to deal with the stressor?
What kinds of things is the client "doing" to deal with the stressor?

**ACTIVATES RESOURCES**
What kinds of personal coping resources is the client activating?
What kinds of family coping resources is the client activating?
What kinds of community coping resources is the client activating?

**SITUATION SPECIFIC**
What does this situation mean to the client?
Has the client experienced a situation similar to this in the past? If so, how was it similar? How was it different?

related situations other than the ones for which they were developed.

Coping, as stated previously, is situation specific, and how any one client copes depends on what that situation means for that individual at that point in time. Coping needs change as the situation changes. Discerning effective from ineffective coping is very risky, for what is helpful to one individual may not be helpful to another. Nurses must realize and respect the individual and personal nature of each coping encounter. To assess coping, the nurse must explore what that particular situation means for that individual at that moment.

Although each situation must be considered as unique, the nurse can use the material in this chapter to guide the assessment and intervention. The box on p. 482 illustrates how the characteristics of coping can guide the assessment phase of the nursing process, and the box below portrays how these characteristics can guide nursing interventions. The case study and care plan that follow illustrate the use of these guides.

---

❖ **CHARACTERISTICS OF COPING AS GUIDE FOR INTERVENTION**

**GOAL ORIENTED**
Is there anything the client can do to change the situation?
Are there any problem-focused coping efforts the client could use?
Is there anything the client can do to change the emotional response generated from the situation?
Are there any emotion-focused coping efforts the client could use?

**PROCESS**
What does the client identify as the stressor?
Has the identified stressor changed?
How does the client appraise the stressor?
  Primary appraisal: Does the client appraise the stressor as irrelevant, benign/positive, stressful?
  Secondary appraisal: What can the client do to cope with the stressor?
    What coping options does the client have?
  Reappraisal: What are the results thus far of coping efforts?
    Has the situation changed as a result of coping?
    Have coping efforts changed as the situation changed?
    What coping efforts will the client continue?
    What coping efforts will the client discontinue?
    What additional coping efforts might the client initiate?

**COGNITIVE AND BEHAVIORAL COMPONENTS**
What kinds of things can the client "think" to help deal with the stressor?
What kinds of things can the client "do" to help deal with the stressor?

**ACTIVATES RESOURCES**
What kinds of personal coping resources can the client activate?
What kinds of family coping resources can the client activate?
What kinds of community coping resources can the client activate?

**SITUATION SPECIFIC**
What does the situation mean to the client?

CASE STUDY: Ms. Buffington, age 58 years, scheduled an appointment with the nurse to discuss her increasing discontent with life. She is one of two children, widowed, and caring for her 81-year-old diabetic mother who lives with her and whose health is rapidly deteriorating. Ms. Buffington works as a librarian at a private school and is concerned that she may have to quit work to care for her mother on a full-time basis. The mother is visually impaired and cannot see well enough to prepare her insulin, and she needs considerable assistance moving through the house. Ms. Buffington administers the insulin, helps her bathe and dress, comes homes to serve her lunch, and returns to her job until late afternoon. Ms. Buffington describes herself as trapped in a situation that can only get worse. She loves to travel yet finds it impossible to get away because of the responsibility of caring for her mother. She has begun having difficulty sleeping through the night, expresses resentment toward her mother, and can envision no plausible solution.

## Assessment

The box, "Characteristics of Coping as Guide for Assessment," was used to guide the assessment. Assessment data are indicated by uppercase letters and are presented in the box on p. 485.

## Plan

Nursing assessment provided the baseline data on which to establish a plan of care. The box, "Characteristics of Coping as Guide for Intervention," was used to guide formulation of the nursing care plan that follows on p. 486.

## Implementation

Because each coping encounter is unique, the nurse began by encouraging Ms. Buffington to share what the situation meant to her and what it was like to care for her mother. The nurse was nonjudgmental and supportive, reassuring the client that it was acceptable to express her feelings and her honest assessment of the situation.

The nurse and client discussed coping efforts as being emotion-focused, i.e., to relieve the unpleasant, uncomfortable feelings generated by the situation, and problem-focused, i.e., to change the situation itself. To provide some immediate relief from the unpleasant feelings (since it would take some time to begin to change the situation), the nurse suggested that Ms. Buffington consider using a stress-reduction technique. The client liked the idea of borrowing travel videotapes from the local library as an emotion-focused coping effort.

Resources for coping were explored. The nurse discovered that the client had a younger sister living 2 blocks away who might be willing to assist in her mother's care. However, Ms. Buffington had always considered it her sole responsibility to provide the mother's care because she was the older of the two siblings. The client was urged to discuss the situation with her sister. Ms. Buffington acknowledged some reluctance to do so but agreed to role-play the situation with the nurse in preparation for the meeting with her sister.

Potential community resources were identified. The client agreed to investigate the services offered by the home health agency and the church. She seemed intrigued and open to the idea of respite care.

Coping efforts that focused on long-term care options for the mother were difficult for Ms. Buffington to consider. She said that she did not want to talk about them at this visit, preferring to explore agencies and services that would enable her to continue to care for her mother at home. The nurse and the client agreed not to discuss long-term residential care at this first visit, but the client did accept some pamphlets and brochures describing long-term care facilities in the area.

**GOAL ORIENTED**

Is client doing something to change the situation? MAYBE. If so, what? SHE EXPRESSES CONCERN THAT SHE MAY HAVE TO QUIT HER JOB AND CARE FOR HER MOTHER.

Is client doing something to change the emotional response generated from the situation? MAYBE. If so, what? SHE EXPRESSES RESENTMENT TOWARD HER MOTHER.

**PROCESS**

What does the client identify as the stressor? HER MOTHER'S INCREASING DEPENDENCY RELATED TO HER DETERIORATING HEALTH.

How does client appraise the stressor?

Primary appraisal: Does the client appraise the stressor as irrelevant, benign/positive, stressful? SHE APPRAISES THE STRESSOR AS STRESSFUL.

Secondary appraisal: What has the client done to cope with the stressor? SHE PROVIDES FOR MOTHER'S BASIC NEEDS, e.g., FOOD, HYGIENE, CLOTHING, SAFETY. SHE ALTERED HER LIFE-STYLE TO ADJUST TO MOTHER'S NEEDS, e.g., COMES HOME AT LUNCH, DOES NOT TRAVEL.

Reappraisal: What are the results thus far of coping efforts? MOTHER'S NEEDS ARE BEING MET, BUT HER HEALTH CONTINUES TO DETERIORATE. THE CLIENT IS HAVING DIFFICULTY SLEEPING.

Has the situation changed as a result of coping? THE SITUATION IS GETTING PROGRESSIVELY WORSE.

Have coping efforts changed as the situation changed? THE CLIENT HAS BECOME INCREASINGLY INVOLVED IN HER MOTHER'S CARE AS HER MOTHER'S HEALTH HAS WORSENED.

What coping efforts has the client continued? ALL.

What coping efforts has the client discontinued? NONE.

**COGNITIVE AND BEHAVIORAL COMPONENTS**

What kinds of things is the client "thinking" to deal with the stressor? SHE IS THINKING ABOUT QUITTING HER JOB.

What kinds of things is the client "doing" to deal with the stressor? SHE HAS CHANGED HER SCHEDULE TO ACCOMMODATE HER MOTHER'S NEEDS.

**ACTIVATES RESOURCES**

What kinds of personal coping resources is the client activating? SHE HAS ADEQUATE FINANCIAL RESOURCES TO PROVIDE FOR HERSELF AND HER MOTHER; HER JOB IS NEARBY SO SHE CAN GO HOME TO PREPARE LUNCH FOR HER MOTHER.

What kinds of family coping resources is the client activating? SHE CANNOT THINK OF ANY.

What kinds of community coping resources is the client activating? SHE CANNOT THINK OF ANY.

**SITUATION SPECIFIC**

What does this situation mean to the client? SHE ADMITS THAT SHE IS BECOMING INCREASINGLY DEPRESSED OVER THE SITUATION. SHE CANNOT SEE ANY SOLUTION, SAYS THAT THINGS CAN ONLY GET WORSE—ESPECIALLY IF SHE HAS TO QUIT HER JOB. SHE FEELS TRAPPED AND RESENTFUL. SHE SAYS THAT THE ONE THING THAT SHE ENJOYS—TRAVEL—IS ONLY A DREAM BECAUSE SHE CANNOT GET AWAY FROM HER MOTHER.

Has the client experienced a situation similar to this in the past? NO; THINGS JUST KEEP GETTING WORSE. If so, how was it similar? How was it different?

# ❖ NURSING CARE PLAN

**CLIENT:** Ms. Buffington

**NURSING DIAGNOSIS:** Ineffective individual coping related to burden of caring for aging parent and perceived lack of control over own life

| GOALS | INTERVENTIONS |
|---|---|
| Ms. Buffington will express her feelings related to her mother and the situation. | ◆ Encourage client to acknowledge and express feelings. Ask the client what it is like to be in the situation and what the situation means to her. <br> ◆ Reassure client that feelings of resentment are not unusual in such situations. |
| Ms. Buffington will initiate one stress-reduction technique. | ◆ Explore potential emotion-focused coping efforts, e.g., travel videotapes, relaxation exercises, imagery. |
| Ms. Buffington will explore ways of sharing the immediate burden of caring for her mother with assistance from her family or community agencies. | ◆ Explore coping resources available from the family, e.g., client's sister who lives 2 blocks away. <br> ◆ Explore coping resources available from the community, e.g., a home health agency that provides respite care, the Episcopal church in which the mother was an active member that provides companionship and support services for the homebound. <br> ◆ Encourage client to activate family and community coping resources. |
| Ms. Buffington will plan an overnight stay out of town next weekend. | ◆ Explore problem-focused coping efforts, e.g., have client negotiate with her sister to come to the house and care for the mother from Friday evening until 6:00 P.M. Saturday. |

❖   **NURSING CARE PLAN—cont'd**

| GOALS | INTERVENTIONS |
|---|---|
| Ms. Buffington will begin to consider options for long-term care for her mother. | ◆ Explore problem-focused coping efforts related to long-term care for her mother, e.g., assist client to identify agencies and services that would help her to continue to care for her mother at home.<br>◆ Encourage and assist client to identify and explore what residential long-term care options are available for her mother. |

**EVALUATION**

Ms. Buffington is able to verbalize her feelings to the nurse and acknowledges feelings of resentment and loss of control over own life. Following this acknowledgment, Ms. Buffington identifies ways to reduce stress and reports daily use of travel videotapes. In addition, she identifies family and community coping resources (e.g., her sister and respite care) and uses respite care resources to help with her mother's care. Over time, Ms. Buffington expresses willingness to investigate one long-term care facility and one home-visit assistance program.

## Evaluation

Ms. Buffington expressed great relief at being able to discuss her feelings about her situation, the burden she experienced, the resentment, the guilt, and the implications related to her job and personal life. She was appreciative of the nonjudgmental atmosphere and supportive environment created by the nurse, which enabled her to discuss her life as she saw it. She revealed that sharing her feelings made her feel so much better that she went to the library immediately after the initial visit with the nurse and borrowed three travel videotapes. She watched two that evening and marveled at the benefits provided by her vicarious adventures to London and Glasgow. She plans to continue borrowing tapes on a regular basis.

Ms. Buffington planned to talk with her sister about her assisting with her mother's care but decided against it, saying that she might do it later. She felt so much better after using the videotapes that she called the home health agency about respite care and arranged for a respite care worker to spend the next Friday night and Saturday with her mother so she can go out 'of town as planned. She said that she simply preferred managing her mother's care without the help of her sister. She did not explore the services offered through the church.

The client learned of other home health services available from the agency that is providing her respite care and believes that some of them will lighten her burden and enable her to continue caring for her mother at home. She did not read any of the pamphlets or brochures from the long-term care residential facilities.

Ms. Buffington described herself as feeling more in control of her life and her future. She and the nurse agreed to meet again after the client returned from her weekend away.

### ❖ SUMMARY

Several definitions of coping were presented, and from them key dimensions or characteristics of coping were identified. Coping is conceptualized as (1) goal oriented, (2) a process, (3) including cognitive and behavioral components, (4) activating resources, (5) situation specific, (6) having emotional and physiological components, and (7) forming the linkage with adaptation. Factors affecting coping are those related to the stressor, the person, and the environment. The unique, dynamic, and extremely personal nature of coping has been highlighted.

Coping is a complex concept; yet it is one that has great utility in the practice of nursing. Currently there are few instruments with which to assess coping in the clinical setting. Hopefully, as nursing research in this area is expanded, additional and more refined tools will be developed to enable a more adequate assessment of coping. With more precise assessment, effective nursing interventions can be developed to assist clients to cope with the stressors in their lives.

### ❖ APPLYING KNOWLEDGE TO PRACTICE

1. Discuss the key dimensions or characteristics of the concept of coping as they apply to the situation of a nurse returning to school.
2. Reflect on your practice, and identify a client who is coping with a stressful situation. Use the key dimensions of coping to analyze the client's response.
3. Identify a research study in a nursing journal that focuses on coping. After reading the study, describe the purpose of the study, identify which dimensions of coping were included, and discuss the nursing implications.

### REFERENCES

Benner, P. & Wrubel, J. (1989). *The primacy of caring.* Menlo Park, Calif.: Addison-Wesley.

Carpenito, L. J. (1987). *Nursing diagnosis.* Philadelphia: J. B. Lippincott.

Commission on Nursing Research. (1980). Generating a scientific basis for nursing practice: Research priorities for the 1980s. *Nursing Research, 29,* 219.

Doenges, M. & Moorhouse, M. (1988). *Nursing diagnoses with interventions.* Philadelphia: F. A. Davis.

Folkman, S. & Lazarus, R. S. (1980). An analysis of coping in a middle-aged community sample. *Journal of Health and Social Behavior, 21,* 219-239.

Gass, K. A. & Chang, A. S. (1989). Appraisals of bereavement, coping, resources, and psychosocial health dysfunction in widows and widowers. *Nursing Research, 38,* 31-36.

Goosen, G. M. & Bush, H. A. (1979). Adaptation: A feedback process. *Advances in Nursing Science, 1,* 51-66.

Jalowiec, A. & Powers, M. J. (1981). Stress and coping in hypertensive and emergency room patients. *Nursing Research, 30,* 10-15.

Lazarus, R. S. & Folkman, S. (1984). *Stress, appraisal and coping.* New York: Springer.

Lazarus, R. S. (1979). *Patterns of adjustment.* St. Louis: C. V. Mosby.

Lazarus, R. S., Averill, J. R., & Upton, E. M. (1974). The psychology of coping: Issues of research and assessment. In G. V. Coehlo, D. A. Hamburg, & J. E. Adams (Eds.), *Coping and adaptation* (pp. 249-315). New York: Basic Books.

McCubbin, H. I. (1979). Integrating coping behavior in family stress theory. *Journal of Marriage and the Family, 41,* 237-244.

McCubbin, H. I., Joy, C. B., Cauble, A. E., Comeau, J. K., Patterson, J. M., & Needle, R. H. (1980). Family stress and coping decade review. *Journal of Marriage and the Family, 42,* 855-871.

McCubbin, H. I. & Patterson, J. M. (1981). *Family stress resources and coping.* St. Paul, Minn.: University of Minnesota.

McFarland, G. K. & McFarlane, E. A. (1989). *Nursing diagnosis & intervention.* St. Louis: C. V. Mosby.

Moos, R. H. & Schaefer, J. A. (1984). The crisis of physical illness. In R. H. Moos (Ed.), *Coping with physical illness* (pp. 3-25). New York: Plenum Medical Book Company.

Panzarine, S. (1985). Coping: Conceptual and methodological issues. *Advances in Nursing Science, 4,* 49-57.

Scott, D. W., Oberst, M. T., & Dropkin, M. J. (1980). A stress-coping model. *Advances in Nursing Science, 3,* 9-23.

Sherman, J. E. (1986). The development of a tool to measure helpful coping behaviors in women whose husbands are acutely critically ill. (Doctoral dissertation, University of Maryland, 1985.) *Dissertation Abstracts International, 46,* 2627B.

Walker, C. L. (1988). Stress and coping in siblings of childhood cancer patients. *Nursing Research, 37,* 208-212.

# 27

# Empowerment

Karen E. Dennis

## OBJECTIVES

*At the completion of this chapter, the reader will be able to:*

♦ **Describe the dynamics of control, including its definitions and types and the advantages and disadvantages of retaining versus relinquishing control.**

♦ **Identify common and distinct mechanisms clients may use for achieving control.**

♦ **Apply the nursing process to empower clients of health care systems.**

Power is a strong and pervasive human need. It is more important to people and more central to understanding their behavior than many health care providers recognize. Across time, philosophers such as Plato and Machiavelli have given a great deal of thought to power, whereas political figures such as Hitler and Stalin have epitomized its feared and fearful side through dominance-submission, police states, and other forms of tyranny. Thus it is not surprising that negative impressions of power prevailed for many years, despite the fact that everyone has a need to influence the people, events, and environments that effect his or her well-being and quality of life. Although it is admirable to have hope, need love, want freedom, and work for peace, it has not been acceptable to need, desire, or seek power. At least, it was not acceptable to admit that need, and those who sought power often did so under the guise of altruism. The evolution of contemporary society, however, has revealed the positive aspects of power, its relevance to people's lives, and the critical role it plays in interpersonal and international relationships. Consistent with that evolution, nurses are breaking through the traditional, stereotyped image of "clients," realizing the many benefits that can accrue when people become active participants in their care, and are attempting to empower clients of health care systems.

## ❖ DEFINITIONS
### Power

*Power* is having impact. It is the ability to take action that regulates or manages other people; it is the ability to effect change or prevent it. Power may include the ability to alter people's thinking, beliefs, and preferences along with their behavior, although sometimes it only alters behaviors, leaving belief systems intact. The base of power consists of all the knowledge, resources, opportunities, acts, and objects one can muster to affect the behavior of others. The means of power include rewards and incentives, promises and threats, coercion, and physical compulsion. As a composite, these statements reveal a cause-and-effect element to power that takes place within an interpersonal situation. In a cyclical manner power must have empowering responses. One's power continues only as long as other people conform to the prescribed pattern. "Power resides implicitly in the other's dependency" (Emerson, 1962, p. 32).

## Control

Often used interchangeably, the terms *power* and *control* have different connotations. Whereas power necessitates an interpersonal situation, control also includes successful manipulation of environmental variables, physical resources, and one's own behavior. Thus control might be considered the overarching concept. In common language, people "control" the lights or the thermostat, with dependency residing in objects that are not human. They also "control" their own anger or anxiety, and other people may not be directly involved. Therefore, and particularly in the case of clients, it is helpful to think of power and control as complementary terms and processes rather than become entangled in the nuances of theoretical definitions.

Control is affecting and directing the environment and the behavior of self and others in ways that further one's objectives. It is not necessary that the person *actually* has control over certain events, but rather that he or she *perceives* to have it (Burger, 1989).

In a classic review of the literature Averill (1973) delineated three types of control: behavioral, cognitive, and decisional.

*Behavioral control* refers to an action that may directly influence or modify the objective characteristics of an event and thus implies direct action on the environment or the activities of others.

*Cognitive control* includes acquiring information, making appraisals about whether the environment is a threat, a challenge, or something neutral, and interpreting the meanings of internal and external stimuli. Cognitive control is possible through the formulation of a cogni-

tive plan, which may change one's own responses such as considering a fearful event as a challenge. By itself, cognitive control exists within the person and has no direct effect on features of the environment or event.

*Decisional control* is having and/or executing a choice among alternative courses of action. It includes either directly choosing among alternatives or making substantial contributions to the decision making of others.

## ❖ UNDERSTANDING THE CONCEPT OF CONTROL

Control may be considered an existential rather than biological need, which develops throughout the maturation process. Infants who are fed when they cry to meet a hunger need achieve three kinds of gratification: (1) relief of hunger, (2) reduced fear that hunger will never end, and (3) the experience of making satisfaction happen. Control, therefore, brings a reward not only because it satisfies a need, but also because it decreases anxiety (Renshon, 1979). The need for control, which originates as an attempt to satisfy other basic needs, leads to a set of beliefs about nature and the world and to a set of behaviors reflective of those beliefs. Knowing someone's belief systems and individual orientation to control increases the ability to understand and predict what a person will think, feel, and do.

## Locus of Control

*Locus of control* refers to an individual's expectancies about the outcomes of actions (Lefcourt, 1981; Rotter, 1966). People with an *internal locus of control* expect that their own behaviors determine outcomes, whereas those with an *external locus of control* expect that luck, fate, or chance are the determining factors. Despite its popularity in research and practice, many fail to note that locus of control refers to an expectation, which is not the same as a need or a desire. For example, a person may not *expect* to win a million dollars in the latest sweepstakes, but the *desire* to win that fortune can be very strong. A client may not *expect* to have 24-hour visiting privileges but may *want* to have a significant other with him or her at all times.

## Personal Causation

More than an expectation, having control is the experience of originating actions and causing things to happen; not having control is the experience of being pushed around (deCharms, 1979). Powerlessness ensues when people believe their actions are not having any effect. The more people expect or want to have control and the more important the outcomes are, the more strongly they will experience powerlessness in circumstances in which there is no control. When placed in an extremely unpleasant environment over which they have no control, individuals eventually lose motivation to initiate any actions that might change things for the better. Over time, they may passively accept and acquiesce to other negative situations as well. With increased passivity come feelings of helplessness, anxiety, and depression (Seligman, 1975).

Recently there has been an increased emphasis on the pleasurable aspects of being in control of and dealing effectively with the environment, independent of the possible satisfaction of other needs achieved thereby. Individuals who have control tend to be healthier, happier, more active, solve problems better, and feel less stress (Wallston & Wallston, 1981; Seligman & Miller, 1979; Strickland, 1978). Nurse researchers have found that middle-aged women who perceived a sense of control engaged in more health promotion behaviors (Duffy, 1988); likewise, clients with spinal cord injuries felt less depressed (Ferington, 1986). In contrast, a low sense of control has been associated with less self-initiated preventive health care, less optimism concerning the efficacy of early treatment, poor self-rated health,

and more illness episodes, bed confinement, and dependence on the physician (Seeman & Seeman, 1983).

An extensive number of studies support the impact that control has on mediating stress reactions. Research findings from studies conducted in laboratory and clinical settings have documented the importance of control in reducing stress-related signs and symptoms such as blood pressure, heart rate, anxiety, and pain (Johnson, 1984). Moreover, these findings were supported whether clients actually had control or only thought that they did, which points to the importance of control perception, along with expectation and desire (Miller, 1980).

## Retaining or Relinquishing Control

Evidence also has accumulated that indicates that having control, particularly behavioral control, may increase stress. There will be times when individuals want to retain control, even fiercely protecting their right to have it, and other times when they want nothing more than to give it away. An explanation for these opposing behaviors is evident in the meaning of the control response for the individual and the meaning of the event. With control, people know they can depend on their own response to minimize danger and therefore believe that the situation will not become so bad that it exceeds a maximum "worst" that they can handle or endure. On the other hand, when people think that others can best guarantee a limit to the maximum worst, they prefer to relinquish control (Burger, 1989; Miller, 1980). Increased control may lead to negative responses when the following occur:

1. The controlling response is difficult to figure out or do (e.g., central venous catheter care for the client who has never been taught how to do the procedure).
2. The increase in perceived control leads to a high level of concern for self-presentation (e.g., the client who fears she will be considered "incom-

petent" if the insulin injection is not done perfectly).

3. The person perceives a decreased probability of obtaining desired outcomes (e.g., the client who believes that inserting her own nasogastric tube would be more, not less, uncomfortable).

4. The increased controllability leads to an increase in attention to the now-predictable but aversive events (e.g., the burned client whose ability to schedule his own debridements makes him focus on his plight even more).

An additional clinical example illustrates situations when a client may prefer to retain or relinquish control. Preferring to control her wet-to-dry dressing change by removing the bandage herself, a postoperative client can regulate the pace to endure better the pulling sensation from tape and gauze that has adhered to the skin. However, she may be grateful when the physician or nurse removes her drain and sutures, knowing that their skill is more deft and experienced than her own, that she can look out the window rather than at her incision, and that she will have a more comfortable experience.

Inherent in having cognitive control is a reduction in uncertainty. When an event is uncertain, it is likely to have vagueness, lack of clarity, ambiguity, unpredictability, inconsistency, varying probability, multiple meanings, and lack of information (Mishel, 1981). Uncertainty hampers cognitive appraisal because the person does not know whether to judge an event as benign, threat, or challenge, and it impedes coping because there is no frame of reference for dealing constructively with that unknown situation. Although information seeking is a logical first course of action, barriers to information exchange in health care systems compromise the effectiveness of this approach. Treatment routines, obscure bureaucratic procedures, impersonal care on the part of staff, and a limited flow of information make it difficult for clients to exercise control during hospitalization (Taylor, 1979). Thus there may be

either prolonged avoidance behavior by trying to ignore or escape from the situation or vigilance by monitoring the situation for cues in an unrelenting manner.

Even though the individual knows when and under what circumstances an event will occur, what it will be like, and what effects it will have does not mean he or she can exercise behavioral control over it. Nevertheless, having more knowledge may enhance the perception of control and facilitate cognitive control so that the person can alter his or her own response to the event, even though the event itself cannot be changed. For example, to deal with functional limitations and emotional downslides, clients with chronic illness have kept a positive frame of reference and warded off feelings of defeat by telling themselves, "It's not that bad; I can handle it" (Forsyth, Delaney, & Gresham, 1984).

## ❖ CLINICAL APPLICATIONS OF THE CONTROL CONCEPT
### Clients' Control: Sources and Solutions

**Outpatient settings.** Studies of obstetrical clients (Shapiro et al, 1983) and neurological clients (Faden et al, 1981) revealed that they preferred far more detail than physicians actually provided. Prenatal clients wanted more information from their obstetricians about the baby, labor, and related health behaviors than they received. Lower social class clients wanted more and obtained less information than those in higher social classes, possibly because other sources of information such as books and childbirth classes were not available to them. Neurological clients wanted to know more about risks associated with their medication and what the possible alternatives were. Their physicians believed that with more information, clients would be less likely to adhere correctly to the regimen and that they would be less confident in the treatment. Reflecting the movement in consumerism, other clients noted they have a right to take some responsibility for medical decision making, and many have challenged medical authority (Haug & Lavin, 1981). Underscoring the impact of individual differences when it comes to control, Krantz et al (1981) observed varying degrees in outpatients' quest for information and their tendency to initiate behaviors related to their health care.

**Long-term care.** Studies in long-term care settings have shown that the facilitation of personal control in the form of responsibility and choice resulted in significantly greater levels of alertness, activity, participation, and a sense of well-being, which had sustained, beneficial physical and psychological effects (Langer & Rodin, 1977; Schulz & Hanusa, 1978). Demonstrating that interventions to facilitate control can be seemingly simple, these residents were given encouragement to take responsibility for themselves, the responsibility of caring for a plant, the choice of a movie night, and the ability to determine the length and frequency of visits from friends. In contrast, caregivers in other nursing homes saw themselves as the predominant decision makers and did not emphasize the availability of choices or options for residents. Even though the caregivers preferred a higher level of self-determination for residents, only in one-to-one or solitary activities did they give away the primary decision-making role, possibly because they saw most residents as incapable of making decisions. Since grooming and eating were identified as areas in which residents had the least control, targeting initial interventions in those two areas might be the most productive (Ryden, 1985).

Relocation from one facility to another presents a profound change to the lives of elderly clients. Many make successful transitions, but others do not. For the elderly who adapted well, a critical factor was not an involvement in choosing the specific new facility, but their ability to make choices within each institution, the social interaction milieu, and the feeling that they had mastery and control over their lives during the crisis of the relocation experience (Lieberman & Tobin, 1983; Pohl & Fuller, 1980).

**Acute care hospitals.** When clients enter a hospital, they face many unknowns: what diagnostic tests will reveal, whether there will be cure or disability, whether there will be pain, disfigurement, a permanently altered life-style, or a combination of all of these or death. Adding to the problem, clients entering a hospital leave behind family, home, and daily routines. Activities usually undertaken with freedom and autonomy are greatly curtailed, and there is an increasing reliance on others for what previously had been done independently. Unique to the hospital is the notion that going to the bathroom is indeed a privilege. There is sure to be an effect on people who are stripped of usual clothing and told when to eat, when to bathe, and when to have visitors. Specific hospital events that studies have shown as stressful to clients are using a bedpan, anticipating a painful treatment or procedure, seeing another client who is very ill, leaving usual work, being away from the family, and the client's own condition or illness (Wilson-Barnett, 1976). Experiences that induced feelings of powerlessness revolved around the health care system's control of time, scheduling, environmental stimuli, and information and a client's alterations in self-concept and roles (Kritek, 1981). Stressful thoughts included thinking about losing sight, hearing, or a kidney or some other organ and those that evolved from a lack of communication and receipt of information (Volicer & Bohannon, 1975).

## Stressful Procedures

Undergoing invasive diagnostic and treatment procedures is a common experience for clients of health care systems. Determining ways to decrease the stressfulness of those events has been the focus of a large volume of research. Studying preparation for and clients' reactions to procedures as diverse as orthopedic cast removal, gynecological examination, cardiac catheterization, dental extraction, and cholecystectomy, numerous researchers across many disciplines, including nursing, have reached similar conclusions. Procedural information that tells clients step-by-step what will happen, sensory information, including the kinds of sensations (e.g., warmth, pressure, dizziness) they will feel, and suggestions of coping behaviors that clients might try before, during, or after the procedure have been the most effective in reducing distress. Across this array of studies, clients who had preparatory information that facilitated their cognitive and/or behavioral control experienced less anxiety and negative mood states, reported less pain, requested fewer pain medications, appeared to be more comfortable, and went home earlier than those who did not receive this type of intervention (Johnson, 1984; Devine, 1983).

## Shared and Distinct Mechanisms for Client Control

**Information: the common and critical theme.** Clients want and need information because it is their right, it helps them deal with uncertainty and the anxiety associated with uncertainty, and it is imperative for developing future plans and making decisions. Having information, particularly that related to their diagnosis, treatment, prognosis, illness severity, and the life-style implications of their disease process, is very important to clients and is critical to the resolution of uncertainty and the development of cognitive control (Dennis, 1987; Mishel, 1983).

Clients with chronic illness particularly tend to seek information that has direct utility in solving issues they perceive as problematic. For example, a client focusing on deformities secondary to arthritis might welcome advice on the nightly use of wrist braces. Attuned to a variety of information sources, clients with chronic illness are particularly receptive to readings, information on self-help groups, and opportunities to talk to other hospitalized clients (Forsyth, Delaney, & Gresham, 1984).

Major categories of informational needs for cancer clients, in order of importance, were disease, personal, family, and social relationships (Derdiarian, 1986). Rated in order as the greatest informational needs within each category were the following:

1. *Disease:* treatment outcomes, prognosis, diagnosis, consequences/results of tests
2. *Personal:* implications for physical and psychological well-being, potential disruptions of plans
3. *Family:* implications for spouse and children, then parents and siblings
4. *Social relationships:* impact on job/career, the future, and leisure activities

Even though these types of information were derived from a study of clients with cancer, they are consistent with the information needs of a more diverse array of medical-surgical clients (Dennis, 1990, 1987; Mishel, 1983, 1981). Therefore health care providers would not be amiss in being sensitive to these topics for other clients as well until further research identifies the informational needs of clients with a wider range of diagnoses.

Despite the importance placed on having information, clients have expressed concern about exclusion from discussions during ward rounds, lack of information about the results of diagnostic tests, the belief that they would not receive information unless they asked for it, inhibitions about asking questions, the perfunctory replies they received when they did ask, and their perceived treatment as objects rather than persons. Clients believed that anxiety and fear are the consequences of poor communication and admitted that a fear of the unknown is a much heavier burden to bear than the full knowledge of their illness, however serious it may be (Reynolds, 1978).

Beyond viewing having information as central to having control, hospitalized clients manifest marked differences in other means for achieving and expressing control. In replicated studies of medical-surgical clients Dennis (1990, 1987) delineated four additional, distinct mechanisms through which clients find control: client role enactment, decision making, personal integrity preservation, and global self-determination. Clients may use these approaches either singly or in combination.

**Client role enactment.** Clients of this type want to have information about diagnostic tests and treatments, but they do not necessarily want to be actively involved in making decisions about these events. They view decision making as the prerogative of health care providers and think they will complicate or impede the process by participating in it. Instead, these clients are concerned about their role as a client, wanting to know what is expected of them and wanting to do things right as a client. It is important for them to know about schedules and routines so that they can be in compliance with them and to do things for themselves as much as possible so as not to "bother" the staff. People in this category need to be known as "good" clients and believe they should be obedient, cooperative, and objective about their illness and that they should expect attention only if they are very ill (Lorber, 1975). Along with their own role enactment, it is important for these clients to know that nurses and physicians will also fulfill the obligations of their roles such as having nurses take action when things are not going right and having physicians give them the information they seek.

**Decision making.** These clients want an active role in making decisions about their care and treatment and are less concerned about having control over activities of daily living and the physical environment. They want to help decide whether or not to have certain diagnostic tests, treatment modalities, and surgery and want to be involved in determining their discharge date. Because their lives and bodies are involved, they want to have a say in what happens. For this type of client, however, being involved does not mean complete decision-making independence. Rather, they are "interdependent-participative," preferring a pattern of shared control (Dennis, 1990; Degner & Russell, 1988). Although additional research is needed to identify personal characteristics of the active decision makers, studies to date suggest that likely profiles include clients with cancer, those who are undergoing a barrage of stressful and invasive procedures, and individuals with chronic illness who have extensive and intimate experience with their disease (Degner & Russell, 1988; Dennis, 1987; Forsyth, Delaney, & Gresham, 1984).

**Personal integrity preservation.** Of all types, these people place less importance on having information about the diagnostic tests, treatments, and/or surgery that constitutes their reason for hospitalization. Instead, they emphasize maintaining independence and the integrity of their personhood. It is particularly important for these individuals to do their own activities of daily living, set their own schedules, and ensure their sense of privacy.

**Global self-determination.** These individuals focus more heavily, but not exclusively, on personal rather than medical concerns. What they experience as hospitalized clients is only one of many components that comprise the scope of their lives. As such, it is important for these clients to have good interpersonal relationships with the people around them and to regulate the amenities of their physical environment. Self-directed and the center of their own universe, they have less regard for knowing about hospital schedules and routines that may impinge on their independence.

## ❖ CONTROL AND THE NURSING PROCESS
### Assessment

**Information.** Assessing a client's need for information is central to evolving an individualized plan of care. An obvious way of determining what a client knows or needs to know is to ask some pointed questions when obtaining the nursing history and again as events unfold

## ❖ LISTENING FOR INFORMATION NEEDS: ASSESSMENT CATEGORIES

**PROCEDURES: DIAGNOSTIC TESTS AND TREATMENTS**

What has been ordered to date
When the test is scheduled
When the treatment(s) will be done
Procedural information
   What will be done
   What sensations to expect throughout the experience
   What the client can do to help in the process
Alternatives
   Purpose
   Expected benefits of each
   Anticipated drawbacks
Impact
   Discomfort
   Dysfunction
   Time and inconvenience
Costs
   Physical
   Monetary

**LIFE-STYLE IMPACT**

Activities of daily living
   Diet
   Functional status and physical activity
   Independence
Interpersonal relationships
   Spouse, children, parents, significant others
Work
   When to expect to return to work
   Limitations not previously imposed

throughout the course of hospitalization or outpatient visits. Results from research on clients' information needs provide a focus. The box on the left lists major areas for assessment and topics within those categories about which the nurse should ask or listen for in the client's response.

Other mechanisms for determining information and control needs have been more typical of research studies than clinical programs, perhaps because most instruments used in research are too long, complex, and trying for clients to complete and health care providers to score. Although it may not be feasible or reasonable to give the client an array of questionnaires on admission, giving one questionnaire early in the hospitalization or selecting several questions from these scales to pose verbally can be insightful. Three of these questionnaires have ease and relevance for clinical use: the Health Opinion Survey (Krantz, Baum, & Wideman, 1981), the Mishel Uncertainty in Illness Scale (Mishel, 1981), and the Multidimensional Health Locus of Control Scale (Wallston et al, 1978). Selected items from each, as presented in the box on p. 499, have been rephrased from the original statements into questions that can be asked verbally.

**Control.** An initial assessment of clients' control orientations may be achieved through asking questions and observing behaviors, although it may take a period of time to develop a clear understanding of individual expressions. The nurse can ask whether the client wants to take an active role by helping to make decisions about his or her care and treatment, but watching the client's behaviors as decisional matters arise may be more insightful. The client who initiates participation in decision making is relatively easy to assess; the client who holds back either may not want the responsibility or may be acting out of deference to what is perceived as the physician's prerogative, not realizing his or her rights in the process. Moreover, the nurse should be alert for clients' comments, questions, and behaviors that reveal a concern for the expected client role, personal integrity preservation (e.g., privacy, independence in activities of daily living), and self-determination.

Very often clients whom staff members classify as difficult behavioral management problems actually may be acting on their thwarted needs for control. For clients who are passively compliant, excessively noncompliant, belligerent, spiteful, aggressive, and/or willfully independent, control may be a major issue. These individuals may be doing the best they can to meet their need for control but lack an understanding of additional strategies that may be more productive and helpful within the strange environment of a health care system. Assessing the real core of the problem rather than labeling clients' actions as "obnoxious be-

❖ **ELICITING INFORMATION NEEDS: SELECTIONS FROM RESEARCH QUESTIONNAIRES REPHRASED FOR VERBAL APPLICATION IN CLINICAL PRACTICE**

**HEALTH OPINION SURVEY**
Do you usually ask the doctor or nurse many questions about what they are doing?
Do you usually wait for the doctor or nurse to tell you about the results of a test rather than asking him or her?
Would you rather have doctors and nurses make the decisions about what is best or have them give you a whole lot of choices?
Do you think it is better to rely on the judgments of doctors (who are experts) than to rely on "common sense" in taking care of yourself?
Do you think that learning how to cure some of your illness without contacting a physician is a good idea?

**MISHEL UNCERTAINTY IN ILLNESS SCALE**
Do you know what is wrong with you?
Have you been told how your illness will be treated?
Is your treatment too complex to figure out?
Is it difficult to know if the treatments or medications you are getting are helping you?
Are you unsure of whether your illness is getting better or worse?
Do you know what is going to happen to you while you are here?
Do you know when things will be done to you?
Do you have questions that have not been answered?
Do the explanations you receive seem hazy?
Do the doctors say things to you that could have many meanings?
Do you receive so much information that you cannot tell what is most important?
Do you think there are so many different types of staff it is unclear who is responsible for what?
Do you know how you will manage after you leave the hospital?

**MULTIDIMENSIONAL HEALTH LOCUS OF CONTROL**
Do you feel as if you are in control of your health?
Do you believe that you can pretty much stay healthy by taking good care of yourself?
Is it what you do that determines how soon you get well again?
Is following the doctor's orders to the letter the best way for you to stay healthy?
Does your family have a lot to do with your becoming sick or staying healthy?
Do you think that good health is largely a matter of good fortune?
Does it seem that no matter what you do, you are likely to get sick?
Does luck play a large part in determining how soon you will recover from an illness?

❖ **Table 27-1**
Potential nursing diagnoses reflecting control-related issues

| Diagnosis: Powerlessness | Issue |
|---|---|
| Coping, ineffective individual | Related to thwarted control need |
| Uncertainty | Related to lack of information |
| Anxiety | |
| Confusion | |
| | |
| Assertiveness | Related to quest for control |
| Aggressiveness | |
| Compliance | |
| Noncompliance | |
| | |
| Concern for | |
|   Independence | Related to quest for control |
|   Privacy | |
|   Interpersonal Relationships | |
| | |
| Alteration in decision-making ability | Related to lack of information, ambiguity of treatment alternatives, unpredictability of life-style impact |
| Resistive behavior | Related to lack of personal control |
| | |
| Anxiety | Related to "proper" execution of expected client role behaviors |

havior designed to give nurses a difficult time" will make major inroads into the first step of developing an appropriate nursing care plan.

## Nursing Diagnosis

Powerlessness is the major nursing diagnosis that deals directly with issues of control, but Coping: Ineffective individuals also could be used to specify the problem (Carpenito, 1989). However, early stages of taxonomy development should not preclude other statements that clearly reflect client's control-related needs and behaviors. Based on the nursing assessment, the nursing diagnoses and problem statements displayed in Table 27-1 are examples of what might be included in the client's care plan.

## Planning and Implementation

Without question, nursing interventions that address the issue of clients' control should be planned according to the assessment that

was made. The goal of nursing care should not be urging people to exercise control but should be helping them retain or relinquish control in accordance with their changing preferences and needs in each of the situations they encounter as a client.

Three major nursing actions that can be more finitely detailed on the care plan are *facilitate, support,* and *advocate.* An example of how these three nursing interventions can be applied to a specific client is provided in the nursing care plan.

**Facilitate: information.** Given the impact of uncertainty and unpredictability on the behavioral, cognitive, and decisional components of control and the pervasiveness of the theme "need to know," facilitating the flow of information should be one of nurses' highest priorities. Because they are with clients every hour of every day, nurses can provide immediate information and feedback. Even though they may not have the specific information that clients want

**NURSING CARE PLAN**

**CLIENT:**   David L.

**MEDICAL DIAGNOSIS:**   Morbid obesity: postoperative gastric stapling

**NURSING DIAGNOSES:**   Powerlessness
Anxiety related to lack of information
Resistive behavior related to lack of personal control

| GOALS | INTERVENTIONS |
|---|---|
| | Facilitate: information<br>Support: decision making<br>Advocate: in the health care system |
| David will speak calmly and with confidence about his treatment and the life-style implications of his surgery. | ◆ Remind health team members to discuss with David the status of his postoperative recovery and laboratory results. |
| | ◆ Encourage David to ask questions, repeatedly if necessary, when he does not know or does not understand anything about his care or when he "just wonders" about something. |
| | ◆ Spend 15 minutes each day to listen, problem solve, and teach David about managing diet, exercise, family relationships, and daily activities at home. |
| David will participate in making decisions about his care and treatment and will initiate actions that maintain his personal integrity. | ◆ Support David's involvement in making decisions and then actively participate in implementing those decisions. |
| | ◆ Encourage David to tell staff members how he wants things done. As he does so, add these requests to this care plan and follow them. |

*Continued.*

# ❖ NURSING CARE PLAN—cont'd

| GOALS | INTERVENTIONS |
|---|---|
|  | ◆ Be alert for privacy needs. Post "Do not disturb" sign on the door during times of personal care and need for emotional quiet. Encourage David to post his own sign as needed. |

## EVALUATION

David discusses changes in his future life-style and diet in a realistic and calm manner. In addition, he makes decisions about his care and maintains personal integrity when, for example, he places a "Do not disturb" sign on his door and then removes it voluntarily when it is no longer needed. When David makes a request for changes in the schedule or routine activities, he displays further evidence of empowerment.

such as a postoperative pathology report or the result of a nuclear medicine scan, nurses can prod the system and question other health team members on the client's behalf. During rounds nurses can remind a client that there was a question he or she wanted to ask or can share a nursing diagnosis with other providers and suggest that they talk to a client about a certain issue. As client advocates and coordinators of care, nurses can educate others to the importance clients attach to having information about their disease, care, and treatment and can encourage everyone to keep clients informed. With the holistic approach to client care, nurses can take the knowledge gained by clients and help them convert it into relevant alterations in life-styles and help them cope with transient or permanent changes in the quality of life (Dennis, 1987).

In the course of disseminating information the necessity of individualization should not be overlooked. The information gaps must be filled without endlessly repeating what is already known, overwhelming the client with torrents of unwanted details, or providing too much information too fast for assimilation. Health care is based on probabilities; it is not an exact science. Health care providers must present information about illness and alternative courses of action in ways that do not simplify the complexity of their own underlying decision-making process but do reflect the probabilistic nature of health care. Clients whose experiences differ from the textbook examples they are given are more likely to experience increased uncertainty and decreased control (Christman et al, 1988).

**Support: decision making.** Since clients have major differences in their orientation to making decisions, nurses may assume various roles in supporting the appropriate involvement. For some individuals nurses may actively promote the client's participation in making decisions of all types and magnitudes, or they very deliberately may not require decisions from a client who does not want and cannot cope with that responsibility. With both types of client, it is imperative not to pose decision alternatives when there clearly is no choice. For example, a seemingly logical and innocent way of individualizing care may be to ask a client if he or she wants a morning or evening bath. Unless the person is completely independent in this activity of daily living, current practice, staffing patterns, and reality may dictate a morning bath, regardless of the spoken preference. To give the client a choice and then not abide by the outcome may have a more adverse impact on control and feelings of well-being than proceeding according to policy and not asking the question at all.

**Advocate: in the health care system.** By understanding the health care system and the individual's control perspectives, nurses are in a prime position to serve as advocates. Nurses' actions such as posting a "Do not disturb" sign on the door to ensure privacy, getting the client separated from a noisy roommate, arranging a different time for a diagnostic test so there is time to rest, and doing a nursing procedure as much as possible in accordance with a person's wishes can make tremendous strides toward helping the client attain or maintain a sense of control. Either speaking out on a client's behalf or actively encouraging him or her to do so can contribute to the client's belief that he or she is more than a hapless victim of a strange health care environment.

## Evaluation

To date no research has been conducted to evaluate whether nursing interventions that foster and support clients' control actually mediate the stressfulness of the total hospitalization experience, facilitate recovery, decrease the length of hospital stay, and soften a reluctance to make initial or return visits to health care providers. Nevertheless, there is promise in the findings that clients who received psychoeducational preparation for surgery were discharged 1 day sooner than those who did not receive this type of intervention (Devine & Cook, 1983).

An empirical lack of knowledge on a global scope, however, should not preclude nurses from evaluating the effectiveness of their interventions in support of clients' control. When evaluating the outcomes of interventions, nurses should remember that the critical element is a link between clients' actions and the type of control mechanisms they prefer to use. Both retaining or relinquishing control can be appropriate outcomes, depending on the circumstances and the individual client.

**Verbal manifestations.** Although there may always be some uncertainty in illness no matter how much information is disseminated, clients who speak with confidence and clarity about their diagnosis, treatment, and life-style implications surely have received and processed the input and added it to their knowledge repertoire. Those who ask increasingly complex questions or even ask questions at all instead of being fearfully reticent are feeling safe in doing so and are becoming more involved in meeting their needs for cognitive control. Clients who share their viewpoints and desires during decision making or listen passively with equanimity may be meeting their individual needs for decisional control. Moreover, as clients perceive their control needs are being met, they may verbalize that they feel more comfortable and less anxious and are being treated like an important person.

**Behavioral manifestations.** Clients who feel in control are likely to assume greater responsibility for their own care, manifest greater independence, and initiate actions that preserve their personal integrity. In the case of a previous example these clients may feel self-assured enough to place their own "Do not disturb" sign on the door rather than hoping the nurse will do it. Client role behaviors may be enacted with more certitude, and there may be less evidence of anxiety, depression, and helplessness.

**Physiological manifestations.** If facilitating control truly mediates the stressfulness of the hospitalization experience, one might expect drops in otherwise elevated blood pressure readings, lower pulse rates, "average" pupil sizes, dry rather than sweaty palms, normal levels of urinary catecholamines, and precise small motor movements. Although these outcome indicators have been used in studies of the relationship between stress and control, they have brought difficulties to researchers and pose even greater problems in the clinical environment. Too many other physiological, psychological, and environmental events besides control contribute to physiological changes. Thus nurses should rely the most on verbal and behavioral manifestations of control to evaluate their interventions while watching physiological patterns that could possibly correspond to them. Such clinical observations of biopsychosocial relationships can lead to carefully designed research studies that improve the knowledge base for nursing practice.

## ❖ SUMMARY

Findings from clinical research and observations from clinical practice have shown that clients do need and want to have control over the people and events that affect their well-being and quality of life, even though they may not be able to identify and articulate those needs on a conscious level. Nurses who have insight into the issues surrounding control and sensitivity toward various patterns of expression will be able to assess the client's control needs, formulate an individualized care plan, and evaluate the successfulness of their interventions. By facilitating the flow of information, supporting decision making, and being an advocate within the system, nurses have the potential to help clients achieve a sense of control during what can be a very vulnerable hospitalization experience.

## ❖ APPLYING KNOWLEDGE TO PRACTICE

1. Think back to one of your "most difficult" clients. Was control an issue? If so,
   a. What control-related needs were at stake, and how was the client manifesting them?
   b. What parameters did you use to reassess those needs?
   c. If you could return to caring for that client, what nursing interventions would you implement to meet the control needs you identified?
   d. How would you know whether or not your interventions were helpful?
2. What might be the most effective means of communicating clients' control-related needs to other members of the health care team in ways that encourage their support?
3. What could happen when a client's control needs clash with the control needs of nurses and physicians? How might you intervene to prevent a "win-lose" scenario?

## REFERENCES

Averill, J. R. (1973). Personal control over aversive stimuli and its relationship to stress. *Psychological Bulletin* 80, 286-303.

Burger, J. M. (1989). Negative reactions to increases in perceived personal control. *Journal of Personality and Social Psychology, 56,* 246-256.

Carpenito, L. J. (1989). *Nursing diagnosis: Application to clinical practice.* New York: Lippincott.

Christman, N. J., McConnell, E. A., Pfeiffer, C., Webster, K. K., Schmitt, M., & Ries, J. (1988). Uncertainty, coping, and distress following myocardial infarction: Transition from hospital to home. *Research in Nursing & Health, 11,* 71-82.

deCharms, R. (1979). Personal causation and perceived control. In L. C. Perlmuter & R. A. Monty (Eds.), *Choice and perceived control,* 29-40. Hillsdale, N.J.: Lawrence Erlbaum.

Degner, L. F., & Russell, C. A. (1988). Preferences for treatment control among adults with cancer. *Research in Nursing & Health, 11,* 367-374.

Dennis, K. E. (1987). Dimensions of client control. *Nursing Research, 36,* 151–156.

Dennis, K. E. (1990). Patients' control and the information imperative: Clarification and confirmation. *Nursing Research, 39,* 162-166.

Derdiarian, A. K. (1986). Informational needs of recently diagnosed cancer patients. *Nursing Research, 35,* 276-281.

Devine, E. C., & Cook, T. D. (1983). A meta-analytic analysis of effects of psychoeducational interventions on length of postsurgical hospital stay. *Nursing Research, 32,* 267-274.

Duffy, M. E. (1988). Determinants of health promotion in midlife women. *Nursing Research, 37,* 358-362.

Emerson, R. M. (1962). Power-dependence relations. *American Sociological Review, 27,* 31-40.

Faden, R. R., Becker, C., Lewis, C., Freeman, J., & Faden, A. I. (1981). Disclosure of information to patients in medical care. *Medical Care, 19,* 718-733.

Ferington, F. E. (1986). Personal control and coping effectiveness in spinal cord injured persons. *Research in Nursing & Health, 9,* 257-265.

Forsyth, G. L., Delaney, K. D., & Gresham, M. L. (1984). Vying for a winning position: Management style of the chronically ill. *Research in Nursing & Health, 7,* 181-188.

Haug, M. R., & Lavin, B. (1981). Practitioner or patient—who's in charge? *Journal of Health and Social Behavior, 22,* 212-229.

Johnson, J. E. (1984). Coping with elective surgery. In H. H. Werley, & J. J. Fitzpatrick, (Eds.) *Annual Review of Nursing Research,* Vol. 2, (107-132.) New York: Springer.

Kritek, P. S. (1981). Patient power & powerlessness. *Supervisor Nurse, 12,* 26-34.

Krantz, D. S., Baum, A., & Wideman, M. V. (1981). Assessment of preferences for self-treatment and information in health care. *Journal of Personality and Social Psychology, 39,* 977-990.

Langer, E. J., & Rodin, J. (1976). The effects of choice and enhanced personal responsibility for the aged: A field experiment in an institutional setting. *Journal of Personality and Social Psychology, 34,* 191-198.

Lefcourt, H. M. (1981). *Research with the locus of control construct.* New York: Academic Press.

Lieberman, M. A., & Tobin, S. S. (1983). *The experience of old age: Stress, coping, and survival.* New York: Basic Books.

Lorber, J. (1975). Good patients and problem patients: Conformity and deviance in a general hospital. *Journal of Health and Social Behavior, 16,* 213-225.

Miller, S. M. (1980). Why having control reduces stress: If I can stop the roller coaster, I don't want to get off. In J. Garber, & M. E. P. Seligman, (Eds.), *Human Helplessness: Theory and Applications,* New York: Academic Press.

Mishel, M. H. (1981). The measurement of uncertainty in illness. *Nursing Research, 30,* 258-263.

Mishel, M. H. (1983). Adjusting the fit: Development of uncertainty scales for specific clinical populations. *Western Journal of Nursing Research, 5,* 355-370.

Pohl, J. M., & Fuller, S. S. (1980). Perceived choice, social interaction, and dimensions of morale of residents in a home for the aged. *Research in Nursing & Health, 3,* 147-157.

Renshon, S. A. (1979). The need for personal control in political life: Origins, dynamics, and implications. In L. C. Perlmuter & R. A. Monty (Eds.), *Choice and perceived control* (pp. 41-63). Hillsdale, N.J.: Lawrence Erlbaum.

Reynolds, M. (1978). No news is bad news: Patients' views about communication in hospital. *Hospital Topics, 1,* 1673-1676.

Rotter, J. B. (1966). Generalized expectancies for internal versus external control of reinforcement. *Psychological Monographs, 80,* (1, Whole No. 609).

Ryden, M. B. (1985). Environmental support for autonomy in the institutionalized elderly. *Research in Nursing & Health, 8,* 363-372.

Schulz, R., & Hanusa, B. H. (1978). Long-term effects of control and predictability-enhancing interventions: Findings and ethical issues. *Journal of Personality and Social Psychology, 36,* 1194-1201.

Seeman, M., & Seeman, T. E. (1983). Health behavior and personal autonomy: A longitudinal study of the sense of control in illness. *Journal of Health and Social Behavior, 24,* 144-160.

Seligman, M. E. P. (1975). *Helplessness: On depression, development, and death.* San Francisco: W. H. Freeman.

Seligman, M. E. P., & Miller, S. M. (1979). The psychology of power: Concluding comments. In L. C. Perlmuter, & R. A. Monty (Eds.). *Choice and perceived control.* Hillsdale, N.J.: Lawrence Erlbaum.

Shapiro, M. C., Nahman, J. M., Chang, A., Keeping, J. D., Morrison, J., & Western, J. S. (1983). Information control and the exercise of power in the obstetrical encounter. *Social Science and Medicine, 17,* 139-146.

Smith, R. A., Wallston, B. S., Wallston, K. A., Forsberg, P. R., & King, J. E. (1984). Measuring desire for control of health care processes. *Journal of Personality and Social Psychology, 47,* 415-426.

Strickland, B. R. (1978). Internal-external expectancies and health-related behaviors. *Journal of Consulting and Clinical Psychology, 46,* 1192-2111.

Strull, W. M., Lo, B., & Charles, G. (1984). Do patients want to participate in medical decision making? *Journal of the American Medical Association, 252,* 2990-2994.

Taylor, S. E. (1979). Hospital patient behavior: Reactance, helplessness, control? *Journal of Social Issues, 35,* 156-184.

Volicer, B. J., & Bohannon, M. W. (1975). A hospital stress rating scale. *Nursing Research, 24,* 352-359.

Wallston, K. A., & Wallston, B. S. (1981). Health locus of control scales. In Lefcourt, H. M. (Ed.). *Research with the locus of control construct.* (pp. 189-243). New York: Academic Press.

Wallston, K. A., Wallston, B. S., & DeVellis, R. (1978). Development of the Multidimensional Health Locus of Control (MHLC) Scales. *Health Education Monographs, 6,* 161-170.

Wilson-Barnett, J., & Carrigy, A. (1979). Factors influencing patients' emotional reactions to hospitalization. *Journal of Advanced Nursing, 3,* 221-228.

# 28 Hope

Patricia M. Grimm

*"For to him that is joined to all the living there is hope."*

ECCLESIASTES 9:4

## OBJECTIVES

*At the completion of this chapter, the reader will be able to:*

◆ Describe the concept of hope.

◆ Identify a model for examining the impact of hope on the individual's experience with acute and chronic illness.

◆ Explore the implementation of the nursing process with persons experiencing a loss of hope, hopelessness.

◆ Describe the past, present, and future trends in hope research.

## ❖ INTRODUCTION OF A CONCEPT

The word *hope* is an integral part of everyday speech and even popular song. Hope and its symbol, the anchor, appear on the state flag of Rhode Island, and even Charlie Brown's dog Snoopy espouses that "a whole stack of memories doesn't equal one little hope." In recent years, increasing attention has been given to the meaning of hope, its relevancy to health and illness, and its importance to the practice of nursing. Hope has been identified as playing an important role in physical and emotional well-being. Weisman (1979) identifies hope as a prerequisite for good coping with the demands and challenges of illness, such as cancer. Frankl (1959) documents situations where the pres-

ence or lack of hope has meant the difference between survival or death. "To hope is a state of being . . . an inner readiness . . . a psychic commitment to life and growth" (Fromm, 1968, pp. 11-12).

Hope has its origins in infancy (Erikson, 1963) and is further elaborated during times of suffering, personal trial, and a state of captivity (Marcel, 1962). "Hope enables human beings to cope with difficult and stressful situations, deprivation, tragedy, failure, boredom, loneliness and suffering" (Travelbee, 1971, p. 77). Illness, either physiological or psychological, can be construed as a time of suffering and personal trial, as well as captivity. The ill individual often faces an unknown future while dealing with the

507

physical and emotional pain of diagnosis, treatment, and life-style changes in the present. Hope ... "presupposes a tragic situation; it is a response to felt tragedy, and is the positive outgrowth of a tragic sense of life" (Pruyser, 1987, p. 465). Bahnson (1975) has identified hope for an emotionally satisfying life as the greatest asset for a patient with cancer. He underscores the importance of nurturing the patient's hope and identifies the maintenance of hope as a primary goal of psychotherapeutic care.

If hope is viewed as an essential ingredient for life and growth, and the positive outgrowth of felt tragedies, such as illness, certainly the profession of nursing needs to be knowledgeable about the meaning of hope, its assessment, and the planning of nursing care designed to support, enhance, and instill hope. The focus of this chapter is to provide such a knowledge base. This discussion begins with the description and definition of hope as found in the literature. This review provides a working definition of hope and explores its relationships with other concepts such as wishing, optimism, denial, and spirituality. Having defined hope, a model for viewing hope in relationship to the impact of illness is presented. The consideration of hope as an important concept for nursing practice follows as the nursing process related to hope is outlined. Finally, the state of the science of hope research is reviewed, and areas in need of further research are identified.

### ❖ HOPE: DESCRIBED AND DEFINED

The concept of hope has appeared in the recorded words of man since Biblical times. Menninger (1975) presents a historical perspective on hope, quoting the words of St. Paul, Martin Luther, Samuel Johnson, and others. To the ancient Greeks hope was evil. Since they believed that fate was unchangeable, hope was viewed as a destructive illusion. More contemporary existential philosophers, such as Nietzche and Sartre, have extended the notion of

hope as being harmful. In contrast, there are many philosophers, poets, religious and social scientists who see hope as an essential internal resource to man. "With hope, man acts, moves, achieves. Without hope he is often dull, listless, moribund" (Stotland, 1969, p. 1).

Lynch (1965) believed that hope has a close bond with imagination, that we have to be able to imagine a future outcome or goal in order to hope. He further clarifies the seemingly paradoxical view of hope as a negative attribute by pointing out that for many people hope means despair. When we say an individual has hope, we are usually also saying that that person is in serious trouble and the implication is he or she has nothing else. Lynch offered a more positive and comprehensive definition of hope:

... the fundamental knowledge and feeling that there is a way out of difficulty, that things can work out, that we as human persons can somehow handle and manage internal and external reality, that there are "solutions" in the most ordinary biological and physiological use of the word, that, above all, there are ways out of illness (p. 32).

He stresses three basic ideas in relation to hope: a future orientation, the difficulty of the present, and a sense of expectation. As noted earlier, his conceptualization is consistent with that of Marcel. Lynch also addresses the interpersonal nature of hope.

### The Interpersonal Nature of Hope

The interpersonal nature of hope has its origins in the work of Erikson (1963). Hope is the outcome of achieving an appropriate balance between trust and mistrust, which is the first developmental task of life. The origins of hope are in early childhood experiences (Lange, 1978). The infant, through his relationship with a significant caregiver, learns to trust others, himself, and the world about him. Such trust is "a global undifferentiated attitude, a contentment and confidence which stems from a deep assumption that life is pleasant and will not become unmanageable" (Thomas, 1978, p. 164). This attitude of trust is the basis of hope. To hope is to trust in oneself and in others in order to facilitate reaching one's goals.

The interpersonal theme of hope is one that is particularly prominent in nursing literature. Limandri and Boyle (1978), using a case study, discussed the effect of pervasive feelings of hopelessness, the factors that affect such a state, and the importance of the involvement of the nurse's hope to patients. Dubrie and Vogelpohl (1980) distinguish between magic hope and hope. "Magic hope, a passive nonhope, is a kind of wishful expectation that another person, or God, or fate, or even time will magically change a situation without one's having to do anything one's self" (p. 2048). Such beliefs may be supportive at first, but in time lead to disappointment and despair. These authors state that although hope is directly related to help from others, patients need to develop hope for themselves separate from these relationships. The relationship helps motivate one to hope, in assisting the patient to set goals, but ". . . one's own activities form a sounder base for hope than reliance on the good will and competence of someone else" (Frank, 1974, p. 137). This individual nature of hope is supported in the writings of Kubler-Ross. She stresses the need to support the patient's realistic hopes, even if they are different from those of others involved (Kubler-Ross, 1977).

Valliot (1970) also placed importance on the interpersonal aspect of hope: ". . . hope reaches out to someone or some One" (p. 8). For her, the interpersonal nature of hope can transcend human relationships and be a relationship with God. "Heagle states the goal of hope is not the things we hope for but the persons one trusts in, the person of God and human persons who represent him" (in Miller, 1983, p. 296). Hope is a personal bond, and the greatest of these bonds, ". . . the one that pro-

vides the most hope, is the bond with God" (Miller, 1983, p. 296). Empirically, Stoner (1982) examined hope among patients with cancer and found a positive association between hope and religiosity, a belief or faith in God. For many individuals, this bond with a higher power is basic to the ability to hope and as such requires nursing's recognition and support.

## Future Orientation and Goals

Returning to Lynch's conceptualization, Travelbee (1971) also viewed hope in terms of future orientation, goals, and expectation. For her, hope is "a mental state characterized by the desire to gain an end or accomplish a goal combined with some degree of expectation that what is desired or sought is attainable" (Travelbee, 1971, p. 77). Travelbee also relates an individual's ability to hope as being based on a balance between trust and mistrust. As discussed earlier, trust in others, oneself, and the environment is the genesis of hope. Travelbee therefore views hope as an interpersonal concept, which is also related to choice, because hopeful people are able to see alternatives to their goals. Hopeful people are also courageous because they are able to realize their fears and weaknesses, yet are able to persevere toward their goals.

Other authors have sought to define hope. Dufault and Martocchio (1985) and Miller (1985) present their respective conceptual models. Dufault and Martocchio suggest a model of hope with guidelines for assessment and intervention. Miller (1985), in defining hope and suggesting hope-inspiring strategies, believes ". . . hope allows the individual to use a crisis as an opportunity for growth" (p. 23).

## A Definition of Hope

From this exploration of the writings on hope, several themes emerge:

Hope implies a future orientation. The difficult present is made tolerable through the anticipation of what is to come.

To hope is to have expectations of the future, and the expectations have the possibility of being met.

Hope implies the setting of future goals in order to enhance the meeting of one's expectations.

To hope is to take action to achieve these goals.

Hope is an interpersonal process. It is created through trust and is nurtured by trusting relationships with others, including God.

In addition, hope can be considered a psychological characteristic of the individual, which has trait and state dimensions. The trait dimension of hope is conceived of as an enduring characteristic of a person (Panagis, 1982). *Traits* are relatively stable individual differences that predispose an individual to respond in a consistent manner (Speilberger, 1970). The trait dimension of hope is designed to see people through adversity, because it can be strategically generated or discouraged (Weisman, 1979). At the same time, hope can be considered as having a *state* dimension, that is, one conceived as varying within the person from situation to situation (Panagis, 1982). States are dynamic and changeable individual differences that are the response to a specific situation (Speilberger, 1970). Although a developmental component of the individual's psychological adjustment, hope is called to the fore by experiences of physical and emotional captivity such as illness (Marcel, 1962).

From a consideration of the literature themes and the identification of hope as a psychological characteristic, with trait and state dimensions, the following definition evolves:

Hope is a psychological characteristic, with trait and state dimensions, characterized by cognitive and affective behaviors which demonstrate an expectant orientation toward the future and the planning of goals and taking of action to facilitate meeting one's future expectations, all with the context of supportive relationships with others.

Later in this chapter this definition will serve as the basis for a discussion of the nursing process with the nursing diagnosis of hopelessness, a loss of hope.

## The Relationship of Hope to Other Concepts

It is important to delineate how hope is the same or different from such related concepts as wishing, optimism, denial, and spirituality. Wishing, according to Travelbee (1971), is not the same as hoping. *Wishing* is to desire the improbable and to know that there is a low degree of possibility of ever obtaining what is wished for. Hope is to desire the possible and to strongly believe that that which is hoped for can and will be obtained. "That which is hoped for is within the range of possibility" (Travelbee, 1971, p. 81). *Optimism* is also not the same as hope. Weisman (1979) stated that false hope masquerades as optimism, an attitude of anticipating the best possible outcome under all circumstances. "Genuine hope does not need denial, because good copers seek and use resources of all kinds. Counterfeit hope only pretends to cope. Actually it covers passivity" (Weisman, 1979, p. 12). Hope is not a form of denial, since true hope is rooted in reality. *Denial* strives to keep from awareness all disturbing events, thoughts, and feelings, while "... in hoping you look at the situation, no matter how negative, to seek out those few remaining positive elements and build on them" (Goleman, 1984, p. 60).

Although hope can have as its orientation secular goals, actions, and relationships, it can also be oriented towards eternal goals, actions, and, as noted earlier, a relationship with God. For many persons, these two perspectives are intertwined. Hope, grounded in a belief in God, allows for a sustaining perspective when one's secular hopes are met with disappointment. Hope, whether for earthly activities or eternal goals, is visualized in terms of a relationship with God and is thus an aspect of an individual's spirituality (Carson, Soeken, & Grimm, 1988).

Hope is also related to spiritual well-being, or a healthy spirit. Banks (1980) defines *spiritual health* or well-being as encompassing four characteristics: (1) a unifying force that integrates physical, mental, emotional, and social dimensions of health; (2) meaning in life that may serve as an inner driving force for personal achievements; (3) a common bond between individuals, which facilitates the sharing of love, compassion and warmth, the performance of unselfish acts, the adherence to a set of ethical principles, and a commitment to God; and (4) individual perceptions or faith that allows the individual to acknowledge the supernatural and experience pleasure. These characteristics of spiritual health encompass the future orientation, goal setting, action taking, and interpersonal relationship components of hope. This apparent relationship between hope and spiritual well-being was supported in a study of healthy adults (Carson, Soeken, & Grimm, 1988). Hope and spiritual well-being were found to be significantly related to each other. This finding implies that hope can be enhanced and maintained by both secular and spiritual approaches tailored to the specific belief system of the individual.

## ❖ HOPE, STRESS, APPRAISAL, AND COPING: A MODEL

Hope has been defined as a psychological characteristic that is both inherent in each person (trait hope) and that can be elaborated upon in response to a specific life event such as illness (state hope). Just how does hope affect an individual's experience with acute or chronic illness? The exploration of a transactional model of stress, appraisal, and adaptational outcomes (Lazarus & Folkman, 1984) may suggest some answers to this question.

As described in Chapter 26, Lazarus and Folkman (1984) present a model of stress, appraisal, and coping that allows for the consideration of hope as an influencing factor in this process. Their model takes into consideration both the characteristics of the person as well as the nature of the stressful environmental event. Psychological stress is defined as ". . . a relationship between the person and the environment that is appraised by the person as taxing or exceeding his or her resources and endangering his or her well-being" (p. 21). The appraisal of the stress is cognitive in nature and asks the questions "Am I affected, in what way, and what can and might I do?"

All appraisal is affected by person and situation factors. *Person factors* are the unique characteristics of the individual that will influence his or her cognition of the stressful event, while *situation factors* are those properties of the encounter with the stressful event that influence that cognitive process. Both person and situation factors create the potential for the event to be appraised as threatening, harmful, or challenging. Depending on the outcome of the appraisal process, the individual chooses specific forms of coping with the specific stress. Illness and its diagnosis and treatment can be considered a stress that leads to cognitive appraisal and coping. Hope, the trait dimension, can be considered one of many person factors that influence this appraisal process. Situation factors identified as influencing the appraisal of illness as a stress would include the various aspects of the specific disease and its treatment. Hope, the state dimension, can also be viewed as an outcome of appraisal and theoretically may influence the coping process and

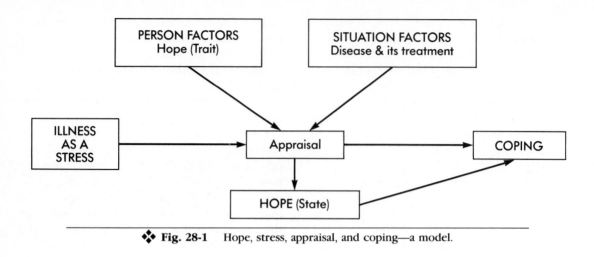

❖ **Fig. 28-1**    Hope, stress, appraisal, and coping—a model.

choice of either effective or ineffective coping strategies. A model of the relationships of hope to stress, appraisal, and coping is presented in Fig. 28-1.

Such a model is an oversimplification of the stress, appraisal, and coping process, but it does serve to identify the potential areas of influence that result from the patient's hope. It is clear that hope theoretically exerts influence at two levels on the individual's ability to cope with the stress of acute or chronic illness. Developmentally, each person brings a certain level of hope (trait) to all daily experiences and to the reaction to the diagnosis of an illness. In addition, the reaction or appraisal itself results in a level of hope (state) in response to the illness experience. Although these two different though complementary dimensions of hope make sense in theory, hope research has not as yet empirically validated such a distinction. Therefore, in discussing the nursing process and hope, only the overall loss or lessening of hope experienced by the individual will be considered, not the separate conceptualizations of trait and state hope.

## ❖ THE CONCEPT OF HOPE AND NURSING PRACTICE

"Hope, like love, transcends all time. It is a friend, a healer, a maker of dreams."

Flavia

Loss of hope, or hopelessness can be experienced by any person, at any time, regardless of health status. However, illness is a challenge to an individual's hope. Life-threatening illnesses such as cancer or AIDS can certainly challenge the individual's ability to maintain hope. Experiencing life-threatening injuries or undergoing major surgical procedures can also tax the maintenance of this important life force. Chronic illnesses, such as cardiovascular or respiratory disease, progressive neurological conditions, or conditions such as post-trauma functional losses and chronic pain may impair the individual's sense of any future goal achievement and may directly impair day-to-day activity. Experiencing a major psychiatric illness, particularly a chronic condition such as severe depression and schizophrenia, leaves the individual with a limited ability to maintain hope without professional help. Hope enhancement may be appropriate for individuals who are experiencing developmental or situational crises. The adaptations required of a family with a new infant or an aging family member may have an impact on the hope of those involved. Research on hope in terms of specific patient groups is presented later in this chapter.

Illness threatens more than the hope of the individual; it also has a major impact on family members and other loved ones. Their ability to hope can be a vital resource for the individual, since hope does exist within the context of supportive relationships with others. In planning the nursing care of patients, the nurse must also consider the hope of those patients' significant others. To enhance or inspire the hope of a supportive family member or friend is to do so for the patient as well.

We as nurses must also examine our own ability to hope both in terms of patients in general and in terms of each specific patient. The ability of any nurse to maintain hope in the face of illness and adversity will depend on the person factors he or she brings to each nursing care encounter, and the situation factors that comprise that patient situation. Obviously, the area of practice specialization will influence the degree to which each nurse is exposed to life-threatening or chronic illness experiences. For example, an emergency room or oncology nurse may be exposed to more hope-challenging situations than nurses working in other areas of practice.

How does the nurse maintain his or her hope in the face of often tragic and apparently hopeless patient experiences? It is imperative that we maintain our future orientation with each patient, even if that future is defined as tomorrow or next week, rather than years from now. We must identify our own goals, both in terms of patient care and for ourselves. Planning activities directed at maintaining the patient's optimal level of health and functioning is essential. This includes preparations for a comfortable death as well as a functional life. We also must continue to identify and carry out activities that help us meet our own personal and professional goals. Lastly, and perhaps most importantly, each nurse must maintain his or her connections with others, such as coworkers, family, and friends. These relationships can provide the nurse with support, so that he or she can then provide such interpersonal support to patients. If a relationship with a higher power, a God, is important to the individual nurse, this source of strength and hope also needs to be nurtured. In summary, intervention with the patient experiencing a loss of hope begins with self-assessment of the nurse's own attitudes and feelings regarding this patient's illness experience and the development of an ongoing plan of hope enhancing self-intervention.

### Hope and Nursing Theory

The concept of hope has not been identified as a major theoretical component of any single nursing theory. Watson (1979), in her formulation of the philosophy and science of caring, does mention the instillation of faith-hope as one of the 10 primary carative factors that form a structure for studying and evaluating nursing as the science of caring. Further elaboration on this carative factor does not specifically address the concept of hope. Certainly hope can be considered an element of caring theory.

Other nursing theories that stress the interpersonal nature of nursing practice and the promotion and enhancement of health for the patient could serve as a framework for the study and understanding of hope as an important concept to nursing. It is interesting to note that in the research literature addressing hope, a spe-

## ❖ ASSESSMENT OF LOSS OF HOPE/HOPELESSNESS

**ASPECTS OF CURRENT ILLNESS AND/OR TREATMENT**

Nature of illness:  chronic, acute, life-threatening

Process of illness: deteriorating, cyclic

Effects of illness:  physical restrictions, cognitive restrictions, social restrictions, short-term and long-term stress

**In terms of future orientation:**

What are the effects of the illness/treatment on the person's future?

What are the person's:

> views about the future?
> feelings about the future?
> values in life?
> time orientation—past, present, or future?

Is the person experiencing a sense of:

> loss of control over the future?
> uncertainty?
> pessimism?
> disrupted continuity between the past, present, and future?
> feeling trapped?

Does the person express:

> having no purpose in life?
> giving up the will to live?
> suicidal thoughts?

Do you observe:  an apathetic manner?

> self-destructive behaviors?

**In terms of setting goals:**

What are the effects of the illness/treatment on the person's ability to identify goals?

What are the person's:

> goals and desires?
> are they realistic?
> strengths and potentials, are they recognized?
> purpose and role in life?
> capabilities for achieving goals?

Is the person experiencing:

> a loss of independence?
> decreased self-esteem?
> no feelings of success or pleasure?
> lack of ambition?
> lack of interest in anything?
> doubts about capacity to achieve goals?
> unachieved goals as failures?

Does the person express:

> self-doubts?
> discouragement with self?
> passivity?

Adapted from Brunger & Grimm, 1986; Carpenito, 1989; Doenges & Moorhouse, 1988; Falsetti-Shanty, 1988; Hickey, 1986; and Miller, 1983, 1985, 1986, 1989.

## ❖ ASSESSMENT OF LOSS OF HOPE/HOPELESSNESS

**ASPECTS OF CURRENT ILLNESS AND/OR TREATMENT—cont'd**

**In terms of identifying the implementing activities:**

What are the effects of the illness/treatment on the person's ability to identify and implement activities?

What are the person's:

  expressed interests, hobbies, daily activities?

  expressed interests in self-care activities?

  problem-solving, decision-making, planning, and organizing skills?

  self-care abilities/activities?

Is the person experiencing:

  lack of interest in activities?

  lack of interest in self-care?

  loss of independence?

  passivity?

  inability to solve problems or make decisions?

Does the person express:

  apathy?

  dependency on others?

  resignation to fate?

Do you observe: decreased activity level, interests?

  decreased self-care?

  apathetic manner?

  increased sleep?

  lack of involvement in care?

**In terms of relationships with others:**

What are the effects of the illness/treatment on the person's relationships with family, friends, caregivers?

What are the effects of the illness/treatment on the person's religious beliefs and spiritual relationships?

What is the person's:

  interest in relationships?

  degree of involvement with others?

  relationship with religion and/or God, and its importance?

Is the person experiencing:

  lowered trust in self and others?

  decreased contact with significant others?

  a recent loss due to death or change in a relationship?

  role changes?

  changes in his/her relationship with God?

Does the person express:

  not receiving help, nurturance, or esteem from others?

  a loss of gratification from roles and relationships?

  a loss of intimacy?

Do you observe:

  a decrease in verbal and nonverbal communication, body language, eye contact
    isolative behavior?

cific nursing theory has not been identified in any discussion of a conceptual framework. This could be considered a limitation of hope research that needs to be addressed in the design of future studies.

## Hope and The Nursing Process

Hope has been described and defined, and a conceptualization of the relationship of hope to the illness experiences of patients has been presented. It is now time to consider the assessment of hope, the planning and implementation of nursing interventions designed to enhance or inspire hope, and the evaluation of such plans. Nursing care of the individual who is experiencing a loss of hope, hopelessness, can be based on the definition of hope presented earlier. The four conceptual components of hope—future orientation, goal setting, action taking, and interpersonal relationships, provide a framework for the nurse's assessment, planning, intervention, and evaluation activities.

**Assessment of hope.** Hope, and its antithesis hopelessness, can be assessed both by observation and interaction with the individual and by use of instruments developed to measure hope. An assessment of hope needs to be an integral part of the nursing care of every patient. Being a subjective emotional state, hopelessness must be validated by the nurse with the individual. It is important to assess behavioral, cognitive, and emotional areas in order to infer that the person is experiencing hopelessness (Carpenito, 1989). The box on pp. 514 and 515 outlines the areas of assessment that must be considered in order to infer the nursing diagnosis of hopelessness.

In order to empirically study hope, several researchers have developed instruments designed to quantify this psychological characteristic. Table 28-1 lists these instruments, their author or authors, and a brief description of each instrument's structure and conceptual

base. All of these measures, with the exception of the Gottschalk Hope Scale, are self-report, pencil and paper measures of hope. One additional instrument frequently used in the assessment of hope is the Beck Hopelessness Scale (Beck, et al., 1974). A summary of the state of the art in the measurement of hope is also presented by Stoner (1988).

In considering which instrument to use as an assessment or research tool, one must consider a variety of factors including one's own conceptual beliefs regarding hope, the purpose of administration, and the respondent group that will be completing the measure. Length and complexity of instruments must be matched to the skills and functional abilities of one's respondent group. For example, a longer, multiple task instrument may be appropriate for a group of well- educated, healthy individuals, while such an instrument may be beyond the cognitive and functional abilities of an elderly group with an average educational level of eighth grade or less. The ability to read is a basic skill required for all self-report measures of hope, and the nurse clinician or researcher must consider alternative approaches when respondents are unable to demonstrate basic reading skills.

**Nursing diagnosis.** A loss of hope has been given the nursing diagnosis of hopelessness. *Hopelessness* can be defined as a sustained subjective emotional state in which an individual sees limited or no alternatives or personal choices available to solve problems or to achieve desired goals and cannot mobilize energy on his or her own behalf to identify goals or explore problem solving (Carpenito, 1989; Doenges & Moorhouse, 1988). In other words, the individual who is feeling hopeless experiences a lack of future orientation, an inability to identify goals for himself or herself, and difficulty in identifying and implementing activities directed at goal achievement. In addition, hopelessness can evolve from changes in, or losses of, significant interpersonal relationships. Con-

❖ **Table 28-1**
Instruments for the clinical and research measurement of hope

| Title and author(s) | Description of instrument |
| --- | --- |
| The Hope Scale<br>  Erickson, Post & Paige (1975) | List of twenty future goals that are ranked: (1) on seven point scale for importance, and (2) percent estimated chance of reaching each goal. |
| Gottschalk Hope Scale<br>  Gottschalk (1979) | Designed for content analysis of verbal samples. Five minute sample is scored for seven content categories by trained technicians. |
| Stoner Hope Scale<br>  Stoner (1982)<br>  Stoner & Kaempfer (1985) | Thirty goal statements representative of three theory-based domains: intrapersonal, interpersonal, and global. Goal statements each ranked on: (1) a four point scale for importance, and (2) a four point scale for probability of realization. |
| Hope Index Scale<br>  Obayuwana, Collins, Carter,<br>  Rao, Mathura, & Wilson (1982) | Sixty item questionnaire requiring yes or no answers to statements reflecting cognitive, affective, or motor component of ego strength, human family support, religion, education, and economic assets. |
| State-Trait Hope Inventory<br>  Grimm (1984, 1989) | Forty item scale, using a five-point Likert format. Separate twenty item state and trait subscales. Items on subscale represent four dimensions of hope found in the literature: future orientation, goal setting, taking of action, and relationships with others, including a relationship with God. |
| Miller Hope Scale<br>  Miller & Powers (1988) | Forty item scale, using a five-point Likert format. Items represent ten critical elements of hope as described in the literature: mutuality-affiliation, sense of the possible, avoidance of absolutizing, anticipation, achieving goals, psychological well-being and coping, purpose and meaning in life, freedom, and reality surveillance-optimism. |
| Nowotny Hope Scale<br>  Nowotny (1986, 1989) | Forty-seven item scale, using a four-point Likert format. Items represent six dimensions: hope is future oriented, includes active involvement, comes from within and is related to trust. That which is hoped for is possible, hope involves other people, or a higher being, the outcome of hope is important to the individual. |

versely, any change in such interpersonal relationships can leave the individual feeling alone, socially isolated, and perhaps hopeless.

Hopelessness is not the same as depression. *Depression* is a broader concept, often a medical diagnosis, which is inclusive of more than just hopelessness. The depressed person may experience hopelessness. However, that person will also demonstrate impaired adjustment, ineffective individual coping, self-concept, and self-esteem disturbances as well as changes in physiological functioning such as alterations in nutrition, sleep patterns, and elimination.

*Grief* and hopelessness are also not the same. The grieving individual may experience hopelessness, but each person experiencing

## ❖ ADDITIONAL NURSING DIAGNOSES RELATED TO LOSS OF HOPE/HOPELESSNESS

> Adjustment, impaired
> Coping, ineffective individual
> Decisional conflict
> Knowledge deficit (specify)
> Powerlessness
> Self-concept disturbance
> Self-esteem disturbance
> Social isolation
> Spiritual distress

hopelessness may not be grieving. Grief is the response to an actual or perceived loss. Hopelessness may result from grief, but as discussed, may also be the outcome of a broader range of experiences than just loss.

Some of the same behaviors considered in order to infer the nursing diagnosis of hopelessness may be seen in individuals with other related nursing diagnoses. The box above lists those diagnoses that have behaviors in common with the diagnosis of hopelessness or are closely related to this diagnosis. The reader is referred to any of the excellent texts on nursing diagnosis for a complete discussion of these related problem areas.

**Planning and intervention.** As noted earlier, the planning and implementation of nursing interventions with the person experiencing hopelessness must begin with a self-assessment of the nurse's ability to hope and the consideration of self-directed interventions. In addition, certain basic intervention principles must be considered. Since hope appears to rely heavily on an interpersonal component, the establishment of a caring, trusting nurse-patient relationship is most important. The nurse must have well-developed interpersonal communication skills, both verbal and nonverbal, when providing nursing care for a person who manifests a loss of hope. If desired by the patient, the ability to provide closeness through active listening, eye contact, and touch can be very therapeutic.

Patience is required because the person who is feeling hopeless may become easily discouraged, withdraw, and become apathetic. The identification of intervention strategies specifically tailored to the uniqueness of each individual's experience and situation requires flexibility and hopefulness on the part of the nurse. For example, the use of techniques such as progressive relaxation and guided imagery may be most helpful for the person who also experiences fear and anxiety. The nursing care plan that follows provides general guidelines for intervening with the person experiencing a loss of hope. Again, more specific goals and interventions need to be mutually identified and tailored to the unique situation of each person.

**Evaluation.** The evaluation of any plan of nursing care is based on the achievement of the stated goals with a person experiencing hopelessness, one would expect to see an increase in future orientation, the development of the ability to identify goals and participate in goal-directed activities, and an improvement in the individual's interpersonal relationships, both in terms of quality and use of available resources. Evaluation must be a mutual process and must occur at prescribed intervals so that achievement of goals can be acknowledged. This provides the person with positive reinforcement regarding his or her ability to set and achieve goals. Thus the evaluation process for these individuals can serve also as an intervention strategy.

# ❖ NURSING CARE PLAN

**CLIENT:**  Jennifer H.

**MEDICAL DIAGNOSIS:**  Chronic back pain

**NURSING DIAGNOSIS:**  Hopelessness related to chronic pain

| GOALS | INTERVENTIONS |
|---|---|
| Jennifer will experience positive expectations about the future. | ◆ Assist with life review and putting life in perspective.<br>◆ Provide opportunities to express feelings about the past and present.<br>◆ Teach relaxation, imagery techniques and other strategies for the management of fear, anxiety.<br>◆ Teach to anticipate daily experiences, savor the moment.<br>◆ Aid in the identification of future experiences and events that can be looked forward to.<br>◆ Discuss reasons for living and meaning of life. |
| Jennifer will demonstrate increased self-direction and autonomy in goal setting and decision-making activities. | ◆ Assist with the identification of and revision of realistic goals.<br>◆ Help in the identification of strengths and potentials.<br>◆ Assist with the identification of activities required for goal achievement.<br>◆ Provide information regarding illness, treatment procedures.<br>◆ Involve in self-care within the limits of ability.<br>◆ Involve in decision-making process regarding care and treatment.<br>◆ Educate regarding problem-solving approaches.<br>◆ Provide positive feedback for areas of success. |

*Continued.*

**NURSING CARE PLAN—cont'd**

| GOALS | INTERVENTIONS |
|---|---|
| Jennifer will use relationship systems, both those already in existence and those that are newly identified. | ◆ Establish a nurse-patient relationship.<br>◆ Assist with communication skills.<br>◆ Involve family members in care and information giving.<br>◆ Support sustaining relationships.<br>◆ Foster attachment with significant others.<br>◆ Provide opportunities for socialization with others.<br>◆ Explore feelings related to losses and changes.<br>◆ Provide teaching regarding the grief process.<br>◆ Review her spiritual beliefs.<br>◆ Support use of prayer.<br>◆ Encourage contacts with clergy and church activities.<br>◆ Discuss appropriate community support systems.<br>◆ Refer her to community resources and encourage contacts. |

**EVALUATION**

Jennifer verbalizes positive expectations regarding the future as evidenced by descriptions of anticipated activities. She sets realistic goals such as cooking a meal or taking a short walk. She becomes more involved with family and friends and begins to attend community and religious events.

## ❖ HOPE AND THE RESEARCH PROCESS

The state of the art of hope research is still in its infancy. It is interesting to note that nurse researchers have been at the forefront in trying to quantify hope and in determining and describing the relationships among hope and other person and situation variables. For the purposes of this discussion, we will again return to the ideas of hope as an influence on appraisal of, or the response to, illness and hope as an outcome of appraisal of illness. The majority of the research has been done with people who have cancer. However, studies involving other patient groups will also be noted.

### Hope as an Influence on Appraisal

This literature consists of studies that focus on concept development, instrument development, or both. Stanley (1978), in order to identify the common elements in the "lived experience" of hope, asked 100 college students to write descriptions of their experience of hope. Through qualitative analysis, a structure of hope, consisting of seven common elements, was defined for healthy young adults. These elements were: expectation of a significant future outcome, confidence in outcome, a quality of transcendence, interpersonal relatedness, experiencing comfortable feelings, experiencing uncomfortable feelings, and action to effect outcome. Similarly, Hinds (1984) interviewed 25 adolescents, using a grounded theory approach to interview analysis, formulated a definition of hope consisting of categories that seemed to form a continuum of degrees: forced effort, personal possibilities, expectation of a better tomorrow, and anticipation of a personal future.

In order to empirically study hope, several authors have developed instruments designed to quantify this psychological characteristic. A discussion of these instruments was presented earlier in this chapter.

## Hope as an Effect of Appraisal

Several researchers have sought to define hope based on the direct assessment of individuals experiencing a specific disease or health impairment. As noted earlier, people with cancer have been the focus of much of this work. Buehler (1975) interviewed 24 people with cancer receiving radiation treatment as well as several members of the patient care staff. She proposed that these patients, after the initial shock of their diagnosis, read social and physical cues of other regarding their illness, and tended to express hope if these cues were hopeful and lacked "dying trajectories."

Using a participant observation approach, Dufault (1981) investigated the phenomena of hope among 22 elderly individuals with cancer over a 2-year period. The outcome of her work was a multidimensional model of hope composed of two spheres—generalized hope and particular

hope—having six common dimensions: affective, cognitive, behavioral, affiliative, temporal, and emotional. Young-Brockopp (1982) sought to evaluate and clarify psychosocial needs that are repeatedly attributed to individuals with cancer and other life-threatening illnesses. Sixty-one patients completed a Q-sort Needs Assessment Inventory, and hope was ranked as a significant need with the hope statements all being placed among the top 10 choices.

Several researchers investigated the relationship of hope to other variables among individuals experiencing cancer. Raleigh (1980) attempted to identify the variables that help physically ill individuals maintain hope. She assessed hope, locus of control, social support, religious or philosophical beliefs, and attribution of meaning of the illness among 45 respondents with cancer and 45 respondents with nonlife-threatening illness. She found no statistically significant relationships among these variables but pointed to the need for a reliable and valid measure of hope.

Stoner and Keamper (1985) interviewed 33 people with cancer to determine the relationships among recalled life expectancy information, phase of illness, and hope. Using the Stoner Hope Scale, they determined that receiving life expectancy information has a significant effect on hope. Using the McGee-Clark Hope Scale, locus of control, hope, and disease-free interval were evaluated among 34 breast cancer patients by Kerber (1987). Hope was found to be significantly and positively related to disease-free interval, with stressful life events being an intervening variable. The relationships among hope, affect, psychological status, and the cancer experience were the focus of Grimm (1989). Hope was assessed using the State-Trait Hope Inventory (Grimm, 1984) with 60 individuals with newly diagnosed breast, lung, colon, and rectal cancer. Hope was found to be high among this sample, and the more hopeful the individual, the more positive their affect was and the less psychological distress was experienced.

Other groups have been the focus of hope

research. Rideout (1986) and O'Malley (1988) both assessed hope among patients with cardiovascular illnesses. Hope, morale, and adaptation in patients with chronic heart failure was the focus of Rideout's study. She determined that the more hopeful the individual, the higher their morale and the better their social functioning. O'Malley examined the relationship of hope to stress after myocardial infarction. This study of a small sample (seven patients) did not reveal any significant relationships.

Additional subject groups have included the elderly (Farran & McCann, 1989), the chronically mentally ill (Brunger & Grimm, 1986), the critically ill (Miller, 1989), and persons with AIDS, AIDS-related complex, and HIV antibodies (Falsetti-Shanty, 1988). A convenience sample of 126 older adults was assessed by Farran and McCann (1989) for stressful life events, social support, hope, personal control, religiosity, mental health, physical health, and activities of daily living. Several causal models of the relationships among these variables were tested, and implications for intervention were implied. Thirty-one chronically mentally ill members of a psychosocial rehabilitation program were assessed by Brunger and Grimm (1986). These participants were found to have a relatively high level of hope, perhaps because of the focus of the psychosocial program: a future orientation, goal setting, action-oriented activities, and interpersonal relationships.

Miller (1989) interviewed 60 persons who had been critically ill to determine what strategies they used to maintain or increase hope while confronted with a life-threatening event. From their responses, the author identified nine categories of hope-inspiring strategies that included cognitive strategies, determination, world view, spiritual strategies, relationships with caregivers, family bonds, control, goals, and miscellaneous strategies. Patient-identified threats to hope were also presented. Similarly, Falsetti-Shanty (1988) determined sources of hope among 65 persons diagnosed with HIV antibodies, ARC, or AIDS. In addition, this group also identified nursing activities that were hope-promoting.

In summary, nursing research pertaining to hope is evolving. Early studies were aimed at concept development, instrument development, or both, and descriptive relationships between hope and other variables. More recently, hope researchers have sought to test conceptual and causal models of hope in relation to health and illness. The present focus appears to be on patient-identified strategies for the enhancement of hope and their perceptions of the activities of caregivers, and the health care system, that threaten or support hope.

## Future Areas for Hope Research

Although continued refinement of the conceptualization and measurement of hope is important, the future direction of research pertaining to this important psychological characteristic needs to be in terms of intervention strategies. Studies must be conducted that will further delineate the person and situation factors that influence hope, so that person and situation-directed intervention approaches for the enhancement of hope can be identified.

Once intervention strategies have been defined, both theoretically and empirically, research examining the implementation of these strategies and their outcomes will be in order. Hope researchers have begun to move toward these goals. The work of Miller (1989) and Falsetti-Shanty (1988) are examples of the future direction hope research needs to take.

## ❖ SUMMARY

This chapter presented an overview of the psychological characteristic hope as an essential ingredient for life and growth and as an important resource for coping with the multiple stresses of illness and its treatment. Hope was defined, and its similarities to and differences from other related concepts were explored. A model for identifying the impact of hope on a person's experience with illness was presented. In discussing the nursing process and hope, the nurse's hope was identified as an important resource in the provision of nursing care. The assessment of a loss of hope, hopelessness, and a nursing care plan designed to enhance or instill hope was presented. Finally, a brief review of the "state of the science" of hope research was provided, with suggestions regarding the future directions for the study of this important psychological resource.

"To hope means to be ready at every moment for that which is not yet born, and yet not become desperate if there is no birth in one's life time."

Fromm, 1968

## ❖ APPLYING KNOWLEDGE TO PRACTICE

1. Think of a patient for whom you have recently cared whom you identified as experiencing hopelessness. What behaviors did you observe? What did this person experience or express that would lead you to infer this nursing diagnosis?
2. In your area of nursing practice, how is the concept of hope, as described here, relevant to patient experiences and nursing care? What intervention approaches, specific to this practice area, might assist patients in maintaining hope?
3. Drawing from your own clinical experiences and observations, identify a research question related to hope.
4. The nurse's hope has been identified as an important resource in patient care. What professional and personal factors might affect the level of your hope? Identify strategies that you might use to maintain your own hope.

## REFERENCES

Bahnson, C. (1975). Psychologic and emotional crises in cancer: the psychotherapeutic care of the cancer patient. *Seminars in Oncology 2*(4), 293-309.

Banks, R. (1980). Health and spiritual dimensions: relationships and implications for professional preparation programs. *Journal of School Health, 50,* 195-202.

Beck, A., Weisman, A., Lester, D., & Trexler, L. (1974). The measurement of pessimism: the hopelessness scale. *Journal of Consulting Clinical Psychology, 42*(6), 861-865.

Brunger, J., & Grimm, P. (1986). *Hope and the chronically mentally ill.* Paper presented at The Eighth Southeastern Regional Conference of Clinical Specialists in Psychiatric Mental Health Nursing. Hilton Head, South Carolina.

Buehler, J. (1975). What contributes to hope in the cancer patient? *American Journal of Nursing, 75*(8), 1353-1356

Carpenito, L. (1989). *Nursing diagnosis: application to clinical practice* (3rd ed.). New York: J.B.Lippincott Co.

Carson, V., Soeken, K. & Grimm, P. (1988). Hope and its relationship to spiritual well-being. *Journal of Psychology and Theology, 16*(2), 159-167.

Doenges, M., & Moorhouse, M. (1988). *Nurse pocket guide: nursing diagnosis with interventions* Philadelphia: F.A. Davis, Co.

Dubree, M., & Vogelpohl, R. (1980). When hope dies—so might the patient. *American Journal of Nursing, 80*(11), 2046-2049.

Dufault, K. (1981). *Hope of elderly persons with cancer.* Doctoral Dissertation, Case Western Reserve University.

Dufault, K., & Martocchio, B. (1985). Hope: its spheres and dimensions. *Nursing Clinics of North America, 20*(2), 379-391.

Erickson, R., Past, R., & Paige, A. (1975). Hope as a psychiatric variable. *Journal of Clinical Psychology, 31*(2), 324-329.

Erikson, E. (1963). *Childhood and society.* New York: Norton.

Falsetti-Shanty, J. (1988). *Level of hope in patients with HIV antibodies, AIDS related complex and AIDS* Unpublished masters thesis. University of Maryland School of Nursing.

Farran, C., & McCann, J. (1989). Longitudinal analysis of hope in community-based older adults. *Archives of Psychiatric Nursing, 3*(5), 272-276.

Frank, J. (1974). *Persuasion and healing.* New York: Schachin Books.

Frankl, V. (1959). *Man's search for meaning.* New York: Simon & Schuster.

Fromm, E. (1968). *The revolution of hope.* New York: Harper & Row.

Goleman, D. (1984). To dream the possible dream: an interview with Shlomo Breznitz. *American Health, 3*(9), 60.

Gottschalk, L. (1979). A hope scale applicable to verbal samples. In L. Gottschalk, *The content analysis of verbal behavior: further studies* (pp. 1-7). New York: SP Medical and Scientific Books.

Grimm, P. (1984). *The state-trait hope inventory: empirical evaluation of an instrument.* Unpublished manuscript University of Maryland School of Nursing.

Grimm, P. (1989). *Hope, affect, psychological status and the cancer experience* (Doctoral Dissertation). University of Maryland.

Hickey, S. (1986). Enabling hope. *Cancer Nursing, 9*(3), 133-137.

Hinds, P. (1984). Inducing a definition of 'hope' through the use of grounded theory methodology. *Journal of Advanced Nursing, 9:*357-362.

Kerber, A. (1987). *Locus of control, hope and disease-free interval.* (abstract). Oncology Nursing Forum supplement, p. 121.

Kubler-Ross, E. (1977). Hope and the dying patient. *Nursing Digest, 5*(2), 82-84.

Lange, S. (1978). Hope. In C. Carlson & B. Blackwell (Eds.). *Behavioral concepts and nursing intervention* 2nd ed. New York: J.B. Lippincott Co.

Lazarus, R., & Folkman, S. (1984). *Stress, appraisal and coping.* New York: Springer Publishing Co.

Limandri, B. & Boyle, D. (1978). Instilling hope. *American Journal of Nursing, 78*(1), 79-80.

Lynch, W. (1965). *Images of hope: imagination as healer of the hopeless.* Baltimore: Helicon Press, Inc.

Marcel, G. (1962). *Homo viator: introduction to a metaphysic of hope.* New York: Harper & Row.

Menninger, K. (1975). Hope. *Menninger Perspective, 5*(4), 4-11.

Miller, J. (1983). Inspiring hope. In J.F. Miller (Ed.), *Coping with chronic illness: Overcoming powerlessness.* (pp. 287-299) Philadelphia: F.A. Davis Co.

Miller, J. (1985). Inspiring hope. *American Journal of Nursing, 85*(1), 22-25.

Miller, J. (1989). Hope-inspiring strategies of the critically ill. *Applied Nursing Research, 2*(1), 23-29.

Miller, J. & Powers, M. (1988). Development of an instrument to measure hope. *Nursing Research, 37* (1), 6-10.

Nowotny, M. (1986). *Measurement of hope as exhibited by a general adult population after a stressful event.* Doctoral Dissertation, Texas Women's University abstract received by personal communication.

Nowotny, M. (1989). Assessment of hope in patients with cancer: development of an instrument. *Oncology Nursing Forum, 16*(1), 57-61.

Obayuwana, A.; Collins, J.; Carter, A.; Rao, M.; Mathura, C. & Wilson, S. (1982). Hope index scale: an instrument for the objective assessment of hope. *Journal of the National Medical Association, 74*(8), 761-765.

O'Malley, P. (1988). Relationship of hope and stress after myocardial infarction. *Heart & Lung, 17*(2), 184-190.

Panagis, D. (1982). Psychological factors and cancer outcome. In J. Cohen, et al. (Eds.). *Psychosocial aspects of cancer,* (209-220). New York: Raven Press, 209-220.

Pruyser, P. (1987). Maintaining hope in adversity. *Bulletin of the Menninger Clinic, 51*(5), 463-474.

Raleigh, E. (1980). *An investigation of hope as manifested in physically ill adult.* Dissertation Abstracts International, *41*(4), 1313-1314B.

Rideout, E. (1986). Hope, morale and adaptation in patients with chronic heart failure. *Journal of Advanced Nursing 11:* 429-438.

Speilberger, Gorsuch & Llushine (1970). *STAT manual for the State-Trait Anxiety Inventory ("Self-Evaluation Questionnaire).* Palo Alto, CA.: Consulting Psychologists Press, Inc.

Stanley, T. (1978). The lived experience of hope: the isolation of discreet descriptive elements common to the experience of hope in healthy adults. *Dissertation Abstracts International, 39*(3), 1212B.

Stoner, M. (1982). *Hope and cancer patients.* University of Colorado, Doctoral Dissertation.

Stoner, M., & Keampfer, S. (1985). Recalled life expectancy information, phase of illness and hope in cancer patients. *Research in Nursing & Health, 8,* 269-274.

Stoner, M. (1988). Measuring hope. In M. Frank-Stromborg (Ed.). *Instruments for clinical nursing research* (pp. 133-140). Norwalk, Conn.: Appleton-Lange.

Stotland, E. (1969). *The psychology of hope.* San Francisco: Jossey-Bass, Inc.

Thomas, S. (1978). Breast cancer: the psychosocial issues. *Cancer Nursing,* Feb. 53-60.

Travelbee, J. (1971). *Interpersonal aspects of nursing.* 2nd ed., Philadelphia: F.A. Davis.

Vaillot, M.C. (1970). Hope: the restoration of being. *American Journal of Nursing, 70*(2), 270-273.

Watson, J. (1979). *Nursing: the philosophy and science of caring.* Boston: Little, Brown & Co, Chapter 1.

Weisman, A. (1979). *Coping with cancer.* New York: McGraw-Hill Book Co.

Young-Brockopp, D. (1982). Cancer patients' perceptions of five psychosocial needs. *Oncology Nursing Forum, 9*(4), 31-35.

# 29 Hardiness

Linda Lindsey Davis

## OBJECTIVES

*At the completion of this chapter, the reader will be able to:*

◆ Describe the three dimensions of personality hardiness.

◆ Integrate hardiness-promoting strategies into the steps of the nursing process.

◆ Identify important areas for future nursing research on hardiness as a health-promoting characteristic of individuals and families.

At some point in life, every individual will encounter a stressful life event, whether it is an unexpected illness or injury, the loss of a loved one or treasured possession, or the challenge of an unanticipated opportunity. Why do some individuals cope effectively with life changes and even use those changes as opportunities for personal growth, while others are seemingly paralyzed by such events? There are many theories about why individuals differ in their abilities to cope with change. Some of these theories may be classified as *situational,* those theories related to the characteristics of the life change encountered; some are *contextual,* related to the conditions under which the life change is experienced; and some are *personal,* those theories concerned with the characteristics of the individual who encounters the life change. Nurse clinicians who work with clients across the life cycle continue to search for personality characteristics that influence an individual's ability to cope and adapt and that are responsive to nursing intervention. This chap-

ter explores the personality characteristic of "hardiness" as a major factor that influences coping and adaptation when stressful life events are encountered. Hardiness characteristics are then integrated into the steps of the nursing process to demonstrate its usefulness in clinical nursing practice.

## ❖ STRESS AND COPING CONCEPTS IN NURSING PRACTICE

Nursing interventions that seek to promote successful individual and family coping have their roots in stress-adaptation theory. Stress has been a frequent topic in nursing literature since the mid 1950s, when Selye published his major work on the general adaptation syndrome. Selye described a *stressor* as an external challenge to an organism and *stress* as the response to that challenge. Selye described the *adaptive response* syndrome as having three stages: alarm/mobilization, resistance, and exhaustion (Selye, 1956). It is important to note that it is not the stressor that is thought to have long-term or lasting effects on an organism; rather, it is the nature of an organism's adaptive response to that stressor that largely determines whether the end result will be harmful or helpful to the organism. Responses that prove to be harmful to the organism are described as *maladaptive*. Maladaptive stress responses have been identified as causal factors in a wide variety of major illnesses including depressive disorders, coronary heart disease, and certain types of cancer. However, the reasons why some individuals exposed to stressful stimuli become ill while others do not remains unclear. One explanation for differential illness rates among individuals experiencing comparable levels of stress is related to the differential coping styles used. (The concept of stress is discussed in depth in Chapter 17.)

*Coping* has been defined as an individual's efforts to master a stressor (Burckhardt, 1987). Coping occurs after the initial appraisal of an event (primary appraisal) and the subsequent appraisal of personal resources that are available to manage that event (secondary appraisal). Coping may be *problem-focused*—directed at solving the problem inherent in a stressful event, or *emotion-focused*—concerned with the feeling responses generated by the event (Lazarus & Folkman, 1984). Studies of factors that influence stress, coping, and adaptation with health crises, chronicity, or convalescence have become major emphasis areas in nursing research literature.

Since Selye's early work on stress and adaptive responses, many social scientists have come to disagree with Selye's stress-adaptive response model, proposing that it represents a somewhat passive, reactive model of human behavior. Instead, cognitive theorists have endeavored to develop stress-coping models that take into account the human potential and capacity to define and shape life by personally choosing to respond in certain ways when confronted with new events. Building on the works of existentialist philosophers such as Kierkegaard and Heidegger, cognitive theoreticians characterize the ability for individuals in contemporary society to assume some measure of personal control over their own life and in some cases to choose their own responses in certain life situations as a more proactive model of coping. Conceptualizations of coping that acknowledge rational decision making and personal choice may be found in the work of several contemporary theoreticians on coping and adaptation. (See Chapter 26.) *Hardiness* is a personality-focused concept thought to influence coping and adaptation through personal decision and choice.

## ❖ THE CONCEPT OF PERSONAL HARDINESS

Suzanne Kobasa, an existential psychologist, proposed that individuals who experience a high degree of stress without falling ill have personality structures that are different from those who become ill as a consequence of a high level of life stress (Kobasa, 1979). According to Kobasa, hardy individuals have three personality characteristics that enable them to cope effectively when they encounter life stress events and still remain healthy. First, the hardy individual has a sense of *commitment*, a purpose and involvement with life, work, others, and self. Second, the hardy individual has a sense of *challenge*, a belief that life changes can represent meaningful opportunities for personal growth. Lastly, hardy individuals have a sense of personal *control*, a belief in their ability to shape and influence the outcomes of their life situations. For hardy individuals, this control means the ability to successfully appraise a stressful event (cognitive control); to make a sound decision from among various possible courses of action (decisional control); and, to choose from a personal repertoire of responses (coping skills). The potential usefulness of the hardiness concept for clinical nursing practice has already been identified in the nursing literature (Bigbee, 1985; Call & Davis, 1989; Keane, Ducette, & Adler, 1985; Lambert & Lambert, 1987; McCranie, Lambert, & Lambert, 1987; Lee, 1983; Pollock, 1986; 1989; Rich & Rich, 1987).

Kobasa (1979) built upon an existential model of coping and adaptation in developing three hypotheses about what happens when hardy individuals encounter stressful life events:

1. Those who view life change as a challenge will remain healthier than those who view change as a threat.
2. Those who feel committed to their life will remain healthier than those who feel alienated.
3. Those who have a greater sense of personal control over what happens in their own life will remain healthier than those who feel powerless.

Kobasa's premise, that individuals who perceive themselves as having more commitment and control in their life and who view change as a personal challenge will be healthier, served as the basis for her descriptive survey of over 800 public utility executives on their health and hardiness levels. Kobasa asked each executive to complete self-scored measures of their perceived stress levels, their history of recent illnesses, as well as measures designed to tap their perceived levels of challenge, commitment, and control. By analyzing responses from 670 completed questionnaires, Kobasa concluded that those executives who reported both high stress levels and low illness levels also perceived themselves to be more in control, more committed, and more personally challenged in their lives. In contrast, executives who reported both high stress levels and high illness levels also reported lower levels of personal control, commitment, and challenge. Kobasa's use of a cross-sectional survey design did not permit clarification of whether the high stress and high illness levels reported by some executives preceded

Stressful life events

+

Personality hardiness

+

Use of selected coping skills

⇩

Stress response

⇩

Health status outcomes

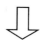 **Fig. 29-1**    The relationship of personality hardiness to stressful life events and health status outcomes.

their personal beliefs that they had less control, commitment, and challenge or resulted from their lessened sense of control, commitment, and challenge. However, these results do suggest that there is a strong link between these three hardiness characteristics, stress, and illness (Kobasa, 1979). Fig. 29-1 demonstrates these linkages.

## ❖ MEASURING HARDINESS

In the initial phases of research on hardy personalities, Kobasa and others have used several instruments from various sources to tap into the hardiness concepts. To measure *challenge,* Kobasa used components from the California Life Goals Evaluation Schedules (Hahn, 1966). the *Vegetative Versus Vigorousness Scale* and *The Need for Adventurousness Scale*

(Maddi, Kobasa & Hoover, 1979) as well as the *Need for Cognitive Structure Scale* and the *Need for Endurance Scale* from the Personality Research Form (Jackson, 1974; Wiggins, 1973). Nowack (1986) has reported using the *Sensation Seeking Scale* (Zuckerman, 1964) to measure challenge. To measure **commitment,** Kobasa used the *Alienation Test* (Maddi, et al., 1979) as well as portions of Gergen and Morse's (1967) Role Consistency Test. To measure **control,** Kobasa and others have used the *Internal-External Locus of Control Scale* (Lefcourt, 1973; Rotter, Seeman & Liverant, 1962), the *Powerlessness Versus Personal Control Scale* and the *Nihilism Versus Meaningfulness Scales* from the Alienation Test (Maddi et al., 1979). Control has also been measured with the *Achievement Scale* and *Dominance Scale* from the Personality Research Form (Jackson, 1974; Wiggins, 1973), as well as the *Leadership Orientation Scale* from the California Life Goals Evaluation Schedules (Hahn, 1966).

Over the past decade, the various methods of measuring hardiness have evolved into a single, unitary measure. Individuals are asked to mark self-scored items on a four-point Likert scale with responses ranging from *a little true,* (scored as a 1) to *completely true* (scored as a 3). Answers that respondents believe are *not at all true* are scored as 0. Examples of individual items on this combined measure include statements such as:

> Changes in routine bother me (challenge item).
> I really look forward to my work (commitment item).
> I usually feel that I can change what might happen tomorrow by what I do today (control item).

This unitary hardiness measure has been factor analyzed to determine the validity of three separate dimensions of hardiness. The measure has been evaluated with various populations for reliability; the three individual scales for challenge, commitment, and control have demonstrated re-

liability coefficients (internal consistency) above 0.70, and the entire 50-item measure has consistently had reliability coefficients above 0.90. Repeated administrations of the instrument over time shows good stability with test-retest correlations above 0.60 (The Hardiness Institute, 1987).

In the past decade, the outcomes of several additional studies of hardiness suggest that the concept has promise for nurse clinicians. In a five-year retrospective study of male executives, Kobasa, Maddi, and Courington (1981) found high hardiness individuals reported significantly fewer illnesses, even when previous health levels were controlled. In a second study using 70 of these same executives, Kobasa, Maddi, Puccetti, and Zola (1985) found hardiness alone accounted for 22% of the variation in illness levels and surpassed all other personal characteristics in its ability to explain variations in illness levels among these executives. In a study of hardiness and coping skills in lawyers, Kobasa (1982) found lower levels of commitment (characterized by high scores on an alienation test) among lawyers to be correlated with their use of more regressive coping skills (e.g., the use of anger and avoidance). Kobasa concluded that individuals with higher levels of hardiness should demonstrate more positive coping skills (more transformational).

In a sample of 193 workers in human service fields who were classified as either personality type A (i.e., exhibiting a hard-driving, competitive, aggressive, time-urgent response style) or B (i.e., exhibiting fewer or none of these behaviors), Nowack (1986) found cognitively hardy Type A individuals experienced less burnout and psychological distress when measured over a 4-month period. Howard, Cunningham, and Rechnitzer (1986) also studied male personality type A subjects to determine whether hardiness was associated with coronary risk factors. These researchers found that individuals with high levels of hardiness (as represented by a high score on a dependence/independence scale) had lower systolic and diastolic blood pressure levels as well as lower total cholesterol and triglyceride levels. There were no differences in the risk factors of personality Type B males who had high or low levels of hardiness, leading the researchers to conclude that hardiness was a "buffer" for the stress-prone type A individuals.

Keane, Ducette, and Adler (1987), focused on hardiness in their study of staff nurses in intensive care units (ICU) in a large university hospital. They compared these ICU nurses with their staff nurse counterparts in general medical and surgical units in the same hospital and found that it was not the setting (ICU vs. general unit) where the staff nurse worked that influenced nurse burnout, it was the level of hardiness. Across all units, staff nurses who felt more challenge, had more commitment, and perceived themselves to have some personal control over their life situation reported lower levels of burnout. Because of the correlational nature of their study, Keane, Ducette, and Adler were unable to determine whether high levels of hardiness caused lower levels of burnout or whether low levels of burnout empowered these staff nurses to feel challenged, committed, and in control.

Rich and Rich (1987) also related levels of self-reported hardiness to the presence of physical, psychological, and behavioral manifestations of work-related burnout among 100 staff nurses. Results showed a significant, negative correlation ($r = -0.39$) between hardiness and burnout; the higher the hardiness in the staff nurse sample, the lower their level of burnout. Rich and Rich found that hardiness alone accounted for 25% of the variance in staff nurse burnout. The combination of years of nursing experience and hardiness accounted for 41% of the variance in burnout scores. The researchers concluded that low levels of hardiness, combined with few years of nursing experience, were strongly correlated with high levels of burnout among this sample of staff nurses.

In a third study of burnout among hospital staff nurses, McCranie, Lambert, and Lambert (1987) also reported higher levels of burnout and higher stress correlated with lower levels of hardiness among their sample of 107 staff nurses. However, their findings revealed that higher hardiness was correlated with higher job stress levels. They concluded that hardiness does not neutralize work-related stresses.

In a fourth study of stress, burnout and hardiness, Topf (1989) found the commitment dimension of hardiness to account for almost 24% of the variation in work-related burnout among 100 critical care nurses. Topf concluded that greater hardiness in these critical care nurses was associated with less stress and burnout.

## ❖ USING HARDINESS CONCEPTS WITH THE NURSING PROCESS

Research on the outcomes of numerous behavioral therapies suggests it may be possible to increase or enhance client levels of hardiness through selected nursing interventions. Maddi and Kobasa (1984) have proposed that hardiness can be learned at any time in life. Nurse clinicians who work with individuals and families across the life cycle can use the nursing process to identify their clients' existing levels of challenge, commitment, and control and to develop interventions that support or enhance high level hardiness as important in the process of coping with stressors.

### Assessment

Kobasa described the hardy individual as one who welcomes challenge, an active change seeker who anticipates new experiences as opportunities for personal growth. Before developing a health care regimen with a new client, a nurse will want to explore the client's feelings about new experiences in general. To explore this characteristic of challenge, the nurse might ask clients about whether they have set routines for activities of daily living and if so, how often they deviate from these routines and whether they see deviations as a welcome change.

When asked about personal routines, a busy accountant responded "Organization and routine are extremely important in my business; I have set routines which I follow every day; deviating from these routines always means confusion and usually means lost time." The nurse clinician seeing this client for diabetic self-care correctly concluded that the client placed a high priority on routine and procedure and less value on novelty and change. Integrating changes into this client's eating patterns subsequently proved difficult because of the client's reluctance to alter many of his firmly entrenched eating habits. Knowing whether clients view life changes as challenges, or as threats to their personal stability is an important component in assessing their hardiness level.

Kobasa also characterized the hardy individual as someone with a high level of life commitment, one who has a sense of involvement in life work, in interpersonal relationships with others and with the self. Committed individuals have a belief in and an appreciation for their own values, skills, and personal goals. In assessing commitment, the nurse might ask clients questions about life, work, and whether personal satisfaction is derived from them. In response to such a question, a young mother of three responded "My work is raising my three children; sometimes it's exhausting but it's still exciting to watch them grow and develop."

A middle-aged computer sales representative responded to the same question with "My job is to be sure that our customers get the hardware and software systems that meet their needs; I look forward to helping customers get the things they need."

An older woman who had just retired from her job as principal in a high school responded to the same question with "My job right now is taking care of just myself, doing all of the things I never had time for before; enjoying the increased freedom and personal interests I always promised myself I'd eventually get to, when I retired." In different ways, all three of these individuals are expressing a strong sense of commitment in their life work and to themselves. According to Kobasa, such individuals will cope more successfully with stressors and be more resistant to illness because they are involved with and committed to mastering life situations.

Identification of a client's personal sense of control may be the most crucial component of hardiness assessment. A perceived level of personal control represents an individual's belief that he or she can accurately assess new situations and correctly choose an effective course of action to solve problems. When asked whether she felt capable of managing the multiple demands of her busy life, a 50-year-old married woman with two teenagers who was simultaneously caring for her aged mother responded

> I have always been able to take care of my own family. For the past 16 years, I have managed a home and two children and a part-time job which I love. The recent death of my father and the need to take on the care of my mother who lives 30 miles out of town has overwhelmed me. I am meeting the needs of others but my own needs are getting lost in the process.

The nurse clinician, a family nurse practitioner who had provided health care services to this client for the last 5 years, believed the client was someone who in the past had been able to successfully control her day-to-day life situation. However, currently she verbalized a personal loss of control and felt immobilized by the expectations placed upon her by others. Based upon this assessment, the nurse practitioner recommended the client join a support group for family care givers of aged parents.

Identify the personal meaning
to be gained from stressful
events and life changes
(the challenge factor)

Make reality-based decisions about
a personal course of action
(the decisional control factor)

Hardy individuals can:

Integrate new experiences into
life work and personal goals
(the commitment factor)

Acquire knowledge to accurately
assess stressful events
and life changes
(the cognitive control factor)

Develop enhanced/new coping
skills as needed
(the coping skill factor)

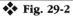 **Fig. 29-2**   Behaviors exhibited by hardy individuals.

## Planning

The literature on the link between stress responses and illness suggests that clients who perceive themselves as personally incapable of managing life changes and stressors are candidates for stress-related illness or accidents. Promoting hardiness in clients who are confronted with illness, injury, loss, or unexpected life situations should be directed primarily at assisting them to see stressful events as having relevant meaning and as providing opportunities for personal growth. When new coping skills are needed, hardiness promotion can also mean providing systematic opportunities for clients to observe successful role models who demonstrate the desired behavior. In addition, clients should have opportunities to demonstrate new behaviors and skills to ensure mastery. Fig. 29-2 shows behaviors and skills typically manifested by hardy individuals that can provide direction for goal-setting during the planning phase of the nursing process.

## Intervention

While the reality of most stressful events can seldom be controlled, clients can learn to change or control behavioral responses to such events. The box that follows gives a list of nursing interventions based on Kobasa's three-dimensional model of personal hardiness that promote hardiness.

❖ **FIVE NURSING INTERVENTIONS DESIGNED TO PROMOTE INDIVIDUAL HARDINESS**

Provide opportunities for clients to explore the potential challenges and commitments inherent in new or stressful events.

Break desired new behavioral responses to be learned into a series of easily mastered subtasks.

Provide clients with relevant role models who can successfully demonstrate the desired behavioral responses.

Structure regular and frequent opportunities for clients to demonstrate their own mastery of the desired behavioral response.

Assist clients in developing self-monitoring skills for personal assessment when new stressful situations are encountered.

### Evaluation

The existential origins of the hardiness construct suggest that clients are the best judges of whether hardiness promotion interventions have been productive in enabling them to cope more effectively. When they encounter stressful events, clients should be encouraged to ask themselves: What meaning can I find in this situation? How can I use this situation for personal growth? What responses are within my personal control? Who else has coped with such an experience and what strategies did they use? Are there new skills I need to learn to cope with this situation? What new skills have I developed as a result of this situation that may be useful in the future?

### ❖ HARDINESS CASE STUDIES

The following case study demonstrates the use of the hardiness concept for individual health promotion.

### Case Study #1: Health Promotion

Cynthia B., a single, 36-year-old woman with a doctoral degree in business administration who teaches management theory at the local, private, liberal arts college came to the HMO for a routine insurance physical. Physical examination revealed no health problems with the exception that Cynthia's weight of 180 lbs. was too much for her 62 inch frame. This weight placed her in a "moderate" risk category for health insurance. Based upon her weight and insurance risk classification, the HMO physician referred Cynthia for the HMO's Self Health Classes, which are managed by the professional nursing staff.

During her first visit, Cynthia recounted her personal desire to lose weight but her belief that her family history of obesity (both parents are overweight) coupled with numerous, unsuccessful previous personal efforts to lose weight likely made participation in classes of little value.

Over the course of several visits, Cynthia and the nurse clinician explored Cynthia's feelings about her weight, her commitment to her work as a teacher, and her long-standing interest in starting her own private consulting business. To Cynthia, her weight began to take on new meaning as a "protective" factor, one which had previously enabled her to avoid exploring her fantasy of going into business for herself. After three weeks of individual sessions, Cynthia elected to join the Monday evening Working Woman's Self Care Group. Weight loss and maintenance in the group averaged 18 pounds per member. Cynthia approached weight loss with her customary need to excel and quickly became the group "expert" on various types of exercise and calorie expenditures.

Over the course of the next year, Cynthia lost and maintained a 35 pound weight loss. She also initiated a private consulting service for small businesses on her own time. She found that the combination of teaching and consulting was more personally rewarding than either would be by itself.

At the request of the nurse who leads the Monday night self care group meetings, Cynthia visits with new groups every 3 to 4 months for what she terms personal "booster sessions" for her own weight loss maintenance and to serve as a mentor to new group members.

The nurse in this situation used hardiness promotion as a unifying principle in working with Cynthia. She diagnosed Cynthia's problem as *unmet needs for personal control as demonstrated in verbalized feelings of inability to manage selected aspects of life and health.* Nursing goals included assisting Cynthia in establishing a sense of control. First, the nurse worked with Cynthia to explore the personal meaning of her excess weight and the potential life changes that weight loss represented to her.

In the early stages of the interaction, the nurse encouraged Cynthia to reframe weight loss activities as a set of subtasks to be mastered. She encouraged Cynthia to apply those general problem-solving skills that she already possessed to master one specific skill in weight loss management: balancing exercise and calorie expenditure. Through the Monday group meetings, she made sure Cynthia had opportunities to meet and talk with other women who were successful weight loss role models. Lastly, the nurse ensured that Cynthia had regular opportunities to continue to model her own, newly mastered techniques for others through her periodic visits with the Monday night groups. A sample of client goals and nursing interventions designed for this client is shown in the following nursing care plan.

## ❖ NURSING CARE PLAN

| | |
|---:|:---|
| **CLIENT:** | Cynthia B. |
| **MEDICAL DIAGNOSIS:** | Moderate obesity (height 5'2", weight 180 lbs.) |
| **NURSING DIAGNOSIS:** | Altered health maintenance related to inability to manage personal health habits |
| | Powerlessness related to lack of control over personal nutrition and exercise programs |

| GOALS | NURSING INTERVENTIONS |
|---|---|
| Establish personal commitment to a sound nutrition and exercise program | Support client in: <br> ◆ Exploring the personal meaning of weight loss/gain <br> ◆ Identifying benefits to be gained from successful weight management <br> ◆ Developing a number of satisfying daily/weekly/monthly personal rewards/incentives for successful weight loss |

*Continued.*

**NURSING CARE PLAN—cont'd**

| GOALS | NURSING INTERVENTIONS |
|---|---|
| Acquire the belief that personal nutrition and exercise program management is a meaningful challenge that can be mastered | Assist client in:<br>♦ Identifying counterproductive diet/exercise habits that need to be changed<br>♦ Developing realistic weight loss goals<br>♦ Breaking the necessary new behavioral changes associated with nutrition/exercise program into easily mastered subtasks |
| Develop the belief that nutrition, exercise, and related health habits are within her ability to control. | Provide client with:<br>♦ Moderate fat, protein, and calorie menu planning<br>♦ Information on diet/exercise groups in her community<br>♦ Opportunities to meet successful role models for changing exercise, nutrition, and fitness habits<br>♦ Opportunities to demonstrate new health habits and coach others involved in similar activities |

**EVALUATION**

Cynthia verbalizes her willingness to make a long-term commitment to a sound nutrition and exercise program to manage her weight. She states the belief that management of exercise and nutrition is a challenge that must be mastered and sets specific weight loss goals. Cynthia demonstrates hardiness behaviors when she manages her own weight loss through low calorie menu planning, participating in regular exercise and using support groups as appropriate.

Some of the intervention strategies shown in the sample care plan are similar to those used by many nurses with their clients. The primary difference is not in the strategies used, but rather in the nursing goals for the client. This nurse clinician did not begin nursing care for this client by establishing goals for a set number of pounds to be lost each week. Rather, the clinician's goal was to enable Cynthia to envision weight loss as a realistic challenge that she could master if broken into a series of more easily managed subtasks. She also wanted to work with Cynthia over time to develop a personal commitment to healthy self care. Finally, the clinician's third goal was to enable Cynthia to believe she had the necessary cognitive and decisional control—as well as the necessary coping skills—to achieve this important aspect of personal health promotion.

According to Wright and Leahey (1987),

family problem solving and coping with illness is greatly influenced by the family perception of the event. The following case study represents application of the hardiness concept by a community health nurse working with a family that is attempting to gain some meaningful perspective on the experience of chronic illness.

## Case Study #2: Health Maintenance

David Kimball is a 52-year-old asphalt worker. David lives with Luann, a 39-year-old data processor for a local hospital. They have a 7-year-old son. A year ago, David was diagnosed as having essential hypertension. He was advised to stop smoking and to reduce his dietary intake of saturated fats because of a serum cholesterol of 240 mg/dl. The physician at the clinic where David goes for health care first prescribed Inderal, 240 mg QD to control his hypertension. Over the course of the past six months David has been hospitalized twice: once for pulmonary pneumonia and once for observation following a work-related accident. At each hospital admission, David's blood pressure has always been above 150 systolic and 110 diastolic. His pulse has remained in the 80 to 90 range. David admitted not being consistent in taking the Inderal because it made him feel "down" most of the time. To reduce drug side effects and improve David's adherence to a medication regimen, the physician changed his medication regimen to Isoptin 240 mg and Dyazide 60 mg QD. Because of the change in David's medications, the physician made a visiting nurse referral.

At the time of the first home visit, the community health nurse initially checked David's blood pressure and briefly discussed the new drug regimen with David and Luann. The nurse then suggested that the three of them explore how David's illness had affected them individually and as a family. Finally, she suggested they discuss their future expectations for the family in managing David's health care. At first, David referred to his health condition as "just a bad piece of luck." Later, he stated that "maybe the pressure problems mean I need to slow down and smell the flowers a bit." Luann thought the changes had been primarily hers, because she now felt compelled to take on the role of being a care giver for David, reminding him to take his medications and attempting to discourage his smoking. Luann also reported that she had learned to do "low-fat cooking" and now was able to plan menus that were low in saturated fats. She saw this new skill as having additional benefits beyond being part of David's blood pressure regimen because it had enabled her to lose 8 pounds as well. However, Luann continued to express feelings of resentment over what she described as having to be the "watchdog" for David's health.

For the remainder of the visit, the nurse worked on focusing with David and Luann on how the family was responding to the illness experience. Neither David nor Luann could identify ways in which their son had been affected by David's illness. Their energies were primarily focused on their own dissatisfactions with each other's behaviors. By the end of the session, David and Luann had agreed to some individual responsibilities; David would take on more responsibility for his medication and smoking behaviors; Luann would continue to manage their dietary patterns.

A week after the first home visit, the community health nurse called David and Luann to find out how they were managing. Both believe they had made progress in managing their own, agreed to responsibilities; however, neither was completely satisfied with the other's behavior. David reported that he felt he was "being nagged"; Luann felt she still tended to fall into the "same old rut of being the responsible one." The nurse suggested that she meet with David and Luann again to discuss additional strategies for managing David's health maintenance program.

**Encouraging family members to discuss a stressful experience is an important step in enabling them to find possible meanings as well as opportunities for growth in the experience. With this family, the community health nurse initially focused on encouraging the couple to verbalize their individual beliefs about the illness experience and their vision of the future as a result of the experience. David's comment about the need to "slow down" likely reflects an effort to find some personal meaning in the experience. Luann's observation about the additional benefits of learning low-fat diet menus also reflects this effort to find personal meaning. However, neither David nor Luann were yet**

able to move beyond their individual concerns to more general, family-level issues. Both continued to express dissatisfaction with their personal control in the situation as reflected in David's comments about "being nagged" and Luann's observation that she is the "watchdog." This couple is obviously experiencing great stress as a response to the onset of a chronic illness for one partner. Whether the problems of communication and control manifested in their interactions are recent or of long-standing duration will require more extensive assessment. The initial nursing diagnosis formulated by the community health nurse was *family turmoil related to onset of chronic illness (hypertension) of the husband and father.* Hardiness promotion with this family must first be focused on enabling this couple to explore their individual issues as relevant factors influencing family problem-solving. Nursing interventions to promote the hardiness of this couple, both as individuals as well as a family unit, would likely require a number of visits, periodic follow-ups, additional referral for individual or family counseling or both.

## ❖ HARDINESS AND SELECTED NURSING THEORIES

Hardiness appraisals and nursing interventions are focused on promoting, enhancing, or sustaining a more proactive coping response when stressful life events are encountered. The concept of hardiness for health promotion and health maintenance is congruent with the assumptions of most major nursing theories. For example, the three dimensions of hardiness can be viewed as aspects of the needs for security and for self-actualization inherent to most of the human need-based theories. The conceptualizations of challenge, commitment, and control lend themselves to assessment as residual stimuli (i.e., the genetic or personality-based characteristics of the individual) depicted in human adaptation theory. The exis-

tential origins of the hardiness concept, which is reflective of a potential for personal action and capability, support assessment of hardiness as part of a self-care agency associated with self-care theory.

## ❖ NURSING RESEARCH ON HARDINESS

There are few studies of hardiness in clinical nursing research literature. Pollock (1986) used an adapted version of Kobasa's hardiness measure, the *Health Related Hardiness Scale* to explore physical and psychosocial adaptation in individuals with three chronic illnesses: heart disease, diabetes, and rheumatoid arthritis. Pollock's findings revealed that hardiness was positively associated with better psychosocial and physiological adaptation for the diabetic subjects. She also found the lowest hardiness control scores to be among those individuals with rheumatoid arthritis, leading her to conclude that clients with this chronic illness were most likely to believe the illness was beyond their personal control. In a second study of hardiness among individuals with chronic illness, Pollock (1989) also related hardiness to the use of specific coping skills by 30 diabetics. She measured diabetic subjects' appraisals of possible outcomes, the type of coping strategies they reported using (problem-focused, emotion-focused, or a mixture of the two), and their perceived levels of hardiness. Pollock found that 56% of the variation in physiological adaptation was explained by a combination of outcome appraisals: harm and benefit, mixed-focused coping patterns, having participated in a patient education program, the use of one emotion-focused coping strategy, and hardiness. Hardiness alone accounted for 11% of the variation in physiological adaptation. Pollock concluded that higher levels of challenge, commitment, and control were related to positive physiological adaptation.

Lambert, Lambert, Klipple, and Mewshaw

(1989), also explored hardiness factors in individuals with a chronic disease. Lambert and colleagues surveyed 122 women with rheumatoid arthritis from one large rheumatology clinic in the Southeast to determine whether hardiness, social support, or both were predictive of psychological well-being in these women when the severity of illness was statistically controlled. The results of multiple correlation analyses showed that almost 44% of the variation in these women's psychological well-being was related to the combination of social support and high levels of personality hardiness. While few in number, these clinical nursing studies demonstrate the links between personality hardiness, stress, and coping previously identified in the literature.

## Limitations in Previous Research

Funk and Houston (1987) have noted the difficulties in comparing outcomes from one hardiness study with another because of the different instruments used to measure hardiness. These authors question the applicability of certain scales in measuring the different dimensions of hardiness. For example, Funk and Houston question whether a low score on an alienation scale is a sound representation for high levels of hardiness commitment. They also question the statistical conclusions drawn from some of the hardiness research studies. In their own hardiness study, Funk and Houston found their findings differed from those of previous researchers when various statistical techniques were applied. Specifically, Funk and Houston found that the statistically significant differences among groups that could be demonstrated with analysis of variance techniques could not be replicated when multiple regression techniques were used.

Other critics of the use of hardiness as a relevant personality variable that influences health and coping suggest that the three characteristics of challenge, commitment, and control may not be equally important or well developed. Hull, Van Treuren, and Virnelli (1987) reviewed results from the various published studies of hardiness and concluded that while commitment and control have been demonstrated to be predictors of health and wellness, challenge has not demonstrated comparable ability. Hull and colleagues suggest that hardiness may actually be only a two-dimensional concept, composed of the individuals' sense of life commitment and personal control.

## Future Hardiness Research

As a potential buffer against maladaptive stress responses, the hardiness concept is in need of further exploration. Nowack (1986) has commented upon the limitations in the work of Kobasa and others because of the overly narrow focus on physical illness symptoms as the exclusive indicator of health status. Rich and Rich (1987) have commented on the limited hardiness research using women subjects. Rich and Rich are among the few researchers who have used the hardiness concept in personality research primarily with women subjects. While they propose that challenge, commitment, and control concepts have relevance, they conclude that research on the relevance of hardiness as a personality characteristic in women needs further clarification. There is also a need to better clarify how hardiness may be different or comparable to other coping factors identified in the literature such as locus of control, motivation, and self-efficacy. For example, the differences between hardiness, a personality-specific concept thought to influence coping, and self-efficacy, a situation-specific concept thought to influence coping (Bandura, 1982), needs to be explored.

Nurse clinicians, researchers, and theoreticians are interested in identifying those personality variables that have the potential to influence individual and family coping when stressful life events are encountered. Previous research on hardiness suggests this three-dimensional concept of an individuals' personality may be positively correlated with effective coping skills and positive health outcomes when stressful events are encountered.

As previously mentioned, it is not clear whether an individual's personal sense of challenge, commitment, and control *subsequently* bring about improved coping or are the *result* of an individual's subjective sense of personal satisfaction when coping strategies used are successful. Previous research has demonstrated links between high levels of personal challenge, commitment, and control and health status. Whether hardiness is a predictor variable or an outcome variable in personal coping remains unclear. Both interpretations have merit for clinical nursing practice and research. If hardiness is a causal factor, influencing coping behaviors and health status, then nurse clinicians will need to focus on developing a broad repertoire of interventions that promote the development of high levels of hardiness in their clients. If a high level of personal hardiness is the result of successful coping, then nurse clinicians could use hardiness measures as indicators of the desirable outcomes for many nursing interventions.

To date, the nursing research on hardiness has been limited primarily to the study of burnout in nurses (Rich & Rich, 1987) and the study of coping skills used by individuals with selected chronic illnesses (Call & Davis, 1989; Pollock, 1986; 1987; 1989; Lambert, Lambert, Klipple, & Mewshaw, 1989). Further research is needed to clarify how the three different dimensions of hardiness are related to each other and whether one is more important in predicting or promoting hardiness in individuals and families. In addition, while Kobasa's third-generation hardiness instrument (Hardiness Institute, 1987) is easy to administer and score, the relative meaning of the scores has not been clarified. Whether there is some "minimal" amount of hardiness that clients need to be able to cope effectively with life change events and stress is unknown. This is an important area for future research if clinicians are to use the hardiness measure in practice.

## ❖ SUMMARY

Clinicians who work with individuals and families across the life cycle may find hardiness to be a useful concept in identifying and intervening with clients who are "at risk" for developing problems with coping and adaptation. Integration of the three hardiness dimensions into the steps of the nursing process provides direction for holistic nursing care with a focus on the long-range goals of strengthening and enhancing client coping and adaptation across many types of stressful situations. Hardiness-promotion as a part of nursing practice could be useful in working with clients experiencing a wide variety of problems including children with developmental difficulties, teen-aged parents, adolescents who must make choices related to smoking, drugs, and sexual behaviors, families in maturational or situational crisis, and families managing predictable life change events such as aging, illness or injury, death of a family member, or becoming a family care giver. The success of many interventions traditionally used by nurse clinicians and researchers may actually be related to the unexamined ability of these interventions to promote effective levels of challenge, commitment, and control in clients when stressful life events are encountered. As a three-dimensional concept derived from the work of existential philosophers and psychologists, the long-term value of hardiness for nursing practice may be in its potential to provide direction for empowering clients to become active agents in shaping their own health and well-being.

## ❖ APPLYING KNOWLEDGE TO PRACTICE

1. Think of a client from your own clinical practice. How would you assess their hardiness?

2. The control aspect of hardiness includes cognitive and decisional control as well as the use of personal control strategies (coping skills). Identify some specific ways in which you could promote these three aspects of personal control and hardiness with a client who has a chronic illness.

3. Hardiness interventions have been used primarily with individual clients. In what ways might hardiness promotion interventions be adapted for use with families in crisis?

## REFERENCES

Bandura, A. (1982). Self-efficacy mechanism in human agency. *American Psychologist, 37,* 122-147.

Bigbee, J. (1985). Hardiness: a new perspective in health promotion. *Nurse Practitioner, 10,* 51, 54-56.

Burckhardt, C. (1987). Coping strategies of the chronically ill. *Nursing Clinics of North America, & 22,* 543-549.

Call, J., & Davis, L. (1989). The effect of hardiness on coping strategies on adjustment to illness in chronically ill. *Applied Nursing Research, 2,* 187-188.

Funk, S., & Houston, B. (1987). A critical analysis of the Hardiness' scale's validity and utility. *Journal of Personality and Social Psychology, 53,* 572-578.

Gergen, K., & Morse, S. (1967). Self-consistency: measurement and validation. Proceedings of the 75th Annual Convention of the American Psychological Association, *2,* 207-208.

Hahn, M. (1966). California Life Goals Evaluation Schedules. Palo Alto, Ca.: Western Psychological Services.

The Hardiness Institute, (1987). The third generation hardiness test. Chicago: The Hardiness Institute.

Howard, J., Cunningham, D., & Rechnitzer, P. (1986). Personality (hardiness) as a moderator of job stress and coronary risk in Type A individuals: A longitudinal study. *Journal of Behavioral Medicine, 9,* 229-244.

Hull, J., Van Treuren, R., & Virnelli, S. (1987). Hardiness and health: A critique and alternative approach. *Journal of Personality and Social Psychology, 53,* 518-530.

Jackson, D. (1974). Personality Research Form Manual, Goshen, NY: Research Psychologists Press.

Keane, A., Ducette, J., & Adler, D. (1985). Stress in ICU and non-ICU nurses. *Nursing Research, 34,* 231-236.

Kobasa, S. (1979). Stressful life events, personality, and health: an inquiry into hardiness. *Journal of Personality and Social Psychology, 37,* 1-11.

Kobasa, S. (1982). Commitment and coping in stress resistance among lawyers, *Journal of Personality and Social Psychology, 42,* 707-717.

Kobasa, S., Maddi, S., & Courington, S. (1981). Personality and constitution as mediators in the stress-illness relationship. *Journal of Health and Social Behavior, 22,* 368-378.

Kobasa, S., Maddi, S. & Kahn, S. (1982). Hardiness and health: A prospective study. *Journal of Personality and Social Psychology. 42,* 168-177.

Kobasa, S., Maddi, S., Puccetti, M., & Zola, M. (1985). Effectiveness of hardiness, exercise and social support as resources against illness. *Journal of Psychosomatic Research, 29,* 525-533.

Lambert, C., & Lambert, V. (1987). Hardiness; Its development and relevance to nursing. *Image, 19,* 92-95.

Lambert, V., Lambert, C., Klipple, G., & Mewshaw, E. (1989). Social support, hardiness and psychological well-being in women with arthritis. *Image, 21,*128-131.

Lazarus, R., & Folkman, S. (1984). Stress Appraisal and Coping. New York: Springer Publishing Co.

Lee, H. (1983). Analysis of a concept: hardiness. *Oncology Nursing Forum, 10,* 32-35.

Lefcourt, H. (1973). The functions of the illusions of control and freedom. *American Psychologist, 28,* 417-425.

Maddi, S., & Kobasa, S. (1984). The Hardy Executive: Health Under Stress. Chicago: Dorsey Press.

Maddi, S., Kobasa, S., & Hoover, M. (1979). An Alienation Test. *Journal of Humanistic Psychology, 19,* 73-76.

McCranie, E., Lambert, V., & Lambert, C. (1987). Work stress, hardiness and burnout among hospital staff nurses. *Nursing Research, 36,* 374-378.

Nowack, K. (1986). Type A, hardiness, and psychological distress. *Journal of Behavioral Medicine, 9,* 537-548.

Pollock, S. (1986). Human responses to chronic illness: physiologic and psychosocial adaptation. *Nursing Research, 35,* 90-95.

Pollock, S. (1989). Adaptive responses in diabetes mellitus. *Western Journal of Nursing Research, 11,* 265-275.

Rich, V., & Rich, A. (1987). Personality hardiness and burnout in female staff nurses. *Image, 19,* 63-66.

Rotter, J., Seeman, M., & Liverant, S. (1962). Internal vs. external locus of control of reinforcement: A major variable in behavior theory. In N.F. Washburne (Ed.), Decisions, Values and Groups. London: Pergamon Press.

Selye, H. (1956). The Stress of Life. New York: McGraw-Hill.

Topf, M. (1989). Personality hardiness, occupational stress, and burnout in critical care nurses. *Research in Nursing and Health, 12,* 179-186.

Wiggins, J. (1973). Personality and Prediction: Principles of Personality Assessment, Reading, MA: Addison-Wesley.

Wright, L, & Leahey, M. (1987). Families and Chronic Illness. Springhouse, PA: Springhouse Corporation.

Zuckerman, M. (1964). Development of a sensation seeking scale. *Journal of Consulting and Clinical Psychology, 28,* 477-482.

# 30 Humor

C. Faye Raines

## OBJECTIVES

*At the completion of this chapter, the reader will be able to:*

◆ **Describe the development of humor theory.**

◆ **Discuss theories of humor.**

◆ **Apply the concept of humor to nursing practice.**

The concept of humor has been described since the times of Plato and Aristotle, indicating its importance as an aspect of human behavior. One of an infant's first reactions is to smile, which is seen as a behavioral indicator of humor. For adults, it serves as a means of establishing camaraderie, relieving tension, and coping with stress. We place a high value on humor as evidenced by the prices we pay to be entertained by comedians and by the fact that we view a sense of humor as an admirable characteristic. Only recently, however, has significant attention been given to either the function of humor in illness or to the use of humor as a treatment intervention. The fact that humor has not been recognized as a nursing intervention may be a result of, at least in part, professional socialization, the type of humor associated with hospitals, and gender-related uses of humor (Ruxton, 1988).

Many health care professionals have tended to view the use of humor in treatment as disruptive and potentially destructive to therapeutic relationships. Patient care is seen as serious business, and professionals who approach it humorously are often suspect. As a result, clinical education in the health disciplines has not included encouragement to use humor. In addition, nursing had its roots in religious orders and the military, which emphasized regimentation and control as well as strict morals and devotion to duty rather than to incongruous and funny things (Fry, 1987). Although great changes have been made in education, neophytes are still inculcated with the outlook that caring for patients is serious business and that joking and laughing are unprofessional.

This professional socialization, combined with a constant exposure to life-threatening situations and strict status differences in the hospital structure, provides an excellent stage for the "gallows" humor often shared by health care providers. This type of humor is a response to stress, and it also serves to strengthen solidarity among professionals (Ruxton, 1988). It establishes group boundaries and is not extended to clients and their treatment.

Gender influences may also contribute to

the lack of recognition of humor as a therapeutic tool among nurses. Research indicates that men are more likely to initiate humor, while women are more likely to react to it. Since most nurses are female, it may be that they are more reserved in the expression of humor (McGhee, 1979).

Positive effects of humor are receiving increased attention. It is now commonly believed that humor is healthy and can serve as an effective means of reducing stress. Increased attention has been devoted to the therapeutic value of humor in both physical and mental illness. The effective use of humor provides a human approach in an increasingly technologically oriented health care system.

---

*LAUGHTER*
*IS THE*
*PRESSURE RELIEF VALVE*
*THAT*
*INSURES SANITY*

---

### ❖ DEFINING HUMOR

Because it is highly subjective, the precise nature of humor has defied exact description. What is humorous to one person may not be to another. However, despite differences in perception about whether a specific situation is funny, humor is usually described as both a cognitive and emotional process. Health care professionals are also beginning to define it as a coping mechanism, a communication skill, and as a tool to promote healing.

The term *humor* is derived from the Latin word for moisture or vapor. Hippocrates believed that the balance of the four chief body fluids—blood, phlegm, yellow bile, and black bile—determined an individual's health and temperament. When the four fluids were in balance, "good humor" resulted, while an imbalance resulted in "bad humor" (Robinson, 1977).

From the Medieval perspective of humor as a balance of body fluids, the definition has developed into a more specific term referring to a quality that produces the amusing, the comic, the laughable, the ludicrous, the witty, and the funny (Flugel, 1954). Webster (1980) defines humor as "that quality which appeals to the sense of the ludicrous and absurdly incongruous" (p. 552). Haig (1986) describes humor as an intellectual process of perceiving and expressing that which is amusing or comical. Similarly, McGhee (1979) defines humor as a "mental experience of discovering and appreciating ludicrous or absurdly incongruous ideas, events or situations; those attributes of an event that make us laugh or lead us to perceive the event as ludicrous or humorous" (p. 10). Eysenck (1972) defines humor in three ways. First, it may be conformity or identification with someone who laughs at the same things as others. Second, it may be described quantitatively as the frequency with which one laughs or smiles. Third, humor may refer to the extent to which one tells funny jokes and amuses others.

Others have focused on humor as a coping mechanism. According to Freud (1903), humor is a coping mechanism that provides a means of reducing tension by expressing hostile or obscene impulses in a socially acceptable fashion. Robinson defines it as a communication form used extensively as a coping mechanism. It is "any communication which is perceived by any of the interacting parties as humorous and leads to laughing, smiling, or a feeling of amusement" (p. 192) (Robinson, 1978). Robinson also indicates that humor is indirect communication conveying messages that are usually emotionally tinged and that might be unacceptable if expressed directly. Simon (1987) provides a comprehensive definition of humor "as a coping strategy based on an individual's cognitive appraisal of a stimulus which results in behavior such as smiling or laughing, or feelings of amusement which lessen emotional distress" (p. 9).

Humor can be either verbal or situational.

Puns, jokes, comic verses, anecdotes, satires, and allegories are examples of *verbal humor,* while practical jokes, impersonation, comedies, tickling, and visual arts are examples of *situational humor* (Moses & Friedman, 1986). Ferguson and Campinha-Bacote (1989) define the following attributes of humor that distinguish it from related concepts: tension reducer, form of therapeutic communication, learning enhancer, and behavioral responses of laughter, smiling, grinning, and shedding tears. They also list empirical referents indicating the presence of humor as smiling, laughing (side splitting laughter, belly laughter, hysterical laughter), grinning, decreased musculoskeletal activity (relaxed intercostal, abdominal, diaphragm, neck, and shoulder muscles), increased heart rate, and increased respiratory rate.

## ❖ DEVELOPMENT OF HUMOR THEORY

Historically, the development of humor theory (Table 30-1) can be traced through three phases: pretheoretical, psychoanalytic, and cognitive (Bellart, 1989; Goldstein, 1976). The pretheoretical stage extended from the time of the Greek philosophers until the early 1900s. It was during this stage that physiologists described temperament as either good or

❖ **Table 30-1**
Development of humor theory

| | |
|---|---|
| Pretheoretical phase | Originated with Greek philosophers |
| | Temperament described as good or bad humor |
| Psychoanalytical phase | Originated with Freud |
| | Humor arises from the unconscious |
| Cognitive phase | Reflects current emphasis on reasons for laughter |
| | Humor is an intellectual phenomenon with affective expression |

bad humor, depending on the balance of body fluids. Some beginning observational studies explored laughing and smiling behaviors.

The second phase of humor research primarily related to Freud's psychoanalytic theory. He believed that humor begins in childhood and arises from the unconscious. He also believed that humor has the potential to transform pain into pleasure. According to Freud's model, humor gives pleasure because it permits temporary gratification of hidden or forbidden wishes (Freud, 1903; Millar, 1986).

The most current phase of humor theory is the cognitive approach. Researchers now seek to understand why people laugh and to identify the effects of humor on attitudes and behavior (Goldstein, 1976; Porteous, 1988). The psychological and social mechanisms of humor and the physiological effects of laughter are being studied, and there is major attention to incongruity, absurdity, and timing (McGhee, 1971; Porteous, 1988; Apte, 1988; Berger, 1976; Kuhlman, 1984; Martin & Lefcourt, 1983). A prevailing theme is that humor is an intellectual phenomenon accompanied by an affective expression.

## ❖ THEORIES OF HUMOR

Throughout history, humor has had both positive and negative connotations. Early Greek philosophers were critical of laughter especially if used too often. Laughter was not seen as compatible with Christian values in the Middle Ages. The Pilgrims disapproved of laughter except when it taught a moral lesson. Some believed it represented a mental disorder. On a more positive note, beneficial aspects of humor, including physical benefits, have also been cited throughout history. These conflicting views of humor as evil versus beneficial were the forerunners of our current theories of humor, which help explain why people laugh (Ruxton, 1988). Superiority theory, incongruity theory, and relief theory provide some insight into the phenomena of humor (Table 30-2).

The *superiority theory* views humor as an

❖ **Table 30-2**
Theories of humor

| | |
|---|---|
| Superiority theory | Humor expresses superiority over others |
| Relief theory | Humor releases energy and acts as a catharsis |
| Incongruity theory | Humor results from juxtaposition of ideas in an unexpected manner |

expression of superiority over others. Often the expressed superiority is used to compensate for feelings of inferiority. Examples include "put down" humor, ethnic jokes, or laughing at oneself when in an embarrassing situation (Simon, 1988b; Ruxton, 1988).

*Relief theory* suggests that laughter results in a venting of nervous energy and acts as a catharsis. Freud theorized that joking brings out suppressed thoughts from the unconscious and that humor serves as a mediating force in expressing those emotions (Morreall, 1983). Psychic energy is required to control socially unacceptable thoughts and feelings, and energy is spared when inhibitions are released through telling a socially sanctioned joke.

*Incongruity theory* (Suls, 1983) emphasizes the cognitive aspects of humor. Incongruity occurs when ideas are juxtaposed or brought together in an unexpected manner. This theory suggests that we laugh when the order governing our lives is disrupted by events inconsistent with our expectations.

None of these three theories completely explain the origin of humor and laughter. However, they collectively add to an understanding of the concept.

## ❖ FUNCTIONS OF HUMOR

According to Robinson (1977), humor serves four functions in health and illness: communicative, social, psychological, and physiological.

## Communication Functions

Humor is a form of indirect communication. When used appropriately, it can assist in establishing a comfortable atmosphere and in neutralizing emotional events. The use of humor may allow clients to release pent-up emotions and express feelings that might be difficult to express more directly (Ruxton, 1988). Humor may also provide a means of moving out of situations or for moving into more serious discussions. There are reports in the literature of the judicious use of humor in psychotherapy as a means of creating an atmosphere of openness and equality (Rosenheim & Golan, 1986; Reynes & Allen, 1987).

## Social Functions

Humor also serves social functions and assists in coping with external pressure. Robinson (1977) describes the sociological uses of humor as establishing relationships, releasing tension from social conflicts, promoting solidarity, providing social control, and managing embarrassing situations. Hospitalized patients find themselves in a rigid structure where normal rules of behavior are altered, their privacy is invaded, and they are placed in a dependent role. Humor can provide a means for coping with embarrassing situations, help reduce tension, and reduce fear of unfamiliar settings. It is a familiar pattern of communication that can be shared in an unfamiliar situation.

Within a cultural group, humor is used to express the culture's concerns, conflicts, and aspirations (Robinson, 1977). Different cultures have developed various forms of institutionalized humor, which are used for social release and regulation. In minority cultures, humor is often used to ward off anticipated attacks (Ferguson & Campinha-Bacote, 1989). For example, Robinson (1977) points out that one way in which the Jewish culture survived years of persecution was to laugh and joke at tormentors. Studies of Native Americans note that humor in ritualistic ceremonies allows the acting out of otherwise prohibited regressive, sexual, and aggressive behaviors (Levine, 1969).

Sociologists report that laughing together forms cohesive bonds within groups and that it is socially contagious (Moody, 1978). Humor assists in establishing rapport and decreases social distance (McGhee, 1979; Moody, 1978; Ferguson & Campinha-Bacote, 1989).

## Psychological Functions

Psychological functions of humor relate to coping with stress through the release of tension and emotions such as anxiety, hostility, and anger (Robinson, 1977). Expressing these emotions can be a significant factor in promoting a feeling of relaxation and well-being. Freud (1903) described humor as an important adaptive, defensive mechanism that saves emotional energy. Stuart and Sundeen (1987) describe psychological functions of humor as promoting insight by bringing repressed material to awareness, resolving paradoxes and aggression, and providing a socially acceptable form of sublimation.

Coombs and Goldman (1973) studied the use of humor by staff in a hospital intensive care unit. They found that the staff commonly used humor to handle the emotional stress of caring for critically ill patients. The use of humor appeared to increase the quality of their performance by reducing the pressure and anxiety of constantly dealing with life-threatening situations.

Dixon (1980) describes the beneficial aspects of humor in dealing with stress. These benefits result from cognitive shifts and changes in affect that accompany those shifts. A shift in perspective allows a distancing from the immediate stress and viewing it from a different angle, thereby reducing it.

Fay (1983) explored the role of humor in stress management through measurements of stress, anxiety, coping, and humor appreciation. Subjects who had more effective coping mechanisms also had the greatest appreciation of humor, while those with the least effective coping strategies displayed a lesser ability to use humor.

Martin and Lefcourt (1983) measured stress, mood, and sense of humor in undergraduate students. They found that five of the six humor interventions used had a significant moderating effect on the relationship between stress and mood. They concluded that in order for humor to moderate the effects of stress, the individual must place a high value on it and must use it in daily stressful situations. This subjective quality helps explain why some clients respond to the use of humor while others do not.

## Physiological Functions

The body's physiological response to humor is a pattern of stimulation and relaxation similar to that produced by physical exercise (Fry & Rader, 1977; Svebak, 1977; Chapman, 1976). Fry (1977, 1979) studied the effects of laughter on heart rate, oxygen levels in peripheral blood, and respiration. He found that laughter increases respiratory activity, oxygen exchange, muscular activity, heart rate, activity of the sympathetic nervous system, and production of catecholamines, which stimulate the production of endorphins. The arousal state produced by laughter is followed by a relaxation state in which respiration, heart rate, and muscle tension return to below normal rates. Blood pressure is also reduced. Fry concluded that laughter produces valuable physiological effects important to physical health. Bellart (1989) describes the effects as "internal jogging." These conditions are thought to be especially beneficial in prevention of heart disease and other stress-related conditions.

One possible mechanism for the positive physiological effects of humor might be through enhancement of immune system functioning. Investigations have focused on secretory immunoglobulin A (S-IgA) as an indicator of immune functioning. S-IgA is the predominant antibody in saliva, tears, and intestinal secretions, and it serves as the primary defense against infections in the upper respiratory and gastrointestinal tracts. There is evidence that some aspects of immune functioning may be depressed after stressful experiences and during illness (McClelland, Alexander, & Marks, 1980; McClelland, Ross, & Patel, 1985; McClelland, Floor, Davidson, & Saron, 1980; Stone et al, 1987; Rogers, Dubey, & Reich, 1979). McClelland and his associates found a negative relationship between epinephrine and S-IgA suggesting that the immunosuppressive effects may be a result of action of adrenal hormones, which are elevated during stress. This reduced immune functioning may make individuals more susceptible to some infections.

Dillon and his associates (1985) studied the effects of humor on the immune system by measuring the concentration of salivary immunoglobulin A (IgA) in a small sample of subjects. They found that salivary IgA concentration increased after their subjects viewed a humorous videotape leading them to conclude that elevated IgA levels were associated with a positive emotional state.

Martin and Dobbin (1988) studied the moderating effect of humor on the relationship between stressors and S-IgA. They reported that college students with a strong sense of humor experienced less disturbance in mood and less impairment in immune functioning following stressful experiences than did their more serious counterparts. They hypothesize that this moderating effect might be exerted in two ways. First, individuals who perceive humor in a situation are less likely to see the situation as threatening and therefore do not respond with as great an increase in sympathetic-adrenal arousal. Second, if individuals are able to derive humor from some aspects of their lives, those pleasant emotions may counteract the unpleasant emotions associated with stress perceptions, thus minimizing sympathetic-adrenal stress arousal, which might result in less impairment of immune functioning.

The affective experience of humor is likely associated with activity of the limbic system and with adequate functioning of the left and right hemispheres of the brain (Goldstein, 1976). Therefore, drugs or disease-related changes affecting processing between the left and right hemispheres can alter humor perception and appreciation.

The previous studies indicate that humor can have positive physical effects. However, the studies are few in number, use small samples, and do not provide conclusive results. Additional studies must be done to definitively demonstrate the relationships among humor, psychophysiological mechanisms, and healing.

## ❖ USE IN PRACTICE

The appropriate use of humor in practice has been discussed by a number of authors (Fry & Salameh, 1987; Leiber, 1986; Nemeth, 1979). Leiber presents three criteria for determining the appropriate use of humor with clients: timing, receptiveness, and content. Situations in which the use of humor is likely to be inappropriate include times of crisis, when the caregiver and client are new to each other, and when humor is at the client's expense.

The effects of humor on healing have been presented in several reports. Norman Cousins (1979) describes the importance of humor in his recovery from both a collagen disease and a myocardial infarction. During his recovery, he routinely viewed "Candid Camera" reruns and Marx Brothers films and reported that laughter gave him periods of pain-free sleep. Tennant (1986) found a positive relationship between recovery rate and humor scores in elderly clients recovering from cataract surgery. Miller (1983) identified humor as one coping strategy in adults with chronic illness. In studying adaptation to physical disability, Lefcourt and Martin (1986) found that disabled people who laughed at disability-relevant cartoons demonstrated more vitality and higher self-concepts than their counterparts. These individuals also had the disability for a longer period of time indicating that a sense of humor might be developed over time and that using humor might not be appropriate in new disabilities. Simon (1988a) found a positive relationship between situational humor and perceived health and between situational humor and morale in noninstitutionalized older adults. Sumners (1988) describes the effective use of humor in the recovery process from addiction.

Some authors discuss setting as a consideration in the use of humor in patient care situations. Some point out that the intensive care unit may be a place in which humor is not appropriate or should be used very cautiously (Leiber, 1986). Others indicate that the use of humor is not necessarily setting-related (Ruxton, 1988). Robinson (1986) found a high incidence of humor interactions in high stress clinical areas. However, staff-client humor interactions did occur more frequently in low stress areas.

The effects of humor on anxiety have also been explored. Nemeth (1979) found that a group of hospitalized clients who were shown a humorous film displayed significantly lower levels of anxiety than groups that were shown a nonhumorous film as well as a control group with no intervention. He proposes that humor serves as a defense mechanism that allows individuals to cope with daily problems. Warner (1984) describes the use of humor in mental health and indicates that it facilitates self-disclosure.

Ruxton (1988) identifies humor intervention as useful in patient teaching as well as situations in which patients are facing life-threatening circumstances, experiencing anxiety over hospitalization, or are in isolation. She reports a project designed to promote the use of humor in patient treatment. The first part of the project included development of an instrument to assess the person's experience with humor. The second part of the project collected data from nurses about their current use of humor. The third part included workshops for nurses to explore experiences with humor and to develop interventions. The fourth part focused on the use of humor as an intervention. Ellis (1978) described humor as a powerful nursing intervention because of its ability to facilitate positive communication.

There are also reports in the literature of the use of humor to enhance the learning process. Leiber (1986) posits that humor can create an environment conducive to the retention of knowledge. She also suggests that laughter serves as an "incentive spirometry" and is an effective tool to assist patients after surgery with coughing and deep breathing exercises.

Robinson (1978) states that when nurses relate appropriate humorous stories while teaching patients, the exchange helps them laugh at their uncertainties and reduces stress, which leads to more effective learning. Moses and Friedman (1986) report positive effects from the deliberative use of humor as a strategy in evaluating nursing students; their results may have implications for patient teaching situations as well.

Although there are a number of indications that humor may be an effective part of a treatment program, there are also a number of cautions that indicate we should not jump to hasty conclusions about its usefulness. Most authors caution that the use of humor is not appropriate in all situations and that it should be used judiciously. Humor can be interpreted by patients as showing a lack of concern or not taking situations seriously, thereby weakening the caregiver-patient relationship. Other concerns relate to the fact that humor is highly subjective and might be misinterpreted, thereby increasing the patient's distress rather than alleviating it. Caution must be taken to avoid "laughing at" the patient. While humor might decrease emotional stress, it might also prevent realistically dealing with problems (Robinson, 1978; Haig, 1986). Humor has also been generally seen as potentially destructive with only very limited usefulness in psychotherapy (Kubie, 1977). Freud (1903) also discussed potentially destructive uses of hostile and obscene humor.

Ruxton (1988) points out that humor cannot cure all ills. But neither does penicillin. She suggests that increasing our understanding of humor as an intervention might provide increased knowledge of the body's response to illness and to life around us. She quotes the response of a patient with cancer to the question, "What has humor done for you?" as:

"It probably has done nothing to appreciably alter the course of my disease, yet through humor I have found freedom. Freedom to be honest, to take risks, to live one day at a time. I've found it's okay to be scared to death every time I have another ache or pain. It has given me a kind of energy to look longer and harder at things and become more creative in my approach to life and living as well as death and dying" (p. 60).

Using humor might not fix all ills, but it is a creative strategy that is worth a try. As Dolan (1985) indicates, it may be that "A good dose of laughter can ease a multitude of ills while causing the most pleasant side effects."

## ❖ USE OF THE NURSING PROCESS
### Assessment

As part of the total assessment of the client, the nurse should assess previous use and current appreciation of humor. A good way to understand clients and their families is knowing what makes them laugh. If the client has used humor in the past, it is more likely to be used as a coping strategy in the current situation. If the client seems to value humor, the nurse may decide to use it as a strategy to help relieve stress and help the client gain another perspective on the problems at hand.

Sample questions that may be included in an assessment related to humor use and appreciation include:

1. How often do you find yourself looking at the humorous side of a situation when dealing with everyday problems?

2. Since you have been ill, do you find yourself using humor more, less, or about the same?
3. Which of the following activities do you find amusing or enjoyable?
   a. watching comedy movies
   b. watching cartoons
   c. watching comedies on television
   d. hearing jokes
   e. telling jokes
   f. reading joke books
   g. being around funny people
4. Does it make you feel better or worse if the people around you have a sense of humor?
5. Can you think of a time when humor has made you feel better?
6. Do you like telling jokes or funny stories?
7. Can you think of a time when humor had made you feel worse?

The nurse needs to be attuned to the situations in which the client uses humor in order to determine if indirect messages are being sent. If the focus is on unpleasant hospital routines or embarrassing situations, it may be an indication that the client is attempting to find out if these are acceptable topics for discussion (Simon, 1988b). Sarcastic or biting humor may indicate a great deal of anger that needs an outlet and may indicate topics that the nurse should explore. Reports of inability to perceive humor in situations that would normally be funny may be an indication of stress or depression.

In addition to direct questions to the client, the nurse can use those answers and personal observations for a complete assessment before using humor as an intervention. Answers are needed to the following questions:

1. What cues have been given that the client would be receptive to humor?
2. What cues have been given that the client would not be receptive to certain kinds of humor or are there are certain areas about which the client is sensitive?
3. Is the client's physical or emotional state

such that humor might be annoying or indicate a lack of caring?

4. What are the specific problems for which a humorous approach could be used?
5. Are there cultural aspects to consider in using humor? Robinson (1977) found that there are differences among Black Americans, Spanish Americans, and Southwest Indian cultures in the use and appreciation of humor. These differences are related to cultural beliefs, beliefs about health, minority group status, degree of acculturation, and socioeconomic status. There are not definite answers to the questions of culture and humor, but it is a factor to consider, especially when the caregiver is from a different group than the client.

## Planning

Planning the use of humor should be based on assessment data. Nursing diagnoses related to anxiety and stress may be especially amenable to humor as an intervention. If the client has used humor in the past to deal with difficult situations, it may be appropriate to use humor in nurse-client interactions. If the nurse cannot provide direct humor intervention because he or she is not a funny person, another strategy can be identified such as pointing out the client's sense of humor to other staff members, providing joke books, or suggesting a funny program that will be on television. The nurse can also allow the client to talk about the things that are personally funny.

Saper (1988) cautions that planning for the use of humor in treatment should be carefully considered before initiation. Physical condition, severity of illness, and the sociocultural status of the clients can easily alter the effectiveness of humorous intervention. Certain situations such as those in which there is a need for decreased sensory stimulation or when laughter might cause physical discomfort are contraindications for humor as an intervention.

## Intervention

The use of humor should be unique to each individual and each situation. It should be used after careful assessment with special consideration given to the client's developmental level, physical condition, and psychological status. Timing is important. If humor is interjected too soon, it may serve as a distancing maneuver. When used as the primary method of interacting with others, humor can also become a distancing maneuver, keeping relationships at a superficial level. Therefore, care should be taken not to overuse it. Only strategies that are appropriate to the setting and the client should be used. A significant factor to consider is the appropriateness of using humor in relation to the client's own condition such as jokes about similar situations as compared to using less personalized humor as a stress reduction strategy. Clients who are particularly sensitive to or embarrassed about their condition are likely to respond better to general rather than more personalized humor.

A suggested menu of strategies for intervention include:

1. Keeping a library of humorous comedy films on the unit if VCRs are available.
2. Telling jokes.
3. Posting cartoons, funny captions, and pictures in places where clients and their families can see them.
4. Providing joke books and humorous story books to clients and families.
5. Wearing costumes for holidays or special occasions.
6. Telling anecdotes about what has happened to others in similar circumstances.
7. Arranging for a clown or storyteller to visit the unit. Children are especially receptive to these situations.
8. Encouraging clients to decorate or name IV poles or other equipment.
9. Inviting comedians and clowns from local high school and college music and theater groups to perform humorous skits.

**NURSING CARE PLAN**

**CLIENT:**  Thomas M.

**MEDICAL DIAGNOSIS:**  Open reduction of patella fracture

**NURSING DIAGNOSIS:**  Moderate anxiety related to change in role function

| GOALS | INTERVENTIONS |
|---|---|
| Mr. M. will experience decreasing levels of anxiety. | ◆ Explore techniques that have reduced anxiety in past. |
| | ◆ Encourage Mr. M. to verbalize his feelings of anxiety, especially related to loss of role function. |
| | ◆ Suggest humorous anxiety reduction techniques that have been effective in the past. |
| Mr. M. will engage in satisfying and amusing activities and behaviors. | ◆ Provide resources that are acceptable to Mr. M. such as comedy shows on television and taped radio shows. |
| | ◆ Move Mr. M. to the dayroom where other clients are located so humorous situations can be shared. |

**EVALUATION**

Mr. M. is able to verbalize anxious feelings regarding loss of role function and reports a decreased anxiety level over time as satisfying humorous activities are identified and used. When Mr. M. is in the dayroom he uses humor with other clients and seems receptive to humor anxiety reduction techniques; the length of time spent in the dayroom indicates that he finds these activities pleasurable.

10. Obtaining audio cassettes of old radio programs such as George Burns and Gracie Allen and Fibber McGee and Molly. These may be played in groups for older clients to provide enjoyment, enhance group interaction, and encourage reminiscence. This strategy also includes individuals who are visually impaired (Simon, 1987).

11. Planning parties for special events such as birthdays. Birthday games are a way of enhancing humor and giving permission for adults to have fun. These types of events can be especially effective in long term care settings where clients know each other.

12. Including humorous stories in stress management classes to encourage anxiety reduction.

### Evaluation

It is important to evaluate the timing, content, and receptivity to humor. Questions to be asked in evaluation include:

1. Does the client appear to be comfortable with the type of humor being used?
2. Does the client appear to be less distressed (physically and/or emotionally)?
3. Has the use of humor resulted in improved communication?

If the intervention was not effective, it is essential to examine why. It may be that the technique was not the correct one for the situation, the content was inappropriate, or the client may not have been ready.

The nursing care plan on p. 550 provides an example of a care plan for a client for whom humorous intervention may be especially effective. Thomas M. is a 55-year-old male who is hospitalized for surgery after sustaining a fracture of the patella while playing tennis. He is healthy otherwise. The nurse completes an assessment of Mr. M. and establishes several nursing diagnoses. Based on the assessment data that indicated that Mr. M. has a good sense of humor, which he often uses in stressful situations, she determines that there is one nursing diagnosis that is especially suited to humor in-

terventions as outlined in the care plan. The selected interventions assist Mr. M. in using a coping strategy that has been effective in the past.

### ❖ NEED FOR ADDITIONAL RESEARCH

Much work remains to be done in order to determine the significance of humor as a client strength and as a treatment method. Questions needing exploration include:

1. What is the impact of humor on the quality of life and recovery from disease?
2. What are the physiological and psychological effects of laughter?
3. What are the indicators of successful humor intervention?
4. What factors contribute to the success of humor intervention?
5. What factors contribute to the failure of humor interventions?
6. Does the use of humor help improve staff morale?
7. What types of humor are the most effective with particular client situations?
8. What are the best measures for determining the effectiveness of humor as an intervention?

### ❖ SUMMARY

The value of humor as a client strength and its use in treatment requires much additional work before definitive answers can be provided. However, there is evidence that when used appropriately humor can be a significant component of care. It is one communication tool that can be useful in the right situation at the right time. It can, however, be overdone as can many other methods of treatment. What is important is that we understand humor, develop skill in recognizing when it is appropriate, and use and encourage it in those situations. It can serve as a means of sharing our humanity in a time of increased technology in health care.

## ❖ APPLYING KNOWLEDGE TO PRACTICE

1. What types of humor intervention would be most appropriate for various age groups?
2. Discuss specific physical conditions in which humor might be contraindicated as an intervention. Identify alternative appropriate interventions.
3. Develop an inventory of specific humor interventions that would be especially appropriate for hospitalized adolescents.
4. Of the three humor theories, which one most closely describes your "sense of humor?" What specific situations, conditions, or circumstances do you find most amusing?

## REFERENCES

Apte, M. L. (1988). Disciplinary boundaries in humorology: an anthropologist's ruminations. *Humor: International Journal of Humor Research, 1,* 5-25.

Bellart, J. L. (1989). Humor: A therapeutic approach in oncology nursing. *Cancer Nursing, 12*(2), 65-70.

Berger, A. A. (1976). Anatomy of the joke. *Journal of Communication, 26,* 113-115.

Chapman, A. J. (1976). Social aspects of humorous laughter. In *Humor and Laughter: Theory, Research, and Implications.* London: Wiley Press.

Coombs, R. & Goldman, L. (1973). Maintenance and discontinuity of coping mechanisms in an intensive care unit. *Social Problems, 20,* 342-355.

Cousins, N. (1979). *Anatomy of an Illness.* New York: Norton Press.

Dillon, K. M., Minchoff, B., & Baker, K. H. (1985). Positive emotional states and the enhancement of the immune system. *International Journal of Psychiatry in Medicine, 15,* 13-18.

Dixon, N. F. (1980). Humor: A cognitive alternative to stress? In I. G. Sarason and C. D. Spielberger (Eds.). *Stress and Anxiety.* (Vol. 7). Washington, D.C.: Hemisphere Publishing.

Dolan, M. B. (1985). A drug you can't overuse. *RN, 11,* 47-48.

Ellis, S. (1978). Humor: The wonder drug. *Nursing Times,* 1792-1793.

Eysenck, H. (1972). Foreword. In J. H. Goldstein and P. E. McGhee (Eds.), *The Psychology of Humor.* New York: Academic Press.

Fay, R. (1983). The defensive role of humor in the management of stress (Doctoral dissertation, United States International University). *Dissertation Abstracts International, 44,* 1219B.

Ferguson, S. & Campinha-Bacote, J. (1989). Humor in nursing. *Journal of Psychosocial Nursing, 27*(4), 29-34.

Flugel, J. (1954). Humor and laughter. In G. Lindzey and E. Aronson (Eds.). *Handbook of Social Psychology,* Reading, MA: Addison Wesley Co.

Freud, S. (1903). *Jokes and the Unconscious.* Translated by J. Strachney, 1961. New York: W. W. Norton and Company.

Fry, W. F. (1977). The respiratory components of mirthful laughter. *Journal of Biological Psychology, 19*(2), 39-50.

Fry, W. F. (1979). Humor and the human cardiovascular system. In H. Mindess and J. Turek (Eds.), *The Study of Humor.* Los Angeles: Antioch University.

Fry, W. F. (1987). Introduction to *Handbook of Humor and Psychotherapy,* W. Fry and W. Salameh (Eds.). Sarasota, Fla.: Professional Resources Exchange.

Fry, W. F. & Rader, C. (1977). The respiratory components of humor and laughter. *Journal of Biological Psychology. 19,* 39-50.

Fry, W. F. & Salameh, W. (Eds.). (1987). *Handbook of Humor and Psychotherapy.* Sarasota, Fla.: Professional Resources Exchange.

Goldstein, J. H. (1976). Theoretical notes on humor. *Journal of Communication, 26,* 104-112.

Haig, R. (1986). Therapeutic uses of humor. *Journal of Psychotherapy, 40*(4), 543-553.

Kubie, L. S. (1977). The destructive potential of humor in psychotherapy. *American Journal of Psychiatry, 127*(7), 861-866.

Kuhlman, T. L. (1984). *Humor and Psychotherapy.* Homewood, Illinois: Dow-Jones-Irwin.

Lefcourt, H. M. & Martin, R. A. (1986). Sense of humor and coping with physical disability. In *Humor and Life Stress: Antidote to Adversity.* New York: Springer-Verlag.

Leiber, D. (1986). Laughter and humor in critical care. *Di-*

*mensions of Critical Care Nursing, 5*(3), 162-170.

Levine, J. (1969). *Motivation in Humor.* New York: Atherton Press.

Martin, R. A. & Dobbin, J. P. (1988). Sense of humor, hassles, and immunoglobulin A: Evidence for a stress-moderating effect of humor. *International Journal of Psychiatry in Medicine, 18*(2), 93-105.

Martin, R. A. & Lefcourt, H. M. (1983). Sense of humor as a moderator of the relation between stressors and moods. *Journal of Personality and Social Psychology, 45,* 1313-1324.

McClelland, D. C., Alexander, C., & Marks, E. (1980). The need for power, stress, immune function, and illness among male prisoners. *Journal of Abnormal Psychology, 10,* 93-102.

McClelland, D. C., Floor, E., Davidson, R. J., & Saron, C. (1980). Stressed power motivation, sympathetic activation, immune function, and illness. *Journal of Human Stress, 6,* 11-19.

McClelland, D. C. Ross, G., & Patel, V. (1985). The effect of an academic examination on salivary norepinephrine and immunoglobulin levels. *Journal of Human Stress, 6,* 52-59.

McGhee, P. E. (1971). Development of the humor response: A review of the literature. *Psychological Bulletin, 76,* 328-348.

McGhee, E.. (1979). *Humor: Its Origin and Development.* San Francisco, W. H. Freeman and Company.

Millar, T. P. (1986). The triumph of reason. *Perspectives in Biological Medicine, 29,* 545-559.

Miller, F. (1983). *Coping with Chronic Illness.* Philadelphia: F. A. Davis.

Moody, R. (1978). *Laugh After Laugh: The Healing Power of Humor.* Jacksonville, Fla.: Headwaters Press.

Morreall, J. (1983). *Taking Laughter Seriously.* Albany, N.Y.: State University of New York Press.

Moses, N. & Friedman, M. (1986). Using humor in evaluating student performance. *Journal of Nursing Education, 25*(8), 328-333.

Nemeth, P. (1979). An investigation into the relationship between humor and anxiety (Doctoral dissertation, United States International University). *Dissertation Abstracts International, 40,* 1378B.

Porteous, J. (1988). Humor as a process of defense: the evolution of laughing. *International Journal of Humor Research, 1,* 63-80.

Reynes, R. & Allen, A. (1987). Humor in psychotherapy: A view. *American Journal of Psychotherapy, 41*(2), 260-270.

Robinson, V. M. (1977). *Humor and the Health Professions.* Thorofare, N.J.: C. B. Slack.

Robinson, V. M. (1978). Humor in Nursing. In C. Carlson and B. Blackwell (Eds.) *Behavioral Concepts and Nursing Interventions.* (pp. 191–210). Philadelphia: J. B. Lippincott Company.

Robinson, V. M. (1986). Humor is a serious business. *Dimensions in Critical Care Nursing, 5,* 132-133.

Rogers, M. P., Dubey, D., & Reich, P. (1979). The influence of the psyche and the brain on immunity and disease susceptibility: A critical review. *Psychosomatic Medicine, 41,* 147-164.

Rosenheim, E. & Golan, G. (1986). Patients' reaction to humorous interventions in psychotherapy. *American Journal of Psychotherapy, 40,* 110-124.

Ruxton, J. P. (1988). Humor intervention deserves our attention. *Holistic Nursing Practice, 2*(3), 54-62.

Saper, B. (1988). Humor in psychiatric healing. *Psychiatric Quarterly, 59*(4), 306-319.

Simon, J. M. (1987). The therapeutic value of humor in aging adults. *Journal of Gerontological Nursing, 14*(8), 9-13.

Simon, J. M. (1988a). Humor and the older adult: Implications for nursing. *Journal of Advanced Nursing, 13,* 441-446.

Simon, J. M. (1988b). Therapeutic humor: Who's fooling who? *Journal of Psychosocial Nursing and Mental Health Services, 26*(4), 9-12.

Stone, A. A., Cox, D. S., Valdimarsdottir, H., Jandorf, L, & Neale, J. M. (1987). Evidence that secretory IgA antibody is associated with daily mood. *Journal of Personality and Social Psychology, 52,* 988-993.

Stuart, G. & Sundeen, S. (1987). *Principles and Practice of Psychiatric Nursing.* St. Louis: C. V. Mosby Co.

Suls, J. (1983). Cognitive processes in humor appreciation. In P. E. McGee and H. H. Goldstein (Eds.). *Handbook of Humor Research.* New York: Academic Press.

Sumners, A. D. (1988). Humor: Coping in recovery from addiction. *Issues in Mental Health Nursing, 9,* 169-179.

Svebak, S. (1977). Some characteristics of resting respiration as predictors of laughter. In A. J. Chapman and H. C. Foot (Eds.). *It's a Funny Thing, Humor.* Oxford: Pergamon Press.

Tennant, K. F. (1986). The effect of humor on the recovery rate of cataract patients. In L. Nahemow, K McCluskey-Fawcett, and P. McGhee (Eds.), *Humor and Aging.* New York: Academic Press.

Warner, S. (1984). Humor and self-disclosure within the milieu. *Journal of Psychosocial Nursing, 22*(4), 17-21.

Webster's *New Collegiate Dictionary* (Ed. 8). (1980). Chicago: Merriam.

# UNIT VI

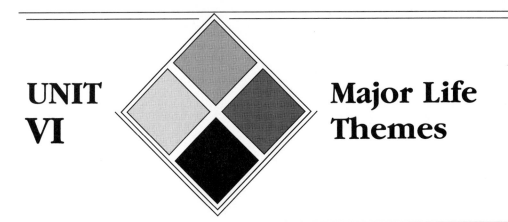

# Major Life Themes

**M**AJOR life themes are issues faced by most individuals and families throughout the life span. These themes are generally universal attributes that are relevant in most client care situations. All individuals and families encounter losses, deal with issues related to their own or their family members' sexuality and aging, and are influenced by parenting as they become parents or relate to their family of origin. Nurses play an integral role in addressing these issues as they work with individuals and families who experience them.

The chapters in this unit describe the concept and incorporate relevant nursing research. Application to nursing practice is facilitated by discussions of normal expectations regarding the concept and potential problems such as sexual dysfunction or parenting problems with a premature or chronically ill child. Discussion questions further illustrate the application of the concept to clinical practice.

# 31 Sexuality

Anna C. Alt-White

## OBJECTIVES

*At the completion of this chapter, the reader will be able to:*

◆ **Differentiate psychosexual development over the life cycle.**

◆ **Describe the Mims-Swenson Sexual Health Model.**

◆ **Apply the Model to client situations.**

Sexuality pervades our very existence. Starting at conception, genetic material determines the sex of an individual. At birth, the first statement or question raised by those in attendance addresses the sexual identity of the infant. These biological and social beginnings are the foundation for the development of an individual's sexuality or the "complex phenomenon that pervades the biological being, sense of self, and relationships with others" (Woods, 1987a, p. 1).

Sexuality, then, should be approached holistically. Yet within the professional literature and the popular press, the focus is primarily on physiological functioning and physical satisfaction (McFarlane & Rubenfeld, 1983). Woods (1987a) further notes that most clinical literature has a narrow focus on sexual dysfunction. Since nurses espouse a holistic approach, they are in a position to address sexual health, or the "positive integration of the somatic, emotional, intellectual, and social aspects

of social beings in ways that are positively enriching and that enhance personality, communication and love" (World Health Organization, 1975, p. 6).

In order to practice holistically, nurses need in-depth knowledge and understanding of human sexuality. Yet the results from a national study of nursing research in sexuality suggest that nurses do not have the requisite education on sexuality (Hott & Ryan-Merritt, 1982). This chapter presents an overview of human sexuality. Initially, psychosexual development is discussed followed by implications for sexuality and nursing practice.

### ❖ PSYCHOSEXUAL DEVELOPMENT

Biological, sociological, psychological, and cultural factors have a role in the development of one's sexuality. The discussion that follows primarily focuses on the influence of biological factors.

## Prenatal Development

Sexual differentiation includes a number of processes. Initially, the first step is fertilization, or the uniting of the ovum and sperm, with the female contributing an X chromosome and the male contributing an X or Y chromosome. Until the fifth or sixth week of prenatal development, the gonad remains undifferentiated, whether genetically male or female. The H-Y antigen, a male specific protein, is most likely responsible for testicular differentiation and hence the development of a male embryo (Pritchard, MacDonald, & Gant, 1985). Further differentiation then occurs through hormonal stimulation from fetal androgens. The female embryo, on the other hand, is not dependent on hormonal stimulation for sexual differentiation (Masters Johnson, & Kolodny, 1985). During the next phase of differentiation, the internal sex structures begin to form. In the male, the Wolffian duct system will develop into the epididymis, vas deferens, seminal vesicles, prostate gland, and ejaculatory ducts. For the female the Müllerian duct system develops into the fallopian tubes, uterus, and upper part of the vagina. Then the external genitalia develop: the penis and scrotum in the male and the clitoris, labias minora and majora, and lower vaginal vault in the female.

The hormones that originate in the gonads also have an effect on the development of the pituitary gland that, in turn, will determine either cyclical hormonal production in women or relatively constant levels of hormonal production in men. Rubin, Reinsch, and Haskett (1981) suggest that these hormonal influences also have an effect on later behavior.

## Infancy and Early Childhood

During the initial years of life, numerous sexual responses and behaviors occur. Infant boys have erections, and vaginal lubrication occurs in girls. Gender identity, the sense that one has of being a male or a female, is established firmly by age 3. Complex influences of biological factors, such as genetics and genital anatomy, verifies the sex of the child for the parents and the way in which they and the rest of society will relate to and socialize the infant. One behavior, parent-infant bonding, arises from the mother's pregnancy and the total dependency of the newborn. This bonding "is the major source for all the infant's subsequent attachments" through which the child develops a sense of self (Klaus & Kennell, 1982, p. 3).

During infancy and early childhood, exploration of the body and self-pleasuring or masturbation is common. As with this behavior, or any other for that matter, parents have the responsibility to teach their children what behavior is appropriate and when and where that behavior is socially acceptable (Masters, Johnson, & Kolodny, 1985). Also, during the preschool years, children learn sex roles and sex role differences through play and observation.

Once a child starts school there is increased modesty and, therefore, less sex play. Friends are primarily of the same sex. The child remains curious about sex and learns vocabulary about sexual body parts and activities. This language may be used for the reaction it elicits from adults.

## Adolescence

The forces that aid in the transition from childhood to adulthood, from approximately ages 12 to 20, require radical adaptation of identity and behavior for the adolescent. The physiological changes are from hormonal stimulation to the pituitary gland that results in the ovaries releasing estrogen and the testes releasing testosterone. As a result, the primary and secondary sexual characteristics develop. Primary sexual characteristics include enlargement and physiological maturity of the internal and external genitalia of both sexes. In the female, secondary sexual characteristics include breast development, growth of pubic and axillary hair, fat deposition in the buttocks and thighs, and broadening of the pelvis. In the male, secondary sexual characteristics include a deepening voice, larger muscle mass, and developing pubic, facial, and body hair.

Along with these changes, important events occur during adolescence. For the female it is menarche, or the first menses, which has an estimated mean age of 12.3 years in the United States (Pritchard, MacDonald, & Gant, 1985). This event may have different meanings to the adolescent ranging from the menses being natural and expected to a traumatic experience (Morrison, Starks, Hyndman, & Ronzio, 1980). For the adolescent male, spontaneous erections occur, often unpredictably, causing concern and embarrassment. The first ejaculation may occur as a nocturnal emission or during masturbation. This experience may elicit a variety of emotions ranging from fear and guilt to pleasure and wonderment (Morrison et al, 1980). For both sexes there is preoccupation with the size of their sexual organs. The female is concerned about the size of her breasts and the male is concerned with the size of his penis. In addition, the adolescent usually has to deal with acne, sweating, and changes in height and weight. All of these experiences produce concerns about body image. Furthermore, adolescents must confront sexual fantasies and thoughts, begin dating and develop intimate relationships, explore lifestyles and sex role behaviors, and decide the extent of sexual activities and relationships (Woods, 1987a).

## Adult Sexuality

Early adulthood lasts from approximately ages 20 to 40. During these years many important life decisions are made. A major decision having an impact on sexuality is developing a value system that predicates the type of and conditions for sexual expression. For example, casual sexual relationships may not occur be-

cause of fear of AIDS, religious values, or lack of satisfaction from such relationships. Another decision is whether or not to make a long-term commitment to another person, which may include marriage and parenting. These decisions also involve acknowledging one's sexual orientation, or the preference for sexual partners of the same sex (homosexuality), opposite sex (heterosexuality), or of both sexes (bisexuality). Other factors include the amount and type of sexual expression and techniques, contraceptive options, and measures to prevent contracting sexually transmitted diseases. Inherent in each of these factors is decision making and learning to give and receive love (Woods, 1984).

Middle adulthood occurs between ages 40 and 60. In some instances, the marital relationship is readjusted if, for example, the couple is without children at home for the first time in years. Other adjustments are necessary because of physiological aspects of aging. For both sexes weight gain and loss of height may occur, as well as changes in skin and hair. Once again, the individuals must adjust to a changing body image.

Traditionally, menopause signifies the end of a woman's fertility. This change is gradual, starting in her thirties with declining fertility, higher rate of miscarriages, decrease in ovulation, and changes in the menstrual cycle before the actual cessation of menses. The amount and frequency of symptoms reported during menopause vary. The 78 menopausal women in Frey's (1981) study reported tiredness, depression, forgetfulness, headaches, irritability, and nervousness as the most frequently occurring symptoms. Yet these women did not view menopause as an illness. Culture influences the perception of menopause. Women from societies that reward them at the end of fertility, or who work outside the home have few or no symptoms. Women from societies that value youth and fecundity or define women's roles as being mother and homemaker have more severe physical and psychological symptomatology (Weg, 1983).

The male climacteric includes a gradual decline in testosterone that accounts for the longer time required to attain an erection. Masters, Johnson, and Kolodny (1985) suggest that males are more susceptible to a midlife crisis because they tend to focus more on sexual performance and capabilities. Once concern is introduced into sexual performance, there is a greater chance for loss of erections or transient impotence. As with menopause in women, "the male climacteric is not uniform or subjectively experienced by all men" (Weg, p. 54).

In late adulthood numerous physiological changes occur that have an impact on sexuality. Changes in estrogen create decreased lubrication and thinning of the vaginal walls, which can make penetration difficult and painful during sexual intercourse and cause bleeding for the female. In the male, the rate of attaining an erection and force of the ejaculate is diminished. The time that an erection can be maintained, however, is lengthened. While the intensity of sensation is diminished for both the male and female, neither enjoyment of the relationship need change nor does sexual activity need to end. When problems do occur, they are often the result of disability, disease, drug side effects, or psychological problems (National Institute on Aging, 1985).

Throughout adulthood, divorce or death of a partner may occur and can have a profound effect on one's sexuality. Ultimately, the individual must decide whether or not to seek and develop new relationships.

Throughout the life cycle numerous biopsychosocial and cultural factors influence an individual's sexuality. The next section discusses implications for nursing practice related to sexuality.

## ❖ SEXUALITY AND NURSING PRACTICE

Two age-old adages apply to sexuality and nursing practice: Socrates' "Know yourself" and Hippocrates' "Above all do no harm." Before assessing client problems relating to sexuality, it is best for the nurse to identify and evaluate her or his own knowledge, feelings, and values about sexuality (see discussion question no. 1). Once a nurse is comfortable with his or her sexuality, the next step is to evaluate knowledge and clinical expertise in order to provide safe and holistic nursing care relating to sexual health. Because sexuality is such a personal and private topic, nurses must know how to approach sexuality issues with clients. One way for nurses to assess their sexual knowledge, attitudes, values, and clinical expertise is to use a model to guide their practice.

In the 1970s Annon (1976a, 1976b) developed the **P-LI-SS-IT** Model for practitioners to use in treating clients with sexual concerns. Each letter or set of letters indicates a level of behavioral treatment: the first three levels encompass brief therapy, and the fourth encompasses intensive therapy. The first level, *permission,* allows a clinician to reassure a client that a behavior is normal and to give permission to continue it. *Limited information* gives clients factual information specific to a particular situation. The next level, *specific suggestions,* is more complex and requires the practitioner to first obtain a sexual problem history to decide on a brief therapeutic approach (1976a). *Intensive therapy* is best left to the clinician specifically prepared to treat sexual problems (1976). With each level, the clinician must have increasing degrees of knowledge, training, and skill. While this model has been used by numerous sexual health practitioners, most nurses do not have the expertise to use it (Mims & Swenson, 1980).

### Sexual Health Model

The Sexual Health Model (Fig. 31-1), based on Annon's work, was specifically developed for nurses to use for self-assessment and for interacting with clients (Mims & Swenson, 1980). Similar to the **P-LI-SS-IT** Model, there are four

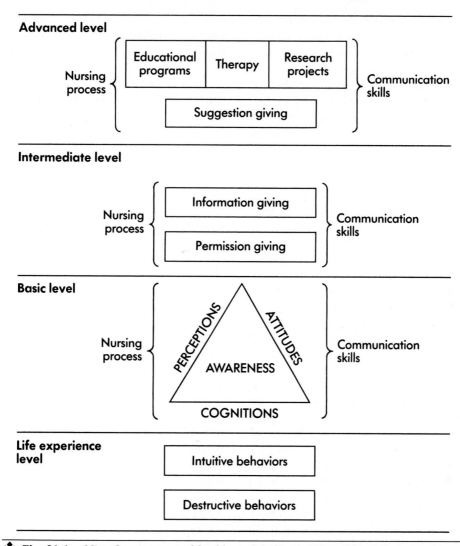

Advanced level

Educational programs | Therapy | Research projects

Nursing process

Suggestion giving

Communication skills

Intermediate level

Information giving

Nursing process

Permission giving

Communication skills

Basic level

Nursing process

PERCEPTIONS    ATTITUDES

AWARENESS

COGNITIONS

Communication skills

Life experience level

Intuitive behaviors

Destructive behaviors

❖ **Fig. 31-1**   Mims-Swenson sexual health model. *(From Mims, F. H., & Swenson, M. (1980). Sexuality: A nursing perspective. New York: McGraw-Hill. Reprinted with permission.)*

ascending levels that build on the previous level and assume greater expertise on the practitioner's part (Mims, 1980). The levels are: life experience, basic, intermediate, and advanced levels. Each level beyond life experiences incorporates the nursing process and communications skills. Each level will be described in detail.

**Life experiences level.** The first level, life experiences, is composed of *intuitively helpful* or *destructive behaviors* that arise from living in a society that constantly provides mixed messages about sexuality (Mims & Swenson, 1980). Individual nurses may instinctively possess accurate and effective behaviors that would enhance client interactions. Destructive behaviors that arise from the fears, myths, stereotypes, and taboos for a given culture can, however, counteract the helpful behaviors. In a survey conducted by Mims and Swenson (1978) with over 100 nursing students, some of the sexual myths that were taken as truth included that most men over 70 are impotent, transvestism is usually part of homosexual behavior, exhibitionists are latent homosexuals, and that after orgasm, women cannot respond to further stimulation. In general, results from numerous studies indicate that nurses need more education about their own or their clients' sexuality, or both (Hott & Ryan-Merritt, 1982).

**Basic level.** Before nurses provide sexual health care, they need to be aware of their own destructive behaviors and obtain the *requisite knowledge* and *clinical expertise.* This occurs at the basic level of the model that uses the nursing process, communication skills, and awareness. *Awareness* is considered to be a necessary component in creating change and is considered requisite to the nurse acknowledging, identifying, and promoting sexual health (Mims & Swenson, 1978). The three elements comprising sexual awareness are cognitions, attitudes, and perceptions. *Cognitions* include knowledge of reproductive anatomy and physiology, sexual development, and psychosocial and cultural influences on behavior (Mims & Swenson, 1978). *Attitudes* are an individual's feelings, values, and beliefs about sexuality. Finally, *perceptions* "are dependent on seeing, hearing, listening and touching skills" (Mims & Swenson, 1978, p. 122). For example, reading the professional literature and enrolling in workshops and classes can increase knowledge and comfort in dealing with sexuality. This is especially true with interactive learning, which includes open discussions, course organization that begins with less sensitive and progresses to more sensitive topics, and practice in dealing with simulated clinical situations (see discussion question no. 2). These activities assist in-

dividuals to be more aware of their own and others' sexuality and how to better use the nursing process and communication skills.

**Intermediate level.** At the intermediate level, the foci are *permission* and *information giving.* This level is similar to Annon's first two levels, permission and limited information, with the addition of the nursing process, communication, teaching, and counseling skills. As previously mentioned, permission giving allows the clinician to reassure a client that thoughts, fantasies, and behaviors that may be a concern are normal. This may include permitting a woman posthysterectomy to express her concern about whether she is still a complete woman now that her uterus has been removed or reassuring a pubescent male that it is normal to have spontaneous erections. As Mims and Swenson (1980) indicated, this process usually begins and is facilitated when a sexual history is included as part of the regular nursing assessment. Through this process, clients can view sexuality as a normal component of their health and learn that sexual concerns can be discussed with the nurse.

The depth of the sexual history will depend on the nurses theoretical and clinical expertise and the individual client situation. No matter what the situation, however, there are a number of basic components to include in the sexual history. In many clinical situations a sexual history is part of the initial assessment, whether it occurs during the first visit in an outpatient setting or during the process of being admitted to the hospital. The logical place to begin a sexual history is after the family and medical history have been completed. Most sexual histories will be brief with a detailed history required only if a problem such as sexual dysfunction exists. Because most nurses do not have extensive preparation in sexuality, the client with problems should be referred to a sexual therapist.

Other considerations are that the same

nonverbal and verbal techniques used for getting a nursing history should be employed with the sexual history. The setting is also critical. Privacy and a quiet place, along with assurance that confidentiality will be maintained assist the client in feeling more at ease and facilitates discussion (Andrews, 1988; Andrist, 1988). After assessing basic demographic characteristics, the nurse will know whether cultural aspects need to be taken into account. Spanish speaking clients and Arabic women, for example, are less likely to discuss sexual concerns than most American women (Andrist, 1988; Krozy, 1978). Other sociocultural aspects to consider are age and gender differences between nurse and client (Krozy, 1978). Some techniques to maximize client comfort are conducting the interview, if possible, when the client is dressed in his or her own clothes. It also helps to use a general, matter of fact approach, use terms familiar to the client, and to structure the interview to first cover less sensitive questions before the more difficult areas. The nurse may find using ubiquitous statements and open-ended questions encourages both discussion and gives the client control over the amount of information that is to be shared (Andrews, 1988; Andrist, 1988; Chapman & Sughrue, 1987; Krozy, 1978). For example, the nurse might begin with a statement like "Many people have concerns about having sexual intercourse following a heart attack," and follow it with something like "What concerns do you have?"

There are other techniques that can be used. The client needs to be informed about the purpose of the sexual history, that some questions will be personal, and that the client does not have to answer all questions. Value-laden statements need to be avoided, such as saying to a young client "You shouldn't be having sexual intercourse unless you are married." Another technique is using reflection in which the nurse returns to an earlier response to a question. For example, the nurse might state: "You mentioned that you sometimes have unpro-

tected intercourse." This statement sets the stage for the practitioner to ask additional questions in order to have enough information to make an accurate diagnosis (Andrews, 1988; Andrist, 1988; Krozy, 1978).

It is important for the nurse to temper any emotional reaction to a client's comment. The nurse needs to accept and not judge the client's behavior so that the information obtained can be used to assess, plan, implement, and evaluate holistic care.

Once the interview begins, some content to cover includes whether or not the client is sexually active, sexual preference, current sexual satisfaction, past problems, problems for the man getting or maintaining an erection and for the woman being aroused and having an orgasm, the effect of the present illness on sexuality (see the Nursing Care Plan), and AIDS risks (Andrews, 1988; Andrist, 1988). After data are collected and the nursing diagnosis made, the nurse may have the expertise to develop a care plan and work with the client. If the nursing diagnosis is potential sexual dysfunction related to recent MI, the nurse could implement the hospital's existing teaching program by showing the client and his or her partner a video about sexuality after a heart attack, answer questions raised by the video or about any other concerns, and provide the client with written material that reinforces or supplements the content presented. If the nurse is uncomfortable presenting this information, it is best that the client be referred to a colleague who has sexual health care expertise.

Detailed sexual education and counseling may prevent sexual dysfunction and facilitate resumption of pre-illness sexual patterns (Shuman & Bohachick, 1987). Sometimes the treatment will require interdisciplinary teamwork. If the diagnosis is, for example, sexual dysfunction (impotence) related to hypertension or diabetes mellitus, the nurse must consult with a physician. The solution may be as simple as changing the medications prescribed to return

# ❖ NURSING CARE PLAN

**CLIENT:** Mildred P.

**MEDICAL DIAGNOSIS:** Breast cancer (just diagnosed by biopsy)

**NURSING DIAGNOSIS:** Altered sexuality related to impending simple mastectomy

| GOALS | INTERVENTIONS |
|---|---|
| Mildred will move through the grieving process for impending loss of her breast | ◆ Assess significance of:<br>  a. psychosocial meaning Mildred attaches to breast.<br>  b. loss of breast as body part.<br>  c. loss of good health.<br>  d. diagnosis to family members.<br>◆ Encourage Mildred to:<br>  a. grieve loss of breast.<br>  b. discuss her thoughts about reconstructive surgery.<br>  c. share her concerns with husband and grown children.<br>◆ Make referrals to community or self-help groups.<br>◆ Follow up with Mildred at 2 to 3 months and 1 year after mastectomy. |
| Mildred will resume prediagnosis level of sexual activity. | ◆ Assist Mildred to accept changes in her body by discussing her reactions to her surgery, being with her, and changing her dressings.<br>◆ Inform Mildred and her spouse that initially they may have decreased interest in sexual intercourse because of fear of injury to incision, the surgery itself, or side effects of chemotherapy or radiation.<br>◆ Encourage Mildred and her husband to share their concerns with one another.<br>◆ Suggest that they can resume sexual intercourse whenever they wish. |

## EVALUATION

Mildred is able to discuss her feelings regarding the loss of her breast with the nurse and her husband. She attends a self-help group and begins to accept the changes in her body. Over time, she is able to return to her prediagnosis level of sexual activity.

normal sexual functioning. On the other hand, if the cause of impotence is diabetes mellitus, it is likely that the impotence will remain and the client and his partner will require assistance to cope, as well as being informed of other methods of sexual pleasure.

Overall, the sexual history can be a valuable learning experience for clients and can provide the nurse an opportunity for teaching and information giving. Andrews (1988) suggests that the process of taking a sexual history facilitates counseling the client through legitimization, empowerment, and universalization. First, with *legitimization,* the nurse's right to ask personal questions is established. The client is *empowered* by retaining control over how much information will be shared.

*Universalization* communicates that there is a range of acceptable sexual behavior. The nurse can facilitate this process by either providing an introductory statement or asking a question indicating acceptance for a particular behavior. While taking a history with someone over 55 years of age, the nurse may state "Many men and women of your age note changes in sexual functioning. What changes have you noticed, and are they a concern?" This question establishes that it is acceptable for older people to have sexual intercourse. The client may also infer that certain physiological changes occur with aging. A man may worry that he needs a longer period of time to get an erection, or a woman may be concerned because of vaginal dryness and irritation during sexual intercourse. The client, however, could also interpret this question to mean the frequency of intercourse. One client may prefer not to have sexual intercourse while another might have intercourse three times or more a week. Regardless, clients need to be aware that either behavior is acceptable and normal.

The previous discussion suggests that the client desires information. The nurse may find after completing the sexual history that the client may not need or want additional information. For example, some gay men seeking AIDS testing may have as much knowledge, if not more, than health professionals about safe sex practices and other facts pertaining to AIDS and HIV infections, so that it is unnecessary to repeat that information. It is important, however, for the nurse to use the nursing process by assessing what services are needed, providing them, and evaluating their effectiveness. Mims and Swenson (1980) also indicate that granting permission can be extended to health professionals, thereby permitting nurses to admit to not knowing everything, to refer situations beyond their expertise, and to not intervene with some clients.

**Advanced level.** The advanced level includes *suggestion giving, educational programs, therapy,* and *research projects.* These services should only be provided by professionals with advanced education and training, such as sexual therapists and counselors. The nurse must have specialized knowledge about specific sexual issues and conditions to use suggestion giving. Typical suggestions include techniques, exercises, positions, and forms of communication to help the client reach sexual satisfaction (Mims & Swenson, 1978; 1980).

Educational programs can be developed by practitioners for any number of issues along either the life cycle or illness/wellness continuums. The audience may be individuals, families, or communities. The post MI teaching program that was previously mentioned could have been developed by an advanced practitioner in conjunction with the nurses in the cardiac care units. The advanced practitioner may also develop research projects examining nurses' sexual knowledge, attitudes, and clinical practice behaviors about sexuality or evaluating whether there is a difference in the level of knowledge, attitudes, and behaviors between clients receiving a new teaching program compared with the existing unstructured program.

A nurse who is a sexual therapist typically is found in obstetric, gynecologic, and psychiatric settings (Woods, 1984). These nurses may use any of a variety of methods: individual practice, co-therapy, marital and family counseling, or group counseling in either private office or clinic settings. The range of problems is extensive and varies from sexual dysfunction issues such as anorgasmia and impotence to the effects of disease processes to sexual abuse and assault (Mims & Swenson, 1980).

**Using the sexual health model.** The Mims-Swenson Sexual Health Model can be used by all nurses to some extent when working with clients, because the model incorporates the nursing process and communication skills. This model can also be used in conjunction with a number of the grand and middle range nursing theories. The theorists who include sexuality as part of their theory or use a developmental approach include Johnson (1980), King (1981), Leininger (1988), Neuman (1989), Rogers (1980), and Watson (1985).

Since sexuality is integral to every person, the nurse must provide basic information and reassurance to the client for life events and potential threats to sexual functioning. An introductory course in human sexuality familiarizes the nurse with structural alterations, physiologic changes, drugs, and body image and self-concept distortions that can have an effect on a client's sexual health.

While it is beyond the scope of this chapter to provide detailed information about all of these concerns, Tables 31-1 through 31-3 and the box on the following pages, summarize various conditions and the effects on sexual health. Table 31-1 summarizes anatomical alterations and their hypothesized disruptions to sexual health for the cardiovascular, genital, and central and peripheral nervous systems. Physiological alterations also can have varying effects on sexuality ranging from a decreased libido to

dyspareunia to impotence as seen in Table 31-2. Medications can have positive and negative impacts on sexuality. Table 31-3 provides this information for common drugs. Finally, various health conditions affect sexuality by altering body image and self-concept. The box lists some of the problems resulting from trauma, surgery, and miscellaneous causes.

Life events not only have an effect on one's sexuality but also potentially on how others perceive that person. Even though the nurse is taught to work with all people using a nonjudgmental manner, there are instances when the nurse's own life experiences and values interfere with the ability to provide holistic care. These issues include abortion, homosexuality, premarital sexuality, and sexually transmitted diseases. The nurse may have difficulty providing optimal care when working with any of these clients. In other instances, some individuals are not considered to be sexual beings by society. Health professionals may need reminders that persons who are developmentally delayed or who have physical or mental disabilities have the same sexual needs and desires as anyone else.

Some life events, such as hospitalization, result in transient changes in sexuality. Most female nurses have encountered the male client who acts seductively. The nurse's usual reaction is anger or disgust, since behaviors like this are not considered to be appropriate. Yet, if the nurse can discuss these behaviors with the client, she is likely to discover that the client acts seductively to confirm his sexuality that has been threatened by the hospitalization and uncertainty surrounding the alteration in health. Sometimes by recognizing and acknowledging that the client's concerns are legitimate, the acting-out behavior will stop. Nursing staff will feel more comfortable with the client and be better able to meet his needs.

❖ **Table 31-1**
Changes in body structure and hypothesized interference with sexual health

| System | Probable mechanism of interference |
| --- | --- |
| **CENTRAL AND PERIPHERAL NERVOUS SYSTEMS** | |
| Spinal cord injury | Disrupts integrity of peripheral nerves and spinal |
| Spinal cord tumors | cord reflexes involved in sexual response (for |
| Herniated disk | example, erection) |
| Multiple sclerosis | |
| Spina bifida | |
| Amyotrophic lateral sclerosis | |
| Tumors of frontal or temporal lobes | May interfere with function of centers controlling |
| Cerebrovascular accident | sexual drive |
| Trauma to frontal or temporal lobes | |
| **CARDIOVASCULAR SYSTEM** | |
| Thrombus formation in vessels of penis | May interfere with blood supply to penis, thus |
| Leriche's syndrome | interfering with erection |
| Sickle cell disorders | |
| Leukemia | |
| Trauma to vasculature supplying sexual organs | |
| **REPRODUCTIVE/SEXUAL SYSTEM** | |
| Prostatectomy, radical perineal | May destroy nerve supply, interfering with sensory |
| Abdominal perineal resection | and motor aspects of sexual response |
| Lumbar sympathectomy | May result in disturbed ejaculation |
| Rhizotomy | May result in impotence, as well as disturbed |
| Absence of penis or penile injury | ejaculation |
| Penectomy | Precludes or discourages intromission |
| Imperforate hymen | |
| Congenital absence of vagina | |
| Pelvic exenteration | |
| Vaginectomy | |
| Obstetric trauma or poor episiotomy | Leaves gaping vaginal opening or painful scarring, |
| Damage to pubococcygeus muscle | thus discouraging intercourse |

From Woods, N. F. (1987b). Intervention for persons with sexual problems. (p 1711). In W. J. Phipps, B. C. Long, & N. F. Woods (Eds.), *Medical surgical nursing: Concepts and clinical practice* (3rd ed.). St. Louis: C. V. Mosby Co.

❖ **Table 31-2**
Physiologic interferences with sexual health

| Physiologic interferences | Hypothesized mechanism of action | Physiologic interferences | Hypothesized mechanism of action |
|---|---|---|---|
| **SYSTEMIC DISEASES** | | Trauma to penis | |
| Pulmonary disease | Debility, pain, and | Vaginal infections | |
| Renal disease | depression probably | Senile vaginitis | |
| Malignancies | interfere with sexual | Vulvitis | |
| Infections | desire and expression | Leukoplakia | |
| Degenerative diseases | | Bartholin's cyst | |
| Some cardiovascular diseases | | Allergic response to vaginal sprays and deodorants | |
| **METABOLIC DISRUPTIONS** | | Vaginitis following radiation therapy | |
| Cirrhosis | Hepatic problems in men | Pelvic inflammatory disease | |
| Mononucleosis | result in estrogen | Fibroadenomas | |
| Hepatitis | buildup from inability | Endometriosis | |
| | of liver to conjugate | Uterine prolapse | |
| | estrogens; similar | Anal fissures, hemorrhoids | |
| | processes occur in | Pelvic masses | Local irritability, damage |
| | women along with | Ovarian cysts | to genitalia, and |
| | general debility | Prostatitis | consequent |
| Hypothyroidism | By depression of CNS | Urethritis | interference with reflex |
| Addison's disease | function, general | | mechanisms involved |
| Hypogonadism | debilitation, and | | in erection and |
| Hypopituitarism | depression, libido may | | ejaculation |
| Acromegaly | be decreased, and | | |
| Feminizing tumors | impaired erectile | | |
| Cushing's disease | abilities in men may | | |
| Diabetes mellitus | result | **MEDICAL OR SURGICAL CASTRATION** | |
| **DISEASES OF THE GENITALIA** | | Orchiectomy | Lowered androgen levels |
| Priapism | Each of these problems | Radiation therapy | depress libido and lead |
| Peyronie's disease | involves damage to | Oophorectomy, adrenalectomy | to impotence, retarded |
| Balantitis | genital organs, which | | ejaculation, or |
| Phimosis | may result in painful | | impaired sexual |
| Genital herpes | intercourse | | responsiveness |

From Woods, N. F. (1987b). Intervention for persons with sexual problems. (p. 1713). In W. J. Phipps, B. C. Long, & N. F. Woods (Eds.), *Medical surgical nursing: Concepts and clinical practice* (3rd ed.). St. Louis: C. V. Mosby Co.

❖ **Table 31-3**
Drug effects on human sexual behavior

| Drug or drug category | Effect | Probable mechanism of action |
|---|---|---|
| Oral contraceptives | Positive | Permits separation of sexual activity from concern about conception |
| Antihypertensives<br>Guanethidine (Ismelin)<br>Reserpine (Serpasil)<br>Mecamylamine (Inversine)<br>Trimethaphan (Arfonad)<br>Spironolactone (Aldactone) | Negative | Peripheral blockade of nervous innervation of sex glands |
| Antidepressants<br>Imipramine (Tofranil)<br>Desipramine (Norpramin, Pertofrane)<br>Amitryptyline (Elavil)<br>Nortriptyline (Aventyl)<br>Protriptyline (Vivactil)<br>Phenelzine sulfate (Nardil)<br>Tranylcypromine sulfate (Parnate)<br>Pargyline (Eutonyl) | Negative | Central depression; peripheral blockade of nervous innervation of sex glands |
| Antihistamines<br>Diphenhydramine (Benadryl)<br>Promethazine (Phenergan)<br>Chlorpheniramine (Chlor-Trimeton) | Negative | Blockade of parasympathetic nervous innervation of sex glands |
| Antispasmodics<br>Methantheline (Banthine)<br>Glycopyrrolate (Robinul)<br>Hexocyclium (Tral)<br>Poldine (Nacton) | Negative | Ganglionic blockage of nervous innervation of sex glands |
| Sedatives and tranquilizers<br>Chlorpromazine (Thorazine, Megaphen)<br>Prochlorperazine (Compazine)<br>Thioridazine (Mellaril)<br>Mesoridazine (Serentil)<br>Chlordiazepoxide (Librium)<br>Diazepam (Valium)<br>Benperidol<br>Phenoxybenzamine (Dibenzyline)<br>Chlorprothixene (Taractan) | Negative and positive | Central sedation; blockade of autonomic innervation of sex glands; suppression of hypothalamic and pituitary function<br><br>Tranquilization and relaxation |

From Woods, N. F. (1987b). Intervention for persons with sexual problems. (pp. 1714–1715). In W. J. Phipps, B. C. Long, & N. F. Woods (Eds.), *Medical surgical nursing: Concepts and clinical practice* (3rd ed.). St. Louis: C. V. Mosby Co.

*Continued.*

❖ **Table 31-3**
Drug effects on human sexual behavior—cont'd

| Drug or drug category | Effect | Probable mechanism of action |
|---|---|---|
| Ethyl alcohol | Negative | Central depression; suppression of motor activity; diuresis |
| | Transiently positive | Release of inhibitions; relaxation |
| Sex hormone preparations<br>Cyproterone acetate<br>Methandrostenolone (Dianabol)<br>Nandrolone phenpropionate<br>(Durabolin) | Negative | Antiandrogenic effects of sexual function; loss of libido; decreased potency |
| Potassium nitrate (saltpeter) | Questionable | Diuresis |
| Cantharis (Spanish fly) | Negative | Irritation and inflammation of genitourinary tract, systemic poisoning |
| Yohimbine | Questionable | Stimulation of lower spinal nerve centers |
| Narcotics and psychoactive drugs | Negative | Central depression; decreased libido and impaired potency |
| Morphine<br>Heroin<br>Cocaine<br>Marijuana<br>LSD<br>Amphetamines | Transiently positive | Release of inhibitions; increased suggestibility; relaxation |
| L-Dopa and p-chlorophenylalanine | Questionable | Improvement of well-being |
| Amyl nitrite | Questionable | Vasodilation of genitourinary tract; smooth muscle relation |
| Caffeine | Questionable | CNS stimulant |
| Vitamin E, selenium | Questionable | Supports fertility in laboratory animals |

❖ **SOME HEALTH PROBLEMS RESULTING IN BODY IMAGE CHANGES THAT MAY RAISE SEXUAL CONCERNS**

**SURGICALLY INDUCED**
Mastectomy
Ostomy
Hysterectomy
Amputation of limb or limbs

**TRAUMATICALLY INDUCED**
Burns
Lacerations, scarring
Amputations

**OTHERS**
Dermatologic disorders
Obesity
Congenital anomalies of sexual organs (for example, absence of penis, hypospadias)
Unusual breast size, including immaturity or hypertrophy

From Woods, N. F. (1987b). Intervention for persons with sexual problems. (p. 1716). In W. J. Phipps, B. C. Long, & N. F. Woods (Eds.), *Medical surgical nursing: Concepts and clinical practice* (3rd ed.). St. Louis: C. V. Mosby Co.

## ❖ SUMMARY

This chapter provided an overview of human sexuality. Psychosexual development, which examines the relationship between biological, psychological, and cultural factors, was presented to illustrate the holistic nature of sexuality over the life cycle. The Mims-Swenson Sexual Health Model provides a mechanism for nurses to evaluate their knowledge, attitudes, and clinical expertise to provide optimal sexual health care for clients. Only through continued reading, education, and workshops can nurses gain the expertise and comfort needed to deal with the complexities of sexual health care.

## ❖ APPLYING KNOWLEDGE TO PRACTICE

1. Keep a diary about your sexuality for at least 1 month. Entries may include personal or professional experiences, cultural influences, or anything else that has had an impact on your sexuality.
2. In the clinical situations that follow use role playing to address sexual health concerns:
   a. Staff nurses have asked you to talk with Bill Jones, a 65-year-old, about the sexual advances he makes toward those involved in his care.
   b. Betty Brown, a 40-year-old homemaker and mother of four children, is 3 days posthysterectomy.
   c. Marcella Smythe, a 16-year-old high school student, thinks she is pregnant.
   d. Robert White, a 30-year-old hospitalized with recurrent infections, has just been informed by his physician that he tested HIV positive.
3. Select a topic that you would like to develop into a sex education presentation for a community group. Use only the resources available at your public library (audiovisuals, children's and adult books).

## REFERENCES

Andrews, S. (1988). Coping with the sexual health interview. *Journal of Nurse-Midwifery, 33,* 269-273.

Andrist, L. C. (1988). Taking a sexual history and educating clients about safe sex. *Nursing Clinics of North America, 23,* 959-973.

Annon, J. S. (1976). *Behavioral treatment of sexual problems: Brief therapy.* Hagerstown, MD: Harper & Row (a).

Annon, J. S. (1976). The PLISSIT model: A proposed conceptual scheme for the behavioral treatment of sexual problems. *Journal of Sex Education and Therapy, 2,* 1-15 (b).

Chapman, J. & Sughrue, J., Jr. (1987). A model for sexual assessment and intervention. *Health Care for Women International, 8,* 87-99.

Fetter, M. P. (1987). Reaching a level of sexual comfort. *Health Education, 18,* 6-8.

Frey, K. A. (1981). Middle-aged women's experience and perceptions of menopause. *Women and Health, 6,* 25-36.

Hott, J. R. & Ryan-Merritt, M. (1982). A national study of nursing research in human sexuality. *Nursing Clinics of North America, 17,* 429-446.

Johnson, D. E. (1980). The behavioral system model for nursing. In J. P. Riehl and C. Roy (Eds.), *Conceptual models for nursing practice* (2nd ed.) (207-216). New York: Appleton-Century-Crofts.

King, I. M. (1981). *A theory of nursing: Systems, concepts, process.* New York: John Wiley and Sons.

Klaus, M. H. & Kennell, J. H. (1982). *Parent-infant bonding* (2nd ed.). St. Louis: C. V. Mosby.

Krozy, R. (1978). Becoming comfortable with sexual assessment. *American Journal of Nursing, 78,* 1036-1038.

Leininger, M. M. (1988). *Transcultural nursing: Concepts, theories and practices* (2nd ed.). New York: John Wiley and Sons.

Masters, W. H., Johnson, V. E. & Kolodny, R. C. (1985). *Human sexuality* (2nd ed.). Boston: Little, Brown.

McFarlane, E. A. & Rubenfeld, M. G. (1983). The need for sexual integrity. In H. Yura and M. Walsh (Eds.), *Human needs III and the nursing process* (185-233). New York: Appleton-Century-Crofts.

Mims, F. H. & Swenson, M. (1978). A model to promote sexual health care. *Nursing Outlook, 28,* 121-125.

Mims, F. H. & Swenson, M. (1980). *Sexuality: A nursing perspective.* New York: McGraw-Hill.

Morrison, E. S., Starks, K., Hyndman, C. & Ronzio, N. (1980). *Growing up sexual.* New York: D. Van Nostrand.

National Institute on Aging. (1985). *Age page: Sexuality in later life* (no. 461-308/200007). Washington, DC: U. S. Government Printing Office.

Neuman, B. (1989). *The Neuman systems model* (2nd ed.). Norwalk, Ct: Appleton and Lange.

Phipps, W., Long, B. & Woods, N. F. (1983). *Medical-surgical nursing: Concepts and clinical practice* (2nd ed.). St. Louis: C. V. Mosby Co.

Pritchard, J. A., MacDonald, P. C. & Gant, N. F. (1985). *Williams obstetrics* (17th ed.). Norwalk, CT: Appleton-Century-Crofts.

Rieve, J. E. (1989). Sexuality and the adult with acquired physical disability. *Nursing Clinics of North America, 24,* 265-276.

Rogers, M. E. (1980). A science of unitary man. In J. P. Riehl and C. Roy (Eds.), *Conceptual models for nursing practice* (2nd ed.) (179-188). New York: Appleton-Century-Crofts.

Rubin, R. T., Reinsch, J. M., & Haskett, R. F. (1981). Postnatal gonadal steroid effects on human behavior. *Science, 211* (20), 1318-1324.

Shuman, N. A. & Bohachick, P. (1987). Nurses' attitudes towards sexual counseling. *Dimensions of Critical Care Nursing, 6* (2), 75-81.

Watson, J. (1985). *Nursing: The philosophy and science of caring* (2nd ed.). Boulder, Co: Colorado Associated University Press.

Weg, R. B. (1983). *Sexuality in the later years: Roles and behavior.* New York: Academic Press.

Woods, N. F. (1984). *Human sexuality in health and illness* (3rd ed.). St. Louis: C. V. Mosby Co.

Woods, N. F. (1987a). Toward a holistic perspective of human sexuality: Alterations in sexual health and nursing diagnoses. *Holistic Nursing Practice, 1*(4), 1-11.

Woods, N. F. (1987b). *Interventions for persons with sexual problems.* In W. Phipps, B. E. Long, and N. F. Woods (Eds.), Medical surgical nursing: Concepts and clinical practice (3rd ed.), (pp. 1707–1722), St. Louis: C. V. Mosby.

World Health Organization. (1975). *Education and treatment in human sexuality: The training of health professionals* (Technical Report Series No. 372). Geneva: World Health Organization.

# 32 ◆ Parenting

Lesley A. Perry

## OBJECTIVES

*At the completion of this chapter, the reader will be able to:*

◆ Discuss the changing patterns of parenting evident in Western society and their impact on family and community life.

◆ Examine the transition to parenthood in terms of developmental tasks, stressful events, role changes, and developing attachment and parent-infant relationships.

◆ Describe parental responses and coping efforts and parent-child relationships when a child is born prematurely or is chronically ill or handicapped.

Parenting fulfills an essential function of society. Traditionally, parenting has involved childbearing and childrearing, which serve the purposes of replacing members and continuing the family and social group's biological and cultural identities. Parenting is defined as ". . . a process by which adult members of society nurture their young. The primary goal of parenting is to prepare children for the roles and responsibilities of the adult world" (Servonsky & Opas, 1987, p. 178). Parenthood involves imposing responsibilities, since the health and development of the child are significantly dependent on the quality of parenting provided. A variety of parent, child, and societal factors influence the parenting behaviors exhibited by parents.

Three basic functions of parenting include ensuring that the child's basic needs are met; providing nurturance, love, and security; and socializing and enculturating the child. The provision of food, shelter, and health and safety measures are fundamental responsibilities that ensure the protection of the young. Nurturance and love lay the basic foundations for the child's development of trust and a sense of self. The child's later ability to form attachments and provide nurturance to others is based on these early experiences. Socialization allows children to learn social roles and expectations and appropriate behaviors and limits in social groups. Cultural values and beliefs are also transmitted through the socialization process (Servonsky & Opas, 1987).

Because of its importance, parenting has been studied extensively. Early investigators focused on parenting attitudes and childrearing techniques. Methods of discipline, feeding, and fostering dependence and independence in children were explored. More recently, parent-infant interactions and nurturing and caregiving activities have been investigated. Interest in parenting behavior has also expanded to include examining the biological basis for parenting, the use of animal models to explain behavior, and cross-cultural studies of parenthood. Explication of the process of parenting serves as a foundation for supporting the development of appropriate parenting skills and behaviors.

This chapter can discuss only a portion of the richness of parenting. The initial section discusses recent changes in patterns of parenting and some factors influencing those changes. The section on transition to parenthood considers the developmental tasks associated with parenting, the stressful nature of new parenthood, maternal role acquisition, the development of attachment, and fathering behaviors. The final section of the chapter explores the demands of parenting in special circumstances, such as when an infant is born prematurely or when a child is chronically ill or handicapped.

## ❖ CHANGING PATTERNS OF PARENTING

The latter half of the twentieth century has seen unprecedented changes in parenting, especially in Western societies. Philosophical, cultural, economic, scientific, and health-related factors have all played a part in changing patterns of parenthood. Increased emphasis on freedom and individual choice, less rigorous sociocultural definitions of gender-specific roles, improved economic conditions for many segments of society, and advances in science and health care have influenced parenthood (Rossi, 1987). Specific demographic trends illustrate the changing picture of family and parenthood. There has been a decrease in the marriage rate, an increase in the age at which people marry, an increase in the divorce rate, and a decrease in the rate of remarriage following divorce (Rossi, 1987). Consequently, for some individuals, parenthood may be delayed until an older age, and many children may be raised in single parent families. Overall, fertility has decreased in the United States. The desire for fewer children, de-

layed marriage and parenthood, and voluntary childlessness have contributed to the decreasing fertility rate (Rossi, 1987). On the other hand, there has been a rise in the rate of teenage pregnancies and in the number of women opting for parenthood without marriage, either out of choice or necessity.

These trends have made parenting an increasingly complex endeavor. The number of households headed by a single adult has increased significantly in recent years. Many more children are being raised in single parent households, the consequences of which include lowered economic status and opportunity, lack of consistent gender socialization from the absent parent, and greater responsibility for adult tasks and decision making placed on the child. The single parent has fewer social contacts, less support from others, restricted opportunity for career advancement, and lowered income. Adolescent parents must frequently contend with their own developmental needs as well as those of their children. Their education may be interrupted or terminated because of the need to care for their infants. Poor educational preparation will constrain their future economic power. Children of adolescents may be adversely affected by the combined developmental, social, and economic limitations of their family situation. Divorce and remarriage often require the blending of two families. Difficulties arising from the process of combining the families and developing a newly integrated and cohesive family unit are a strain on parenting and marital functions.

Other recent developments involve the other end of the age spectrum. Educational experiences have extended adolescence into the age group of the twenties. Children pursuing higher education and graduate study are often dependent on parents for support and housing. In addition, economic factors or divorce may force once independent children to resume living in the parental home. Thus, parenthood may be extended further into the child's young adulthood than ever before. The relationships between older adolescents and young adults and their parents have received little attention to date. How parenting changes during this period is an interesting topic.

Improved health and longevity has increased the number of older adults in the U.S. population. Chronic health problems may restrict the degree to which the elderly person can maintain independence and manage his or her own care. Adult children may need to assume a role in caring for their elderly parents. The degree of involvement necessary and the timing of that requirement in the childbearing and childrearing cycle of the adult child will have a bearing on the adult's parenting function. Caring for an elderly parent as well as young children may be an enormous stress for the family. How the dual responsibilities to parent and children is managed and the resources and supports available are important areas to examine.

The changing patterns and trends addressed in the preceding paragraphs focus on the impact these trends have at the individual and family levels. Rossi (1987) notes that there are also consequences at the societal level. Because of smaller family size and the smaller number of women who bear children, there is less involvement of adults in the general society involved in childrearing activities. Adults spend a greater proportion of their lives in activities and concerns that are unrelated to parenting and children. Childrearing is one means of increasing social integration, since families with children tend to be more involved in community activities and institutions. Rossi suggests that as a result of the decline in the focus on parenting and childrearing, social and community integration may suffer. In addition, a lack of concern for child welfare may result in the needs of parents and children receiving a low priority in public policy agendas (Rossi, 1987, pp. 44-45). Support for parenting, then, is a challenging task that requires action at the

individual, family, community, and societal levels.

## ❖ TRANSITION TO PARENTHOOD

Transition to parenthood is often viewed from three perspectives. Parenthood may be considered a normal developmental event, a stressful life event, and an event requiring transition to a new role. The study of parenthood and the processes that occur as men and women become parents is of significant interest to clinicians and researchers. Understanding parenting may assist nurses in the selection and timing of appropriate interventions.

### Parenthood as a Developmental Event

Viewing parenthood from a developmental perspective requires consideration of the developmental history of families. As much as individuals experience developmental tasks and phases, so too do families encounter a series of events, changes, and adaptations over the course of their existence. Duvall (1977) described the *family life cycle* as a series of eight stages through which families progress. Specific to each stage are developmental tasks that must be accomplished by the family so that family functions and goals can be fulfilled (Table 32-1).

Parents, as individuals, progress through developmental stages and must accomplish individual developmental tasks parallel to family developmental stages and tasks. Erikson (1963) identifies three developmental stages affecting adults. The task of young adulthood is establishing *intimacy,* or the capacity for commitment and affiliative relationships with others. Adulthood involves the stage of *generativity,* which is primarily concerned with establishing and guiding the children of the next generation. Maturity has as its task confirming *ego identity,* or finding acceptance and dignity in one's own life. Duvall (1977) identifies individual developmental tasks for mothers and fathers, depending on the stage of family in the family life cycle. Mothers in childbearing families, for example, have as their developmental tasks reconciling conflicting conceptions of their roles as wife, mother, and individual person; accepting and adjusting to the stresses and pressures of young parenthood; learning to care for infants and young children confidently and competently; establishing and maintaining healthful practices for children and family; providing opportunities for realizing the full potential of the child's development; sharing the responsibilities of parenthood with their partner; maintaining a satisfying relationship with their partner; adjusting to the practical realities of life, such as finances, housing, and planning for the future; maintaining a sense of personal autonomy; and developing a sense of

❖ **Table 32-1**
Duvall's eight stage family life cycle and family developmental tasks

| Stage | Family life cycle stage | Family developmental tasks |
|-------|------------------------|----------------------------|
| I. | Beginning families (married couples without children) | ◆ Establishing a mutually satisfying marriage<br>◆ Adjusting to pregnancy and the promise of parenthood<br>◆ Fitting into the kin network |
| II. | Childbearing families (oldest child birth through 30 months) | ◆ Having, adjusting to, and encouraging the development of infants<br>◆ Establishing a satisfying home for both parents and infant(s) |
| III. | Families with preschool children (oldest child 2 1/2 to 6 years of age) | ◆ Adapting to the critical needs and interests of preschool children in stimulating, growth—promoting ways<br>◆ Coping with energy depletion and lack of privacy as parents |
| IV. | Families with school age children (oldest child 6 to 13 years of age) | ◆ Fitting into the community of school-age families in constructive ways<br>◆ Encouraging children's educational achievement |
| V. | Families with teenagers (oldest child 13 to 20 years of age) | ◆ Balancing freedom with responsibility as teenagers mature and emancipate themselves<br>◆ Establishing postparental interest and careers as growing parents |
| VI. | Families launching young adults (first child leaving home through last child leaving home) | ◆ Releasing young adults into work, college, marriage with appropriate rituals and assistance<br>◆ Maintaining a supportive home base |
| VII. | Middle-aged parents (empty nest to retirement) | ◆ Rebuilding the marriage relationship<br>◆ Maintaining kin ties with older and younger generations |
| VIII. | Family during retirement and aging (retirement to death of both spouses) | ◆ Adjusting to retirement<br>◆ Closing the family home or adapting it to aging<br>◆ Coping with bereavement and living alone |

From Duvall, E.M. (1977). *Marriage and family development.* New York: J. B. Lippincott, pp. 144, 179.

family. Fathers have similar developmental tasks to accomplish. They, too, must clarify their roles as husband, father, and individual; learn child caretaking skills; participate in fostering the child's development; maintain a satisfying relationship with their partner; take part in developing a sense of family; maintain a sense of self; and assume responsibility for supporting the family (Duvall, 1977, pp. 224-229).

Viewing parenthood and families from a developmental perspective is useful as a guide for assessing particular families and their needs. Developmental stages and tasks can serve as an organizing framework for planning interventions, since they allow nurses to anticipate and prepare families for the roles, tasks, and usual stresses they will need to master in a particular stage. Stage models, however, have their drawbacks. Frequently, they have been developed from anecdotal data, with little empirical evidence to either support or refute the behaviors and stages described. Not all parents or families fit the stage model. Friedman (1986) notes that the theory of family developmental stages often fails to take into account the unusual events or nonnormative stressors encountered by families and "can be criticized for its assumption of homogeneity (its lack of adequate attention to family diversity), its middle-class bias, its assumption of stability within each stage, and its lack of explaining the processes that occur between stages that allows families to change" (p. 59). If nurses are cognizant of these deficiencies, they can make appropriate use of developmental stages in evaluating needs of the parents and families for whom they care.

## Parenthood as a Stressful Experience

Becoming parents is a stressful experience for many families. The addition of a new family member brings many changes, both to individuals within the family and to family functioning. Changes occurring include decreased time for oneself and spouse; increased household and child care tasks; diminished social interactions, particularly with friends and community groups; changes in sleep patterns and daily schedules; and increased financial obligations. Responsibilities and tasks within the family system must be reorganized to accommodate the increased demands of the new member. If this is the first child for the parents, there are new roles to be learned, and other roles must be reshaped. Relationships both within and outside the family are readjusted and modified by the birth of a new baby.

The *nature of the stress* associated with parenting, factors contributing to or moderating stress, and parental coping efforts have been explored. Walker (1989b) examined the mediating role of perception of stress and the buffering effects of a health-promoting life-style on the development of maternal identity in mothers of new babies. Mothers were found to have a high level of global-perceived stress, the mean for the mothers exceeding the national norms for all subgroups with the exception of disabled or ill persons. Maternal employment and mothers' perceptions of infant "difficultness" were associated with perceived stress, with mothers who worked full-time, and mothers of difficult infants perceiving higher levels of stress. Perceived stress was found to predict maternal identity. Higher levels of stress had a negative impact on maternal identity. Health promoting life-style did not serve as a buffer to perceived stress in this group of mothers.

Because it was not possible to specify any cause and effect relationships in the first study, Walker (1989a) conducted a longitudinal analysis with the original group of mothers 6 months later. In examining maternal employment as a stressor, employment status, perceived stress, and the health promoting life-styles of self-actualization and interpersonal support were found to be predictive of maternal identity 6 months later. When examining infant difficulty as a stressor, maternal education, perceived stress, and the health promoting life-style of self-actualization were the significant contributors to maternal identity 6 months later. Only two factors contributed significantly to perceived stress at 6 months: initial levels of perceived stress and the number of children in the family.

Cronenwett and Kunst-Wilson (1981) discussed the role of *social support* in the stress associated with transition to fatherhood. Because men are becoming more involved and more active in the parenting role than before, greater role conflict among the roles of worker, husband, and father may be anticipated. Cronenwett and Kunst-Wilson propose social support as an important factor in decreasing role conflict and associated stress. Four types of social support are pertinent to assisting the father's transition to the parenting role: emotional, instrumental, informational, and appraisal support. Emotional support is most usually available from the spouse or partner. However, the mother's emotional reserves may be taxed by the birth of the baby, and she may be the recipient of support rather than being able to dispense it. Other sources of emotional support for the father are needed. Flexibility and control in the work situation are important instrumental supports. Friends and relatives, as well as the spouse, are sources of instrumental, informational, and appraisal support. However, social expectations or traditional sex role socialization may not allow the father to take full advantage of their assistance (Cronenwett & Kunst-Wilson, 1981).

Crnic, Greenberg, Ragozin, Robinson, and Basham (1983) studied the effects of *stress and social support* on mothers of premature and full-term infants. Their findings support the important role that stress and social support play in parenting behaviors and parent-infant interactions. Mothers with greater social support and less stress reported greater general satisfaction with life and greater pleasure and satisfaction in their role as parent. Support from a spouse, partner, or friends was significant in influencing satisfaction with the parenting role. Stress played a

significant role in mothers' sensitivity to their infants' cues and in the clarity of infant cues and responsiveness to the mother. Mothers experiencing greater stress were less sensitive to their infants' cues. In return, greater maternal stress resulted in decreased clarity of infant cues and less infant responsiveness to maternal behavior. Social support was found to have a moderating effect on infant behavior. Infants of mothers with greater support were more responsive and showed more positive affective behaviors.

It is apparent that numerous factors contribute to the stress associated with the transition to parenthood. Also of interest is how parents cope with this stressful experience. Ventura (1982, 1986) studied the *coping* behaviors and patterns of parents. Parents identified specific coping behaviors as being more helpful than others. Helpful behaviors were identified as: "doing things with (the) child, maintaining family stability, trusting one's partner, being a parent to the baby, investing in the child, and being thankful" (Ventura, 1982, p. 271). Mothers found more of the coping behaviors helpful than did fathers. Fathers reported only one behavior (involvement in social activities) to be more helpful than mothers (Ventura, 1982). Ventura grouped the individual coping behaviors into several coping patterns. These patterns were: seeking social support and self-development; maintaining family integrity; being religious, thankful, and content; and being responsible. Mothers found seeking social support and self-development and being religious, thankful, and content as more helpful than did fathers. These differential coping patterns are not unexpected, but should not be discounted when planning interventions. (For further discussion of coping, see Chapter 26.)

## Maternal Role Acquisition

Transition to the maternal role is an important developmental and life event. Mercer (1985) defines *maternal role acquisition* as "... a process in which the mother achieves competence in the role and integrates the mothering behaviors into her established role set, so that she is comfortable with her identity as a mother" (p. 198). The process of maternal role acquisition progresses through four stages (Mercer, 1981). In the *anticipatory stage,* the prospective mother begins to learn the expectations of the maternal role. The birth of the infant heralds the *formal stage* in which the mother's role behaviors are influenced by the formal expectations and precepts of others. Ultimately, the mother encounters situations or events in which the formal expectations or rules are inadequate. The mother develops distinctive approaches, which constitute the *informal stage* of role acquisition. As the mother adapts her own personal style to enacting maternal role behaviors and becomes increasingly comfortable and confident in her style, she enters the final or *personal stage* of role acquisition. This final stage culminates in the development of maternal identity.

*Maternal identity* is the personal relationship that the mother develops with a specific child. The development of maternal identity follows a similar process as that of maternal role acquisition. The pregnant woman may construct an ideal image of herself as a mother. Following the birth of the baby, the mother begins to view herself less as the expert or idealized mother and more as one with the infant. As the mother becomes more intimately acquainted with the individual infant, she is able to differentiate her maternal self from the infant, and she establishes a more reciprocal relationship with the infant (Rubin, 1984). The development of the maternal identity and the attachment process with the child are two inextricable aspects of the same process. Walker, Crain, and Thompson (1986a) describe maternal identity as ". . . constructing a reciprocal relationship in which mothers establish both linkages and boundaries between themselves and their infants" (p. 68).

A number of factors may influence the process of role acquisition and the development of maternal identity. Mercer (1981) identified several factors, including maternal age, self-concept and other personality characteristics, perceptions of the birth experience, maternal health status, infant temperament and other infant characteristics, social support, and cultural and socioeconomic factors. Mercer (1985) studied the process of maternal role attainment in first-time mothers during the first year. Four maternal role attainment behaviors were studied to determine if these behaviors varied over time or were influenced by maternal age. Mothers in three age groups (15-19 years, 20-29 years, and 30-42 years) were interviewed at 1, 4, 8, and 12 months. All four role behaviors were found to differ over the course of the year. Mothers felt more positive about their babies at 4 months than at any other time during the first year. Their gratification with the maternal role reached its highest point at 4 months and decreased slightly at 8 months. Teenage mothers' gratification continued to decrease at 12 months, while 20- to 29-year-old mothers' gratification increased and 30- to 42-year-old mothers' gratification remained about the same. Maternal competency behavior increased between 1 and 4 months and fell slightly at 8 and 12 months. While teenage mothers exhibited this same pattern, they scored consistently lower than older mothers in competency behaviors. Ways of handling irritating child behavior changed over time, with maternal responses becoming more positive from 1 month to 8 and 12 months.

Walker, Crain, and Thompson (1986a, b) studied maternal identity, mothering behaviors, and maternal role acquisition in both primiparous and multiparous mothers during the postpartum period. Mothers showed increased self-confidence in care of the baby and more positive attitudes about themselves between birth and 4 to 6 weeks postpartum. However, their attitudes toward their babies were less positive at 4 to 6 weeks than immediately after birth. Multiparas were more confident than primiparas in infant care activities and expressed more positive attitudes toward themselves and their babies than did primiparas. Walker et al. (1986b) also examined whether these subjective components of maternal roles were related to behavioral indicators of maternal role attainment. Maternal attitudes toward self at the time of the birth of the baby were positively related to the mothers' demonstrated sensitivity and responsiveness to the baby during feeding at 4 to 6 weeks. For primiparas, the mothers' self-confidence in infant care at 4 to 6 weeks was positively related to sensitivity during feeding.

These studies highlight the development of mothering attitudes and behaviors over the course of the first year. It is clear that mothers' feelings of regard for themselves and their infants, self-confidence, and competency change over time as they become better acquainted with their infants and the demands of motherhood. Maternal age and parity are influential factors in developing the maternal role. Other research has demonstrated that the infant is a powerful partner in developing reciprocal relationships. While these studies did not examine the contribution of the infant to the mothers' attitudes and feelings, it is likely that the developing infants' behaviors were influential and may also help to explain differing findings at the different time periods.

## Attachment and Parent-Infant Relationships

The early work of Bowlby (1958) explored the concept of *attachment* from an ethnographic perspective. Specific attachment behaviors, the primary purpose of which were to provide protection for the child, were identified. These behaviors are sucking, clinging, following, crying, and smiling. In later works, Bowlby (1969, 1982) expanded on his theory of attachment. The hallmark of attachment behavior is described by its purpose and its specificity. The behaviors have as their purpose maintaining or restoring proximity to the mother. The infant

develops individual recognition of the mother and exhibits differentiated behaviors toward her. Bowlby described a variety of attachment behaviors. *Orienting behaviors,* such as gazing, tracking, and fixating on the mother's face and rooting and sucking help to orient the infant to the mother. *Signaling behaviors,* such as smiling, crying, babbling, and vocalizing serve to alert the mother and bring her into closer contact with the infant. *Contact behaviors,* such as grasping, clinging, embracing, following, and clambering up, are used to achieve and maintain contact.

Attachment behaviors infer the existence of an attachment and may be used as indicators of attachment. Ainsworth (1973) defined attachment as "an affectional tie that one person forms to another specific person, binding them together in space and enduring over time" (p. 1). Attachment develops as a result of parent-infant interaction and the development of reciprocal relationships. Klaus and Kennell (1982) explored the development of the parents' bond with their infant. They postulated the existence of a sensitive period immediately after birth during which parental contact with the newborn infant is crucial in establishing the basis for attachment. Specific events important to the development of the mother's bond with her infant were identified. These events include planning for the pregnancy, confirming the pregnancy, feeling fetal movement, labor and birth, seeing and touching the infant after birth, and providing care for the infant. Klaus and Kennell recommended significant changes in the existing health care practices to assist parents to bond with their infants. The presence of a supportive companion (spouse, partner, or friend) during labor and the birth process provides the mother with reassurance and encouragement. This practice also allows the partner to be more involved in the birth process and to share the first interaction with the new infant. Allowing the parents privacy and the opportunity for an extended period of contact (preferably skin-to-skin contact) with the infant immediately after birth were recommended to enhance the development of attachment. These practices have been widely adopted and are now commonplace in most hospitals and birthing centers.

The development of attachment is a complex process of reciprocal interactions between infant and caregiver. Barnard (1978) identified the conditions necessary for effective parent-infant interaction as clear cues emitted by both infant and parent, sensitive responses by the parent to the infant's cues, infant responsiveness to the parent's care, and a supportive environment. Pressler (1990) elaborates on these factors in her review of the attachment literature. Caregiver sensitivity is composed of three aspects: emotional availability, sensitive responsiveness, and consistency of responsiveness. *Emotional availability* denotes warmth and affection, which is readily available to the infant. *Sensitive responsiveness* incorporates contingency in responding to infant needs, initiating behavior based on infant signals, pacing one's behavior with the infant's state and behavior, and avoiding interrupting and overstimulating or understimulating the infant. *Consistency of responsiveness* means predictable behaviors occurring over time. (See Table 32-2.)

 **Table 32-2**
Areas to assess in parent-infant relationships

| Child characteristics | Parent-characteristics |
|---|---|
| Infant state | Tactile contact |
|   Quiet sleep |   Touching, stroking |
|   Active sleep |   Holding |
|   Quiet awake |   Enfolds infant |
|   Active awake |   Comforts infant |
|   Crying | Visual contact |
| Infant temperament |   Establishes eye contact |
|   Activity level |   *En face* positioning |
|   Rhythmicity of behavior |   Expressive face with infant |
|   Soothability | Auditory stimulation |
|   Adaptability |   Talks to infant |
|   Intensity of response |   Sings |
|   Distractibility |   Laughs |
|   Attention span and persistence |   Soothing sounds |
|   Distress to approach or limitsVisual contact | Playful interactions |
|   Establishes eye contact |   Engages infant in appropriate play |
|   *En face* positioning |   Enjoyment of play |
|   Expressive face with infant | Emotional availability |
| Care-eliciting behaviors |   Readily available warmth and affection |
|   Physical appearance | Sensitive responsiveness to infant's cues |
|   Crying |   Contingency of response |
|   Smiling |   Initiates behavior based on infant's signals |
|   Vocalizations |   Paces behavior with infant state and behavior |
|   Grasping, clinging, following | Consistency and predictability of response |
| Behavioral organization | |
|   Infant behaviors and responses are organized | |
|   Develops predictable schedule of sleep, feeding, activities | |
| Clarity of cues | |
| Responsiveness to parents | |

## Fathering Behaviors

Fathers were forgotten figures until relatively recently. Their general lack of availability in health care and research settings, as well as cultural and social expectations and norms, contributed to the obscurity of fathers' contribution to parenting and childrearing. Recognition of the importance of fathers to the developing child has sparked a growing body of literature and research on fathering.

Changes in the social and economic environment have led to an increased role for fathers in child care and childrearing. The women's movement, the need for two-income families, and changing cultural definitions of appropriate sex role behavior have provided increased opportunity for fathers to become involved with their children. The degree of paternal involvement has been examined in terms of interaction, availability, and responsibility (Lamb, Pleck, Charnov, & Levine, 1987). While there is considerable variation in the amount of time and degree of responsibility reported, it is interesting to note the customary degree of paternal involvement. Paternal interaction or the direct contact the father has with his children is reported to range from 15 minutes to 2 1/2 hours per day. Fathers' interactions are about a third of mothers' interactions, but they increase when the mother is employed and also with older children. Availability, or the fathers' accessibility to the child, regardless of whether or not interaction occurs, shows a similar pattern. Fathers are reported to be available to children from 1.75 to 4 hours daily (Lamb et al., 1987). Responsibility or taking charge of the care of and arrangements for the child is still the primary purview of the mother. For many fathers, caretaking is a discretionary activity.

Despite these low figures, there is evidence that paternal involvement has increased (Lamb et al., 1987; Rossi, 1987). How much fathers are involved is influenced by a variety of factors, including motivation to become involved, perceived or real lack of child care skills, support

from significant others, and institutional factors, such as employment practices (Lamb et al., 1987). Nursing is in a particularly favorable position to provide interventions that will increase fathers' child care skills and influence social support for fathers.

Differential responsiveness of mothers and fathers to infants has been postulated. There has been some attempt to argue for a biological basis for increased receptivity in mothers to infants' signals. Evidence from animal models, citing hormonal influences, has been advanced in support of this notion (Lamb et al., 1987). However, studies indicate that fathers exhibit sensitivity and responsiveness to infant cues and behaviors. First-time fathers responded to crying infants with an affectionate and comforting touch. Infants who were awake but not crying elicited more stimulating touch behaviors from fathers. Affectionate talking was more likely to occur with boys and with infants who were awake or crying (Jones & Lenz, 1986). Further support for fathers' sensitivity to infant cues comes from a study of physiological responses during father-infant interactions. Specific cardiovascular responses (increased systolic and diastolic BP and increased heart rate) were noted during the interaction period. Of particular interest is the finding of increased diastolic BP during interaction with a crying infant, which persisted into the postinteraction period (Jones & Thomas, 1989). Since these physiological responses are not under conscious control, it is apparent that paternal sensitivity to the infant is present. Differential socialization of men and women is a more likely explanation for differences in parental behavior found between men and women (Lamb et al., 1987).

As with mothers, fathers' early interactions with the infant serve as a basis for attachment (Klaus & Kennell, 1982). Greenberg and Morris (1974) use the term *engrossment* to describe the emotions and behaviors exhibited by fathers at the birth of their infants. Fathers demonstrate awareness of their newborn through looking at, touching, and noting the distinct features of the infant. They regard their infant as perfect and focus on the infant. Fathers describe their response to the birth of their infant as a "high" and exhibit elation and an increased sense of self-esteem (p. 520). While the care-taking function of fathers tends to be limited, fathers do interact with and develop attachment to their children. However, differences in style of parental behavior between mothers and fathers have been noted. Fathers are more likely to respond to gross motor activities, use intermittent physical and social stimulation, and engage in physical play activities (Lamb et al., 1987). Despite differences in parental style, father-infant attachment does occur.

## ❖ PARENTING IN SPECIAL CIRCUMSTANCES

The birth of a preterm, ill, or handicapped infant may disrupt or make more difficult the usual parenting process. The stress and demands of a child with special needs also places additional stress on the developing role of a parent. The impact a preterm, ill, or handicapped child has on parents is examined in the following section.

### Parenting the Preterm Infant

The premature birth of an infant initiates a variety of difficulties and potential problems. Both short-term and long-term consequences result from a preterm birth. These consequences affect both infant and parents and play a significant role in the interaction between the two.

Prematurity is defined as gestational age of less than 37 weeks or birth weight of less than 2500 grams. Due to the immaturity of various body systems, the premature or low birth weight (LBW) infant is subject to numerous physiological problems and complications that threaten the infant's physical well-being and survival. The infant's health status generally requires special care in a neonatal intensive care unit (NICU), ranging from several weeks to several months. This set of circumstances has an impact on the parents and their ability to begin the parenting role in numerous ways. Parents are seldom prepared for the birth of a preterm infant. They may experience shock and grieve for the loss of their idealized child. The first week is a particularly stressful time for parents (Trause & Kramer, 1983). The fragility of the infant's health and the concern for survival make this event a crisis situation for the parents. Adding to the stress and anxiety experienced by the parents is the unfamiliar environment of the NICU and the appearance of the infant. The variety of equipment and interventions necessary to support the infant's functions are overwhelming to parents. The small size and characteristic appearance of premature infants may be frightening to those unfamiliar with them. Parents benefit greatly by orientation to the NICU environment, explanation of the infant's characteristics and behaviors, and information about the child's health and progress.

Subsequent weeks may be characterized by periodic crises as the infant experiences a variety of complications or setbacks. Parents' anxiety is again heightened by these episodes. As the threat of the infant's death diminishes, parents begin to focus on other worrisome aspects. The financial drain of the prolonged and specialized care required by the infant is a frequent source of stress. Parents may also be concerned about the infant's long-term health problems and their ability to provide care for the infant. As the time for discharge of the infant approaches, parents may again experience a high level of stress as they confront the task of caring for the LBW infant without the support of the hospital staff and environment. Brooten, Gennaro, Brown, Butts, Gibbons, Bakewell-Sachs, and Kumar (1988) found that mothers experienced greater anxiety and depression around the time of the infant's discharge from the hospital than they did several months after discharge. Multiparous mothers and mothers of infants who had longer hospitalizations experienced more depression at discharge than other mothers.

The opportunity for parents to begin attachment to their infant can be disrupted or delayed. The early separation of infant and parents and the limited physical contact necessitated by the infant's health status and supportive devices interfere with the attachment process. In addition, LBW infants may not exhibit the usual attachment behaviors that help draw the parents to them. These early experiences have implications for attachment during infancy and the child's ability to establish intimate relationships later in life.

The developing parent-infant relationship is dependent on mutual engagement of parent and infant in responsive, reciprocal, and contingent interactions. The interaction of parents and LBW infants is made more difficult by the unique characteristics and behaviors of the preterm infant and the parents' responses to and perceptions of their infant. LBW infants display a number of characteristics that are not typical of full-term infants. Infant state, behavioral organization, and temperament are salient factors in the infant's behavior. Preterm infants tend to be less alert, more difficult to arouse, and less attentive to visual and auditory stimuli. Their behavioral organization is less mature and more likely to be disorganized and unpredictable. Preterm infants have limited behavioral repertoires and do not send clear behavioral cues. A weak cry, limited energy, and behavioral disorganization combine to make the infant's distress signal unclear. Preterm infants tend to be more irritable, fussy, and difficult to soothe (Magyary, 1984; Ramey, Bryant, Sparling, & Wasik, 1984).

The infant characteristics, coupled with the parents' grief, stress, and anxiety, and the limitations imposed by the NICU environment are serious deterrents to establishing mutually rewarding parent-infant interactions. Evidence exists that the difficulties encountered in early interactions can persist well into infancy. Preterm infants experience later developmental problems in the areas of perceptual-motor, cognitive, and social development (Ramey et al., 1984; Schraeder, 1986). Mothers of preterm infants have been found to differ from mothers of full-term infants in their interactions with and response to their infants during the first 6 months (Magyary, 1984). Mothers of preterm infants showed higher levels of activity in initiating and continuing interactions than mothers of full-term infants. They also tended to provide more constant stimulation to the infant, while full-term mothers provided stimulation more contingently based on infant behaviors. The preterm infants tended to be less responsive, exhibited negative affect, and were less likely to initiate interactions with their mothers than were full-term infants. Some mothers continued an intrusive, noncontingent style of interacting with their infants into later infancy or became less responsive to their infants. However, other mothers are able to develop a more contingent and responsive pattern of interaction with their babies. The change to a more rewarding interchange is likely to be a result of the increased skill of the mother in reading the infant behaviors and to the increased maturity and developmental abilities of the infant (Magyary, 1984).

The parents' perception of their LBW infant may interfere with their ability to respond appropriately to the infant. The infant's characteristics, behavior, and history of health problems may lead the parents to view their child as vulnerable. The perception of vulnerability can cause parents to lower their expectations for the child and to behave accordingly. The infant responds to the parents' behavior and reinforces their notion of vulnerability and lower expectations. This "self-fulfilling prophecy" can adversely affect the parent-infant relationship (Stern & Hildebrandt, 1986).

Parenting a LBW infant is no easy task. Many factors such as those described above conspire against the establishment of mutually satisfying parent-infant relationships. Further complications arise from the circumstances with which premature births are associated. LBW infants are more likely to be born to adolescent mothers, mothers from low socioeconomic environments, and mothers who lack prenatal care (Ramey et al., 1984). In many respects, these mothers have greater stresses and fewer resources with which to meet the demands of caring for a LBW infant. Interventions that focus on providing supportive relationships, improving parental social competence with their infants, increasing understanding of child development, and improving use of available resources have proven effective in supporting positive parent-infant relationships and development (Barnard, Magyary, Sumner, Booth, Mitchell, & Spieker, 1988; Beckwith, 1988; Osofsky, Culp, & Ware, 1988).

## Parenting a Chronically Ill or Handicapped Child

Estimates of the number of children affected by chronic illness range from 10% to 15% of all children in the United States. Approximately 1% to 2% of children are severely affected by chronic illnesses (Hobbs, Perrin, & Ireys, 1985). Survival rates for a number of chronic illnesses have increased as a result of advances in medical science and health care. Improved technology and systems of care have enhanced children's ability to survive trauma, premature birth, and other previously fatal diseases. Despite improved survival, the resulting chronic health problems or handicapping conditions may impose significant demands on the parents and families of the affected children.

The birth of an infant with a physical or mental disability often precipitates a crisis situation for the parents. Parents begin developing ideas of what their child will be like before the birth of the infant. When the reality of the infant (such as the birth of an ill or handicapped child) fails to match the parents' ideal or fantasized image, significant adjustment is required on the part of the parents (Horan, 1982; Romney, 1984; Zamerowski, 1982). Romney (1984) identifies as a developmental task of parenting the need "to resolve the discrepancy between the ideal and real infant" (p. 8). The greater the discrepancy between the real and the ideal, the greater the difficulty in completing this task. Parents experience mourning for the loss of the fantasized infant while attempting to integrate the handicapped child into their own sense of identity as a parent and a family (Romney, 1984; Zamerowski, 1982).

Parents experience a variety of emotions and responses to the birth of a handicapped infant. Shock, numbness, disbelief, and denial are often initial responses of parents. Parents may feel overwhelmed and helpless in light of the obstacles facing them. Feelings of sadness, grief, anxiety, anger, guilt, and blame are frequently present (Horan, 1982; Romney, 1984; Zamerowski, 1982). Fortier and Wanlass (1984) described five stages through which families of handicapped children progress following diagnosis: impact, denial, grief, focusing outward, and closure. Families are affected in behavioral, affective, sensory, interpersonal, and cognitive aspects. The *impact stage* begins when the diagnosis is disclosed to the family. This period is one of anxiety and disorganization. Parents may display behaviors of agitation or appear dazed and lethargic. Physiologic symptoms usually associated with anxiety, such as nausea, diarrhea, and feeling faint, may be experienced by the parents. Cognitive processes may be disrupted and parents may appear to be disoriented and confused. Denial follows soon after the impact of the diagnosis is felt. The *denial stage* may provide parents with temporary protection from becoming overwhelmed and allow them the opportunity to absorb the situation incrementally. Hope is sustained by denial and is necessary to assist parents in their day-to-day functioning. However, protracted denial is usually considered to be maladaptive. Parents may shop around for a new diagnosis or cure during this stage. They may engage in wishful thinking and avoid anyone or anything that would contradict their view of events.

During the *grief stage,* parents may experience sleeplessness, crying, and fatigue. The feelings of anger, helplessness, guilt, and blame are most evident during this stage. Parents may begin to doubt their abilities to cope with the situation and manage care of the child. The question of why this happened often arises, and parents may engage in a search for the cause or the meaning of the situation. Parents feel isolated, as if they were the only ones experiencing this event. Following the expression of grief, the parents are often ready to direct their *focus outward*. They may have regained some confidence in themselves and have more energy to devote to beginning coping efforts. Fortier and Wanlass (1984) view this stage as a period when parents are most open to intervention. Parents are ready to seek information, discuss options, and make plans for the care of the child. The final stage, *closure*, is the beginning of the mobilization of efforts to deal with the child's problem. Increased family cohesion and acceptance of the situation are positive outcomes of this stage (Fortier & Wanlass, 1984).

While much of the literature and professional interventions focus on the crisis period surrounding diagnosis of a serious illness or handicap, continued support for parents after this period is frequently lacking. Parental grief and other emotional responses do not necessarily disappear when the initial crisis period is over. Rather, many parents experience chronic sorrow, the periodic resurfacing of feelings of loss and grief throughout the life of the child. Damrosch and Perry (1989) examined whether the adjustment patterns of parents of children with Down Syndrome reflected the experience of chronic sorrow. Significantly different patterns of adjustment were found for mothers and fathers. Eighty-three percent of the fathers in the study described their adjustment as gradual and steady. Sixty-eight percent of the mothers, on the other hand, described their adjustment as a chronic, periodic crisis. Often the periodic crises are precipitated by developmental or situational events. The child's failure to meet a developmental milestone, such as walking, talking, or going to school at the appropriate age may trigger a grief reaction in the parent. The onset of a health problem or deterioration in

the child's health may also precipitate a reevocation of the parents' fears, sorrow, and grief.

Because of the improved outlook for many chronic diseases, parents are faced with long-term management of the illness and related care for their child, as well as performing parenting functions. Numerous stresses are present when raising a chronically ill or handicapped child. Parents may experience increased feelings of distress and lower self-esteem, especially for mothers (Goldberg, Marcovitch, MacGregor, & Lojkasek, 1986). There may be a lowered sense of parental competence and satisfaction in the parenting role, particularly for fathers (Cummings, 1976), increased strain in the marital relationship (Barbarin, Hughes, & Chesler, 1985; Hymovich & Baker, 1985), and increased concern with financial matters (Hymovich & Baker, 1985; Kazak & Marvin, 1984). How well parents manage the situation depends on a number of factors. McCubbin and McCubbin (1987) have described the process by which families handle stressful situations. The multiple stresses and responsibilities inherent in usual family life are complicated by the demands of caring for a chronically ill or handicapped child. These stresses may accumulate or "pile up" and increase the difficulty experienced by the parents in managing the situation. How the parents perceive their situation, including how they view the particular stressors or demands and their ability to deal with them, is an important aspect of the parents' response. The resources available to parents and their ability to use the existing resources or develop new ones is also a significant factor. Resources may include personal strengths and skills, financial or material assets, social supports and services available from other family members, friends, professionals, and community members and organizations. Lastly, the coping behaviors or strategies used to manage the stresses and demands associated with parenting a chronically ill or handicapped child are of critical importance in the parents' adaptation.

Numerous studies have examined the coping strategies used by parents of children with chronic illnesses or handicapping conditions. These studies provide a rich description of how parents cope. Barbarin et al. (1985) described the coping strategies used by parents of children with leukemia. The most frequently used strategies were acceptance, problem solving, optimism, emotional balance, and information seeking. The strategy used least frequently was help seeking. Fathers tended to use denial more than mothers, while mothers were more likely than fathers to use religion and information seeking as coping strategies. McCubbin (1989) identified three coping patterns used by parents of children with cerebral palsy: family integration, cooperation, and an optimistic definition of the situation; maintaining social support, self-esteem, and psychological stability; and understanding the health care situation through communication with other parents and consultation with the health care team. Gibson (1986), using McCubbin and McCubbin's family stress and adaptation model, studied coping in parents of children with cystic fibrosis. Coping behaviors that emphasized doing things as a family, strengthening family relationships, and maintaining a positive outlook on life were found to be the most helpful approaches. Understanding the health care situation was also cited as being very helpful. Mothers engaged in behaviors to strengthen family integration more frequently than fathers. Damrosch and Perry (1989) also found significant differences in how mothers and fathers of children with Down Syndrome coped. Mothers reported using all coping behaviors more frequently than did fathers. The coping strategies most frequently used by mothers were cognitive restructuring, wish-fulfilling fantasy, information seeking, and expression of negative affect. Fathers cited cognitive restructuring, wish-fulfilling fantasy, and information seeking as their most frequently used coping behaviors.

Darling and Darling (1982) identified normalization as the most important task of parents of handicapped children. Normalization is an important coping strategy for parents and has benefits for the affected child and other children in the family. Children, both handicapped and nonhandicapped, need to engage in usual childhood activities and events. Appropriate developmental progression is aided by the process of normalization. Knafl and Deatrick (1986) describe normalization as a cognitive process in which the handicap is acknowledged but the implications or significance of it are minimized. Parents' efforts to normalize the situation may include carrying out usual parenting behaviors, attempting to make the child's appearance as normal as possible, identifying and avoiding embarrassing situations, avoiding contact with other families with a handicapped child, and controlling information about the child's condition. While some of these strategies may appear to be counterproductive to help seeking and social support, it is important to recognize their existence and the role they play in parents' ability to manage their child's illness or handicap. Normalization is important in the areas of discipline, sibling relationships, school experiences, and how parents deal with repeated hospitalizations for health problems (Scharer & Dixon, 1989).

A variety of factors influence how parents cope. It is evident that fathers use different coping strategies than mothers. Undoubtedly, different socialization patterns and social norms influence the coping strategies developed. Other factors that affect parents' coping include the severity of the child's illness or handicap (McCubbin, 1989), the marital relationship (Barbarin et al., 1985), whether it is a single parent family or a two-parent family (Gibson, 1986; McCubbin, 1989), the number of children in the family, and the age of the affected child (Gibson, 1986). It is important that these factors be considered when assessing parents' coping abilities and planning interventions.

## ❖ THE NURSE'S ROLE

Nurses are in a position to help parents adapt to their roles and support them as they strive to accomplish developmental tasks. Interventions designed to promote and enhance

**Table 32-3**
Nursing interventions to foster development of adaptive parenting

| Goals | Nursing strategies |
|---|---|
| Facilitate the development of supportive relationships. | ◆ Establish therapeutic, helping relationship to support parents' development of adaptive parenting behaviors.<br>◆ Actively listen to parents—reflect, clarify, and restate ideas.<br>◆ Validate parents' positive actions. Offer praise, encouragement, and positive feedback. Discourage maladaptive parenting behaviors.<br>◆ Act as a sounding board.<br>◆ Assess social support available.<br>◆ Help parents identify and develop additional sources of social support. |
| Improve parental social competence with their infants. | ◆ Assist parents to identify infant cues and responses to parents.<br>◆ Identify for parents the effect of their behaviors on the infant.<br>◆ Serve as a role model for parents in interacting with infant.<br>◆ Establish parent support groups. |
| Increase parents' understanding of child development. | ◆ Provide information on developmental milestones and expectations.<br>◆ Use tools such as the Brazelton Neonatal Assessment Scale and the Denver Developmental Screening Test to demonstrate accomplishments.<br>◆ Demonstrate infant and child care skills.<br>◆ Use a variety of teaching approaches, including one-on-one teaching, group sessions, pamphlets, books, and videotapes.<br>◆ Provide anticipatory guidance for the next developmental level. |
| Improve use of available resources. | ◆ Refer parents to appropriate health and social services.<br>◆ Help parents rehearse contacts with other providers of health or social services.<br>◆ Act as an advocate for families. |
| Support the use of adaptive coping strategies for parents coping with the stresses of parenthood. | ◆ Provide information about the stresses being encountered by the parent.<br>◆ Help parents to explore alternatives for dealing with problems or stressors.<br>◆ Actively listen to parents and allow parents to express feelings.<br>◆ Assist parents to use social support resources.<br>◆ Teach new skills needed by parents to manage the situation. |

adaptive parenting are presented in Table 32-3.

## ❖ SUMMARY

Parenting is a complex task that is influenced by both the characteristics of the parent and the child and the ongoing transactions between them. Social norms and expectations, social support, and the personal and social resources available to parents affect how the parenting role is enacted. Societal pressures and changes greatly influence how the parenting role is perceived and supported. The development of beginning parenting skills and early parent-child interactions are a prime time for nursing interventions directed toward strengthening the parents' capabilities and competencies. Periods of crisis or stress, such as those associated with the birth of a preterm infant or the diagnosis and ongoing care of chronically ill or handicapped child, are opportune periods for nurses to support and assist parents with their task.

## ❖ APPLYING KNOWLEDGE TO PRACTICE

1. Identify, from your clinical practice or your personal experience, a family experiencing the birth of a new baby. Discuss the following areas in relation to this family:
   a. Identify areas of stress for the parents of the new baby. What strategies did they use to cope with the stress? What supports were available to the parents?
   b. Describe behaviors of both parents and infant that indicated developing attachment relationships. How much involvement did the father have in this family?
   c. Discuss nursing interventions that assist parents in adjusting to the parenting role and support the development of positive parent-infant interactions and attachment.
   d. Identify resources available in your community to support the parenting role in beginning families.
2. Describe a family who has experienced the birth of a preterm infant. What initial responses did this family exhibit?

   a. Describe the parent and infant characteristics that impeded development of attachment in preterm infant-parent relationships.
   b. Discuss what interventions were successful in promoting positive parent-infant interactions and enhancing the infant's development.
   c. Identify resources in your community that assist families with preterm infants.
3. Describe the responses of parents when a child is diagnosed with a chronic illness or handicapping condition.
   a. Discuss what coping behaviors or strategies you have observed in families who have a chronically ill or handicapped child. Were there differences in the strategies that mothers and fathers used? Which strategies did you think were most helpful for parents?
   b. Identify what factors in your clinical setting support or hinder parents' coping.

## REFERENCES

Ainsworth, M. D. S. (1973). The development of infant-mother attachment. In B. M. Caldwell & H. N. Ricciuti (Eds.), *Review of child development research* (Vol. 1, pp. 1-94). Chicago: University of Chicago Press.

Barbarin, O. A., Hughes, D., & Chesler, M. A. (1985). Stress, coping, and marital functioning among parents of children with cancer. *Journal of Marriage and the Family, 47,* 473-480.

Barnard, K. E. (1978). *Nursing child assessment training instructor's leaning resource manual.* Seattle: University of Washington, School of Nursing.

Barnard, K. E., Magyary, D., Sumner, G., Booth, C. L., Mitchell, S. K., & Spieker, S. (1988). Prevention of parenting alterations for women with low social support. *Psychiatry, 51,* 248-253.

Beckwith, L. (1988). Intervention with disadvantaged parents of sick preterm infants. *Psychiatry, 51,* 242-247.

Bowlby, J. (1958). The nature of the child's tie to his mother. *International Journal of Psychoanalysis, 39,* 350-373.

Bowlby, J. (1969). *Attachment and loss. Vol. 1. Attachment.* New York: Basic Books, Inc.

Bowlby, J. (1982). *Attachment and loss. Vol 1. Attachment.* New York: Basic Books, Inc.

Brooten, D., Gennaro, S., Brown, L. P., Butts, P., Gibbons, A. L., Bakewell-Sachs, S., & Kumar, S. P. (1988). Anxiety, depression, and hostility in mothers of preterm infants. *Nursing Research, 37,* 213-216.

Crnic, K. A., Greenberg, M. T., Ragozin, A. S., Robinson, N. M., & Basham, R. B. (1983). Effects of stress and social support on mothers and premature and full-term infants. *Child Development, 54,* 209-217.

Cronenwett, L. R. & Kunst-Wilson, W. (1981). Stress, social support, and the transition to fatherhood. *Nursing Research, 30,* 196-201.

Cummings, S. T. (1976). The impact of the child's deficiency on the father: A study of fathers of mentally retarded and of chronically ill children. *American Journal of Orthopsychiatry, 46,* 246-255.

Damrosch, S. P. & Perry, L. A. (1989). Self-reported adjustment, chronic sorrow, and coping of parents of children with Down Syndrome. *Nursing Research, 38,* 25-30.

Darling, R. & Darling, J. (1982). *Children who are different.* St. Louis: C. V. Mosby Co.

Duvall, E. M. (1977). *Marriage and family development* (5th ed.). New York: J. B. Lippincott.

Erikson, E. H. (1963). *Childhood and society* (2nd ed.). New York: W. W. Norton & Company, Inc.

Fortier, L. M. & Wanlass, R. L. (1984). Family crisis following a diagnosis of a handicapped child. *Family Relations, 33,* 13-24.

Friedman, M. M. (1986). *Family nursing: Theory and assessment* (2nd ed.). Norwalk, Conn.: Appleton-Century-Crofts.

Gibson, C. H. (1986). How parents cope with a child with cystic fibrosis. *Nursing Papers/Perspectives En Nursing, 18,* 13-24.

Goldberg, S., Marcovitch, S., MacGregor, D. & Lojkasek, M. (1986). Family responses to developmentally delayed preschoolers: Etiology and the father's role. *American Jouranl of Mental Deficiency, 90,* 610-617.

Greenberg, M. & Morris, N. (1974). Engrossment: The newborn's impact upon the father. *American Journal of Orthopsychiatry, 44,* 520-531.

Hobbs, N., Perrin, J. M., & Ireys, H. T. (1985). *Chronically ill children and their families.* San Francisco: Jossey-Bass Publishers.

Horan, M. L. (1982). Parental reaction to the birth of an infant with a defect: An attributional approach. *Advances in Nursing Science, 5,* 57-68.

Hymovich, D. P. & Baker, C. D. (1985). The needs, concerns and coping of parents of children with cystic fibrosis. *Family Relations, 34,* 91-97.

Jones, L. C. & Lenz, E. R. (1986). Father-newborn interaction: Effects of social competence and infant state. *Nursing Research, 35,* 149-153.

Jones, L. C. & Thomas, S. A. (1989). New fathers' blood pressure and heart rate: Relationships to interaction with their newborn infants. *Nursing Research, 38,* 237-241.

Kazak, A. & Marvin, R. (1984). Differences, difficulties and adaptation: Stress and social networks in families with a handicapped child. *Family Relations, 33,* 67-77.

Klaus, M. H. & Kennell, J. H. (1982). *Parent-infant bonding.* St. Louis: C. V. Mosby Co.

Knafl, K. A. & Deatrick, J. A. (1986). How families manage chronic conditions: An analysis of the concept of normalization. *Research in Nursing and Health, 9,* 215-222.

Lamb, M. E., Pleck, J. H., Charnov, E. L., & Levine, J. A. (1987). A biosocial perspective on paternal behavior and involvement. In J. B. Lancaster, J. Altmann, A. S. Rossi, & L. R. Sherrod (Eds.), *Parenting across the lifespan: Biosocial dimensions* (pp. 111-142). New York: Aldine De Gruyter.

Magyary, D. (1984). Early social interactions: Preterm infant-parent dyads. *Issues in Comprehensive Pediatric Nursing, 7,* 233-254.

Mercer, R. T. (1981). A theoretical framework for studying factors that impact on the maternal role. *Nursing Research, 30,* 73-77.

Mercer, R. T. (1985). The process of maternal role attainment over the first year. *Nursing Research, 34,* 198-204.

McCubbin, M. (1989). Family stress and family strengths: A comparison of single- and two-parent families with handicapped children. *Research in Nursing and Health, 12,* 101-110.

McCubbin, M. & McCubbin, H. (1987). Family stress theory and assessment: The T-double ABCX model of family adjustment and adaptation. In H. McCubbin & A. Thompson (Eds.), *Family assessment inventories for research and practice* (pp. 3-32). Madison, Wisconsin: University of Wisconsin.

Osofsky, J. D., Culp, A. M., & Ware, L. M. (1988). Intervention challenges with adolescent mothers and their infants. *Psychiatry, 51,* 236-241.

Pressler, J. L. (1990). Promoting attachment. In M. J. Craft & J. A. Denehy (Eds.), *Nursing interventions for infants and children* (pp. 4-17). Philadelphia: W. B. Saunders Company.

Ramey, C. T., Bryant, D. M., Sparling, J. J., & Wasik, B. H. (1984). A biosocial systems perspective on environmental interventions for low birth weight infants. *Clinical Obstetrics and Gynecology, 27,* 672-692.

Romney, M. C. (1984). Congenital defects: Implications on family development and parenting. *Issues in Comprehensive Pediatric Nursing, 7,* 1-15.

Rossi, A. S. (1987). Parenthood in transition: From lineage to child to self-orientation. In J. B. Lancaster, J. Altmann, A. S. Rossi, & L. R. Sherrod (Eds.), *Parenting across the life span: Biosocial dimensions* (pp. 31-81). New York: Aldine De Gruyter.

Rubin, R. (1984). *Maternal identity and the maternal experience.* New York: Springer Publishing Company, Inc.

Scharer, K. & Dixon, D. M. (1989). Managing chronic illness: Parents with a ventilator-dependent child. *Journal of Pediatric Nursing, 4,* 236-247.

Schraeder, B. D. (1986). Developmental progress in very low birth weight infants during the first year of life. *Nursing Research, 35,* 237-242.

Servonsky, J. & Opas, S. R. (1987). *Nursing management of children.* Boston: Jones & Bartlett.

Stern, M. & Hildebrandt, K. A. (1986). Prematurity stereotyping: Effects on mother-infant interaction. *Child Development, 57,* 308-315.

Trause, M. & Kramer, L. (1983). The effects of premature birth on parents and their relationship. *Developmental Medicine and Child Neurology, 25,* 459-465.

Ventura, J. N. (1982). Parent coping behaviors, parent functioning, and infant temperament characteristics. *Nursing Research, 31,* 269-273.

Ventura, J. N. (1986). Parent coping, a replication. *Nursing Research, 35,* 77-80.

Walker, L. O. (1989a). A longitudinal analysis of stress process among mothers of infants. *Nursing Research, 38,* 339-343.

Walker, L. O. (1989b). Stress process among mothers of infants: Preliminary model testing. *Nursing Research, 38,* 10-16.

Walker, L. O., Crain, H., & Thompson, E. (1986a). Maternal role attainment and identity in the postpartum period: Stability and change. *Nursing Research, 35,* 68-71.

Walker, L. O., Crain, H., & Thompson, E. (1986b). Mothering behavior and maternal role attainment during the postpartum period. *Nursing Research, 35,* 352-355.

Zamerowski, S. T. (1982). Helping families to cope with handicapped children. *Topics in Clinical Nursing, 4,* 41-56.

# 33 Loss

Shirley A. Murphy ◆ Beverly A. Osband

## OBJECTIVES

*At the completion of this chapter, the reader will be able to:*

◆ **Define key concepts: attachment, loss, bereavement, grief, and mourning.**

◆ **List common characteristics of all loss experiences.**

◆ **Apply the nursing process to one unique loss experience.**

Loss as a major life theme can be understood as one reflects on the expressions of its meaning throughout history. Artists, musicians, writers, philosophers, and scientists have documented the effects of loss on individuals, families, and communities. Throughout this chapter we emphasize the experience of loss and how its meaning guides clinical nursing practice. One goal of the chapter is to convey that loss is a common universal phenomenon. We use the life span perspective to point out ordinary loss events, because these events pose considerable challenges in adaptation. The second and major goal of the chapter is to communicate the concept of loss as a unique or extraordinary experience, which makes assessment and intervention a sensitive and individualized process between the nurse and client. We present clinical research findings and case examples that illustrate varied human responses within the same individual over time and among persons experiencing the same event at the same time. This chapter has four major sections: (1) loss as

a universal human experience; (2) loss as a theoretical construct; (3) factors that affect loss experiences, assimilation, and resolution; and (4) clinical nursing applications.

## ❖ LOSS AS A UNIVERSAL HUMAN EXPERIENCE
### Common and Unique Qualities of Loss

Themes of separation and loss are threaded throughout the life cycle, beginning with birth as the newborn infant is separated from the mother and ending with death as relationships undergo permanent physical separation. In between these two entry and exit events, life's ordinary experiences with separation and loss are essential for learning the meaning of personal autonomy and developing a sense of mastery over life experiences. Normative losses associated with growth and development, such as one's first day of school, leaving home, and marriage, all link gains with loss. However, common losses not linked with gains, at least initially, include loss of one's job, loss of friends through relocation, and the multiple losses that occur with divorce. The most profound loss one can experience is the death of a person who is loved. The family and sociocultural environments provide an important context for learning how to cope with life changes, which include both gains and losses and are unique to each individual.

According to Benoliel (1985), "the extent to which a given experience of loss is *major* for an individual depends on a combination of circumstances and contingencies: (a) the significance of the attachment to the individual and its special meaning, (b) the degree to which the relationship is replaceable, (c) the amount of personal and social disruption produced by the loss, (d) the vulnerability level of the person in terms of time in the life cycle when loss occurs, and (e) the nature of the surrounding situation—supporting or nonsupporting of the person" (p. 222).

### Loss Experiences in Western Culture

There are few cultural norms for handling loss. The exception is death. The history of civilization confirms that the most profound loss one experiences is the death of a valued other. Although the universality of death is recognized, it is kept as remote and impersonal as possible. Blauner (1966), in a provocative paper, *Death and Social Structure,* wrote that mortality in modern society rarely interrupts the business of life. The consequences of "modern death control" as Blauner called it, are that persons may die alone and that there is less emphasis on a formal period of mourning. The expectation that the bereaved return to normal activities of living as quickly as possible after the death of a significant other increases the social distance between the living and those who have died. Thus death is pushed further and further out of the minds of the living. While other losses such as the loss of a job or divorce

may seem less shattering than death, these losses are profound to those experiencing them. Yet the grief process that follows is often unrecognized.

### ❖ LOSS AS A THEORETICAL CONSTRUCT
### Definition of Key Terms

The grief and loss literature uses several key words that have complex meanings and that may have different meanings for the lay person and the professional. The following definitions will clarify the meanings of these words as they commonly occur in the professional literature. Contrary to some usage, the terms are *not* interchangeable.

**Attachment:** reflects the propensity of human beings to develop strong affectional bonds to particular others (Bowlby, 1980; Osterweis, Solomon, & Green, 1984).

**Loss:** is a state of being deprived of something that was once available and important and now is gone (Benoliel, 1982). Loss may be physical/tangible or symbolic/psychosocial. A divorce, job change, or demotion may represent symbolic changes that are often not recognized as a loss.

**Bereavement:** the fact of loss through death (Osterweis et al, 1984); the state of having suffered a loss (Rando, 1984). Bereavement entails ongoing change and adjustment in every aspect of life including role relationships, social interactions, and economic factors (Murphy, 1983).

**Grief:** the feeling (affect) and certain associated behaviors, such as crying—also sorrow, anxiety, agitation, sleeplessness, lack of interest in things, frequent gastrointestimal complaints, loss of appetite, and seriously impaired social functioning (Osterweis et al, 1984). Grief is an *intrapersonal, affective* reaction to loss (Murphy, 1983). Grief is a *process,* not a *problem.* It is an essential and healthy coping response to loss; however, it is difficult to describe "typical" grief because of the diversity of behaviors among individuals. Apparent absence of grieving (Bowlby, 1980), extreme and prolonged social isolation, and suicidal ideation are atypical and are a basis for professional intervention (Lindemann, 1944).

**Mourning:** the *social* expression of grief, including mourning rituals and associated behaviors.

The reader is likely to be familiar with Kubler-Ross's stages of grief (denial, anger, bargaining, depression, and acceptance), which are commonly used by health professionals and the general public to understand human responses to loss. Kubler-Ross's conversations with dying persons have been a significant catalyst for bereavement research, and most importantly, her work has made discussion of death and dying more acceptable in our society. However, we do not apply the Kubler-Ross model in this chapter. Our rationale is as follows: (1) the stages have remained descriptive (i.e., no testable hypotheses have evolved to guide research); (2) the stages apply only to grief response, yet research on major loss events have demonstrated that they are too complex to be explained by affective factors alone; and (3) the final stage, acceptance, suggests that this stage can be observed in a limited period of time, which is true for terminally ill clients from whom the model originated. In contrast, bereavement research findings have shown that resolution following the death of a significant other is rarely achieved in a matter of months. For these reasons, two alternative theoretical perspectives are offered to guide the nursing process.

## Theoretical Perspective: Tasks of Mourning

Worden (1982) wrote that both cognitive and affective efforts are required to assimilate loss experiences. The four *tasks* of mourning are to (1) accept the reality of the loss, (2) experience the pain of grief, (3) adjust to the environment in which the deceased is missing, and (4) withdraw emotional energy and reinvest it in another relationship. Nurses can be involved in facilitating all four tasks by using the therapeutic communication skills of listening, clarifying, validating, and summarizing; by giving permission to grieve and explaining that the grieving process is painful but normal and necessary; and by teaching coping skills to manage the third and fourth phases. Moreover, there is demonstrated need to educate the general public regarding the tasks of loss assimilation. Recent research documents the lack of understanding of human responses to loss through examples of inappropriate remarks and behaviors of well-intentioned persons toward bereaved family members, friends, and colleagues (Davidowitz & Myrick, 1984).

## Theoretical Perspective: Transition Theory

A *transition* is defined as "a passage or change from one place or state or act or set of circumstances to another" (Tyhurst, 1957, p. 150). A transitions perspective offers a useful way to conceptualize human responses to loss.

Transitions are of three basic types: maturational, situational, and health-illness. *Maturational transitions* are sometimes called developmental and occur at key points in the life cycle. *Situational transitions* occur as a result of a stressful life event that at least temporarily taxes ones resources. *Health-illness transitions* occur when changes need to be made to manage a chronic illness. These types of transition frequently overlap in the experiences of human beings and are commonly accompanied by both important losses and gains, and most importantly, require adaptation to significant life change. For example, one maturational transition, the passage from adolescence to young adulthood, involves the development of both the young person and his or her parents. A discrete event within the transition, leaving home, provokes feelings of both gain and loss from both generations and may have elements of situational and health/illness transitions. Pennebacker (1988) studied college freshmen who reported to university health facilities for illness. He found that those who could disclose their feelings and draw cause and effect relationships between leaving home and their illness responses coped better with loss and change.

Crucial to understanding the concept of transition are the following: (1) one's assumptions or structures of meaning enable one to understand the world and to interpret his or her experiences in it; (2) assumptions shape behavior; (3) events, especially uncontrollable and unpredictable ones such as death, challenge or change assumptions, undermine meaning of the world and one's place in it, and lead to perceptions of stress; (4) change encompasses not only external circumstances, but more importantly, self-perceptions; (5) stresses associated with loss and change require passage of time to cope with change and incorporate role and identity change, and require several kinds of support.

## ❖ TRANSITION DIMENSIONS: FACTORS AFFECTING LOSS EXPERIENCES AND THEIR ASSIMILATION/RESOLUTION

According to Schlossberg (1981) and others, three dimensions are essential to predict adaptations (the fourth dimension) to transitions and to assist individuals through transitions. These dimensions shown in Fig. 33-1 are the nature of an event or nonevent and the significance of its meaning to the individual involved, the attributes of the individual, and the resources and support available and used. Factors associated with an event and its meaning to the individual include the anticipation, type, timing, onset, and duration of the event, the perception of impact of the event on relationships, routines, assumptions, and roles. Factors associated with the individual include age, gender, ethnicity, state of health, psychosocial competence, socioeconomic status, beliefs and values one holds, and previous experience with a similar transition. Factors associated with resources and supports include composition of social network and resources and options avail-

| Loss event Dimension | Person Dimension | Resources and support Dimension |
|---|---|---|
| Type of loss | Age | Characteristics of social network |
| | Gender | |
| Timing in life cycle | Ethnicity | Availability of: |
| | Health Status | Support |
| | Coping/Efficacy | Resources |
| Details re: Impact | Socioeconomic status | |
| | Value orientation | |
| | Previous loss experience | |

Adaptation

Degree of success in managing transition

❖ **Fig. 33-1**   Assessment data needed for each loss transition dimension.

able. Adaptation depends on one's perceptions and one's resource and deficit balance. These factors have also been identified as central to the stress, coping, and health outcome process. At the end of this section we present studies pertaining to loss and demonstrate how transition perspective is used for assessment and intervention purposes.

## Transition Dimension: Characteristics of the Loss Event

**Types of loss.** Four major types of loss that can occur at any phase of the life cycle are (1) loss of aspects of self, (2) loss of context that defines one's reason for being (3) loss of meaningful interpersonal relationships, and (4) loss of valued objects. These are not mutually exclusive as shown in the examples provided.

The *loss of an aspect of the self* has many manifestations, may have a gradual or sudden onset, and may be temporary or permanent. Our first example portrays the loss of self in normal aging. Decremental losses include sensory losses (hearing, vision, taste), cognitive losses (short-term memory, confusion), physical losses (mobility, energy), and psychological losses (sense of worth, sense of future). A second example pertains to chronic illness. Persons with schizophrenia and Alzheimer's disease experience varying levels of awareness and express perceptions of depersonalization, self-derision, hopelessness, and guilt associated with burdens they place on family and caregivers. Significant others also experience loss as shown in our example of Catanzaro's research on p. 604.

*Loss of context* that defines one's reason for being occurs as a result of role loss. The loss of work, an achieved role, is an example of how the same loss is experienced very differently among persons the same age (cohort) at the same time. According to George (1980), retirement poses a threat to identity and social adjustment for some, making the return to work

after retirement common across all socioeconomic strata. Professionals who return to work do so because of the significance or value work holds for them.

A second role loss involves ascribed family roles and demonstrates unique responses over time to an event experienced more than once. The following brief case history illustrates this point.

Mr. and Mrs. K. were bereaved parents who participated in an intervention study conducted by the first author. The intervention was directed towards needs of parents whose adolescent and young adult children died suddenly following an accident. The K's daughter, 18 at the time of death, died instantly after her car was hit by a truck. The parents' gender responses were unique. Mr. K. was unable to function effectively at work whereas Mrs. K. found it helpful to be out of the home and at her work site. The K's lost an infant 15 years earlier to SIDS. Their grief was compounded as they became aware that they had not yet resolved the previous loss of a child.

*Loss of meaningful personal relationships* are major stressors that tax the coping capacities of those involved. Nurses frequently must assist clients to accept what cannot be changed, facilitate finding meaning, and teach coping skills. Common examples of these loss experiences are divorce among parents of dependent children and the death of a spouse, child, or parent.

*Loss of valued objects* frequently accompany forced relocation among the elderly and among victims of catastrophic loss. In Murphy's study of victims of a natural disaster, persons who lost their homes and belongings reported only moderate recovery, and their scores on a standardized measure of mental distress remained higher than comparison group scores, even 3 years after the event.

Group losses are increasingly receiving the attention of clinicians and researchers, partly because of the unique opportunity for assessment and intervention that promotes mutual self-care. Like individual losses, recent studies of group loss have shown that assimilation, accommodation, or recovery from loss is much more difficult than previously thought. Examples of group losses are victims of disaster, holocaust, war, and caregivers who share responsibility and concern for clients who die. The latter has important implications for groups of nurses who care for persons with AIDS, cancer, and trauma, clients who are more likely to die than other clients. Nurses and caregivers must also grieve and assimilate the loss.

**Timing of loss.** Timing in the life cycle and the perceived scope of the loss have been found to affect resolution. Deaths that occur "off time" and deaths of children and young or middle-aged adults are considered to be untimely as are those that are premature, unexpected, or calamitous (Weisman, 1973). Many consider that it is particularly difficult to achieve resolution following untimely or unnatural death (Rynearson, 1987). The perceived scope of the loss, whether through death, divorce, or illness, has implications for resolution. Rosen (1985) and Bank and Kahn (1982) note that the death of a sibling results in multiple losses for surviving children, regardless of age at the time of the loss. Role relationships are lost, familiar family roles must be renegotiated, and perhaps most significantly, bereaved parents are lost to the surviving children in the sense that they may be unavailable for parenting for some time following the death.

Wallerstein (1983), in her longitudinal study of children of divorce, notes that the long-term or "sleeper" effects of divorce are becoming apparent only many years after the event. In Wallerstein's study, children of divorce, as they entered adulthood, seemed to have difficulties with identity development, commitment to relationships, and achievement of goals 10 to 15 years after their parents divorced more often than their peers from intact families. Researchers are continuing to study the timing of divorce and its effects on children.

When loss is anticipated, a person may be in a better position to deal with the loss both cognitively and emotionally. However, in her studies of parental grief following the death of a child from cancer, Rando (1983) found that where loss is anticipated, particularly if there is a prolonged period of terminal illness, the outcome for survivors is worse.

Literature on developmental transitions and anticipatory guidance suggests that nurses have primary roles in preparing individuals, families, and community groups for predictable events and in providing interventions after unpredicted stressful events to prevent further negative effects of loss. The following example of nursing research demonstrates the impact of current innovation in nursing practice. Mishel and Murdaugh (1987), by careful nursing observations, identified the need for their study of family members and clients who underwent heart transplantation. A major finding they discovered was the unrealistic expectations family members held for "normal recovery" of the client. The authors described the sense of loss that emerges and how it was accommodated in the following excerpt of a published report: "The belief in a normal life is gradually eroded and the partner becomes *aware* of the necessity to redefine the term *normal*" (p. 335). The coping strategy used by spouses is defined by Lazarus and Folkman (1984) as emotion-focused coping (described in Chapter 26) and is one coping strategy taught to clients and families following loss.

## Transition Dimension: Characteristics of the Person

Individual factors include one's age, gender, ethnicity, health status, coping strategies, socioeconomic status, value orientation, and previous experiences with loss. While the grief response is unique to each individual, studies suggest that there are some characteristics of a person that are associated with increased likelihood of problems in grief resolution. In their critical bereavement literature review, Osterweis and colleagues (1984) cited the following findings:

1. Following bereavement, males over 75 had a statistically significant increase in mortality, especially in the first 12 months, though the rate continues to be higher for up to 6 years.
2. Substance use (alcohol, cigarettes, tranquilizers) increases among the bereaved, particularly if they were already using the substances.
3. Depressive symptoms are common among bereaved persons in the early months following the loss, though among bereaved spouses, between 10 to 20% reported continued feelings of depression up to a year later.
4. Among risk factors for a poor outcome following loss are poor physical health, alcoholism and substance abuse, and perceived lack of social support.
5. Studies suggest that perceived adequacy of social support and remarriage following spousal loss are associated with better bereavement outcomes.
6. Among bereaved children, the following have been observed to be associated with poor outcome:
   a. Loss of a parent or sibling before age 5 years or during adolescence.
   b. Preexisting psychological or emotional problems in all children.
   c. Conflicted relationship with the deceased person.
   d. Parents who become dependent on a child following a loss.
   e. Lack of or failure of parent(s) to make use of family and community support services.
   f. Perceived multiple losses following death, which are associated with lack of stability in the home and inconsistent or unavailable parenting.
   g. Lack of knowledge about death.
   h. Sudden, unexpected death.
   i. Death caused by suicide or homicide. (McClowry, Gilliss, Martinson, 1989; Martinson, Davies, McClowry, 1987; Osterweis et al, 1984; Rosen, 1985).

In their long-term follow-up study of siblings who had lost a brother or sister to cancer, Martinson and associates (1987) found that children whose parents valued them as unique individuals, who did not compare them unfavorably to the dead sibling but rather spoke with pride of the child for who he or she is, and who were in no way made to feel guilty for the sibling's death, had higher self-concepts than the norm. Other characteristics of families who seem to do better following the loss of a child include open communication among family members, redistribution of roles within the family and not assigning one child to take on the role of the deceased, and availability of and use of supports within the family and community (McClowry et al, 1989).

## Transition Dimension: Mediating Factors

Despite its appearance in hundreds of studies in the past decade, much remains to be learned about social support. Except for the mutual support group movement, very little is known about help seeking following major loss, or about *who* provides *what kind* of support at *what time* and for *how long*. Some of the most needed areas of research are the analysis of helpful and unhelpful transactions, particularly between bereaved persons and supportive others and the costs and benefits of being a primary support person (Davidowitz & Myrick, 1984; Lehman, Wortman, & Williams, 1987).

Mutual support shows promise as an effective strategy to mediate the effects of loss on health and well-being for several reasons. First, primary support persons become depressed and exhausted and may not be effective support providers throughout the transition. Second, group involvement with others whose plight is similar is very powerful. Group participants learn that the concerns and pain they are experiencing are shared by others. Thus these similarities provide the impetus for discussion on how to manage what has happened (Osterweis et al, 1984).

### Transition Dimension: Assimilation/Resolution of Loss

The problems in defining resolution of loss lie within how individuals experience and progress through the tasks of grief. Whether using the Kubler-Ross model or Worden's (1982) tasks of mourning, the ultimate goal for the bereaved person is to accept or adjust to the loss. What does it mean to accept, adjust to, resolve, or integrate a loss into one's life? Worden (1982) states that resolution is subjectively defined. Some losses are never completely resolved, yet emotional energy is invested elsewhere.

With respect to some losses, this seems a reasonable process. If one loses a job and finds another, it is reasonable to imagine withdrawing energy from the old work while putting time, effort, and interest into the new position. The same may be said of moves from one locale to another, necessitating the development of new friendships and other relationships. Over time, one may stay in touch with past relationships, but with time, one invests in new ones.

Problems arise, however, when one considers the resolution of losses through death. The parental loss of a child, a child's loss of a parent, and spousal loss are all losses through death that challenge the notion of resolution, adjustment, and acceptance. There are several reasons for this difficulty. Perhaps the most compelling is the nature and meaning of the relationship. Marris (1974) has observed that it is not so much the loss that is difficult, but the meaning of the lost relationship that mitigates against a willingness to withdraw from the lost relationship and invest in another.

Among bereaved parents, there is fear that to withdraw from the relationship with the dead child is to make it seem as if the child had never been. For the child who loses a parent, the loss is one that has ramifications for the child's long-term development (Rando, 1986). A young child depends upon his or her parents for protection and nurturing and for security in an uncertain world. The loss of a parent seriously threatens the child's developing sense of self and may lead to dependency and clinginess in later relationships and a tendency toward anxiety when threatened with separation (Parkes & Weiss, 1983).

With time, the bereaved individual is generally able to give up internalized roles related to the deceased person and develops new ones. Memories of the deceased no longer elicit overwhelming feelings of sadness and pain as they once did.

In summary, a variety of factors affect one's ability to resolve a loss, including the nature of the loss, whether it is death, divorce, or loss of self in terms of identity or physical losses, which occurs with aging or illness. In addition, age at the time of loss, the perceived preventability of the loss, and availability and use of family and community systems all figure in resolution following loss.

### ❖ CLINICAL APPLICATIONS: LIFE CYCLE PERSPECTIVE

As already indicated, loss affects people differently depending in part on where they are in the life cycle. To a large extent the effect is a function of the developmental tasks a person faces at different stages of the life cycle in relation to the meaning that the loss has.

## Childhood and Loss

Much of what we understand about the effects of loss in childhood comes from the work of Bowlby (1980) who looked at the phenomenon of attachment and loss in children with an awareness that early childhood experiences of loss seemed to influence the way people dealt with loss in later life.

For the infant who is developing a sense of trust (vs. mistrust) (Erikson, 1963), the responsiveness of caregivers to cries for food, dry diapers, cuddling, and warmth will determine the extent to which the infant perceives the world as a good place and himself or herself as worthy of the attention of others. The first experiences of loss have to do with the frustration of these basic needs (Benoliel, 1985). At this stage the child is also learning something about his or her own self-efficacy. The child whose cries consistently meet with success in terms of need satisfaction develops a sense of efficacy. By contrast, the consistent frustration of needs by neglectful or disinterested caregivers is thought to teach the child that he is ineffectual in getting his needs met (Seligman, 1975). In later life, these early experiences appear to influence the grief response following various types of loss.

## Adolescence and Loss

For the adolescent, the development of identity (vs. role diffusion) is a central task (Erikson, 1963). While earlier experiences that have built a sense of self-efficacy are still important, the adolescent who is in the process of separation and individuation seems particularly vulnerable to loss. In their extensive review, Osterweis and associates (1984) noted that adolescent boys who lose their fathers are at risk for depression. However, other studies (Balk, 1983; Martinson et al, 1987) suggest that if home life was good before a death, adolescents seemed to make very good adjustments.

## Research Summary: Death of a Parent in Childhood or Adolescence

**Introduction.** Sandler, Gersten, Reynolds, Kallgren, and Ramirez (1988) developed an empirically based intervention for bereaved children. Of primary concern to the investigators were factors that affected psychological adaptation over time to the death of a parent. They studied 91 bereaved children between the ages of 8 and 15. A control group of children were matched on age, gender, and neighborhood.

**Risk assessment.** Bereaved children were found to be at risk for depression, conduct disorder, and anxiety. There were no significant reductions in these risk factors 30 months following the death of a parent. Next the investigators determined several additional environmental risk factors: an insufficient caretaking environment, negative life events since the death of the mother or father, and demoralization of the remaining parent.

**Intervention.** Sandler and associates (1988) developed a family bereavement program that included two components: a family grief workshop composed of three informational support sessions and a family advisor program that supplemented peer emotional support to the bereaved parent and children. The problem-focused and emotion-focused (see Chapter 26 for descriptions of these terms) intervention is currently being tested for its effectiveness in reducing risk.

## Adulthood and Loss

For young adults between the ages of 26 and 40, the central developmental tasks have to do with generativity (vs. stagnation) (Erikson, 1963), tasks that revolve around achievements including those related to family (childbearing

# ❖ NURSING CARE PLAN

**CLIENT:** Susan B., 28-year-old schoolteacher

**CLINICAL DESCRIPTION:** Susan's mother, Jane, died 2 weeks ago following a prolonged illness with metastatic breast cancer. Jane died at home where she had been cared for by Susan (her only child) and a hospice team, consisting of a nurse, an aide, a social worker, in consultation with a physician. Susan is presently living in the family home because she gave up her apartment 1 year ago to live with and care for her widowed mother. Since her mother's death 2 weeks ago, Susan is finding it difficult to sleep through the night, waking frequently to check on her mother, only to remember that she is dead. Susan has requested "something to help me sleep." She is also finding it difficult to concentrate at work and reports feeling anxious. Susan returned to work 3 days after her mother's funeral.

**SUPPORT SYSTEMS:** No siblings; Several elderly aunts and uncles; Fiancé, John A.; Several friends at work and in church

**NURSING DIAGNOSES:** Acute grief response associated with mother's recent death
Sleep disturbance associated with acute grief response
Difficulty concentrating and feelings of anxiety possibly related to acute grief response.

| SHORT-TERM GOALS | NURSING INTERVENTIONS |
| --- | --- |
| Susan will accept the reality of her mother's death over the next several weeks | ◆ Provide Susan with opportunity to talk about her mother's illness and death. |
| Susan will know some common manifestations of acute grief | ◆ Discuss with Susan some common manifestations of acute grief including: sleep disturbance, preoccupation with the image of the deceased, sighing, rapid heart rate and sensations of physical pain—sometimes in the area of the stomach or in the chest. |

## ❖ NURSING CARE PLAN—cont'd

| LONG-TERM GOAL | NURSING INTERVENTIONS |
|---|---|
| Susan will be able to experience her grief as a healthy response to a serious loss. | ◆ Reassure Susan that while everyone grieves differently, what she is experiencing is a normal part of acute grief—she is not sick or crazy.<br>◆ Explore with Susan how it was for her when her father died. |

**EVALUATION**

On a short-term basis, Susan expresses recognition that her current difficulty in sleeping is a normal response to her recent loss. Over the next few weeks, she is able to recognize additional responses to grief that she is experiencing without becoming alarmed. She exhibits a beginning acceptance of the reality of death when she talks about her mother in the past tense and reports fewer occurrences of waking to care for her mother. She gives up internalized roles related to her mother and begins to develop new ones as she moves toward resolution of the loss. On a long-term basis, Susan will incorporate coping strategies learned with this loss into future experiences of loss.

and childrearing), and occupation. Loss that threatens family relationships, whether that of a child or spouse, seriously threatens the accomplishment of adult developmental goals. Physical changes that result from illness or accidents also have the capacity to frustrate a sense of accomplishment. Previous experiences with loss, a sense of self-efficacy, and the availability of support systems will influence how an adult responds to loss. Resolution of a loss occurring in young adulthood is illustrated in the nursing care plan.

### Research Summary: Death of a Child in Middle Adulthood

**Introduction.** Lehman, Wortman, and Williams (1987) studied 41 bereaved parents whose children died as a result of a vehicular accident. All children were under 18 years of age and living at home at the time of the accident. Data were also collected from 41 matched controls.

**Risk Assessment.** Risk factors identified among the parents up to 7 years following the accidents were: lowered self-esteem, depression, impaired role performance, and divorce.

**Intervention.** Murphy (1990) used the risk factors identified by Lehman and others (1987) to design a preventive intervention to ameliorate the effects of parental loss. The intervention consisted of a 6-week program of informational support and emotional support program based on these risk factors. The intervention was tested with experimental and control groups. Paper and pencil test results, parent, and group leader evaluations of the type and timing of the intervention demonstrated therapeutic effectiveness and will be tested with a sample of 200 parents over time. Longitudinal data will be collected and analyzed to determine whether risk reduction effects can be maintained.

### Aging and Loss

In later adulthood and for the elderly person, there is a greater expectation that a spouse or friends will die. At this stage, loss of one's independence, health, mobility, and often the resulting loss of possessions as one may need to enter a nursing home appear to constitute multiple losses to which the elderly are particularly vulnerable (Benoliel, 1985; Osterweis et al, 1984).

### Research Summary: Chronic Illness in a Spouse

**Introduction.** Catanzaro (1990) studied 67 marital dyads in which one member was diagnosed with multiple sclerosis and the other member assumed the major caretaking role of the affected spouse. The spouses were interviewed separately, and some standardized measures were used to determine outcomes.

**Risk assessment.** Two high-risk groups were identified. The most severely affected

group in the sample was women under 50 years of age whose husbands were diagnosed with progressive neurological disease. They reported the highest rates of depression, lowest rates of self-esteem, more social isolation, and were more inclined to take full responsibility for caretaking than other groups in the study. The second most severely affected group was men over 50 years of age. Their responses were expressed outwardly in the form of anger and frustration.

**Intervention.** A supportive intervention is currently being designed for testing by Catanzaro. The plan includes mutual support with aged peers who need assistance with caretaking and recognizing their own needs.

### ❖ NURSING PROCESS APPLICATION When Loss is not the Presenting Problem

**Loss history.** Whenever a nurse begins a new relationship with a patient or client, it is essential that a loss history be incorporated into the initial assessment. The approach and specific questions will vary with the age of the person, but documentation of significant losses should become a permanent part of that person's written record.

With respect to children, the nurse will want to know whether the child has experienced any significant losses and what the child's understanding is of the loss. McCowan (1988) developed the "Childhood Death Awareness Inventory." When using this tool, the nurse can systematically record data regarding experiences the child has had with the death of another (whether a pet, a friend, or a relative); the rituals the child has experienced around loss; beliefs the child has about death; what the parents or others have told the child about death; and supportive measures that were found to be helpful. While this inventory relates specifically to death, similar kinds of questions can be asked with respect to other transitions that are occurring in the child's life including those related to school, peers, and family.

In working with adults, it is equally important to obtain information regarding significant losses. Asking an opening question such as "Since we last talked, have there been any major changes—losses or gains—in your life?", provides the client with an opportunity to share important information with the nurse. It is important to note, however, that the way one asks questions may influence the completeness of the data obtained. For example, when interviewing a woman of childbearing age, it is more informative to ask if she has ever been pregnant and if so, how many pregnancies she has had and how many live children she now has. These questions quickly establish whether there have been miscarriages, stillbirths, or children who have died. These questions are far more informative than simply asking, "How many children do you have?" Men are less likely than women to be asked about losses related to childbearing, yet they are also affected by such losses. Again, a general inquiry about life transition—gains and losses—may provide an avenue for obtaining important information during assessment. It is also essential to ask specifically about use of alcohol, cigarettes, and other drugs, since increased use has been noted among persons coping with loss.

If a loss has occurred, it is essential to obtain information about when and how the loss occurred, whether it was anticipated or unexpected, and how activities of daily living (Carnevali, Mitchell, Woods, & Tanner, 1984) are now as compared to before the loss. Lindemann's (1944) study of grief reactions showed that following the death of a significant other, survivors are likely to experience a variety of symptoms including changes in sleep, appetite, gastrointestinal function, ability to concentrate, and relations to others. Somatic complaints frequently prompt one to seek health care in the period following a loss; however, without

an adequate loss history an important causative factor for the symptoms will be missed.

**Nursing diagnoses.** In developing nursing diagnoses related to loss, it is helpful if the nurse first explores with the client how the loss has affected everyday life. Exploring common behaviors related to sleeping, eating, work, and social life in comparison to such behaviors before the loss will allow the nurse first to develop some hypotheses about the areas of concern and later to develop accurate diagnoses that clearly reflect the client's needs (Carnevali et al, 1984). While it is tempting to provide sample diagnoses, these will prove of little value in practice inasmuch as the diagnosis should be specific to the client's actual problem. The diagnosis should reflect what the client is experiencing and the etiology or cause of the problem. Care planning, implementation, and evaluation would be based on assessment of functional behaviors listed above.

## When Loss is the Presenting Problem

**Assessment.** Fig. 33-1 shows the specific data to be obtained following a loss perceived to be problematic by oneself or concerned others. Since grieving is a painful but manageable process by most persons, only about 10% will seek professional assistance. The data in the loss event dimension is usually easily obtained by encouraging the person to "tell their story." After listening carefully, the nurse should validate what issues are important to the individual. In the individual dimension, the nurse should obtain specific data on coping. What problem-focused and emotion-focused strategies are being used? To what extent are they working? Finally, what supports are available? Is there a match between what is needed and what is available? The nurse should inquire about assistance that is perceived as nonsupportive as well as supportive and what can be changed to improve hurtful encounters. Assessment of risk, referral, and specific interventions can be planned around data collected. Signs of atypical adjustment such as the apparent absence of grieving or the opposite extreme effects, such as prolonged clinical depression or inability to find meaning in the loss should be noted, and plans for referral should be made.

**Intervention.** Recommended intervention would be further evaluation, referral for individual counseling, or referral to a mutual support group. Precise interventions are difficult to specify because, for the most part, assimilation and finding meaning are done cognitively and affectively by the individual. The assessment interview usually is therapeutic in itself. Often clients will remark, "this is the first time anyone has listened to me."

**Evaluation.** Evaluation is a neglected area in both research and clinical practice. Replication of studies is highly desirable. Evaluation in clinical practice is difficult because of short inpatient stays and lack of funds to follow up clients who participate in community-based programs.

## ❖ SUMMARY

This chapter emphasized that loss is both a common and unique experience. Theoretically, loss can be best understood as a major life transition that must be grieved and assimilated over time. A life cycle perspective, a transitions framework, and research-based examples were used to describe loss experiences. The importance of obtaining a loss history from all persons was emphasized. Finally, the nursing process was used to exemplify the kind of data needed for assessment, risk identification, and potential interventions to assist persons who have difficulty managing loss.

## ❖ APPLYING KNOWLEDGE TO PRACTICE

1. Explore some personal loss experiences with another member of your class after both of you have read this chapter.
   a. What vulnerabilities were apparent at what point(s) in your life cycle? (i.e., did you have multiple major losses as a child, adolescent, or young adult?)
   b. Trace the process you used to find meaning in the loss and its assimilation into your life experience.
   c How did you know when the loss was "resolved"?
2. Also with another member of your class, select one of the research-based examples of loss described in the chapter on pp. 601 and 603. Construct a brief case history of an individual. Have your partner become the client and you the nurse. Conduct a loss history or an assessment interview and record data obtained. Plan two priority interventions based on the data. Now switch roles and repeat the process.

**REFERENCES**

Balk, D. (1983). Effects of sibling death on teenagers. *The Journal of School Health, 53*(1), 14-18.

Bank, S.P. & Kahn, M.D. (1982). *The Sibling Bond.* New York: Basic Books, Inc.

Benoliel, J.Q. (1982). *Women and loss: The many faces of grief.* (221-233) In: G. Hongladarom, R. McCorkle, N.F. Woods (Eds.). *The Complete Book of Women's Health.* Englewood Cliffs: Prentice-Hall Publishers.

Benoliel, J.Q. (1985). Loss and adaptation: Circumstances, contingencies, and consequences. *Death Studies, 9,* 217-233.

Blauner, R. (1966). Death and social structure. *Psychiatry. Journal for the Study of Interpersonal Process, 29,* 378-394.

Bowlby, J. (1980). *Loss: Sadness and depression.* New York: Basic Books.

Carnevali, D., Mitchell, P.H., Woods, N.F., & Tanner, C.A. (1984). *Diagnostic reasoning in nursing.* Philadelphia: J.B. Lippincott.

Catanzaro, M. L. (1990). Transitions in midlife adults with long term illness . In S.A. Murphy (ed.) Holistic Nursing Practice, (4)3, 65-73.

Davidowitz, M. & Myrick, R. D. (1984). Responding to the bereaved: An analysis of "helping" statements. *Research Record, 1,* 35-42.

Erikson, E. (1963). *Childhood and society.* (2nd ed) New York: Norton.

George, L. K. (1980). *Role transition in later life.* Monterey, CA: Brooks-Cole, 55-76.

Kalish, R. A. (1981). *Death, grief, and caring relationships.* Monterey, CA: Brooks-Cole, 235-254.

Lazarus, R. S. & Folkman, S. (1984). *Stress, appraisal and coping.* New York: Springer.

Lehman, D. R., Wortman, C. B., & Williams, A. F. (1987). Long-term effects of losing a spouse or child in a motor vehicle crash. *Journal of Personality and Social Psychology, 52,* 218-231.

Lindemann, E. (1944). Symptomatology and management of acute grief. *American Journal of Psychiatry, 101,* 141-148.

Marris, P. (1974). *Loss and change.* London: Routledge & Kagan Paul.

Martinson, I. M., Davies, E. B., & McClowry, S. (1987). The long-term effects of sibling death on self-concept. *Journal of Pediatric Nursing, 2,* (4), 227-235.

McClowry, S., Gilliss, C. L., & Martinson, I. M. (1989). The process of grief in the bereaved family. In Gilliss, C L., Highley, B. L., Roberts, B. M., Martinson, I. M. (Eds.) *Toward a Science of Family Nursing.* (pp. 216-225). Reading: Addison-Wesley Publishing Company.

McCowan, D. (1988). When children face death in a family. *Journal of Pediatric Health Care, 2*(1), 14-19.

Mishel, M. H. & Murdough, C. L. (1987). Family adjustment to heart transplantation: Redesigning the dream. *Nursing Research, 36,* 332-338.

Murphy, S. A. (1983). *Theoretical perspectives on bereavement.* In: P. Chinn (Ed.), *Advances in Nursing Theory Development.* (191-206). Rockville, MD: Aspen Systems (pp. 191-206).

Murphy, S. A. (1990). Preventive intervention *Image—Journal of Nursing Scholarship. 22(3), 174-179. Preventive intervention following accidental death of a child.*

Osterweis, M., Solomon, F., & Green, M. (1984). *Bereavement—Reactions, Consequences, and Care.* Washington, D.C.: National Academy Press.

Parkes, C. M. & Weiss, R. S. (1983). *Recovery from bereavement.* New York: Basic Books.

Pennebaker, J. W. (1988). Confiding traumatic experiences and health. In S. Fisher and J. Reason (eds). *Handbook of life stress, cognition, and health.* (671-684). New York: Wiley,

Rando, T. A. (1983). An investigation of grief and adaptation in parents whose children have died from cancer. *Journal of Pediatric Psychology, 8*(1), 3-20.

Rando, T. A. (1984). *Grief, dying and death—Clinical interventions for caregivers.* Champaign, IL.: Research Press Company.

Rando, T. A. (1986). *Parental loss of a child.* Champaign, IL: Research Press Company.

Rosen, H. (1985). Prohibitions against mourning in childhood sibling loss. *Omega, 15*(4), 307-316.

Rynearson, E. K. (1987). Psychotherapy of pathologic grief—Revisions and limitations. *Psychiatric Clinics of North America, 10*(3), 487-499.

Sandler, I., Gersten, J. Reynolds, K., Kallgren, C., Ramirez, R. (1988) In: Gottlieb, B. H. (Ed.). *Marshalling social support—Formats, processes & effects.* (pp. 53-83). Newbury Park, CA: Sage.

Schlossberg, N. K. (1981). A model for analyzing human adaptation to transition. *The Counseling Psychologist, 9,* 19-36.

Seligman, M. E. P. (1975). *Helplessness: On depression, development, and death.* San Francisco: W. H. Freeman.

Tyhurst, J. (1957). *The role of transition states—including disasters—on mental illness.* Symposium on Preventive and Social Psychiatry. Washington, D.C.: Walter Reed Army Institute of Research, 149-169.

Wallerstein, J. (1983). *Children of divorce: Stress and developmental tasks.* In: Garmezy, N. & Rutter, M. (Eds.). *Stress, Coping and Development in Children.* (pp. 265-302). New York: McGraw Hill Book Company.

Weisman, A. (1973). Coping with untimely death. *Psychiatry, 36,* 366-379.

Worden, J. W. (1982). *Grief counseling and grief therapy.* New York: Springer.

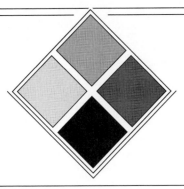

# 34

# Aging

Eleanore L. McCann ◆ Mary E. Soja
Joan L. Creasia

## OBJECTIVES

*At the completion of this chapter, the reader will be able to:*

◆ Describe the demographics and theories of aging.

◆ Discuss physiological, psychological, and sociological changes that commonly occur in aging and identify nursing interventions related to these changes.

◆ Describe health alterations in aging individuals and nursing interventions to address them.

◆ Identify services and agencies of benefit to older adults.

Aging is a process that defines the life cycle. It is natural and progressive, beginning at conception and ending at death. Aging occurs not only physically but also psychologically, socially, and spiritually and encompasses transitions from one life stage to another.

This chapter provides an overview of the later stages of life as a basis for the delivery of nursing care. Brief discussions of the demographics of the aging population and theories of aging are followed by more detailed descriptions of changes and transitions that occur later in the life cycle. Selected health alterations that commonly occur in the older adult are also described. Implications for nursing practice and associated interventions are highlighted throughout. Finally, services and agencies that can benefit older adults are identified.

## ❖ THE PROCESS OF AGING

Mechanisms involved in the aging process are growth, development, decline, dying, and death. These mechanisms operate at all age levels and, consequently, not only in utero but even in later life, a person continues to grow and develop. Aging is not a stagnant segment of life but is an ever-evolving, dynamic process with unlimited potential for actualization. Fig. 34-1 illustrates the concept of aging as a lifelong process.

Aging in the early part of life progresses rapidly and is viewed as a very positive process. Babies become toddlers, preschoolers, and finally teenagers. Aging in young adulthood and middle age, although not as dramatic as in early life, is also apparent, especially in the area of psychosocial development. In later life, changes

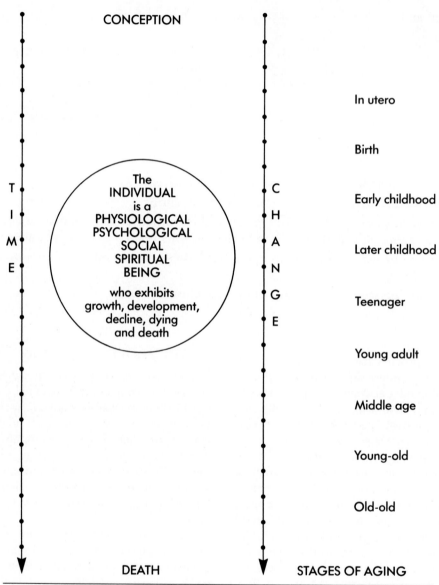

CONCEPTION

In utero

Birth

Early childhood

Later childhood

Teenager

Young adult

Middle age

Young-old

Old-old

The
INDIVIDUAL
is a
PHYSIOLOGICAL
PSYCHOLOGICAL
SOCIAL
SPIRITUAL
BEING
who exhibits
growth, development,
decline, dying
and death

T
I
M
E

C
H
A
N
G
E

DEATH                    STAGES OF AGING

❖ **Fig. 34-1**   The concept of aging across the life span.

related to aging occur more slowly and are often more subtle. Unfortunately, in our society, attitudes toward this stage of the aging process are not always positive. Robert Butler (1969), former director of the National Institutes on Aging, uses the term *ageism* to define societal bias against people based on age. It is similar to racism or sexism, but in this instance, it is a type of discrimination that will eventually be experienced by all.

The precise moment when later life begins is vague and undefined. People have different ideas about when a person is "old" or "mature" or a "senior citizen." Based upon political and economic definitions, the U.S. government has determined that later life begins at age 65. For some people, physical changes that indicate old age may not be seen until well into the seventies. A person who is still active and contributing to society may not consider himself old at age 80.

For the purpose of studying people in later years, arbitrary age categories have been established. The U.S. government has divided the older population into the young-old, 65 to 74; the old, 75 to 84; and the old-old, 85+. The young-old are usually relatively healthy, self-sufficient, independent, and experience freedom from tasks of middle age, such as employment and childrearing. In contrast, the old commonly manifest more health problems and are in greater need of assistance. While some of the old-old may still be self-sufficient, many need help with their daily activities. This latter group is the fastest growing segment of the U.S. population. In 1980, there were 2.3 million adults 85 years of age and older. In 2030, the number is projected to increase to 9.2 million as the post-World War II baby boomers "come of age" (U.S. Bureau of the Census, 1989).

## ❖ KEY TERMS

Comprehensive nursing care requires an understanding of the process of aging regard-

less of the setting where care is delivered. Not restricted to long-term care facilities, gerontological nursing is also practiced in acute care and community-based settings. To differentiate geriatrics from gerontology and relate these concepts to nursing, key terms are defined in Table 34-1.

## ❖ DEMOGRAPHICS

In all industrialized nations, the number of older adults is increasing. Currently in the United States, approximately 12.2% of the population is at least 65 years of age. Between 1980 and 2020, the total U.S. population is expected to increase 32%, while those 65 years of age and older will increase 103% (U.S. Bureau of the Census, 1989).

In the older age group, females outnumber males, since women usually outlive men by several years. It is estimated that a woman who is currently 65 will live another 18.6 years, while a man who is currently 65 will live another 14.8 years (American Association of Retired Persons, 1987). Women tend to outlive their husbands, and in 1980 there were approximately five times as many widows as widowers. (This is partially explained by the fact that widowers are more likely to remarry than are widows.)

The old-old usually have had less formal education than other age groups. Many of these people who grew up in urban areas went to work after the sixth or eighth grade, and for those who grew up in rural areas, education was not easily accessible. In contrast, the young-old population are more likely to have completed 12 years of education.

Most older people are capable of living independently within the community, either self-maintaining or with minimal support. Only 5% of the entire over-65 population are in institutions, either on a temporary or permanent basis. However, when the 85+ group is examined separately, 22% are in institutions. Most older adults live in their own homes, although they

❖ **Table 34-1**
Terminology associated with aging

| Term | Definition |
| --- | --- |
| GERONTOLOGY | A branch of knowledge dealing with aging, it is concerned with the effects of time on human development. It focuses on all aspects of aging (not merely problems) and acknowledges the possibility of continued growth of the whole person. It addresses various aspects of later life such as physical, psychosocial, economic, legal, spiritual, etc. The term is derived from the Greek, *geros*, meaning old men. |
| GERIATRICS | The branch of health care science (medical and nursing) that is concerned with the study of age, aging, health problems, disease, diagnosis, and treatment of disorders (physical and psychosocial) of older adults. |
| GERONTOLOGICAL NURSING | The scientific study and care of older adults that can occur in any setting and assists older adults to reach and maintain optimal, total functioning. |
| GERIATRIC NURSING | The care of older adults, primarily the ill aged in a medical setting. It is concerned with diseases of older persons for the purpose of assisting them to return to a higher level of functioning or to arrive at a peaceful death. |
| GERONTIC NURSING | Term suggested by Gunter and Estes (1979) that states that a gerontic nurse specializes in the total care of the older adult, which is not limited to illness or scientific principles but encompasses caring, maintenance of wellness, coordination, nurturance, and comfort using basic nursing methods and specialized knowledge. |

may also reside in apartments, retirement communities, congregate housing, hotels, boarding houses, or with relatives or friends (Matteson & McConnell, 1988). Women are more likely to live alone than are men; almost 41% of older women live alone in contrast with 15.6% of older men (U.S. Bureau of the Census, 1989).

Economic status varies widely. In 1987, 12.2% of older adults lived below the poverty level (U.S. Bureau of the Census, 1989). It is somewhat deceiving to compare the average net worth of all U.S. households ($32,667) with the net worth of over-65-year-old households ($60,266) (U.S. Bureau of the Census, 1989) since much of the older person's net worth is nondisposable (e.g., the cash value of a house

purchased many years earlier). Although the median income for older adults is steadily increasing, social security benefits continue to be a major means of support. Thus, after retirement, there is usually a decline in income. Even if the basic cost of living remains stable, reduced income may necessitate substantial lifestyle changes. In addition, more and more of a person's income is likely to be spent on health care or personal services. Those that are at high risk for being classified at poverty or near poverty levels are females, blacks, and those over the age of 75.

From this brief demographic view of older adults, the significance of these statistics on the need for and use of health care in later life is clear. As a person grows older, more health care is needed when there are fewer economic and personal resources available.

### ❖ THEORIES OF AGING

A number of people, from ancient times to the present, have proposed theories concerning the cause of aging and how to curtail it. No theory is all encompassing and universally accepted and although each theory has merit,

each also has limitations. An awareness of the prevalent theories of aging assists the nurse to better understand later life development and social interactions. The nurse can then draw from this knowledge base to plan and administer nursing care.

Theories of aging can be categorized as biological, psychological, and social. Selected theories are briefly described in Table 34-2, since an in-depth discussion is not within the scope of this chapter.

❖ **Table 34-2**
Theories of aging

| Classification | Theory | Main proposition |
|---|---|---|
| **Biological Theories of Aging** | | |
| Gene-Based Theories | Somatic Mutation | Random, spontaneous alterations in DNA or changes resulting from chemicals or radiation cause abnormalities in chromosomes and in cellular replication. As the cells replicate, the abnormalities are maintained and eventually lead to a decrease in cell function and death. |
| | Programmed Aging | A purposeful sequence of events is written in the genes that leads to age changes and determines an individual's life span. |
| Organ-Based Theories | Immunological | The ability of the immune system to produce antibodies decreases with age and the system becomes less able to discriminate between self and nonself. Normal cells are viewed as "foreign" and are damaged or destroyed, leading to an increase in autoimmune diseases and dysfunction that is associated with aging. |
| | Neuroendocrine | Loss of neurons and endocrine cells increases with age. Any decrease in function has a cascading effect on all aspects of the body and predisposes the person to age-associated changes and diseases. |
| Physiological Theories | Free Radical | Free radicals are molecules or atoms with an unpaired electron and, hence, are highly reactive. They are the result of metabolic processes and lead to damage of the cell membrane over time. Lysosomes of the cell interact with the damaged membrane producing an insoluble residue called lipofuscin. This substance accumulates in aging cells, leading to decreased cell function and disease. |

*Continued.*

❖ **Table 34-2**
Theories of aging—*cont'd*

| Classification | Theory | Main proposition |
|---|---|---|
| **Biological Theories of Aging—*cont'd*** | | |
| Physiological Theories—*cont'd* | Cross Link or Collagen | Molecular structures that are normally separate become linked or bonded with aging and become immobile, thereby damaging DNA and leading to mutation or cell death. When it occurs in collagen tissues, the result is a decrease in elasticity, solubility, and permeability, which leads to most changes associated with aging. |
| Other Theories | Evolutionary | After an organism has propagated, it is no longer useful; old age is superfluous and death results. |
| | Wear and Tear | Aging is the result of the accumulated stresses, strains, and injuries to an organism, which eventually is unable to repair or replace the damaged cells. |
| **Psychosocial Theories of Aging** | | |
| Behavioral Theories | Disengagement | States that older people become less interested in events around them and develop ego conservation and increased self-interest. The older adult withdraws from social interaction and roles; society allows and encourages this. If the older adult and society do not mutually withdraw, desynchronization occurs (Cumming & Henry, 1961). |
| | Continuity | Views personality as becoming more pronounced as one ages and as influencing one's life satisfaction regardless of role activity (Neugarten, Havighurst & Tobin, 1968). |
| | Activity Theory | Postulates that if older adults maintain optimal levels of social activity, this will lead to life satisfaction. A person's well being and happiness is achieved by activity, rather than by withdrawal (Lemon, Bengston & Peterson, 1972). |
| Developmental Theories | Developmental Tasks | Proposes that life is a series of tasks to be learned. If the tasks are well learned, satisfaction and reward result. If the tasks are poorly learned, the person has difficulty and social disapproval results. Later life is not perceived as a stagnant process but as a dynamic stage (Havighurst, 1972). |
| | Developmental | Recognizes that certain defined tasks have to be accomplished in later life (Peck, 1968). |

*Continued.*

❖ **Table 34-2**
Theories of aging—*cont'd*

| Classification | Theory | Main Proposition |
|---|---|---|
| | **Psychosocial Theories of Aging—*cont'd*** | |
| Psychological Theories | Freud | Focus is primarily on early life experiences and how these influence later life (1963). |
| | Jung | Building on Freud's ideas; the later part of life has the purpose of self-development and actualization (1976). |
| | Erikson | After life review, the person should reach self-acceptance, dignity, and ego integrity leading to satisfaction. If life has not been acceptable, it results in self-disgust and despair (1963). |
| Social Theories | Life Transitions | "Passages" have to be successfully experienced for progress to occur (Lowenthal, 1977; Sheehy, 1976). |
| | Exchange | Individuals continue interacting with each other as long as each gains from the exchange. As the adult ages, there is a perceived loss of power and a resultant decrease in socialization (Vaillant, 1977; Wentowski, 1981). |

## ❖ DIMENSIONS OF AGING

Comprehensive assessment of older adults requires knowledge of the numerous changes that typically occur in later life in order to differentiate between normal and abnormal manifestations. These changes can be classified as physical, psychological, and/or sociological. Selecting appropriate assessment and intervention strategies is facilitated by an appreciation of these dimensions of aging.

### Physical Manifestations

The rate and extent of physical change varies considerably from person to person. At some point, each body system begins to decline, requiring special considerations in assessing the client and in planning and administering nursing care. Table 34-3 lists common physical manifestations of aging that may result in physiological alterations and some associated nursing interventions.

## Psychological and Sociological Considerations

As a person progresses through developmental stages and life transitions, the composite of life experiences contributes to the uniqueness and individuality of the older adult. Valuable insight can be gained by assessing psychological and sociological aspects of the individual and his or her environment. The data can then be used as the basis for choosing nursing interventions that are appropriate and effective. Selected psychosocial changes related to aging are presented in the following section.

**Personality and coping.** Most older adults retain the same personality and coping styles they demonstrated when they were younger. *Personality* reflects the way an individual perceives and responds to life events and is illustrated by such characteristics as self-esteem, moods, values, and facial expressions. *Coping,* or the ability to minimize stress and master threatening conditions, is

*Text continued on p. 623.*

**Table 34-3**
Physical changes occurring in later life

| Normal changes | Nursing implications |
|---|---|
| **I. INTEGUMENTARY SYSTEM** | |
| A. Decreased subcutaneous fat layer resulting in decreased effectiveness as a thermal insulator. Loss of subcutaneous supporting tissue causes thinning of skin leading to folds, lines, wrinkles, and slackness. | A. Be aware of environmental temperature: not too & hot or too cold.<br>B. Increase padding on soles of shoes. Handle skin with care to avoid trauma, as with tape or restraints. Be aware of body image changes. Encourage good grooming. |
| B. Loss of skin turgor; loss of elasticity; sagging due to gravitational pull. Skin usually the first structure to show the most obvious changes of aging. | |
| C. Decreased mitotic activity and slowing of regenerative capacity. | C. Avoid trauma; know wound healing may take a longer time. |
| D. Increase of benign and malignant neoplasms. | D. Teach person to have any unusual skin lesion checked. Encourage surgical removal, if indicated. Encourage person to avoid overexposure to sun and use sun screens. |
| E. Decreased function of subaceous glands. Increased dryness (xerosis) of skin with cracking may allow entry of microorganisms. | E. Use lotions; use less hot water and soap. Prevent chapping; apply lotions over wet skin. |
| F. Loss of pigmentation over parts of the body due to decrease of melanocytes; produces aging pallor. Increased pigmentation clustering on exposed areas, such as face and hands. | F. Be aware of body image changes. Discourage use of expensive bleaching creams. Teach proper use of cosmetics and sun screens. |
| G. Hair distribution changes: male pattern baldness; less or no hair on lower extremities, trunk, axillae, pubic area; increased female facial hair. Increased coarseness of hair in nose, ears, and eyebrows, especially males. Hair loss begins in males about age 30; in females after menopause. | G. Be aware of body image changes. Understand the use of wigs, hair pieces. Recommend using a depilatory for females. Teach proper grooming and use of cosmetics. |
| H. Graying of scalp hair genetically determined; whites tend to gray earlier than blacks. Decreased hair follicle size with lighter, finer hair on scalp. Reduced activity and number of melanocytes causing loss of color and graying. | H. Understand possible use of tints or wigs. Teach proper grooming and hair care. |
| I. Decreased nail growth with changes in nail composition causing increased thickness, brittleness, and dull yellow appearance with longitudinal ridges. | I. Discuss nail care with proper trimming and filing. |

*Continued.*

❖ **Table 34-3**
Physical changes occurring in later life—*cont'd*

| Normal changes | Nursing implications |
|---|---|

### I. INTEGUMENTARY SYSTEM—*cont'd*

| | |
|---|---|
| J. Increased vessel fragility. May cause spontaneous rupture of subcutaneous vessels resulting in ecchymosis and senile purpura. Atrophy of epidermal arterioles impairing vasomotor mechanisms for temperature regulation; unable to dissipate heat or conserve heat. | J. Avoid trauma; teach about safety factors and possible environmental hazards. Be aware of environmental temperature and need for protective layers of clothing, either warm or cool. |
| K. Possible change in sensory nerve perception. | K. Teach to carefully test water and heating pad temperatures. Check feet for injury or trauma. |
| L. Atrophy of sweat glands. | L. Observe for inability to cope with heat. |

### II. RESPIRATORY SYSTEM

| | |
|---|---|
| A. Nose enlargement due to continued growth of cartilage. | A. Be aware of body image changes. |
| B. Increased calcification of costal cartilage, decreased mobility of chest wall with decreased pulmonary function. More muscle work required to move air. More reliance on use of diaphragm. More sensitivity to abdominal pressure, such as after a large meal or lying flat. | B. Recognize that the person may be less able to deep breathe and clear airway. Prevent bedrest or immobility when possible. May need to be placed in sitting position, especially after meals. May need to eat smaller, more frequent meals. |
| C. Trachea and bronchioles may become calcified and stiffen. Alveoli become smaller, more shallow, with decreased surface and volume. | C. Encourage deep breathing for bedrest patients. Observe for signs of oxygen deficit. Avoid smoking, air pollution. |
| D. Increased anterior-posterior diameter of chest; change in expansion capacity with decreased vital capacity and increased residual volume. "Senile" emphysema with hyperresonance and distant breath sounds. | D. Provide good body alignment and proper positioning for chest expansion. Avoid chest restraints, if possible. Astute chest assessment with auscultation. |
| E. Decreased blood flow to the pulmonary circulation and decreased oxygen diffusion capacity. Arterial oxygen tension decreases with aging. | E. Check laboratory reports for blood gases. Observe for signs of oxygen deficit. |
| F. Decreased ability for airway clearance as a result of decreased ciliary action to remove secretions and inhaled particles. | F. Avoid smoking and air pollution. Consider need for suctioning. Prevent pulmonary infection. |
| G. Decreased cough reflex; less effective as a result of decreased muscle strength. | G. Assist with coughing by increasing abdominal pressure with pillow. |

*Continued.*

**Table 34-3**
Physical changes occurring in later life—*cont'd*

| Normal changes | Nursing implications |
|---|---|

### III. CARDIOVASCULAR SYSTEM

A. Heart may become smaller and be less effective as a pump, thus decreasing cardiac output. May result in left ventricular hypertrophy, which is age-related.

B. Decreased cardiac muscle strength and contractility causing decreased output and decreased ability to respond to increased output demands during stress; decreased cardiac reserve.

C. Heart valves may become thicker and less flexible causing ineffective closure. Valves may have increased fibrous tissue and calcium deposits.

D. Decreased elasticity of blood vessels causing increased systolic blood pressure. Decreased arterial compliance may lead to increased load on the left ventricle. Possible increased incidence of varicosities.

E. Decreased effectiveness of baroreceptors; decreased venous valve competency in lower extremities; may lead to decreased cerebral perfusion from lowered blood pressure and cause dizziness and falls.

F. Increased peripheral resistance and decreased vessel size with possible increase of blood pressure.

G. Apical pulse location may be slightly misplaced as a result of changes in chest configuration; may shift to left lateral position or sixth left intercostal space.

A. Encourage exercise within person's limitations. Encourage walking and swimming rather than jogging.

B. Allow for longer recovery periods after exercise or stress.
Check pulse rate before, during and after exercise.
Be aware of effects of blood loss and excessive fluid administration on heart function.

C. Check for signs of congestive heart failure. Auscultate for abnormal heart sounds.

D. Accurate blood pressure readings.
Instruct about need for blood pressure monitoring.
Observe tissue perfusion, especially in extremities.
Use elastic stockings when indicated.

E. Teach to stand up slowly to allow for compensation of blood to brain during postural change.

F. Teach need for frequent blood pressure checks. Teach need for medication compliance with hypertension.

G. If apical heart rate not audible, move stethoscope slowly over to the left lateral position or down to sixth left intercostal space.

### IV. GASTROINTESTINAL SYSTEM

A. Impaired mastication because of gum disease and loss of teeth, ill fitting dentures, or temporomandibular joint stiffness and pain.

A. Teach importance of dental care.
Promote good oral hygiene, especially before and after meals.
Observe denture fit.
Consider possible pain medication 1/2 hour before meals to decrease jaw pain.

❖ **Table 34-3**
Physical changes occurring in later life—*cont'd*

| Normal changes | Nursing implications |
|---|---|
| **IV. GASTROINTESTINAL SYSTEM—*cont'd*** ||
| B. Decreased salivation; drier mucous membranes. Decreased sense of smell may reduce secretory action. | B. Encourage fluids with food if not contraindicated. Discuss benefits of thorough mastication of food. Recommend use of artificial saliva. Avoid very dry foods. |
| C. Decreased number and acuity of taste buds causing less appetite; increased need for stronger flavors to stimulate taste. Use of dentures may decrease some taste sensation. | C. Encourage use of nonsodium seasonings or salt substitutes, sugar substitutes, and spices and herbs in cooking. |
| D. Decreased gag reflex. | D. Place person in upright position when eating or during tube feedings. Encourage person to chew thoroughly and take time while eating. Be aware of potential for choking. |
| E. Decreased mobility and strength of esophagus causing delayed emptying, irritation, and dilation. Presbyesophagus leads to decreased or uncoordinated peristalsis and decreased sphincter functioning and relaxation. | E. Instruct that smaller, frequent meals may be more easily digested. Encourage person to eat slowly. Be aware of possibility of substernal fullness after small amount of food taken. |
| F. Decreased digestive enzymes, hydrochloric acid, and pepsin. | F. Expect that person may complain of indigestion. |
| G. Decreased gastric motility; peristalsis less intense and frequent, causing delayed gastric emptying time. | G. Recognize that person may feel full after meals. Smaller, frequent meals may be better than three large meals. |
| H. Decreased abdominal muscle tone; may have difficulty contracting muscles for defecation. | H. May need to use external pressure over abdomen to assist with defecation. Body image change as abdomen becomes slack. |
| I. Decreased liver and gall bladder function. Possible decreased drug metabolism. | I. Note route of drug metabolism and possible adverse reaction and overdose. Observe for fatty food intolerance. |
| J. Decreased external sphincter sensitivity and reflex. | J. Check for constipation or incontinence. |
| **V. MUSCULOSKELETAL SYSTEM** ||
| A. Loss of lean muscle mass. Decrease in number and size of muscle fibers. Atrophy of muscle leads to loss of agility, strength, and function, especially seen in dorsal side of hands, upper arms, legs, and buttocks. | A. Be aware of strength loss. Check for fatigue. Teach about energy conservation. |

*Continued.*

**Table 34-3**
*Physical changes occurring in later life—cont'd*

| Normal changes | Nursing implications |
| --- | --- |

### V. MUSCULOSKELETAL SYSTEM—*cont'd*

| Normal changes | Nursing implications |
| --- | --- |
| B. Replacement of tissue by fatty deposits. | B. Be aware of body image changes. Be aware that fat soluble medications may need to be given in higher doses. |
| C. Decreased joint activity and mobility. Cartilage erosion with direct contact of bone on bone; mineral deposits. Synovial fluid becomes more viscous. Large weight-bearing joints show greater wear and stiffness. Ligaments may calcify. | C. Recognize decreased ability to accomplish ADL and need for more time to do ADL, especially in morning. Discuss need for medical care and possibly medication. |
| D. Demineralization of bone; loss of calcium leading to porosity or loss of density, especially in vertebral bodies, and femur. Bone loss seen more frequently in women, but occurs later in men. | D. Recognize potential for spontaneous fracture; need for safety awareness to prevent falls. Teach need for increased calcium in diet, starting earlier in life. Encourage walking. |
| E. Compacity of bone and cartilage, especially vertebrae causing a shortening of stature; loss of height and exaggeration of curvatures results. | E. Promote good posture and body mechanics. |
| F. Wide stance, shorter, smaller steps, and slower gait to maintain balance as a result of decreased proprioception. | F. Recommend safety measures to avoid falls. Discuss use of canes, walker, or both for stability. Encourage use of supportive shoes instead of house slippers. |

### VI. NEUROLOGICAL SYSTEM

| Normal changes | Nursing implications |
| --- | --- |
| A. Gradual degeneration and atrophy of nerve tissue causing decreased nerve acuity and impaired sensation; decrease in number of brain cells after age 50. | A. Discuss need for increased safety measures to prevent accidents. |
| B. Decreased nerve transmission with decreased reaction to stimuli; all neurological responses are slowed. Decreased frequency of impulse transmission and decline in speed of response. | B. Recognize need for more intense stimuli, such as touch, sound, light, taste. Recognize need for more time for processing stimuli and responding to it. |
| C. Kinesthetic senses less efficient; impaired position senses; decreased vibratory senses in extremities. | C. Discuss need for stability; use of walkers, canes. Recommend safety measures to prevent falls. |
| D. Slower thought processes with need for greater time computation but not necessarily decreased intellectual capacity. | D. Decrease complex situations requiring quick judgements. More time needed for decision making. Use simple instructions and reinforcement techniques. |
| E. Decreased cerebral perfusion. | E. Observe for signs of oxygen deficit. |

❖ **Table 34-3**
Physical changes occurring in later life—*cont'd*

| Normal changes | Nursing implications |
| --- | --- |

### VII. SENSORY

A. Decreased sense of smell and taste.

   A. Discuss safety factors: smoke detectors, check for spoiled foods, etc.
Teach awareness of body odors, overuse of perfume.

B. Decreased hearing. Difficulty in hearing consonants and high frequency tones. Decreased sound discrimination. Increased sensitivity to noise and loudness. Possible ossification of bones in middle ear; increased dryness of cerumen.

   B. Understand need for lower pitched voice with forceful presentation; avoid shouting, which distorts sound. Use stethoscope for hearing aid.
Check ears for impacted cerumen.
Encourage audiology testing.
Teach maintenance and proper use of hearing aids.
Be aware of medicines that are ototoxic.

C. Decreased pupil size, peripheral vision and accommodation to light and dark. Increased light required to produce same sensation. Decreased lens elasticity and near vision; development of lens with decreased color differentiation; decreased tearing and increased dryness of eye; eversion and inversion of eye lids; possible increased intraocular pressure.

   C. Avoid going abruptly from light to dark.
Decrease glare, especially fluorescent lighting.
Use colors, such as red or orange, and avoid pastels.
Use artificial tears.
Discuss need for reading glasses.
Encourage annual visual checkups.
Use greater wattage light bulbs.

### VIII. RENAL SYSTEM

A. Kidneys become less effective in disposing of waste products and maintaining homeostasis; reduced renal blood flow leading to decreased glomerular filtration rate.

   A. Observe intake and output carefully; possible medication retention with drug toxicity.
Be aware of possible dehydration or fluid and electrolyte imbalance, even after short periods without food and fluids.

B. Decreased number of functional nephrons causing diminished tubular reabsorption and renal concentration.

   B. Observe for renal failure when body stressed by illness.
Monitor lab reports and urine characteristics.

C. Decreased size and tone of bladder musculature with incomplete emptying and urinary retention.

   C. Check for bladder distention.
Discuss need for frequent urination and possible need for bladder training.

D. Increased urinary retention because of enlarged prostate gland in males.

   D. Assess urinary stream, bladder emptying, and bladder distention.

E. Stress incontinence in females because of loss of sphincter muscle control possibly because of difficult labors and deliveries in early adulthood. Poor musculature from childbearing causing cystocele/rectocele/uterine prolapse.

   E. Be aware of body image change.
Keep dry and control odor.
Observe for cystocele, rectocele, or uterine prolapse. Assess for urinary tract infection.
Teach Kegel exercises.

*Continued.*

❖ **Table 34-3**
Physical changes occurring in later life—*cont'd*

| Normal changes | Nursing implications |
| --- | --- |

### IX. REPRODUCTIVE SYSTEM

A. Decreased hormone production for both males and females.

B. Male: Decreased testosterone causing atrophy of testes and decreased sperm production: Active sperm present in ejaculates, but may be 50% of that of younger men.
Decreased penis size. Slower, weaker reaction during intercourse. Decreased, delayed achievement of full penile erection. Decreased frequency of ejaculation. Refractory period after intercourse may be from hours to days.
Increase in connective tissue in prostrate causing hypertrophy. Possible increase in breast tissue.

C. Female: Estrogen production from peripheral conversion of androgens in adipose tissue, and adrenal glands. Decreased estrogen and progesterone production by ovaries with atrophy of vulva, vagina, uterus, and ovaries. Decreased vaginal lubrication. Relaxation of musculature. Atrophy of glandular, supporting breast tissue.

D. Possible change in libido; slower response to stimuli.

A. Discuss effects of hormonal changes.

B. Understand change in body image.
Recognize need for health teaching about body changes.
Note possible need for partner counseling for understanding and time allowances.
Discuss expression of sexuality in various ways, such as gentle touch.

Teach need for annual rectal exams.

C. Understand change in body image.
Provide health teaching about changes.
Note possible need for counseling of partner.
Discuss need for lubrication with a water soluble product before intercourse.
Recommend supportive bra.

D. Provide health teaching about need for time.
Be aware that some medications may affect sexual functioning.

### X. IMMUNE SYSTEM

A. Decreased immune functioning.

B. Decreased ability to destroy mutant cells; decreased antibody response.

C. Decrease in red bone marrow and increase in yellow, fatty marrow.

A. Be aware of increased potential for infection.

B. Be aware of increase in autoimmune diseases and/or cancer in later life.

C. Understand possible tendency for anemia or reduced red blood cell production.

### XI. METABOLIC SYSTEM

A. Slower metabolic rate with reduction of oxygen consumption.

B. Decreased ability to adapt rapidly to stress and maintain homeostatic regulatory mechanisms; increased time needed to regain equilibrium.

A. Understand that person may feel cooler and need more protective clothing.

B. Allow time for adaptation and adjustment to physical and psychosocial changes; recovery periods take longer.

❖ **Table 34-3**
Physical changes occurring in later life—*cont'd*

| Normal changes | Nursing implications |
|---|---|
| **XI. METABOLIC SYSTEM—*cont'd*** | |
| C. Glucose tolerance curve tends to be higher than younger adult. | C. Be aware that urinary glucose test less reliable and slightly higher blood sugars may be normal in nondiabetic older adult. |
| D. Decreased ability to generate body heat. Temperature regulating mechanism less efficient.<br>May have little or no temperature change with infection.<br>Normal temperature of older adult may be less than 98.6° F; may run lower than 98° F; temperature of 99° F may indicate an elevation. | D. Keep environment comfortable for older adult, about 75° F to 78° F.<br>Observe for other signs and symptoms of infection besides an elevated temperature. |
| E. Less muscle mass and subcutaneous tissue may diminish heat generation.<br>Thinning of skin and less superficial circulation may lead to hypothermia. Shivering may occur later in older adults and is less effective in producing warmth. | E. Observe for hypothermia in cold weather. Advise layered clothing. |
| F. Decreased ability to perspire impairs the body's cooling system. | F. Observe for heat stroke or hyperthermia in hot weather. Provide fans or air conditioning when needed. |
| G. May have decreased pain perception or referred pain. | G. Observe for other signs and symptoms of illness. Administer pain medication judiciously. |

strongly influenced by these personality traits. The nurse can learn a great deal about an individual's previous methods of coping by listening to his or her experiences.

Both personality and coping may be temporarily challenged by the multiple losses and transitions experienced by older people such as the death of a spouse, relatives, or close friends, loss of social status, income and prestige as a result of retirement, and physical losses. The individual's perception of these events and the meaning assigned to them influences his or her coping style. While some older adults might cope with these changes by keeping busy and socially involved, others might withdraw from social interaction altogether. Temporary melancholy related to such losses is not unusual, but the nurse should recognize that persistent sadness might be a sign of clinical depression for which further intervention is indicated.

**Memory.** Memory is divided into three time frames: remote, immediate, and recent. *Remote memory* is the recall of things learned many years earlier. Most older adults have excellent remote memories. *Immediate memory* involves asking the client to repeat such things as numbers that were given a few seconds earlier. Immediate memory is also seldom impaired in normal aging. *Recent memory,* or the ability to recall facts or retrieve information presented more than a few minutes earlier, is usually reduced in older people (Hogstel, 1988). Older adults may require more time to recall the information but if given adequate, unpressured opportunity, they should be successful.

*Reminiscing* is a process involving remote memory. Detailed reminiscing near the end of life has sometimes been described as "life review," a mechanism to maintain oneself because of the threat of death. Reminiscence helps to increase self-esteem by contributing to a feeling of self-worth as the person re-

views accomplishments and reconciles disappointments. The nurse can gain valuable insight into past times and life events of the older adult by using reminiscing as an assessment tool and, at the same time, demonstrate caring and support by willingness to listen to the memories of elder clients. The nurse can suggest that families use a videotape recorder to record the reminiscences of the older adult in order to provide a lasting family history.

**Intelligence and learning.** In general, older people who are physically and mentally healthy do not show signs of decreased intelli-

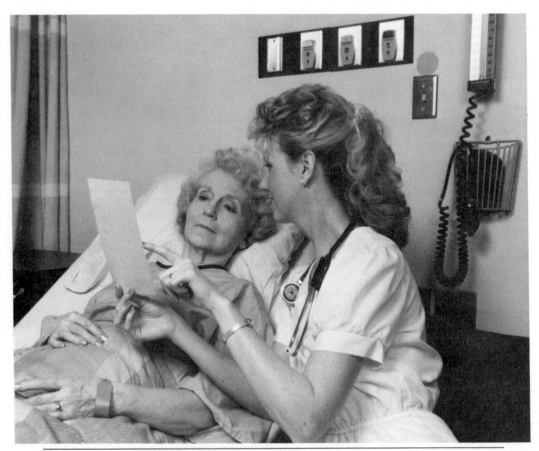

❖ **Fig. 34-2** The nurse teaching the older adult about medications. *(Photo courtesy of Ann Hendrich RN, MSN, CEN, Methodist Hospital in Indiana, Inc.)*

gence in later years. *Fluid intelligence,* which is related to the neurophysiologic status of the individual and emerges as creative and innovative behavior, does seem to decline with time. *Crystallized intelligence,* on the other hand, which is related to education and enculturation and uses past experience as a criterion for problem solving, continues to grow until just before death (Ebersole & Hess, 1990).

Individual differences in learning capacity may be a result of external factors such as motivation, attitudes, perception, and situational components rather than physiologic decline (Hogstel, 1988). Other manifestations common in the older adult that interfere with efficient learning include an increased tendency to respond to extraneous stimuli and a decline in problem-solving skills and organizational ability. If given a little more time than the younger person, the older person can process information well. It follows, then, that successful learning of new information by the older person is enhanced if it is meaningful, self-paced, and presented in an environment free from distraction. These considerations have implications for nursing practice when health teaching is indicated for the older adult (Fig. 34-2).

**Spirituality.** Some theories of aging postulate that as people grow older, they become more introspective and reflective and less concerned with the material aspects of the world. Spirituality or religion frequently becomes more meaningful in later life. To gain a sense of a person's spiritual dimension, the nurse must listen carefully and observe for cues. The initial interview with a client should include questions about the client's religious preferences and practices, especially those that affect health care. Exploration of the client's perception of his or her state of wellness and how illness, suffering, and loss are viewed provides further insight into the client's spiritual dimension. With some clients, adverse circumstances are viewed as punishment, testing of one's faith, or a way of redemption. Others may view them simply as a part of life.

Evidence of religious commitment can also be gained by observing for the presence of religious literature, articles or art work, visits from clergy or spiritual advisors, or overt religious practices. From these observations, the nurse can begin to talk with the client about spirituality and listen for cues that reflect the client's thoughts and feelings. Is the client building upon a past spiritual base? Is spirituality a means of support or a source of conflict? Does the client have concerns about the meaning of aging, loneliness, and death? Are the person's losses overwhelming? Is the person angry at God or a formal religion? Is the person questioning his dignity and life's worth? Does the person feel spiritual distress?

Nursing interventions should vary to meet the individual's spiritual needs. The box on p. 626 lists some nursing interventions that promote or support the client's spirituality.

**Retirement.** The cessation of work, or retirement, is anticipated differently by each individual. Some people look forward to a leisurely, less structured life while others fear isolation and boredom. For those who wish to remain active in more structured situations, the nurse might suggest substituting continued activity, such as volunteer work to maintain morale and a sense of self-worth. To get the most enjoyment out of leisure time, middle-aged people should be encouraged to cultivate hobbies and interests that can be more fully developed in later life. High "life satisfaction" ratings are more common among older people who are socially active and involved.

Upon retirement, most older adults are eligible for social security benefits. However, many people must rely on additional financial resources such as a pension or personal savings to maintain their standard of living. Some financial advisors suggest that people save 5% of their income during their thirties, 10% during their forties, and 15% or more after age 50.

## ❖ NURSING INTERVENTIONS TO MEET SPIRITUAL NEEDS

---

Assisting the individual with a life review to identify positive aspects and to help resolve negative ones.

Confirming the person's worth, dignity, and value of past life.

Identifying past sources of spiritual strength and trying to use these in the present situation.

Determining whether the use of music, such as familiar religious songs, provides special meaning or support.

Reading religious or philosophical material, such as scripture or poetry.

Talking about past religious ceremonies that had special meaning and how these can be sources of comfort.

Encouraging use of prayer or praying with the client, allowing time for private devotions.

Contacting the person's clergy or spiritual advisor and working together with the client.

Encouraging and helping to arrange for the person to continue religious practices and attend services if desired. (Often attendance of services decreases in later life because of problems of poor health, physical immobility, and lack of transportation; lack of attendance does not mean decreased interest.)

Discussing fears of dying and death with the client if desired and helping the client distinguish between them.

---

People who retire at age 62, instead of waiting until age 65, have a 20% reduction in social security benefits. The reduction will gradually rise to 30% after the year 2000. (Weiner, 1989).

In 1978, federal legislation raised the retirement age to 70. For reasons of personal identity, self-esteem, or financial need, many people maintain part-time jobs after they retire. Before age 70, there are limits on a person's annual earnings; for every dollar earned over the limit, there is a reduction in social security benefits. At age 70, however, a person may return to full employment, since earnings are penalty free.

**Support systems.** Although social networks usually decrease in size in later years, family and friends remain important sources of support. Often, lifelong friendships remain intact and offer a source of mutual help and companionship. Peer relationships, such as the emotional bonds two widows provide for one another, are also important support systems. In addition, family networks offer new and often satisfying roles for the older adult such as grandparent or great-grandparent.

Relatives satisfy many of the needs of the elderly and help them maintain independence as long as possible (Kohut, Kohut, & Fleischman, 1987). When indicated, the nurse can conduct a family support system assessment to determine the extent and availability of family resources, which can be tapped to assist the older person. This assessment focuses on the extended family and includes determination of its size, economic resources, frequency of involvement, type of assistance offered, other demands on the family, and recent stresses (Ebersole & Hess, 1990).

**Caregivers.** Many older adults are supported economically, socially, physically, or psychologically by their families as long as possible. A large part of direct care is often provided by the older person's daughter or other female relative. Most of these caregivers are in their forties and fifties. Sociologists term them the *sandwich generation* because they are sandwiched between raising children, usually teenagers, and caring for aging parents. Many of them must work to help support both. Some employers now recognize that care for older adults is becoming as commonplace as child care and are allowing caregivers some time off work with no penalty for "dependent care."

Typical roles established in long-term relationships may undergo transition, because illness in later years forces a role reversal between family members. With increased life expectancy, a daughter in her seventies may be caring for a mother in her nineties. Similarly, a passive, dependent spouse may be forced to assume care responsibilities for an ill mate. Many times, such role reversals require support, encouragement, and reinforcement from the nurse so that the caregiver will not be totally overwhelmed by the responsibilities of the new role.

Stress from the demands of the caregiver role and multiple demands of family and employment increases the potential for abuse of older people. It is estimated that 1 out of 25 older adults is moderately to severely abused annually but that only 1 in 5 cases are reported (Select Committee on Aging, 1985). Steinmetz (1988) conducted extensive interviews with 104 caregivers of elderly kin and found that 23% used physically abusive methods at some time to control the older person. Abusers often live in the same household with the older person; approximately 40% are spouses and 50% are children or grandchildren (Taber & Ansello, 1985). The typical abused person has greater cognitive impairment and is more dependent on the caregiver than nonabused elderly. A history of family dysfunction or violence and caregiver stress contribute to the incidence of elder abuse. (Refer to Chapter 24 for a further discussion of abuse.)

The nurse who visits the client at home should assess both the client and the caregiver. Feelings of anger, frustration, anxiety, or unwarranted guilt that may be expressed by the care-giver must be dealt with in the plan of care. Caregiver support groups are available in many communities, and a referral to such a group might prove helpful in cases where caregiving is a particularly stressful experience.

## ❖ HEALTH PROMOTION IN LATER LIFE

Nursing involvement in health promotion of the older person includes conducting a comprehensive assessment of the client and environment, identifying problem areas, making recommendations to effect behavioral or environmental change, taking necessary actions to protect the client and promote health, identifying needed resources, and initiating referrals.

Several aspects of prevention and maintenance are important nursing concerns in the health care of the older adult. Among these are attention to nutrition, exercise, accident prevention, oral health, foot care, and drug therapy.

### Nutrition

A balanced and adequate diet is required to maintain the structural and functional integrity of the body in later years. However, nutritional assessment of the older client often reveals inadequate nutritional status. Elders are most commonly deficient in the intake of protein, calcium, iron, and vitamins C and A. Nutritional deficiencies can result in such disorders as anemia, osteomalacia, Korsakoff's syndrome, cognitive impairment, and skin breakdown. Various dietary restrictions, such as a low sodium or a low cholesterol diet, can reduce the appetite by changing the flavor of foods. Men who live alone are at greater risk for nutritional deficiencies than other groups, possibly because of a lack of skill or motivation to plan and prepare meals.

Dehydration is also a fairly common problem with the older adult and may be attributed to a variety of factors. Difficulty with mobility can prevent the client from obtaining adequate fluids on his or her own. Clients who take diuretics may mistakenly restrict fluids to control urinary incontinence or frequency. Fever or hot weather can increase the need for fluids. Additionally, there is an age-related insensitivity of the hypothalamus to thirst (Matteson & McConnell, 1988). The nurse should be alert to the usual symptoms of dehydration as well as to early and more subtle findings such as disorientation, anorexia, or constipation. Nursing intervention in the form of teaching, arranging for scheduled fluid intake, or placing fluids in a convenient location may be indicated.

Altered nutrition in the elderly can be attributed to a number of physiological factors, psychosocial factors, or both. Physiological factors include physical limitations, diminished taste acuity, secondary effects of drug therapy, poor dentition, decreased secretion of enzymes, dysphagia, and gastrointestinal disturbances. Psychosocial factors are multiple and varied and include ethnic customs, beliefs, and attitudes, lifelong food preferences, social isolation, altered mental status, lack of transportation, and insufficient funds. In addition, environmental conditions such as inclement weather or fear for personal safety may prevent the older person from going to a supermarket. Some alternatives available to many clients include community health programs such as congregate meals at a senior citizen's center, food stamps, home-delivered meals, and nutritional education.

The importance of a thorough nursing assessment as a prerequisite to resolving nutritional problems cannot be overemphasized. A dietary history can provide insight into lifelong eating patterns. The physical or mental ability of a client to prepare meals can best be assessed by observing in the home setting or by talking with the family. For certain mechanical difficulties, the nurse can recommend supplemental, high-nutritional snacks or "finger foods" for people with limited mobility. Observing the

caregiver during feeding of the older person can help to identify other problems such as poor positioning or feeding too fast.

A multidisciplinary approach such as consultation with a nutritionist and occupational, physical, or speech therapists might prove helpful to the nurse if the nutritional problem is particularly difficult. The nurse should obtain a detailed record of the client's oral intake during a "three day calorie count" so it can be evaluated by the multidisciplinary team. If all else fails, a debilitated client may have to be hospitalized or admitted to an extended care facility for ongoing nutritional therapy.

### Exercise

Physical activity is important to maintain good health in later years. Benefits of regular exercise include weight control, improved cardiopulmonary function, increased muscle strength, greater joint flexibility, and increased mental alertness. Moderate exercise such as walking, swimming, dancing, or golf is recommended for the older adult, unless a disease condition restricts activities.

Many older people participate in regular exercise programs to promote physical fitness. Group exercise programs or walking or hiking clubs are doubly beneficial because they provide social contacts as well as exercise. "Mall walkers" clubs, established in shopping malls in Virginia, have grown to over 1800 members and are especially appealing because they offer protection from inclement weather and uneven terrain. In addition, registered nurses coordinate activities and provide health programs such as blood pressure screening and weight control (Moore, 1989).

For older adults who have limited mobility or are confined to a chair, simple exercises can be done in a sitting position. Active and passive exercises for the client on bedrest are important to prevent contractures and maintain joint mobility. The nurse may wish to consult with physical and occupational therapists to determine an appropriate exercise program for a particular individual.

## Accidents

Accidents are one of the leading causes of death in the older age group. The mortality rate from accidents increases with advancing age, and recent data indicate that individuals age 65 and older account for 72% of all fatal falls, 30% of pedestrian fatalities, and 29% of deaths from burns and fires (Rossman, 1986). According to Tidieksaar and Kay (1986), only 50% of older people who fall will be alive 1 year later. Predisposing factors include deficits in sight, hearing, equilibrium, and reaction time. Numerous conditions such as medication side effects, neurological problems, arthritis, peripheral vascular disease, cardiac arrhythmias, urinary urgency and incontinence, and generalized debility increase the risk of accidents. Osteoporosis is associated with hip, wrist, and vertebral fractures, with women over 75 suffering more than 1 million hip fractures each year. These alarming statistics and multiple risk factors underscore the importance of accident prevention as a top nursing priority.

**Accident prevention in the home.** Eischer and associates (1989) described accident prevention in the home as "geri-proofing" the household. This includes using good lighting, removing all loose throw rugs, tacking down loose carpet edges, installing grab bars, and placing a nonslip bathmat in the tub or shower. Floors should not be highly waxed, and all stairways must have handrails. Shoes are preferable to loose slippers. Assistive devices such as a raised bath stool or toilet seat are also helpful since many older people have difficulty rising from a low position. Burns can be prevented by lowering the temperature setting on the hot water heater, installing well-maintained smoke detectors, posting reminders about the dangers

of careless smoking, and clearly marking stove burners so one can readily tell if they are on or off. It is important to recognize that although the nurse might recommend preventive measures such as these, their implementation may be constrained by resistance, resentment, or economic limitations of the elder.

There are a variety of other circumstances that could lead to accidents in the older age groups. Leaky space heaters or furnace flues can increase the risk of carbon monoxide poisoning. People involved in "do-it-yourself" home repair are at risk for falls from ladders or chairs and injuries from special equipment such as saws and woodworking devices. Older people are especially vulnerable while working around farm machinery. The nurse must increase the older adult's awareness of these hazards and outline measures to prevent accidents.

As a safety measure, older individuals should have someone check on their well-being every day. This can be done by telephone. Some retirement communities have signs that can be placed on the apartment doorknob each morning such as, "Good morning, I'm fine." Another alternative is wearing a personal monitor device that can be activated to notify the police or fire station of an emergency. Monitor alarm systems or emergency "pull cords" to contact someone if the person needs help may also be available.

**Accident prevention in health care settings.** The prevalence of falls in health care settings is a serious nursing problem that jeopardizes life, limb, and quality of care. Falls have raised health care costs by resulting in complications that prolong hospitalization. One consistent finding is that clients fall frequently when they try to get out of bed for elimination needs unassisted.

Some hospitals have developed a "high risk fall prevention program." At one hospital every client is assessed for risk factors upon admittance. Certain risk factors are allotted points,

## ❖ HIGH-RISK FALL PROTOCOL

| | Date |
|---|---|
| Level I— | |
| Identify patient with armband, dots | |
| Call light in reach | |
| Bed in low position | |
| Siderails up | |
| Night light left on (evening/night shift) | |
| Non-slip footwear when ambulating | |
| Level II—(above interventions plus:) | |
| Bathroom light left on (evening/night) | |
| Elimination needs checked every 1–2 hours | |
| Ambulate with assistance only | |
| Level III—(above interventions plus:) | |
| Bed Check® monitor (# of alarms) | |
| | |
| Patient education delivered to: | |
| Patient | |
| Family or sitter | |
| Safety device—specify type: | |
| Skin condition under device clear and intact | |
| Circulation check (color, temperature, sensation) | |
| Device removed: ROM/skin care done | |
| Turn at least every 2 hours (if can't turn self) | |
| Rounds done every (    ) hour/s | |
| Initials | |
| Comments: Document below if protocol discontinued. Document consultations. | |

❖ **Fig. 34-3** Nursing interventions recommended for fall prone patients—part of a high-risk fall protocol flow sheet. *(Courtesy of Ann Hendrich RN, MSN, CEN, Methodist Hospital of Indiana, Inc.)*

the points are added, and the nurse determines what interventions are indicated to help prevent a fall. An unpublished study by Hendrich and colleagues (1989) demonstrated that the highest risk factors for clients who fell were depression (identified by the nurse's assessment, a medical diagnosis, or a recent history of depression) confusion, and a history of previous falls. Other risk factors included being over 65, general weakness, decreased mobility, and abnormal elimination needs, such as diarrhea or urinary urgency.

Some nursing interventions recommended for fall-prone clients are listed in Fig. 34-3. The list is part of a high-risk fall protocol flow sheet used for nurses' charting. The "dots" referred to under *Level 1* are colored symbols posted outside the client's room indicating that the client should be checked frequently.

Another device used to prevent falls is the Bed-Check monitor. The monitor is attached to a pressure-sensitive pad placed under the linen on the client's bed. An alarm sounds when the client attempts to get out of bed without help. Restraints can often be avoided if the alarm from the monitor is answered quickly. Morton (1989) describes a similar program that reported a 60% reduction in client falls over a 5-year period. One manufacturer of hospital beds now has special "sensor strips" built into the bed that can serve the same purpose as the described alarm system. Another hospital has installed a video monitoring system in four client rooms that requires a monitoring technician who alerts the nursing staff if a client tries to get out of bed without help (Krueger, Manon, & Wenzel 1989).

If restraints are necessary to protect a client from injury, they must be checked frequently. Potentially fatal complications such as strangulation by a vest restraint have been documented.

## Oral Health

Maintenance of healthy oral structures does not stop after early maturity. *Gerodontics* (dental care of older adults) is critical to increase the pleasure of eating, enhance the function of the taste buds, improve the appetite, prevent pathology and pain, help with speech, and maintain cosmetic appearance and self-image. Prevention and treatment are key factors in avoiding periodontal disease and tooth loss in older adults. Semiannual dental visits are needed to remove calculus and plaque around the teeth. Dental visits are also recommended for early detection and treatment of oral problems, even if the person is edentulous. Loss of teeth is not a normal part of the aging process and, with today's increased emphasis on pre-

ventive dentistry, the use of fluoride, and improved diets, fewer older people can expect to experience major dental problems.

**Oral problems and nursing intervention.** Some of the major problems of the oral cavity that occur with aging are degeneration of periodontal structures, neoplasia, xerostomia (dry mouth), decreased number of and function of taste buds, and ill-fitting dentures. Tooth loss in later life is usually a result of gingivitis, receding gums, infection, or development of caries. Replacement with partial plates and dentures may or may not be satisfactory and, even when they fit well, never truly function as well as one's own teeth. With age, there is a recession of gingival tissue from the teeth, which allows for exposure of the root or softer part of the tooth. Food particles can build up in pockets between the gums and roots leading to plaque formation, infection, and "root caries." The development of periodontal disease increases with age and is the most significant dental problem in later life.

Reabsorption of bone in the jaw may also cause problems with the proper fitting of dentures, since the shape of the bony alveolar ridge changes and is less able to withstand the pressure of dentures. Ill-fitting dentures cause friction, and people are reluctant to wear them because of pain and embarrassment. Frequently, ill-fitting dentures can be easily relined by a dentist to enhance a person's chewing ability and comfort.

In addition to periodontal disease, older adults, especially smokers and frequent users of alcohol, are more susceptible to neoplasia and should be checked for the presence of oral tumors. Not all growths in the oral cavity are malignant but still need to be examined; the possibility of leukoplakia, epidermoid, and basal cell carcinoma exists, and these require immediate treatment. Dark bluish spots occasionally seen under the tongue are varicose veins and are not to be confused with neoplasia.

Older adults often experience xerostomia, which can range from being mildly uncomfortable to very distressing. A dry mouth lessens lubrication for mastication and food breakdown, decreases the dilution of sugars and cleansing action for removal of food particles, predisposes to impaired fitting of dentures, and decreases the ability to articulate. Xerostomia may be caused by the production of a thicker, more viscous saliva or a decreased salivary production resulting from dehydration, disease, surgery, radiation therapy, or medications. Dryness can be alleviated by taking frequent sips of fluids (if not contraindicated), chewing sugarless gum, sucking on sugarless hard candy, using saliva substitutes, and doing frequent oral care with toothettes and mouth rinses. If xerostomia impairs suction for dentures to fit properly, they can be sprayed with noncholesterol vegetable oil or artificial saliva spray to help adherence to the palate.

Daily oral hygiene, including brushing the teeth and flossing between the teeth and under the gumline, should be encouraged to maintain healthy oral structures. Dentures should be cleaned and brushed just as regular teeth. If clients are unable to do their own oral care and there is potential for aspiration, the nurse can use a suction toothbrush, one with regular bristles and a hollow handle that can be attached to suction. This brush allows for more vigorous care than using a softer toothette.

Nursing assessment of oral structures can reveal problems that need referral. This is also a good opportunity for the nurse to teach about good oral hygiene and to stress that pathology in older adults may not produce pain until the later stages. Therefore, seeking dental care only when pain occurs may be more costly than routine semiannual checkups.

## Foot Care

Attention to foot care becomes more important to prevent immobility and loss of independence as one grows older. Foot problems can result in pain and deformity, leading to impaired walking, and possibly necessitating the use of assistive devices or even confinement to bed. The feet are often neglected until a serious problem arises.

The older person's feet should be checked daily. The client may be able to do this with the aid of a mirror or may require the help of another person, such as a family member, nurse, or podiatrist. Of particular concern is the structure of the foot and the condition of the skin and toenails. Symptoms such as discoloration, edema, or pressure areas should be reported and treated immediately.

**Foot problems and nursing intervention.** While foot problems in later years may be the result of normal changes of aging, they may also be indicative of pathology. Some problems seen in later life and suggested interventions are presented in Table 34-4.

## Drug Therapy

As people age, they are more likely to develop multiple chronic health problems and occasional acute illnesses that require drug therapy. Although older adults make up 12% of the U.S. population, it is estimated that they consume 25% of the prescribed medications and even more of the over-the-counter drugs. In addition, they experience 50% of the adverse reactions (Covington & Walker, 1984). Until recently, geriatric pharmacology was not considered a specialty. Research on drug therapy was typically conducted with healthy, young male adults. Dose determination and effects for elderly persons with multiple health problems were not taken into consideration. There is still a relative lack of information about the effects of drugs on older adults, but health care providers now recognize that as people age, drug tolerance changes. Dosages must be modified for each individual.

Nonchemical means of treatment should be considered for some conditions before drug

❖ **Table 34-4**
Foot problems and nursing interventions

| Possible foot problems | Suggested interventions |
| --- | --- |
| Aging skin of feet: dry, thin, loss of subcutaneous tissue; itching, burning, skin breakdown. | Wash with mild soap and tepid water. Dry carefully, apply lotion. Use protective padding as indicated. |
| Decreased circulation of lower extremities, both arterial and venous. | Assess for impaired circulation. Check pulses, skin color, temperature, and integrity. Suggest avoiding activities that constrict blood flow, such as use of garters, crossing legs, or use of tobacco. Encourage walking or swimming, if feasible, to increase circulation. |
| Joint disease with enlargement and deformity, pain, and decreased range of motion. | Depending upon etiology, use of medication, physical therapy, exercise, or surgery. Instruct to wear sturdy, comfortable, well-fitting shoes and to avoid wearing soft house slippers during the day. |
| Decreased neurological function with decreased sensation in feet; increased vulnerability from unnoticed trauma; unawareness of foot placement. | Assess feet daily for early detection of injury or pressure areas; tactile and vibratory assessment to detect lack of kinesthetic sensation. Instruct to wear foot coverings at all times and to not go barefoot. |
| Pressure and friction areas leading to formation of corns and calluses (benign hyperkerotic lesions that become painful and disabling). | Treat by soaking in warm, mild soapy water and buff with emery board. Use protective padding as indicated. Recommend properly fitting shoes and podiatry consultation for persistent problems. Discourage "bathroom surgery" or caustic "over-the-counter" drugs causing further skin damage. |
| Ingrown toenails. | Suggest cutting nails straight across taking care not to allow spicules to remain at the corners, which become imbedded in the soft tissue. |
| Infections: bacterial, viral, or fungal. Fungal infections may cause toenails to become thick and discolored; hypertrophied nails can place pressure on soft, underlying tissue causing pain, ulceration, and tissue necrosis. Viral infections may result in wart formation. | Use antiinfective agents and prescription drugs for local application; oral antifungal drugs are discouraged because of their lowered tolerance and possible hepatic toxicity in older adults. Discourage "over-the-counter" medications. May require surgical treatment. |

therapy is used. For example, constipation may be relieved by increasing fluids, fiber, and exercise, thus eliminating the need for a daily laxative. Sometimes a medication is given to pacify the family or nursing staff rather than to truly help the client.

**Issues related to drug therapy.** The elderly are generally less physically tolerant of drugs, less capable of metabolizing them, and more susceptible to drug reactions and side effects. Unfortunately, many adverse drug reactions (ADR) are not readily identified, because they can mimic changes seen in aging such as forgetfulness, mild confusion, weakness, and general malaise. Ototoxic drugs can damage the eighth cranial nerve, and resultant deafness may be blamed on the aging process. The nurse should consider the possibility that such conditions could be the result of drug toxicity, drug-food interaction, or drug-drug interaction. Consultation with a pharmacist about these possibilities might be warranted.

Another danger with drug therapy in later life is *polypharmacy* or the ingestion of multiple medications within a 24-hour period. Frequently the older adult sees several physicians, each prescribing medications without knowing what others have given the individual. In addition to prescription drugs, the client may also be taking over-the-counter drugs, which can compound the problem. The hazards of polypharmacy are an increased risk of ADR, increased potential for administration error, and decreased levels of compliance as the elder attempts to control unpleasant side effects by omitting or reducing medication doses. The use of drugs can be the cause of conditions leading to hospitalization or nursing home admission of older adults.

**Physiological changes affecting drug therapy.** As a person grows older, *pharmacokinetics* (drug absorption, distribution, binding, receptor site sensitivity, biotransformation, and excretion) are typically altered. Physiological changes in the gastrointestinal tract, circulation, body mass, fluid content, and serum proteins can all alter the response to medication. Of great significance is the decreased hepatic and renal efficiency that commonly occurs with age, affecting the metabolism and excretion of drugs and resulting in an increase in the amount of active, free drug in the body. Consequently, older adults usually require less of a drug to obtain an optimal effect. It is best to start with the lowest dose possible and gradually increase

the medication to obtain the optimal effect.

Drug administration may be affected by physiological changes in the form of sensory deficits. A person may have presbyopia and not be able to read label instructions. Cataracts interfere with the ability to see clearly, and color vision changes may interfere with correctly identifying pills by color. Hearing impairment can prevent the client from correctly understanding verbal instructions concerning medication.

**Nursing considerations.** Obtaining a thorough and accurate drug history is an extremely important aspect of drug therapy. The nurse can obtain this history from the client or caregiver by addressing such questions as:

1. What medications are currently being taken, both prescribed and over-the-counter? What medications have been taken in the past? (Be certain to include salves, ointments, and patches.)
2. What is the extent of knowledge of the client and/or caregiver about these medications?
3. Where are the drugs purchased and does the client have easy access to the pharmacy?
4. Is the client able to afford the medications without doing without other necessities?
5. Where are medications kept? Are they out of the reach of children and away from excessive heat, light, and moisture?
6. Has the client experienced side effects and if so, how has the client dealt with them?
7. Have the medications altered sexual functioning?
8. What home remedies are used?

A history provides insight regarding the need for health teaching and counseling, as well as determining drug effectiveness and possible ADR. The therapeutic effects of the drug regimen must be assessed frequently, since drug administration frequency and dose may need to be altered. Drug therapy should be reviewed daily for acute inpatients, monthly in extended care facilities, and at least every 3 to 6 months in a home setting.

It has been shown that the more complex the drug regimen is, the more chance there is for administration error. Therefore, simplifying the drug regimen for the elder, such as once-a-day doses rather than multiple doses if feasible, can reduce error and increase medication adherence. Proper education and sufficient time for teaching and understanding of the drug regimen can also decrease administration errors and seems to improve compliance. As older adults frequently value good health, they are usually motivated to take medications if they understand their purpose. It is important to remind the client not to stop or alter the dosage of drugs without consulting the physician.

To facilitate correct medication administration, the nurse might suggest setting up medications for a day or a week at a time. Various methods can be employed such as putting morning, afternoon, and evening medications in color coded cups, using an empty egg carton, using a plastic box with dividers, or purchasing a weekly medication box that can only be opened in sequential order. Thus the client is reminded to take the correct drug at the correct time, and all of the drugs can be accounted for.

## ❖ HEALTH ALTERATIONS

Health alterations experienced by the older adult include variations in mental status and physical functioning. Mental states discussed here are depression, confusion, delirium, and dementia. Physical conditions or symptoms that merit special consideration in the elderly are pain, fever, and altered elimination patterns.

### Depression

*Depression* is a state of lowered self-esteem accompanied by feelings of hopelessness and helplessness (Burnside, 1988). Depression in older people is frequently associated with the numerous losses that accompany aging as well as the felt effects of societal devaluation. Symptoms of depression include sadness, insomnia, anorexia, weight loss, retarded movement, lethargy, fatigue, and slowed thoughts. Often mistaken for dementia, the major difference between the two disorders is that *depression* is a disturbance of mood, while *dementia* is a disturbance of cognition resulting from brain dysfunction. A medical evaluation is warranted to determine whether the symptoms of depression might be caused by a reversible medical condition or drug side effects.

There is a risk of suicide with any severe depression. The incidence is particularly alarming in the older age groups, with the incidence being 10 times that of the population average (Ebersole & Hess, 1990). As a group, white males have the highest suicide rate in the nation, and it increases significantly with age. An examination of the 1986 death rate from suicide in the 85+ year old group reveals that the suicide rate for white males was 66.3 deaths per 100,000 people. By comparison, the 85+ black male suicide rate was 17.9 per 100,000 people. For all 85+ women, the death rate from suicide was 4.7 per 100,000 (National Center for Health Statistics, 1989). Thus, depression in the elderly has potentially serious consequences, and the nurse should refer the client to a psychiatric nurse specialist or physician if the depression does not lift or if suicidal ideation is expressed.

The depressed older person can be treated with antidepressants, which should result in improvement in 2 to 3 weeks (Gomez and Gomez, 1989). The person must be advised that there is a delay in the therapeutic response to the drug and that the medication should be continued, even if it initially seems to be ineffective. Since orthostatic hypotension is one of the most common and most serious side effects of antidepressant therapy, an awareness of the increased potential for falls is indicated. Group therapy, family therapy, and electroconvulsive therapy are other modes of treatment for depression in older people.

## Cognitive Impairment

Cognitive impairment is not the inevitable result of the aging process. When it is present, it varies in severity and duration. Organic or physiological confusion may be of short or long duration. The short duration experience is known as *acute or reversible brain syndrome* and may be divided into *delirium* and other reversible causes. Cognitive impairment of long duration is termed *dementia* and was previously known as chronic or irreversible brain syndrome. Cognitive impairment resulting from psychiatric disorders will not be covered in this discussion.

**Confusion and delirium.** Confusion is a global term that includes both reversible and irreversible types of cerebral dysfunction (Ebersole & Hess, 1990). *Confusion* is a state of disorientation or a disturbance of consciousness in the sense that awareness of time, place, or person is unclear. It is estimated that 30% to 40% of individuals referred with memory disturbances have treatable confusion (Calkins, Davis, & Ford, 1986).

An acute confusional state is often termed *delirium.* The onset is usually rapid and the duration relatively short when compared with dementia. The individual may exhibit perceptual disturbances, alteration in psychomotor activity, disorientation, disturbance in sleep, and incoherent speech. One hypothesis as to the cause of delirium is an excess of dopamine and a deficiency of acetylcholine in the brain (Hackett & Cassen, 1987).

Acute confusional states can be precipitated by a variety of factors. Hypoxia, or decreased oxygen to the brain, as a result of pul-

monary or cardiovascular disease, is a fairly common cause of confusion in the elderly client. Drug toxicity, as previously discussed in this chapter, is another common cause. Fever, dehydration, electrolyte imbalance, and hypoglycemia can also produce confusion as can an elevated blood urea nitrogen (BUN) in renal disease and blood ammonia in liver disease. As many of these are reversible or treatable conditions, it is especially important that the nurse monitor laboratory studies closely for abnormal findings that might explain the confused state. In addition, stress related to physiological, psychological, and environmental factors can precipitate confusion. Symptomatic treatment of these conditions frequently reverses the confusion.

Most organic confusion is periodic and becomes worse at night, especially if the person is in a new environment. *Sundowning,* a confused state that worsens at night, may be caused by factors that decrease cerebral blood flow such as dehydration, cardiac conditions, and medications. Identification and treatment of these factors and implementation of activities that can promote orientation to the environment are indicated. The shock of relocation to a strange environment can be diminished if the nurse explains what to expect ahead of time and repeatedly reorients the elderly client after the relocation. In these situations, nursing measures should be aimed at assuring a comfortable and safe environment and using reality orientation approaches as necessary. The issue of whether nurses should wear uniforms or "street clothes" in an institutional setting is an interesting one, since the uniform may serve as an external cue to reality orientation for the confused client.

The extremes of sensory deprivation and sensory overload may also contribute to confusion. Elderly clients in isolation because of a communicable disease are at risk for confusion resulting from sensory deprivation, especially if the nurse and visitors do not make an effort to

❖  **Table 34-5**
Factors contributing to confusion with nursing goals and interventions

| Cause | Nursing goals | Suggested interventions |
| --- | --- | --- |
| Strange environment | Provide environmental cues. | Repeated orientation. Use clocks, watches, daily calendar. Nurses wear uniforms. |
| Sensory impairment | Improve sight and hearing. | Put on client's glasses and hearing aid as needed. Speak clearly. |
| Sensory deprivation | Provide cognitive, environmental, social, and tactile stimulation. | Reinforce recent events. Provide light, turn on T.V. when appropriate. Use therapeutic touch. Encourage family to visit. |
| Loss of control and independence | Provide choice when possible. | Determine client's previous routine. Ask simple questions. Wait for answers. |
| Immobility | Provide mobilization. | Encourage activity whenever possible. |
| Disruption of elimination patterns | Prevent constipation and urinary retention | Encourage fluids, determine client's previous routine. Assess elimination needs. Try to keep on previous elimination schedule. |
| Pain | Relieve pain. | Change client's position. Use therapeutic touch. Use medications cautiously and check client's reaction carefully. |
| Sensory overload and sleep deprivation (especially in critical care units) | Provide periods of decreased light, quiet, and sleep. | Organize nursing care to decrease interruptions for the client. State one request at a time. Avoid taking client to "busy places," such as the nurses' station during the day. |

provide social contact. Conversely, "busy" places such as a critical care unit with lights on, monitors beeping, and 24-hour activity can also aggravate a confused state. These and other factors that contribute to confusion and respond favorably to nursing intervention are summarized in Table 34-5.

Conducting a thorough assessment of the confused elderly client can provide some insight into the nature and extent of the confused state. There are several mental status exams available, but before selecting one, its reliability and validity for use with the older age group should be ascertained. Several brief questionnaires are in common use. The Mini-Mental State Examination is a particularly useful one (see the box that follows). Lacking access to these, assessing for orientation to person, place, time, and recent events can be easily accomplished. Nursing progress notes should describe the client's behavior, noting specific responses that illustrate confusion.

## ❖ "MINI-MENTAL STATE"

| *Maximum* Score | Score | |
|---|---|---|

### ORIENTATION

| 5 | ( ) | What is the (year) (season) (date) (day) (month)? |
| 5 | ( ) | Where are we: (state) (county) (town) (hospital) (floor). |

### REGISTRATION

| 3 | ( ) | Name three objects: One second to say each. Then ask the client all 3 after you have said them. Give one point for each correct answer. Then repeat them until he learns all three. Count trials and record.<br>Trials |

### ATTENTION AND CALCULATION

| 5 | ( ) | Serial 7's. 1 point for each correct. Stop after 5 answers. Alternatively spell "world" backwards. |

### RECALL

| 3 | ( ) | Ask for the 3 objects repeated above. Give 1 point for each correct. |

### LANGUAGE

| 9 | ( ) | Name a pencil, and watch (2 points)<br>Repeat the following "No ifs, ands or buts." (1 point)<br>Follow a 3-stage command:<br>   "Take a paper in your right hand, fold it in half, and put it on the floor<br>     (3 points)<br>Read and obey the following: |

### CLOSE YOUR EYES (1 POINT)

Write a sentence (1 point)
Copy design (1 point)
_____ Total score
ASSESS level of consciousness along a continuum _____

*Alert Drowsy Stupor Coma*

### INSTRUCTIONS FOR ADMINISTRATION OF
### MINI-MENTAL STATE EXAMINATION

### ORIENTATION

(1) Ask for the date. Then ask specifically for parts omitted, e.g., "Can you also tell me what season it is?" One point for each correct.
(2) Ask in turn "Can you tell me the name of this hospital?" (town, county, etc.). One point for each correct.

From Folstein, M. F., Folstein, S. & McHugh, P. R. (1975). Mini-mental state: A practical method for grading the cognitive state of patients for the clinician. *Journal of Psychiatric Research, 12,* 189-198. Reprinted with permission.

❖ **"MINI-MENTAL STATE"**—*cont'd*

---

### REGISTRATION

Ask the patient if you may test his memory. Then say the names of 3 unrelated objects, clearly and slowly, about one second for each. After you have said all 3, ask him to repeat them. This first repetition determines his score (0–3) but keep saying them until he can repeat all 3, up to 6 trials. If he does not eventually learn all 3, recall cannot be meaningfully tested.

### ATTENTION AND CALCULATION

Ask the patient to begin with 100 and count backwards by 7. Stop after 5 subtractions (93, 86, 79, 72, 65). Score the total number of correct answers.

If the patient cannot or will not perform this task, ask him to spell the word "world" backwards. The score is the number of letters in correct order. E.g., dlrow = 5, dlorw = 3.

### RECALL

Ask the patient if he can recall the 3 words you previously asked him to remember. Score 0–3.

### LANGUAGE

*Naming:* Show the patient a wrist watch and ask him what it is. Repeat for pencil. Score 0–2.

*Repetition:* Ask the patient to repeat the sentence after you. Allow only one trial. Score 0 or 1.

*3-Stage command:* Give the patient a piece of plain blank paper and repeat the command. Score 1 point for each part correctly executed.

*Reading:* On a blank piece of paper print the sentence "Close your eyes," in letters large enough for the patient to see clearly. Ask him to read it and do what it says. Score 1 point only if he actually closes his eyes.

*Writing:* Give the patient a blank piece of paper and ask him to write a sentence for you. Do not dictate a sentence, it is to be written spontaneously. It must contain a subject and verb and be sensible. Correct grammar and punctuation are not necessary.

*Copying:* On a clean piece of paper, draw intersecting pentagons, each side about 1 in., and ask him to copy it exactly as it is. All ten angles must be present and 2 must intersect to score 1 point. Tremor and rotation are ignored.

Estimate the patient's level of sensorium along a continuum, from alert on the left to coma on the right.

---

#### Scoring of Mini-Mental State Examination

| | |
|---|---|
| 0–17 | Severe impairment |
| 18–23 | Mild impairment |
| 24–30 | No impairment |

NOTE: If the client has a noncognitive deficit such as blindness, it may be expected that a total possible score (in this case) would be less than 30. Therefore, an adjustment in scoring is indicated.

**Dementia.** *Dementia* refers to a progressive loss of memory, judgment, language skills, and appropriate behavior. For 60% of clients with dementia, the cause is Alzheimer's disease and related disorders. Cerebral multi-infarct dementia accounts for another 15% to 25%. The remainder is a result of miscellaneous causes such as brain tumors, normal pressure hydrocephalus, or thiamine deficiency Korsakoff's dementia. The estimated prevalence of dementia increases from 1% in people under age 60 to 5% in those age 65, 20% in people age 80 and 50% in those age 90 (Calkins, Downs, & Ford 1986). Although the disease processes that cause dementia are irreversible, some improvement is possible in a person's daily activities.

*Alzheimer's disease.* Alzheimer's disease is a pathological condition that is progressive and irreversible, eventually causing dementia and presenting major challenges for families and health care professionals. Although the rate of decline varies considerably from person to person, Alzheimer's disease follows an inevitable degenerative course, generally leading to death in 5 to 15 years. The burden on the caregiver and family unit is particularly severe. The most troublesome areas are memory disturbances, catastrophic reactions (overreaction to minor stresses), demanding behavior, and nocturnal wandering (Burnside, 1988). A multidisciplinary approach to client care is especially important to assist the family of the individual with Alzheimer's disease. Referral to caregiver support groups has proved extremely helpful to decrease the level of stress in both the family and caregiver.

In a research study by Cleary and associates (1988), a reduced stimulation unit for the care of clients with Alzheimer's disease and related disorders was evaluated. With reduced stimulation, weight loss was curtailed, agitation was diminished, restraint use was reduced, and wandering no longer was a concern of staff or other patients. The principles of a reduced stimulation unit are being applied by many

extended care facilities. In addition, the techniques of reality orientation, remotivation, and validation therapy are all useful nursing care measures.

The following case study illustrates the problems presented by a client with Alzheimer's disease and highlights nursing diagnoses and associated nursing interventions.

*CASE STUDY OF MRS. JONES WITH EARLY ALZHEIMER'S DISEASE.*
Mrs. Jones, a 71-year-old widow, has symptoms of memory loss, poor judgment and attention span, disorientation, and apathy. She lives with her daughter, who had taken her to the family physician 7 months previously, and he could find nothing wrong. Her daughter brought Mrs. Jones to the physician again because her mother's symptoms now included "wandering away from home" and increased memory loss.

The family physician referred Mrs. Jones to a neurologist who performed several tests to rule out reversible causes of mental impairment, including magnetic resonance imaging (MRI). He explained to Mrs. Jones and her daughter that the probable diagnosis of Alzheimer's disease is a matter of exclusion to rule out other diseases. Mrs. Jones' daughter was upset, and the neurologist recommended that a community health nurse visit the family.

When the nurse arrived at Mrs. Jones' home, she conducted a family assessment. She found that Mrs. Jones' 51-year-old daughter was divorced with grown children and that she wanted to keep her mother at home with her as long as possible. She did have a part-time job, which presented her greatest concern, because she was afraid to leave her mother alone. Nursing diagnoses and interventions for Mrs. Jones are presented in the box on p. 641.

## Pain

Pain is a universal, complex symptom that is psychosocial as well as physical in nature.

## ❖ NURSING DIAGNOSES AND INTERVENTIONS TO MEET THE NEEDS OF MRS. JONES AND HER DAUGHTER*

A. ALTERATIONS IN THOUGHT PROCESS
  1. Compensate for Mrs. Jones' memory loss by providing a structured, consistent physical setting, schedule, and routine.
  2. Provide reality orientation.
  3. Provide calendars, signs, labels, and lists.

B. ALTERATIONS IN FAMILY PROCESSES
  1. Assist family in role changes such as a role reversal with parent and child.
  2. Understand loss of the person the client once was.
  3. Advise daughter to plan for future regarding legal matters.
  4. Inform family of respite care, which may include in-home help, nursing care, or day care.
  5. Inform family of a local and national support group.

C. POTENTIAL FOR INJURY
  1. Protect from dangers of wandering: locked doors, bells, sensors may be necessary, especially at night.
  2. Discourage cooking, driving, smoking, and other potentially dangerous activities.
  3. Lock knives and guns to prevent accessibility to client.

D. ALTERATIONS IN SENSORY PERCEPTION
  1. Recognize client's inability to differentiate sensory input—may not be able to identify common objects.
  2. Offer support when client confuses a family member with another person.

E. IMPAIRED VERBAL COMMUNICATION
  1. Use short, simple sentences.
  2. Give one request at a time.
  3. Allow time for thought processing and response.
  4. Don't expect client to comprehend complex conversations.

F. ALTERATION IN NUTRITION: LESS THAN BODY REQUIREMENTS
  1. Maintain nutritional status with a high calorie, high protein diet if client is losing weight because of increased activity.
  2. Encourage small frequent feedings and finger foods, which can be carried as client walks.

G. SELF-CARE DEFICIT
  1. Allow client to do as much for herself as able for as long as possible.
  2. Use leading techniques "to get client started," which sometimes helps with activities of daily living (ADLs).

H. DEFICIT IN DIVERSIONAL ACTIVITIES
  1. Encourage walking in moderation for physical activity.
  2. Recognize that music often has a calming effect; clients may remember the words to songs long after other memory is lost.
  3. Provide access to a television or other diversional activities.

I. SLEEP PATTERN DISTURBANCE
  1. Promote normal rest and sleep patterns by keeping client physically active during the day.
  2. Encourage short naps, especially if client is pacing.
  3. Consult physician regarding a safe hypnotic if necessary.

  The nurse also identified more potential nursing diagnoses to consider as Mrs. Jones' condition worsened:
  a. ALTERATION IN THOUGHT PROCESSES
    (1) Assess and evaluate the need for psychotropic drugs.
  b. IMPAIRED PHYSICAL MOBILITY
  c. IMPAIRED SKIN INTEGRITY
  d. INCONTINENCE
  e. ALTERATIONS IN FAMILY PROCESSES
    (1) Inform family about long-term care facilities.

*The authors wish to thank Judy Pollmann, R.N., Director, Nursing Educational Service, Saint Joseph Hospital, Lexington, Kentucky, for these suggestions.

Although pain has been the focus of a great deal of research, the mechanisms of pain in later life are not fully understood. Whether the pain threshold increases or not has yet to be proven, but the pain response is altered in the older adult. It is possible that older adults perceive pain differently, process pain signals more slowly, or respond more slowly to peripheral pain.

When pain is experienced, the older individual might describe vague feelings of discomfort rather than specific, demarcated pain. Even with the presence of serious pathology, such as a myocardial infarction, pneumonia, or an "acute abdomen," some older people experience little or no discomfort. This altered pain response is potentially hazardous, as it masks warning signs of pathology, delays seeking health care, causes health care providers to underestimate its importance and leads to misdiagnosis.

Older adults' attitude toward pain varies and is manifested by their reaction to the pain experience. Pain from joints and muscles is common, sometimes resulting in frequent complaints and earning those individuals the reputation of being chronic complainers. Conversely, older adults often accept pain as an expected symptom of aging, a normal part of growing old and not worth mentioning. Denial of pain, because of a fear of being examined, treated, or hospitalized is another common response.

The older person has diminished reserve capacities, both physical and psychological, to cope with pain. With a decreased ability to adapt, the fatigue and stress of pain may overwhelm body systems in the attempt to maintain equilibrium, resulting in further illness and even death. A common psychological occurrence associated with pain, especially if chronic, is depression. Since lack of pain expression does not necessarily mean lack of pain, it is also important to evaluate other signs and symptoms that might be associated with pain, such as an increased pulse rate, decreased socialization, anxiety, restlessness, and confusion.

Management of pain can be facilitated by determining how the client has dealt with pain in the past and what measures have proven successful. Providing support to decrease anxiety, fear, feelings of loneliness, and powerlessness is an important nursing intervention. Use of nonchemical means such as heat, cold, massage, change in position, or relaxation techniques should be tried initially or in conjunction with medication. If it is necessary to treat the pain with medication, the lowest dose possible should be used to avoid serious adverse effects.

## Fever

Basal temperature tends to decrease with each decade, and it has been shown that healthy older adults have an average body temperature approximately one degree below the "normal" of 98.6°F. Thus, if a fever occurs in later life, it is likely to be less prominent than in a younger person and cannot be determined by comparison against the assumed norm of 98.6° F. An older person who registers a temperature of 99° F, especially after age 75, probably has a fever (Burnside, 1988).

Common causes of fever in older adults are dehydration, hyperthermia, myocardial infarction, cerebral vascular accident, pulmonary emboli, neoplasia, and infection. The two most common causes of fever from infection are urinary tract and pulmonary infections. Infections can be difficult to recognize because, even if severe, there may be little temperature elevation. Some older clients with culture-proven bacteremia are afebrile, and even leukocytosis can be markedly less than expected with infection (Rossman, 1986). Diagnostic studies should be done if an older person has even a mild fever of undetermined origin, since it may be indicative of serious pathology.

Signs and symptoms of fever in older adults are restlessness, confusion, altered pulse or respiratory rates, dizziness, headache, or just generally "not feeling well." As with younger clients, nursing interventions include fluids, cool sponge baths, a cool environment, and antipyretics. It is important not to cool older people too quickly, however, as they may not be able to readily adapt to rapid changes in body temperature.

### Altered Elimination Patterns

As people grow older, elimination patterns begin to vary. Because of physical changes mentioned in Table 34-1, older adults may have problems with urinary frequency, incontinence, or constipation.

**Urinary frequency and incontinence.** A decrease in bladder capacity from approximately 500 cc to 250 cc can result in frequency, urgency, and nocturia. Although it may be annoying to the older person, it is not uncommon to empty the bladder several times each night and to urinate frequently during the day.

*Urinary incontinence* is defined as the involuntary passage of urine, overflow leakage, or both from a distended bladder, regardless of the amount. The problem of urinary incontinence should not be seen as an inevitable result of the aging process, since it affects only 3% of older men and 12% of older women who are noninstitutionalized (Gioiella & Bevil, 1986). However, it is often the causative factor for institutionalization.

There are various classifications of incontinence, such as stress, urge, and neurogenic. Among the predisposing factors are urinary tract infections, diabetes, medications, vascular accident, impaction, retention, confusion, immobilization, or environmental inadequacies. Consequences of incontinence include social isolation, disrupted personal relationships, embarrassment, and skin irritation. People are hesitant to discuss incontinence and do not realize that it is a common problem that is often treatable or manageable.

A thorough physical assessment and good health history can provide insight regarding the nature and extent of the problem. A chart, detailing such information as frequency, time, precipitating factors, urinary stream characteristics, environment, medications, and intake and output amounts, is useful in analyzing an incontinence problem. A physical exam may reveal problems such as diabetes or atrophic vaginitis, which can be treated. A urinalysis can detect the presence of a urinary tract infection; the incidence of chronic urinary tract infections greatly increases in older people and is a significant causative factor in incontinence.

Interventions vary with etiology and can be medical, surgical, or nursing-focused. Nursing interventions include behavior modification, bladder retraining with positive reinforcement, pelvic floor muscle exercises, and ensuring easy access to toilet facilities. Protective clothing, such as incontinence briefs or pads, can be used. For men, collecting devices such as external catheters and leg urinals are available. Drugs, such as diuretics should be scheduled to control urination as much as possible, especially at night. Good skin care with perineal products helps to avoid tissue breakdown and decreases and controls body odor. Psychological support is important to encourage the client to continue social contact.

**Constipation and fecal incontinence.** Constipation is probably one of the most frequent complaints of older adults. Many older adults believe they must have a bowel movement every day or their "systems will be poisoned." True *constipation* is defined as a decrease in the frequency of stools and not merely difficulty in passing stool (Burnside, 1988). A decrease in peristalsis and lack of abdominal muscle strength as well as other physical changes of later life contribute to constipation (see Table 34-1). Additional factors include the use of certain medications, amounts, and types of food and fluids, environmental setting for elimination, personal hygiene habits, and patterns of daily exercise.

It is important to rule out the possibility of pathology as a causative factor for constipation. Subsequently, the nurse can determine a person's usual elimination pattern and plan interventions. If satisfactory, past patterns of elimination should be supported and continued. Encouraging foods and fluids such as bulk-forming products, fresh fruit and vegetables, and warm liquids in the morning to stimulate the gastrocolic reflex may be effective in alleviating constipation.

Medications are often implicated as causative or contributing factors to constipation. Medications such as sedatives or tranquilizers can decrease the client's awareness of the need to defecate or affect his or her ability to get to the bathroom. Avoiding the chronic use and abuse of irritant laxatives is strongly advised. If needed, stool softeners or bulk laxatives can be used. Increasing dietary fiber might eliminate the need for laxatives altogether.

A bowel training program can be effective in preventing and treating constipation. It is important to establish a pattern of activities that promotes a routine time for defecation. This may also help the client become more aware of rectal sensations that indicate the need for a bowel movement.

Environment is a crucial factor to consider in managing constipation. The nurse should raise these questions: Can the bathroom accommodate a wheelchair if needed? Is the area easily identified or well-marked? Are facilities easily accessible and free from obstacles? Are they safe, private, and well-lighted? What is the distance to toilet facilities? It has been suggested that the toilet should not be more than 30 feet away in a clinical setting. If a client is unable to use a bathroom, a bedside or chairside commode should be obtained. Other considerations are the placement of toilet handrails, the need for an elevated toilet seat, and the availability of night lights.

The problem of fecal incontinence can be even more devestating than urinary incontinence and often leads to decreased self-esteem, an altered self-concept, impaired social relationships, and institutionalization. Fecal incontinence has various etiologies such as pathology of the rectum or anus and cognitive or neurological impairment. Identifying the causative factor is the first step in managing this problem. Fecal drainage resulting from fecal impaction with overflow must not be confused with diarrhea but should be recognized as severe constipation and treated as such.

## ❖ SPECIAL SERVICES FOR OLDER ADULTS

There are a variety of services designed for older adults that address some of the special needs and problems discussed earlier. These include residential facilities, long-term care institutions, community-based programs, and home health care. In addition, there are governmental programs and national organizations that represent the welfare and interests of older adults. To assist the nurse in providing appropriate counseling, education, and referral, a sample of these services is described.

### Places of Residence

Retirement communities are available for people who can live independently. These communities offer benefits such as safety, group activities, and transportation to shopping areas. Some provide a common eating area for one or more meals a day. A limited number of these apartment communities are subsidized by the government, which helps to reduce the monthly cost for older adults on small fixed incomes.

Some large retirement communities have additional arrangements for "assisted living." Help is available for activities such as bathing and administering prescription medications.

Some communities have a third section for "health care" where long-term nursing services are provided.

Additional alternative living arrangements include shared housing and congregate living sites. Careful investigation of these living arrangements is warranted before a knowledgeable decision about their suitability can be made.

### Day Care

Adult day care centers are becoming more common, allowing the family member to work while providing a place for the older adult to stay. These centers offer supervision and care for older citizens who are unable to stay safely at home by themselves. Other resources, such as respite care, can provide relief to family members from the responsibility of caregiving for short periods of time. Respite care may be provided in the home by volunteers, paid caregivers, or in institutions for extended periods of time.

Senior citizen centers help to meet the socialization needs of the older adult. They range from facilities that provide several programs and services to those that provide only a congregate meal program. Many senior centers offer health screening, legal assistance, counseling, and educational and recreational programs. Senior citizen centers are sponsored by public, church, or community groups.

### Long-term Care

Long-term or nursing home care provides total care for the person who can no longer remain in an acute care hospital or be cared for by the family. Most long-term care facilities provide care for individuals on three levels: skilled care, intermediate care, and sheltered or domiciliary care. (Sheltered care is similar to the "assisted living" arrangement described above.)

Long-term care facilities have undergone dramatic changes over the last few years to accommodate the transfer of increased numbers of clients from acute care hospitals. Rather than providing only custodial care, rehabilitation services are now offered, and many clients are eventually discharged to their homes.

### Home Health Care

As the length of stay in acute care hospitals decreases, comprehensive discharge planning is essential to effectively coordinate care after discharge. Home health care agencies provide a variety of treatment, follow-up, and support services to individuals in their homes. Nurses provide skilled care and often coordinate the efforts of the multidisciplinary health team after discharge. Nonprofessional caregivers assist with activities of daily living. Homemaker services, which includes such tasks as cleaning, laundry and meal preparation, are also available through some agencies.

### Governmental Resources

A number of federal and state programs have been established to address the health and economic needs of older adults. Since 1935, Social Security retirement benefits have been available to many elders. An amendment to the *Social Security Act,* Medicare legislation was enacted in 1965 as an acute care health insurance program for individuals 65 years of age and over who receive Social Security benefits. *Medicare Part A* reimburses for acute care hospitalization and, with very specific justification and for limited periods of time, hospice care and skilled health care provided to older people in the home and long-term care settings. However, Medicare A does not provide full coverage of health care costs for most older adults. *Medicare Part B* is an additional federal plan that the eligible older adult may select. It covers, in part, the cost of physician services and outpatient care such as diagnostic tests, physical and speech therapy, and medical supplies. If older adults elect to carry Part B, they must pay a premium for that coverage. Additional private insurances, often called "Medigap" policies, have been designed to cover deductibles and other non-Medicare A and B reimbursed services. The cost may be high, and provisions and limitations of these policies are often complex. Careful investigation is recommended before purchasing. The older person may require assistance in understanding the language of the policy and may also need help in filling out the complex insurance forms to obtain reimbursement for services and prescription drugs.

Part of the same Social Security Amendment as Medicare, *Medicaid* is a publicly funded medical assistance program for low-income people. Older adults can qualify for benefits if they have limited financial assets and meet the income eligibility requirement. Medicaid covers deductibles, premiums, and services not reimbursed by Medicare. Administered at the state level, eligibility requirements vary from state to state.

In 1974, the *Supplemental Security Income (SSI) Amendment to the Social Security Act* was passed, which provides supplemental money for older adults who have inadequate resources. SSI may also qualify the recipient for additional services such as food stamps and Medicaid. These benefits have served to improve the health and welfare of older Americans with limited incomes, but there is still a significant segment (12%) of the older population that is living below the poverty level and who have limited access to health care (see Chapter 7 for a further discussion of health care financing).

The *Older American's Act* of 1965 provided for the establishment of Agencies On Aging (AOA). Each state has Agencies on Aging whose responsibility it is to coordinate and plan services for older people at the local level. There are approximately 600 area Agencies on

Aging, and these organizations are often good places to begin the process of investigating and identifying for the elderly resources. Subsequent amendments to The Older American's Act provide for multipurpose senior centers and a broad range of services focusing on nutrition, transportation, social, legal, educational, and recreational needs.

## National Organizations and Services

The largest organization representing the older American is the American Association of Retired Persons (AARP). It has numerous functions ranging from advocacy in the legislative arena to promoting volunteerism. It offers a variety of legal services, discounts, tours, and educational events. The National Council of Senior Citizens, the Grey Panthers, the National Retired Teacher's Association, and the National Caucus on the Black Aged are additional organizations that advocate legislative changes to benefit older adults and special interest groups.

## ❖ SUMMARY

Aging is a lifelong process that encompasses transitions from one life stage to another. This chapter focused on aging as a concept and examined changes people experience in later life. A thorough assessment is basic to planning, implementing, and evaluating comprehensive nursing care to meet needs that arise as a result of these changes.

It is important to be mindful of the positive aspects of aging that are often overlooked (Palmore, 1989). Older adults have acquired wisdom through years of experience, and they have developed a stable value system that they feel free to express. Retirement from work releases time and energy for them to do what they choose. Many older adults have effective family and community support systems and enjoy new roles as grandparents and great-grandparents.

In summary, the following quotation by Randall (1977) epitomizes the dignity and diversity of older Americans and the survival skills necessary to reach old age:

Beyond our numbers we have the new dimensions of length in that many more of us are living much longer than we ever expected to do; and we also have depth, a new awareness of ourselves as people who count as members of our society ... We have diversity in the membership of what society calls "older Americans." We have all races, creeds, colors, and cultures to call upon ... Most of all we have the dimension of experience in living through the radical changes of this century and discovering that we have the ability and flexibility to cope with change—with success. An eminent psychiatrist at a meeting once asked recently whether older people can learn. The reply was "of course we can, or how otherwise would we have survived at all."

Courtesy of *The Gerontologist*

## ❖ APPLYING KNOWLEDGE TO PRACTICE

1. Describe a client for whom you have provided care in terms of:
   a. the biological and psychosocial theory or theories of aging that are most applicable and explanatory.
   b. the physical and psychosocial changes that are evident.
   c. nursing diagnoses and appropriate nursing interventions needed to maintain health and prevent illness.
   d. services required for ongoing comprehensive care.
2. Discuss economic issues confronting the aging population in the United States. What solutions could you propose to your legislators to address these issues?
3. Given that the number of older adults is expected to continue to increase, what will be the impact on the health care system by the year 2020?

## REFERENCES

American Association of Retired Persons (1987). A Profile of older Americans. Washington, D.C.: AARP.

Burnside, I. (1988). *Nursing and the aged* (3rd ed.). New York: McGraw-Hill.

Butler, R. (1969). Age-ism: Another form of bigotry. *The Gerontologist, 9,* 243-246.

Calkins, E., Davis, P. J., & Ford, A. B. (1986). *The practice of geriatrics.* Philadelphia: W. B. Saunders Co.

Cleary, T. A., Clamon, C, Price, M, R Shullaw, G. (1988). A reduced stimulation unit: Effects on patients with Alzheimer's disease and selected disorders. *The Gerontologist, 28*(4), 511-514.

Covington, T. R. & Walker, J. I. (1984). *Current geriatric therapy.* Philadelphia: W. B. Saunders Co.

Cumming, E. & Henry, W. (1961). *Growing old.* New York: Basic Books, Inc.

Ebersole, P. & Hess, P. (1990). *Toward healthy aging* (3rd ed.). St. Louis: C. V. Mosby Co.

Eischer, J. E., O'Dell, D., & Gambert, S. R. (1989). Typical geriatric accidents and how to prevent them. *Geriatrics, 44*(5), 54-56, 66-69.

Erikson, E. H. (1963). *Childhood and society* (2nd ed.). New York: W. W. Norton & Co.

Folstein, M. F., Folstein, S., & McHugh, P. R. (1975). Mini-mental state: A practical method for grading the cognitive state of patients for the clinician. *Journal of Psychiatric Research, 12,* 189-198.

Freud, S. (1963). *The standard edition of the complete psychological works of Sigmund Freud* (24 vols.). London: The Hogarth Press Ltd.

Gioiella, E., & Bevil, C. (1985). *Nursing care of the aging Client.* Norwalk, CN: Appleton-Century-Crofts.

Gomez, G. & Gomez, E. A. (1989). Dementia? or delirium? *Geriatric Nursing, 10*(3), 141-142.

Gunter, L. & Estes, C. (1979). *Education for gerontic nursing.* New York: Springer Publishing Co.

Hackett, T. P. & Cassen, N. H. (1987). *Handbook of general hospital psychiatry* (2nd ed.). Littleton, MA: PSG Publishing Co.

Havighurst, R. (1972). *Development tasks and education.* New York: David McKay, Co.

Hendrich, A. L. et al. (1989). [Analysis of risk factors for predicting falls]. Unpublished data.

Hogstel, M. O. (1988). *Nursing care of the older adult* (2nd ed.). New York: John Wiley & Sons.

Jung, C. (1976). The stages of life. In J. Campbell (ed.). *The portable Jung* (pp. 3-22). New York: Viking Press. (Translated by RFC Hull.)

Kohut Jr., S., Kohut, J. J., & Fleishman, J. J. (1987). *Reality orientation for the elderly* (3rd ed.). Oradell, N.J.: Medical Economics Books.

Krueger, G. M., Mahon, D., & Wenzel, K. R. (1989). Preventing falls with closed circuit monitoring. *American Journal of Nursing, 89*(5), 646.

Lemon, B., Bengston, V., & Peterson, J. (1972). An exploration of the activity theory of aging: Activity types and life satisfaction among in-movers to a retirement community. *Journal of Gerontology, 27*(4), 511-523.

Lowenthal, M. (1977). Toward a sociological theory of change in adulthood and old age. In J. Birren, & K. Schaie (eds.). *Handbook of the psychology of aging,* (pp. 116-127). New York: Van Nostrand Reinhold Co.

Matteson, M. A. & McConnell, E. S. (1988). *Gerontological nursing: Concepts and practice.* Philadelphia: W. B. Saunders Co.

Moore, S. R. (1989). Walking for health: A nurse managed activity. *Journal of Gerontological Nursing, 15*(7), 26-28.

Morton, D. (1989). Five years of fewer falls. *American Journal of Nursing, 89*(2), 204-205.

National Center for Health Statistics (1989). *Health, United States, 1988* (DHHS Pub. No. PHS 89-1232). Washington, D.C.: U.S. Government Printing Office, March.

Neugarten, B., Havighurst, R., & Tobin, S. (1968). Personality and patterns of aging. In B. Neugarten (ed.), *Middle age and aging* (pp. 173-177). Chicago: University of Chicago Press.

Palmore, E. (1979). Advantages of aging. *The Gerontologist, 19*(2), 220-223.

Peck, R. C. (1968). Psychological developments in the second half of life. In B. Neugarten (ed.), *Middle age and aging* (pp. 88-92). Chicago: University of Chicago Press.

Pollmann, J. (1989). [Alzheimer's disease: Overview of the disease process.] Unpublished paper.

Randall, O. A. (1977). Aging in America today: New aspects on aging. *The Gerontologist, 17*(1), 6-11.

Rossman, I. (1986). *Clinical geriatrics* (3rd ed.). Philadelphia: J. B. Lippincott Co.

Select Committee on Aging (1985). *Elder abuse: A national disgrace* (U.S. House of Representatives Publication No. 99-952). Washington, D.C.: U.S. Government Printing Office.

Sheehy, G. (1976). *Passages: Predictable crises of adult life.* New York: E. P. Dutton & Co.

Steinmetz, S. (1988). *Duty bound: Elder abuse and family care.* Newbury Park: Sage.

Taber, G. & Ansello, E. F. (1985). Elder abuse. *American Family Physician, 32*(2), 107-114.

Tidieksaar, R., & Kay, A. D. (1986). What causes falls? A logical diagnostic procedure. *Geriatrics, 41*(12), 32-50.

U.S. Bureau of the Census (1989). *Statistical Abstract of the United States: 1989.* Washington, D.C.: U.S. Government Printing Office.

Vaillant, G. (1977). *Adaptation to life.* Boston: Little, Brown & Co.

Weiner, L. (1989). How to afford retirement. *U.S. News and World Report, 10*(7), 55-64.

Wentowski, G. (1981). Reciprocity and the coping strategies of older people: Cultural dimensions of network building. *The Gerontologist, 21*(6), 600-609.

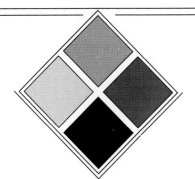

# Index

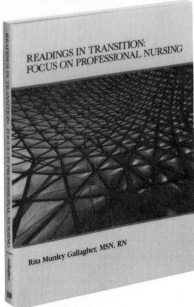